THE

DATE DUE

The Shambhala Encyclopedia of YOGA

Georg Feuerstein

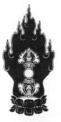

SHAMBHALA

Boston & London

2000

SHAMBHALA PUBLICATIONS, INC.
Horticultural Hall
300 Massachusetts Avenue
Boston, Massachusetts 02115
www.shambhala.com

© 1997 by Georg Feuerstein

9   8   7   6   5   4   3   2   1

FIRST PAPERBACK EDITION
Printed in the United States of America
⊗ This edition is printed on acid-free paper that meets the
American National Standards Institute Z39.48 Standard.
Distributed in the United States by Random House, Inc.,
and in Canada by Random House of Canada Ltd

Library of Congress Cataloging-in-Publication Data
Feuerstein, Georg.
The Shambhala encyclopedia of yoga / Georg Feuerstein.—1st ed.
p.   cm.
Includes bibliographical references.
ISBN 1–57062–555–7 (alk. paper)
1. Yoga—Dictionaries.
BL1238.52.F47   1997
181.45′03—DC20   96-42066
CIP

Contents

Preface

YOGA IS AN immensely rich and highly complex spiritual tradition, with a history that is now thought to extend over at least five millennia. It comprises a great many approaches, schools, teachers, texts, practices, and technical vocabularies. In view of its sheer versatility and protracted history, Yoga must be counted as the world's foremost tradition of psychospiritual transformation. Despite the numerous books available on Yoga, very few reflect that astounding richness. Over the years, I have endeavored to convey some of the splendor and subtleties of the diverse yogic paths in my various publications.

The present encyclopedia is another effort to give an authentic portrayal of the Yoga tradition and to unlock its wealth and perhaps some of its secrets for Western practitioners, historians of religion, and Indologists. There are several dictionaries of Yoga in existence, but these are either too obscure and not readily available or inadequate and unreliable. In the former category belongs the *Yoga Kośa*, compiled by Swami Digambarji and Dr. Mahajot Sahai (Lonavla, Poona, India: Kaivalyadhama S. M. Y. M. Samiti, 1972). While this compilation contains many valuable and detailed references, its scope is limited, and its organization is such that only Sanskritists can access it and benefit from it. Another noteworthy publication is Dr. Ram Kumar Rai's *Encyclopedia of Yoga* (Varanasi, India: Prachya Prakashan, 1975). Like the *Yoga Kośa*, this compilation lists the entries in Sanskrit alphabetical order and is therefore relatively inaccessible to the lay reader. Also, the selection of concepts is rather uneven and the descriptions are occasionally digressive. Neither dictionary contains English entries or cross-references. Among the popular dictionaries, mention must be made of Ernest Wood's *Yoga Wisdom* (New York: Philosophical Library, 1970). This book has only some three hundred entries, which are not always accurate. Slightly bigger but suffering from the same shortcomings is Harvey Day's *Yoga Illustrated Dictionary* (London: Kaye & Ward, 1971).

The idea of preparing an encyclopedia of Yoga that would combine comprehensiveness with accessibility occurred to me in the early 1980s. After plans for a large-scale work failed to materialize, a somewhat abbreviated version was issued under the title *Encyclopedic Dictionary of Yoga* (New York: Paragon House, 1990), which received the Outstanding Academic Book of the Year award for 1991 from *Choice*, a publication for librarians. When the first edition had been sold out, Shambhala Publications, to my delight, offered to reissue my work in the present thoroughly revised and greatly expanded form. This new edition is a gratifying realization of my original goals of comprehensiveness and accessibility.

This encyclopedia, now comprising well over two thousand entries, is arranged and written in such a way that, despite the wealth of detail given, it will inform rather than overwhelm the lay reader, while at the same time providing valuable references for the professional Yoga researcher and historian of religion. While this compilation can usefully be consulted in conjunction with the technical dictionaries mentioned above, several unique features make it an encyclopedia rather than a mere glossary or dictionary. First, each entry is carefully defined and cross-referenced (as indicated by asterisks before words that appear as separate entries), allowing the reader to follow pertinent conceptual linkages. Second, a number of orientational entries furnish the reader with overviews of the most significant aspects of the Yoga tradition, such as its history, psychology, or major branches. Third, the entries are all in English alphabetical order and, moreover, include key words in English, with references to their Sanskrit equivalents or other relevant Sanskrit concepts. Finally, many entries cite, or even quote, the most important original sources, thereby emphasizing the vitality of Yoga's scriptural legacy and, it is hoped, inspiring the reader to examine the originals more closely. Altogether, this encyclopedia is intended to provide a selective but representative range of concepts sufficient to give an authoritative coverage of the many aspects of Yoga theory and practice and to provide valuable guidelines for further study or research.

I would like to express my heartfelt thanks to all those many friends, colleagues, and correspondents who over the years have furthered my interest in Yoga and spiritual traditions in general. I have already named most of them in my previous books. Here I specifically wish to thank Prof. Subhash Kak and David Frawley for providing the stimulus for my complete reappraisal of ancient Indian history (and thus also the earliest history of Yoga) and for coauthoring with me *In Search of the Cradle of Civilization*; David Dykstra for laboring on a multimedia version of this encyclopedia; Matthew Greenblatt of *Inner Directions* magazine and my swami friends of *Hinduism Today* magazine for generously providing me with photographs and illustrations to choose from; Yogacarya B. K. S. Iyengar for his loving moral support and the unexpected gift of a statue of Patanjali (photo on p. 217); Kendra Crossen and Larry Hamberlin for their editorial labor of love; Samuel Bercholz for his vision as a publisher; and my wife, Trisha, for contributing her various skills to the original version of this book and not least for her steadfast love and support.

Ever since my first encounter with the world of Yoga at the age of fourteen, Yoga has claimed my attention again and again, both personally and professionally. I am greatly indebted to the masters of ancient and modern times, who have taught me much through their writings. I like to think of this encyclopedia as a token of my deep appreciation and gratitude, and as a contribution to keeping the tradition of authentic Yoga alive.

Readers wishing to contact me or receive information about my research and teaching programs may write to me in care of the Yoga Research Center, P.O. Box 1386, Lower Lake CA 95457, or by E-mail: yogaresrch@aol.com. The center can also be reached by telephone at (707) 928-9898 or by fax at (707) 928-4738. Programs include the bimonthly newsletter *Yoga World*, correspondence courses, and a series of publications.

Georg Feuerstein
Yoga Research Center

NOTE ON TRANSLITERATION
AND PRONUNCIATION

FOR THE CONVENIENCE of the lay reader, I have adopted a simplified system of transliterating Sanskrit words. Of the various diacritical marks used by scholars to indicate Sanskrit sounds, I have retained only the macron (the dash over the vowels *a*, *i*, and *u*). This sign indicates that a vowel is to be lengthened in pronunciation. For instance, the word *rāja* in *rāja-yoga* is to be pronounced *rahjuh*.

In Sanskrit, most vowel sounds have an open pronunciation, similar to the open vowels of Italian. For example, the *o* in *yoga* is pronounced somewhat like the long *o* in *go*, not like the short *o* in *log*. Likewise, the long *ī* in *īshvara* is pronounced like the *i* in *unique*, not like the *i* in *island*. The short *i* in *bindu* is pronounced like the *i* in *pin*. The word *kundalinī*, which occurs frequently in this encyclopedia, is pronounced *koonduhlinee*, with all vowels except the final *i* being short (the difference between long and short *u* is not as great in Sanskrit as in English).

The Sanskrit language has no *th* sound; rather, *th* represents an aspirated *t* sound. Thus the *th* in the term *hatha-yoga* is pronounced like the *th* in *hothouse*, not like the *th* in *breath* (a common mispronunciation in Western Yoga circles). Similarly, all other consonants combined with an aspirated *h*—*bh*, *ch*, *dh*, *gh*, *jh*, *kh*, and *ph*—are pronounced with a distinct *h* following the initial consonant. Thus the word *phala* is pronounced not *fala* but *p-hala*.

The letter *c* represents the sound *ch*, as in the word *church*. Thus the word rendered here as *cakra* is pronounced *chakra* (the spelling that has made its way into English dictionaries). This system of transliteration avoids confusion with the aspirated *ch* sound (as in *Chāndogya-Upanishad*), which would otherwise have to be rendered as *chh*.

The spelling *sh* is used for both the retroflex *ṣ* and the palatal *ś*, with the following exception: the letter *s* alone is used in the honorific *Sri* (pronounced *shree*) in names such as *Sri Aurobindo* and in the name *Sivananda* (pronounced *Sheevanunduh*). Macrons are omitted in the names of modern personages who have chosen not to use them in the West (for example,

Swami Muktananda). The familiar English spelling *Swami* (not *Svāmin*) is used in personal names.

As in German and Latin, Sanskrit nouns have different endings depending on case (syntactic function). Nouns are given here in the noninflected stem forms; these sometimes differ from the nominative forms often encountered in English-language writings about Yoga. Hence the familiar *yogi* appears here as *yogin, mahatma* as *mahātman,* and so on.

Again for the convenience of the lay reader, I have separated compound words into their individual stems; these hyphenated spellings do not reflect the vowel changes associated with such compounds. Thus *Yogakundalyupa-nishad* appears as *Yoga-Kundalinī-Upanishad.* In cases where letters are al-tered in Sanskrit when they are written together (following the so-called *sandhi* rules), the compound spelling is included in parentheses; the main entry *ācārya-upāsana,* for instance, is followed by the parenthetical spelling *ācāryopāsana.*

Introduction

YOGA IS ONE of the most remarkable accomplishments of human ingenuity and surely one of the most fascinating creations of spiritual aspiration. It is India's mature answer to the universal question "Who am I?"—a question that, sooner or later, will impinge on any self-inspecting individual. Our modern science-oriented civilization has all but ousted spirituality and deeper existential questioning. Religion has to a large extent become synonymous with morality, and the mystical—or true spiritual—impulse has been all but forgotten.

Hence in our century millions of sensitive Western men and women have turned to the East for spiritual nourishment and guidance. In their quest, many have discovered Yoga and been greatly enriched by that encounter. For some, Yoga has strengthened their native faith, particularly among more open-minded Christians. For others, it has led to a spirituality that transcends ideological leanings, as far as that is possible. A few have taken the plunge into the doctrinal structure of Hinduism.

Yoga, as understood here, is an esoteric tradition within the versatile religious culture of Hinduism. It is one of the world's oldest and most continuous branches of spiritual inquiry and, second only to shamanism, the longest and most intense experiment of the human spirit. The purpose of the yogic experiment has been to explore not the behavior of matter but the properties and very limits of consciousness. For the Indians realized that consciousness has primacy over matter—a notion that is gradually being resuscitated through new revelations in physics and parapsychology. What is more, the yogic experiment is continuing even today. India's creeping secularization notwithstanding, the adepts and schools of Yoga have so far held their own. More importantly, Yoga has definitely arrived in the West and is undergoing a promising revival at the hand of creative Western teachers of this ancient discipline.

The history of Yoga encompasses some five thousand years, as compared to two thousand years for Christianity and not quite three centuries of "modern" secular civilization. Its taproots lie in archaic shamanism, and its long evolution is tied to the gradual unfolding of the plural cultures of India, notably Hinduism, Buddhism, and Jainism. As I have shown in my book *Yoga: The Technology of Ecstasy*, which traces the history of the various branches and schools of Yoga, the earliest protoyogic ideas and practices are to be found in the sacred canon of Hinduism—the *Vedas*. Mystical and psychocosmological speculations are present already in the *Rig-Veda*, a collection of hymns "seen" by the *rishis* of yore. Until recently, the consensus of scholarly opinion assigned this hymnody to the era of about 1200–1500 BCE. New research has revealed this date, which has always been rather arbitrary, to be far too late. There is now strong evidence for placing the *Rig-Veda* into the third millennium BCE, with portions of it possibly going back to the fourth millennium BCE and earlier still. Also, the subsequent literature (originally orally transmitted, like the four Vedic collections), which forms an integral part of the Vedic canon, has been dated back by at least a whole millennium. Thus the oldest *Brāhmanas*, previously thought to have been created between 900 BCE and 1200 BCE, are now considered to belong to the early second millennium BCE, possibly even the late third millennium BCE. This historical reevaluation, which is discussed in the entries *Aryan invasion theory* and *Rig-Veda*, has also considerably extended the chronology of Yoga.

In addition to the Rig-Vedic references to Yoga, speculations and practices of a protoyogic type can also be found in the *Atharva-Veda*. This hymnody abounds in magical incantations but includes hymns of a metaphysical and spiritual import as well. It is regarded as being slightly younger than the *Rig-Veda*, though the beliefs and practices mirrored in the *Atharva-Veda* may be as old as or even older than those of the Rig-Vedic hymns.

These early endeavors to explore the possibilities of the human spirit form the nucleus for the diversified psychotechnology that has come to be associated with the name Yoga. Strictly speaking, though, they are characteristic of the tradition of asceticism (*tapas*), which marks the dawn of religion and spirituality in India. Like the shaman, the ascetic (*tapasvin*) aspires to gain control over the powers (or deities/divine energies) animating the universe. He makes himself endure all kinds of hardships to steel his will and generate the inner energy or "heat" (*tapas*) necessary to control the hidden forces of nature through the medium of magic.

By contrast, the *yogin* is primarily (and ideally) concerned with the transcendence of the ego, the deities, and the world as a whole. His great guiding ideal is liberation, variously styled *moksha*, *mukti*, *kaivalya*, *apavarga*, and *nirvāna*. What is liberation? There is no unanimity among the different schools of esotericism. However, their answers are sufficiently similar to provide us with a workable definition: Liberation is the condition of radical, conscious freedom from the bonds of the conditional personality with its ingrained habit patterns, relative unawareness, and fundamental lovelessness.

It is, at the same time, the condition of pure Consciousness, unaffected by the fluctuations of the mind—one's ever-changing opinions and moods.

Fundamental to liberation is the shift from the ego identity to the Self identity: The liberated adept (*mukta-siddha*) no longer experiences his or her body-mind as an impenetrable boundary of awareness. Rather, standing firmly in pure Consciousness (*cit*), the adept experiences the body-mind as arising in that Consciousness. Regardless of the different metaphysical positions that have been elaborated in the course of the long evolution of Yoga, this pure Consciousness—the transcendental witness (*sākshin*)—is the common denominator. It is called *ātman* ("Self") in the Sanskrit scriptures. It is our innermost essence, just as it is the deepest foundation of the cosmos.

This Self cannot be experienced, since it is not an object but the ultimate subject. It can, however, be realized. That is to say, a person can "awaken" as that Self. Self-realization is widely held to be utterly blissful. But this is only to say that it is the antithesis of the ordinary ego identity, which, because of its inherent limitation in space and time, is inevitably associated with the experience of pain and suffering. Self-realization is not pleasurable, for pleasure—like pain—is something only the ego personality can experience. The Self does not get caught up in experiences. It simply notices ("witnesses") their occurrence in the body-mind, rather as the peak of a high mountain abides forever above the good and bad weather of the lower regions.

All this does not mean, however, that the Self-realized sage is an unfeeling monstrosity. On the contrary, Patanjali, the founder of Classical Yoga, describes such a sage as being acutely sensitive, "like an eyeball." The reason for this sensitivity is best summed up in the words of the Latin poet: *Homo sum, humani nihil a me alienum puto*, "I am human; I consider nothing human to be foreign to me."

The Yoga adept arrives at Self-realization only after a long struggle with the human condition. In the course of that personal ordeal, he or she has to face all the numerous liabilities and weaknesses associated with being human. Having transcended them by transcending the ego, the adept can now look upon others with compassion, understanding that those who are still struggling with themselves and with existence at large are also on a journey of both self-discovery and Self-discovery. Even though others' pace may be slow and hesitant, and they may not even be aware of their journey, they too are already liberated, already free. Of course, the sage no longer exclaims, *Homo sum*, "I am human," but rather, *Aham brahma asmi*, "I am the Absolute, the transcendental Self." Yet with the adept's transcendence of the human condition comes the capacity to empathize with those who persist in identifying with the body-mind rather than the Self.

Observing their confusion, uncertainty, and physical and mental suffering, the sage feels compelled to communicate the gospel of humanity's essential freedom. Alas, the noise of our technological civilization has deafened our ears to the gentle but persuasive song of the bearers of wisdom of bygone ages and of our own time.

Despite its noblest discovery of the eternal Self beyond the vicissitudes of the body-mind, the tradition of Yoga has retained many features of the antecedent tradition of asceticism. Thus the *yogin* is typically celebrated as a possessor not only of wisdom but also of paranormal powers (*siddhi*). To the ordinary Indian, he is a knower and a miracle worker, or thaumaturgist. This is in keeping with what we know of other spiritual traditions. Holiness and power go hand in hand. Even the mature *yogin* who has not yet realized the Self is thought to possess mysterious abilities beyond those of ordinary mortals. But the practitioner of Yoga is frequently warned not to abuse these powers, and sometimes even not to use them at all, lest they distract the seeker from the spiritual goal.

The exercise of power of any kind is fraught with danger, since it is apt to feed the ego and lure it away from the great ideal of liberation, which essentially consists in ego transcendence. Once the Self is realized, powers of all kinds are said to become spontaneously available, without endangering the adept's hard-won freedom. The genuine *yogin* will always treat the paranormal powers and power in general with great circumspection. The *yogin*'s prime motive is constantly to step beyond the self, until the Self is realized. When the Self is finally realized, there can be no misuse of power, just as there can be no fall from grace. Self-realization, if true, is forever.

In most schools of Yoga, Self-realization means the realization of the singular Self (*ātman*), the universal essence of Selfhood. This is a suprapersonal event, for the Self exists beyond the particular configuration of one's personality. It is the same Self in all beings. This idea is fundamental to the various schools of Advaita-Vedānta, or Hindu nondualism. In its formative phase, Yoga was closely aligned with the ramifying metaphysical tradition of Vedānta, as expounded in the *Upanishads*. The oldest scriptures of this literary genre, dating to about 1500–1000 BCE, teach a pantheism, or better, panentheism: There is only one Reality, which is experienced as the multiform cosmos by unenlightened beings. Through proper initiation (*dīkshā*), renunciation (*samnyāsa*), and meditation (*nididhyāsana, dhyāna*), the spiritual aspirant can realize the prior singular Reality beyond the mind and the senses.

That Reality is not only the ultimate ground of objective existence or *brahman*; it is also a person's true identity, the transcendental Self or *ātman*. The idealist doctrine of the identity of the *brahman* with the *ātman* is the quintessential notion common to all Upanishadic or Vedantic thought. The

Yoga tradition evolved out of these metaphysical speculations and their attendant spiritual disciplines.

Yoga was originally also most intimately associated with the Sāmkhya tradition, which is marked by a realist philosophy with a strong cosmological bent. Sāmkhya is concerned with defining the categories of existence, as they emerge in hierarchic order out of the perennial world ground called *prakriti* ("procreatrix"). Beyond the world ground and its psychomaterial evolutes stands the primal Self, the *purusha*, or pure Consciousness. Vedānta, Yoga, and Sāmkhya together formed the intellectual milieu of Upanishadic times—the milieu into which Gautama the Buddha and also Vardhamāna Mahāvīra were born.

The Buddha's teaching, which has sometimes been looked upon as a pragmatic version of Yoga, is founded in a rejection of metaphysical speculation, especially the notion of an eternal Self (*ātman*). The Buddha emphasized practical discipline—his noble eightfold path to liberation—to countermand the ever-present tendency to theorize about spiritual life rather than to engage it. As is clear from the schools of Mahāyāna and Vajrayāna Buddhism, however, metaphysics proved ineradicable even within Buddhism, though it has always been tested in the fire of actual practice.

A similar practice-oriented approach characterizes the teaching of Vardhamāna Mahāvīra, the founder of historical Jainism. Vardhamāna, an older contemporary of the Buddha, is thought to be the last in a long line of fully enlightened teachers. The Jaina path does indeed contain features that appear to be very ancient. In later times, some Jaina masters even spoke of their teachings as a form of Yoga.

Both Buddhism and Jainism had a strong influence on the further evolution of Yoga, particularly in its philosophical formulation under Patanjali, who probably lived in the second century CE.

Yoga is first clearly spoken of as a spiritual method in the *Katha-Upanishad*, which was probably composed in the sixth century BCE or earlier. This work propounds what is called *ādhyātma-yoga*, the "Yoga of the inmost self," by which the sage may come to know the great god hidden in the cave of the heart. Then, in the fourth or fifth century BCE, the anonymous composer of the *Bhagavad-Gītā*—the New Testament of Hinduism—made a unique attempt at integrating the various yogic approaches then current. Most importantly, the *Gītā* introduced the ideal of devotion (*bhakti*) to the Divine as a superperson (*purusha-uttama*), thus instituting the path of *bhakti-yoga*, which quickly gained great popularity.

Nevertheless, it was Patanjali's *Yoga-Sūtra* (Aphorisms of Yoga) that gave Yoga its classical form as one of the six philosophical "viewpoints" (*darshana*) of Hinduism. Patanjali's work was very influential, since it proffered valuable definitions of the fundamental concepts of the yogic path; his metaphysical dualism, however, was never looked upon favorably within mainstream Hinduism. Although Patanjali's school came to be regarded as the preeminent philosophy of Yoga, many other yogic schools continued to exist and flourish alongside it.

These nonclassical schools of Yoga retained their Vedantic (nondualist) foundations and over time led to the fascinating developments of Postclassical Yoga, which shows a marked Tantric influence. Tantrism (or Tantra), which originated in the early common era and gathered momentum in the sixth century CE, is a pan-Indian syncretistic movement that greatly transformed Hinduism and Buddhism and to a lesser extent also Jainism. Because of its enormous breadth, Tantrism is difficult to define. It is more a cultural style than a philosophy, and from the outset purported to be the teaching for the dark age (*kali-yuga*), which supposedly commenced with the death of Krishna (traditionally fixed at 3006 BCE).

In simplified terms, Tantrism translated the ancient panentheistic intuition that the world arises in the all-encompassing Being into ritual action and a deep philosophical understanding. It elevated the age-old popular belief in the Divine as feminine power, or *shakti*, to a metaphysical principle of the first order. This resulted in a certain reevaluation of the female gender in society, but primarily it led to a reappraisal of the body as a manifestation of the Divine and thus as a positive instrument for attaining liberation.

An important tradition within Tantrism is the Siddha movement, dating back to the sixth century CE. A *siddha* is a spiritual adept who has attained perfection (*siddhi*) through a transubstantiated body endowed with all kinds of paranormal powers (*siddhi, vibhūti*). Out of this tradition of "body cultivation" (*kāya-sādhana*) grew the various schools of the forceful Yoga (*hatha-yoga*). The origins of *hatha-yoga* are quite obscure but are traditionally connected to the name of Goraksha, a tenth-century master.

The teachers of *hatha-yoga* have created important manuals, some of which are still extant. These show an astonishing arsenal of techniques for manipulating the life force (*prāna*) in the human body, primarily by means of breath control and mental concentration. The underlying idea behind these practices is that a strong and healthy body is needed to gain liberation, or enlightenment, and to manifest its paranormal effects. In the course of time, not a few *hatha-yogins* lost sight of the spiritual goal of this tradition and focused more on its therapeutic and prophylactic aspects, or exploited it as a means for cultivating paranormal abilities. Hence *hatha-yoga* fell into disrepute especially among the more educated classes of the Hindu and Buddhist societies, which tend to favor a more meditative and intellectual approach.

There are today several million people outside India who practice one or the other form of Yoga—from the physical exercises of *hatha-yoga* to the mental disciplines of *rāja-yoga*; from the mysterious *kundalinī-yoga*, which seeks to control the vast psychospiritual energy of the body, to the seemingly glamorous but difficult orientation of *tantra-yoga*, with its manipulation of the sexual drive; and from the approach of the heart favored in *bhakti-yoga* to the conscious execution of actions, which is the essence of *karma-yoga*.

Many Yoga practitioners are simply in search of health, beauty, longevity, and a more meaningful life. Medical research on *hatha-yoga* has shown that many of its techniques are remarkably potent therapeutic instruments. They can not only restore health to an ailing body but also slow, to some extent, the aging process and even reverse some of its baneful effects. Meditation is demonstrably a wonderful tool for cultivating equanimity. Perhaps the best-known approach is that of Transcendental Meditation (TM), which was introduced to the West by Maharshi Mahesh Yogi in the late 1960s. Behind this designation lies an ancient method, the meditative recitation of sacred sounds known as *mantra-yoga*. Research on TM practitioners has shown that they derive many kinds of physical and mental benefits from this method. Some of the findings and conclusions have possibly been somewhat exaggerated but, in substance, they have confirmed what *yogins* have claimed for many centuries, namely, that Yoga is a powerful transformative approach.

Modern research on Yoga has also brought home the fact that the *yogins* were first-class experimenters with a keen understanding of the interaction between consciousness and the body. Many aspects of Yoga practice still await open-minded scientific exploration, and undoubtedly many surprises lie in store for researchers and practitioners alike.

In the meantime, Yoga has become part of the cultural kaleidoscope of the Western world. This prompted C. G. Jung, among others, to caution against any simplistic adoption of Eastern traditions. His warning is certainly valid, because mere imitation cannot produce constructive and beneficial results. Yet Jung's assessment was somewhat lopsided, springing from his own European bias. While there clearly are many differences between the Western and the Indian cultures, and therefore between the underlying personality structures, these differences are not radical. That is to say, there are no insurmountable constitutional differences between Westerners and Indians. However variegated humanity may be, the same basic physical, emotional, intellectual, and spiritual capacities are shared by all human beings.

It is true, however, that Western practitioners of Yoga are not always sufficiently informed about the distinct cultural milieu that has given birth to Yoga. Hence what we encounter as Yoga in the West is often merely one or another unfortunate popularization that distorts the intention behind Yoga and no doubt also diminishes the effectiveness of the original methods and approaches. Beginning students are therefore advised to make every effort to inform themselves about the authentic tradition of Yoga before embarking on any approach or before choosing a teacher or instructor. My various books and also the present work contain ample material for this kind of preliminary study. In fact, I venture to suggest, they can serve even more mature travelers on the yogic path as trustworthy companions.

An important question for the serious student of Eastern traditions is whether the initiatory nature of authentic Yoga is a possibility for Westerners. Traditional Yoga is typically transmitted by a qualified teacher (*guru*). Can Westerners benefit from a practice involving a *guru*? There is no way of answering this question briefly without running the risk of inviting misunderstanding or reinforcing existing prejudices, whether they be for or against the figure of the *guru*. I have addressed this question in some depth—from a historical, psychological, and experiential point of view—in my book *Holy Madness*. The only advice worth giving in this context is to use good common sense and to trust one's bodily felt wisdom, and to continue to do so throughout one's discipleship.

Yoga has survived for over five millennia, mainly through being skillfully adapted to different historical and cultural contexts. There is every indication that it will continue to be with us for a long time. It seems desirable to try to understand it so we can benefit from the cumulative wisdom of its practitioners in our modern quest for self-definition. This encyclopedia is an attempt to make such a better understanding possible, both for practitioners of Yoga and for others who care to comprehend this tradition as part of the complexity of our pluralistic society.

GENERAL ORIENTATION

THIS ENCYCLOPEDIA COVERS a considerable amount of information about the Yoga tradition, and most of the key words are in Sanskrit. Nevertheless, its arrangement makes it readily accessible to the nonspecialist. Important concepts are thoroughly cross-referenced in English, and a number of entries furnish valuable overviews, containing references to specific subcategories. Thus the reader unacquainted with Yoga may profitably begin by consulting the following entries: *Hinduism, Yoga, History of Yoga, Indus-Sarasvati civilization, Psychology, Progress, Body, Sexuality,* and *Cosmos.* These entries contain sufficient cross-references to guide the reader to the next level of accessing this encyclopedia.

An asterisk (*) before a word indicates that the term can be found as a separate entry. To avoid unnecessary duplication, I have used an asterisk only on the first occurrence of a term in each paragraph of an entry. No asterisk precedes a term whose entry is a simple cross-reference, although an asterisk may precede a term whose entry lists several cross-references, thus serving as a nexus of related concepts. Thus "*posture" leads one to the entries for *āsana, bandhā, mudrā, nishadana,* and *pītha.*

THE
SHAMBHALA
ENCYCLOPEDIA
OF YOGA

A

ABANDONMENT. In ancient India there was a prominent trend toward leaving the conventional world and living an ascetic life in the seclusion of forests and caves. This movement of world renunciation (called *tyāga* or *samnyāsa*) started at the time of the earliest *Upanishads*, which are a reflection of this emerging ideal, and soon grew strong enough to become a social problem. In response, the Hindu lawgivers invented the ideal of the stages of life (*āshrama*). According to this social model, a person has to complete the student (*brahmacārin*) and householder (*grihastha*) stages before retiring from the world. See also *vairāgya*.

ĀBHĀSA ("shining"), a term used in Vedantic *Yoga to denote the appearance of reality rather than *Reality itself. According to *Advaita Vedānta, the appearance of the finite world is illusory, but the philosophical schools of *Shaivism regard the world as a real appearance, i.e., a manifestation of the *Divine. See also *māyā, vivarta*.

ABHĀVA ("nonbeing"). Already in early *Vedic times, the sages of India were pondering the philosophical question of why there is something rather than nothing and what the nature of nothing might be. Thus in the *Rig-Veda* (10.129) the seer-poet (*rishi*) raises the question of what existed prior to the emergence of the world. Cf. *bhāva*; see also *asat, shūnya*.

ABHĀVA-YOGA ("Yoga of nonbeing"), a compound found in some of the *Purānas.

The *Kūrma-Purāna* (2.11.6), e.g., understands it thus: "[That approach] in which one contemplates [one's] essence as void and [yet] all-illuminating, and by which one beholds the Self, is called the Yoga of nonbeing." A similar definition is given in the *Linga-Purāna* (2.55.14), where it is said to effect the *mind's extinction (*citta-nirvāna*). The *Shiva-Purāna* (7.2.37.10), again, explains it as that in which the *world is contemplated without any perception of *objects. This appears to be the equivalent of "supraconscious ecstasy" (*asamprajnāta-samādhi*). Cf. *bhāva-yoga*.

ABHAYA ("fearlessness"). Fear is integral to individuated human existence. As the ancient *Brihad-Āranyaka-Upanishad* (1.4.2) puts it: "Fear arises when there is an other." Fearlessness is the fruit of perfect *Self-realization, or *enlightenment (*bodha*), i.e., the recovery of nonduality. Cf. *bhaya*.

ABHAYA-MUDRĀ ("seal of fearlessness"), one of the classical hand gestures found in the iconography of Mahāyāna *Buddhism and *Tantrism; used by *adepts to dispel fear (*bhaya*) in others. All fear is groundless, for our true nature is the single Being, in which there is no otherness and which is unalloyed bliss (*ānanda*). In iconography, the fear-dispelling gesture is also known as *abhaya-hasta* (*hasta* meaning "hand"). See also *mudrā*.

ABHICĀRA. See Magic.

1

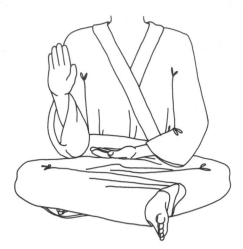

Abhaya-mudrā, hand gesture of bestowing fearlessness

ABHIJÑĀ ("knowledge"), a Buddhist term denoting knowledge acquired by paranormal means. Traditionally, six *abhijñās* are known: "divine eye" (*divya-cakshus*), "divine ear" (*divya-shrotra*), knowledge of another's mind (*para-citta-jnāna*), recollection of former lives (*pūrva-nivāsa-anusmriti*), direct experience of paranormal powers (*riddhi-sakshāt-kriyā*), and knowledge of the end of life (*āshrava-kshaya-jnāna*). See also *bala, siddhi, vibhūti*.

ABHIMĀNA ("pride"), one of the functions of the "inner organ" (*antahkarana*), or psyche. It must be overcome through the insight that one is not identical with the ego personality. See also *darpa*.

ABHINANDA. See Gauda Abhinanda.

ABHINAVA GUPTA (b. ca. 950 CE), the most renowned scholar and *adept of Kashmiri *Shaivism, demonstrating that intellect and spiritual virtuosity are not necessarily in conflict; regarded as an *incarnation of *Shesha and widely hailed as a miracle worker. He left behind numerous writings, the most famous being the voluminous *Tantra-Āloka* ("Luster of *Tantra"), a systematic presentation of the teachings of the *Kaula branch of *Tantrism. His contributions to metaphysics are as significant as those he made to *aesthetics. Legend has it that at the end of his life he went into a remote cave with 1,200 of his disciples, never to be seen again.

ABHINIVESHA ("will to live"), one of the five causes of affliction (*klesha*), according to *Classical Yoga. *Patanjali observes (*Yoga-Sūtra* 2.9): "The thirst for life flowing on by its own nature is rooted even in the sage." Ultimately, *abhinivesha* springs from spiritual ignorance (*avidyā*), whereby a person wrongly identifies with the body and becomes subject to the survival instinct. See also *trishā*.

ABHISHEKA ("sprinkling"), the ritual of baptism, explained in the *Kula-Arnava-Tantra* (17.52) as that which removes the "I" sense (*aham-bhāva*) and fear (*bhīti*) and sprinkles blessed water, inducing *bliss and trembling (*kampa*). This practice is often used in yogic ceremonial contexts, particularly in *Tantrism. It is a ritual of empowerment, a form of initiatory baptism, by which the aspirant's spiritual endeavors are blessed. The term is also used to denote initiation in general. According to the *Shata-Patha-Brāhmana* (5.4.2.2), *abhisheka* brings forth the recipient's inner luster and power. It also specifically denotes the state ritual of anointing a king, particularly the coronation of emperors. Furthermore, the "sprinkling" of sacred images is widely practiced, whereby the image is infused with divine power or life, bringing the deity it represents into the material realm. Milk, oil, and other liquids are also used in addition to water.

The *Tantric scriptures know of eight forms or levels of consecration: (1) *shakta-* ("empowering"); (2) *purna-* ("full"); (3) *krama-dīksha-* ("gradual initiatory"); (4) *sāmrājya-* ("paramount"); (5) *mahāsāmrājya-* ("greatly paramount"); (6) *yoga-dīkshā-* ("yogic initiatory"); (7) *purna-dīkshā-* ("fully initiatory"), or *virāja-grahana-* ("resplendent capturing"); and (8) *parama-hamsa* ("supreme swan") consecration. See also *dīkshā*.

ĀBHOGA ("experience," from the root *bhuj*, "to eat" or "to enjoy"), the consumption of the world whether through the physical *senses or through the *mind.

ABHYĀSA ("practice"), or practical application; one of two essential aspects of spiritual life, the other being dispassion (*vairāgya*), or renunciation. The *Yoga-Bhāshya* (1.12) compares the *mind, or psyche, to a stream that can flow in two directions. One starts with spiritual ignorance and ends in evil (i.e., *rebirth), the other starts with discrimination and ends in what is good (i.e., *liberation). The latter is governed by renunciation, which checks the outflow of *attention toward worldly objects, and the practice of discrimination (*viveka*), which opens higher evolutionary possibilities. The *Shiva-Samhitā* (4.9), a late *hatha-yoga* text, declares: "Through practice comes perfection; through practice one will attain liberation."

ABHYĀSA-YOGA, yogic practice or practical Yoga. This compound is particularly common in *Epic Yoga.

ABHYĀSIN ("practitioner"), a synonym for *yogin or *sādhaka. The feminine form is *abhyāsinī*.

ABILITY, PARANORMAL. See *bala, siddhi, vibhūti*.

ABLUTION. See *abhisheka, snāna*.

ABSOLUTE. All spiritual traditions of India recognize the existence of an ultimate, transcendental *Reality, though different schools propose different conceptions of it. Most are agreed that the Absolute is without qualities and is supramaterial, supraconscious, and suprapersonal. All these traditions insist that the Absolute is identical to the very essence of the human being, the *Self, and is realizable as such by transcending the *mind. However, they offer different speculations about the relationship between the Absolute and that innermost essence. The most radical solution is that of *Advaita Vedānta, which sees no distinction whatsoever between the Absolute (*brahman*) and the essential aspect of the psyche, the transcendental *Self (*ātman*). In *Classical Yoga, however, many such essential Selves (*purusha*) are supposed to exist, and one of them is unique in that it has never been, nor will ever be, subject to the illusion of embodiment. That special Self is called the "Lord" (*īshvara*), the equivalent of *God in *Patanjali's Yoga. In the nondualist schools, however, the Lord (as the Creator) has no ultimacy. Usually called *Brahma or *Prajāpati, he is merely a long-lived deity (*deva*) or a mental projection upon the Absolute.

ABSORPTION. The ability to allow *attention to become absorbed in the object of contemplation is fundamental to all schools of *Yoga. Meditative absorption (*dhyāna*) is a more advanced stage of concentration (*dhāranā*), because of the degree of sensory inhibition that is involved. See also *bhāvanā, laya, nididhyāsana*.

ABSTINENCE. The voluntary disciplining of the sexual drive is an important practice in most traditional schools of spirituality, including *Yoga and *Tantra. It is considered a primary means of accumulating psychospiritual energy in the *body, which is then employed to focus the *mind on spiritual goals. See also *brahmacarya*, Chastity, Sexuality.

ABUDDHA ("unawakened"), in some schools of *Preclassical Yoga, the transcendental ground of nature (*prakriti*), as opposed to the transcendental *Self, which is called *budhyamāna*. See also *aprati-buddha*.

ACALA ("Unmoving"), an epithet of *Shiva.

ĀCĀRA ("conduct"), behavior in general; also, any specific approach to *Self-realization. Thus in *Tantrism an important distinction is made between a "right-hand approach" (*dakshina-ācāra*) and a "left-hand approach" (*vāma-ācāra*). In the *Kula-Arnava-Tantra* (2) seven ways of life are distinguished, in ascending order: (1) the *veda-ācāra* (the Vedic way of rituals); (2) the *vaishnava-ācāra* (the way of the *Vishnu worshipers); (3) the *shaiva-ācāra* (the way of the *Shiva worshipers); (4) the *dakshina-ācāra* (the right-hand way); (5) the *vāma-ācāra* (the left-hand way); (6) the *siddhānta-ācāra* (the doctrinal way); and (7) the *kula-ācāra* (the way of *kula*, which is the feminine principle, or *shakti*). The *kula-ācāra* is hailed as the most excellent and most secret of all approaches to *Self-realization. See also Kaula school.

ĀCĀRYA ("preceptor"). *Yoga is traditionally an initiatory teaching, handed down from *teacher to *disciple by word of mouth. The preceptor is a teacher who may or may not have the function of a *guru*, or spiritual guide. Sometimes the two terms are used interchangeably. The *Brahma-Vidyā-Upanishad* (51–52) distinguishes three kinds of preceptor: the prompter (*codaka*), the awakener (*bodhaka*), and the bestower of *liberation (*moksha-da*). The *Mahābhārata* (12.313. 23) likens the preceptor to a ferryman and his knowledge to a ferry. See also *upā-dhyāya*.

ĀCĀRYA-SEVANA ("service to the preceptor"), sometimes considered among the practices of self-discipline (*niyama*). See also *guru-sevā*, *sevā*.

ĀCĀRYA-UPĀSANA (*ācāryopāsana*, "veneration of the preceptor"). Because of the central importance given to the *teacher in the yogic tradition, all schools emphasize that the pupil (*shishya*) must assume a reverential attitude toward the teacher, without which spiritual *transmission cannot occur. The person of the teacher serves as a means of self-transcendence for the disciple. This must not be confused with adulation, though at times *guru-yoga* has suffered from this kind of excess. According to the *Bhagavad-Gītā* (13.7), veneration of the preceptor is a manifestation of wisdom (*jnāna*). See also *guru-bhakti*, *guru-sevā*, *sevā*.

ACCOMPLISHED (OR ADEPT'S) POSTURE. See *siddha-āsana*.

ACIT ("unconscious"), in the metaphysical system of *Rāmānuja, the counterpoint to the ultimate *Consciousness, or *reality. Like Consciousness (*cit*), *acit* is an eternal principle. It forms the *body of the Divine and is dynamic and in a state of perpetual flux. It comprises *nature (*prakriti*), the pure being (*shuddha-sattva*), and time (*kāla*).

ACTION. The spiritual practitioner (*yogin, *sādhaka) is expected to know how to act in the world in accordance with the higher principles of the *cosmos. For the *adept, right action is action that is not only morally sound (i.e., virtuous or meritorious) but also conducive to spiritual growth, or *progress. Otherwise, action is karmically binding; i.e., it reinforces spiritual blindness (*avidyā) and thus leads to reincarnation. In Sanskrit, the word for "action" and the *fate created by action is the same, *karman (or karma in the nominative case).

Action became a subject of keen philosophical inquiry in India with the early *Upanishads and notably with the *Bhagavad-Gītā. The fundamental existential question "What must I do?" is closely connected to the question "Who am I?" For the Upanishadic sages and later also for the *yogins, human action is played out in the finite realms of conditional reality, and it cannot touch the transcendental *Self, or *Reality. The sense that "I" act is an illusion, and so are, in the final analysis, the consequences of "my" actions. Upon *enlightenment, actions are experienced as simply arising, without there being an ego identity. See also karma-yoga.

ACTIVATOR, SUBCONSCIOUS. See samskāra.

ACTOR or AGENT. The conditional ego personality (*jīva, *ahamkāra) presumes itself to be the performer of *actions, which, according to *Classical Yoga, *Classical Sāmkhya, and *Vedānta, is an illusion. In the view of the former two systems of thought, the transcendental Self (*purusha) is merely a spectator or witness (*sākshin) or passive enjoyer (*bhoktri) of the experiences of the finite human personality. The Self apperceives the contents of

*consciousness with perfect indifference. By virtue of its inherent *purity, however, it acts as an attractive force in the evolutionary play of *nature, and this accounts for the gradual uplifting of individuals and whole world cycles (*yuga).

In contrast to the aforementioned systems, Kashmiri *Shaivism assumes the *Self to be the ultimate agent (*kartri). The Self, as *Shiva, is absolute, self-existent, free, unborn (*aja), eternal, and beginningless. Yet it is also supremely conscious, and in its consciousness or awareness lies its agency: it is the knower (jnātri), the knowing subject, behind all knowledge (*jnāna). It is the creative principle par excellence, and the Self's (or Shiva's) activity (*kriyā) is utterly spontaneous, effortless, and blissful (*ānanda). This aspect of Shiva is called *shakti, the feminine creative principle.

ADAMANTINE POSTURE. See vajra-āsana.

ADARSHANA ("nonvision"), a synonym for *avidyā. Cf. darshana.

ADBHUTA ("marvelous"), one of the nine sentiments (*rasa) acknowledged in Sanskrit *aesthetics. It springs from the sense of wonder (vismaya).

ADBHUTA-GĪTĀ ("Marvelous Song"), a Sanskrit composition ascribed to Guru *Nānak.

ADEPT. The accomplished spiritual practitioner, who has climbed to the top of the ladder of spiritual life, is not only a master of the disciplines but, above all, a master (*svāmin) of his or her own self-body-mind. An adept is generally considered to be an *enlightened being, one who has awakened from the "dream" of conventional life and has realized the Self (*ātman). Such a being is known as a *siddha or *mahā-siddha. See also sādhaka.

ĀDHĀRA ("support" or "prop"), any of several places in the *body on which the *yogin focuses his *attention not only to discipline the mind but also to harness the body's psychosomatic energy (*prāna). Sometimes six, nine, and even sixteen such supports are distinguished. The set of sixteen is frequently presented as comprising the following body parts: thumbs, ankles, knees, thighs, prepuce, genitals, navel (*nābhi), *heart, neck, throat (*kantha), palate (*talu), nose (*nāsa), spot between the eyebrows (*bhrū-madhya), forehead (*lalāta), *head, and the "brahmic fissure" (*brahma-randhra) at the crown of the head.

The word ādhāra is also used specifically to indicate the lowest of the bodily centers (i.e., the *mūlādhāra-cakra). See also cakra, desha, marman.

ĀDHĀRA-SHAKTI ("support power"), a common synonym for *kundalinī.

ADHARMA. The word *dharma has a great many different meanings, and so does a-dharma. Generally speaking, the latter word stands for "lawlessness" or "anomie," indicating a lack of virtue or righteousness, as well as moral and spiritual chaos. In the *Bhagavad-Gītā (4.7) *Krishna declares that he incarnates in every age (*yuga) to stamp out lawlessness and reestablish the spiritual order on earth. Lawlessness creates demerit (*apunya), or disadvantageous *karma, which in turn gives rise to an unfavorable rebirth. Adharma must be overcome by the cultivation of dharma, but ultimately, both must be transcended through enlightenment.

ĀDHIBHŪTA ("pertaining to the elements"). In the *Bhagavad-Gītā this term refers to the perishable (*kshara) manifestation of the Imperishable (*akshara). See also ādhidaiva, ādhyātman.

ĀDHIDAIVA, lit. "pertaining to the deities (*deva)," i.e., to one's *destiny, which is thought to be governed by higher powers. In some contexts, this word refers to the transcendental *Self. See also ādhibhūta, ādhyātman.

ADHIKĀRA ("qualification"). The transmission (*shakti-pāta) of spiritual knowledge and *power requires that the *student be truly qualified to receive what is given. The unqualified person was traditionally supposed to be excluded from such transmission, since it could damage him or her, as well as the *teacher.

ADHIKĀRIN ("qualified [aspirant]"). The various traditions of *Yoga resort to all kinds of criteria for determining who is a qualified practitioner (*sādhaka), i.e., a competent person who is worthy of being initiated and instructed in the great esoteric lore of *liberation. Thus in the *Shiva-Samhitā (3.16–19) a positive frame of mind, or *vishvāsa, is said to be the primary qualification. This is followed by faithful application to practice, veneration of the teacher (*ācārya-upāsana), impartiality, sense restraint, and a moderate *diet.

According to this *hatha-yoga scripture (5.10ff.), the weak (mridu) aspirant is unenthusiastic, foolish, fickle, timid, ill, dependent, ill-mannered, and unenergetic. He is considered fit only for *mantra-yoga, or the recitation of empowered sounds (*mantra). The mediocre (madhya) aspirant, on the other hand, is endowed with even-mindedness, patience (*kshamā), a desire for virtue (*dharma), *kind speech, and the tendency to practice moderation in all things. He is considered capable of practicing *laya-yoga, or the dissolution of the mind through meditative *absorption.

The exceptional (adhimātra) aspirant shows such qualities as firm understanding, an aptitude for meditative absorption (*laya), self-reliance, liberal-mindedness, bravery, vigor, faithfulness, the willingness to worship the teacher's "lotus feet" (both literally and figuratively), and delight in the practice of *Yoga.

The extraordinary (adhimātratama) aspirant, who may practice any type of *Yoga, demonstrates the following thirty-one virtues: great energy, *enthusiasm, charm, heroism, scriptural knowledge, the inclination to practice, freedom from delusion (*bhrānti), orderliness, youthfulness, moderate eating habits, control over the senses (*indriya-jaya), fearlessness (*abhaya), *purity, skillfulness, liberality, the ability to be a refuge for all people, capability, stability (*sthairya), thoughtfulness, the willingness to do whatever is desired by the teacher, patience (*kshamā), good manners, observance of the moral and spiritual law, the ability to keep his struggle to himself, *kind speech, *faith in the *scriptures, the readiness to worship the *Divine and the *guru (as the embodiment of the Divine), knowledge of the vows (*vrāta) pertaining to his level of practice, and lastly, the active pursuit of all forms of Yoga.

ADHVAN ("road" or "pathway"), in Kashmiri *Shaivism, any of the three types or categories of existence called *tattvas. The three pathways of manifestation or creation (*sarga) are the pure (*shuddha), the mixed (mishra), and the impure (*ashuddha). The first comprises the five highest categories of existence, consisting of *shiva ("benign"), *shakti ("power"), *sadā-shiva ("eternally benign"), *īshvara

("lord"), and sad-vidyā ("real wisdom"). The second pathway comprises the seven intermediate ontic categories, consisting of *māyā and the five *kancukas, as well as the *purusha, called *anu in Shaivism. The third pathway consists of the twenty-four categories familiar from the *Sāmkhya tradition, which is *prakriti and its evolutes.

Adhvan also refers to the six paths by which a spiritual practitioner (*sādhaka) can pursue the highest goal of *liberation. According to *Abhinava Gupta, these are: (1) the primordial sound or *nāda (here called *varna), which is manifested through the action of *prāna-shakti with the *guru's help; (2) recitation of various kinds of *mantra; (3) the approach of knowledge as inherently self-luminous by means of the ten *padas; (4) discovery of the true nature of the five *kalās underlying various levels of existence; (5) discovery of the underlying unity of the thirty-six categories of existence (*tattva), and (6) realization of the transcendental matrix of the 118 worlds (bhuvana), or realms of existence, on various levels of *creation.

ADHYĀROPA ("implanting," from the root ruh), a key concept of *Vedānta, referring to the act of attributing qualities of the unreal (i.e., the illusory realm of finite existence) to *Reality. See also adhyāsa, māyā.

ADHYĀSA ("superimposition"), a fundamental notion of *Advaita Vedānta, referring to the false attribution of qualities to a given reality—specifically, projecting finite qualities on the *Absolute. The most common simile used to explain this imposition is that of an illusory snake being projected on what is really a rope. See also adhyāropa, māyā.

ĀDHYĀTMAN ("pertaining to the self"), the innermost Self (*ātman), or one's essential nature. See also *ādhibhūta*, *ādhidaiva*.

ADHYĀTMA-PRASĀDA ("clarity of the inner self"), a term used in the *Yoga-Sūtra* (1.47) to describe an elevated state of consciousness arising at the highest level of the suprareflexive (*nirvicāra*) *ecstasy, when the *mind is as clear as the sky over Northern India in autumn.

ĀDHYĀTMA-VIKĀSA ("spiritual unfolding"), the blossoming of those qualities or aspects of the human personality that draw the *practitioner closer to the transcendental *Reality or *Self. See also *vikāsa*.

ADHYĀTMA-YOGA ("Yoga of the inner self"), a phrase that first occurs in the *Katha-Upanishad* (1.2.12): "Realizing through *adhyātma-yoga* the *God (*deva*) who is primordial, difficult to see, hidden, entered, stationed in the cave, and dwelling in the deep, the sage abandons [both] excitement (*harsha*) and grief (*shoka*)." *Adhyātma-yoga* was taught by the saintly Dāda of Aligarh and was introduced into Great Britain in 1929 by Dāda's disciple, the learned Hari Prasad Shastri, founder of Shanti Sadan in London.

ĀDHYĀTMIKA ("pertaining to the self"), often used in the sense of "spiritual," as in *ādhyātmika-shāstra* or "spiritual teaching."

ĀDI-GRANTH ("First Book"), or **GRANTH SĀHIB** ("Book of the Lord"); the sacred scripture of the adherents of *Sikhism, compiled by Guru Arjun (Sanskrit: Arjuna), the fifth teacher. Its date of completion is traditionally said to be August 1604 CE. It is a central object of veneration in every Sikh temple. One third of its almost 6,000 hymns is from the pen of Guru Arjun, while the remaining compositions stem from the four preceding *gurus*, the ninth *guru* (Tegh Bahadur), and other noted teachers of Hindu and Sufi devotionalism (*bhakti*).

ĀDINĀTHA ("Primal Lord"), an appellation applied to the original teacher of the *Kaula or *Nātha tradition, identified with *Shiva himself, who is held to be the first great adept (*mahā-siddha*) in the long line of master teachers (*ācārya*).

The title *ādinātha* is also given to *Rishabha, the first of the twenty-four enlightened teachers, or "ford makers" (*tīrthankara*), of *Jainism.

ADITI ("Unbounded"), a *Vedic goddess who, among other things, stands for the vast expanse of the sky. In the *Yajur-Veda* Aditi is invoked as the supporter of the earth and the sky and as the wife of *Vishnu. She had eight sons, of whom she cast away Mārtānda, the solar deity. In later epic *mythology, however, she is addressed as Vishnu's mother, who gave birth to twelve sons (the *Ādityas), including Vishnu and *Indra. In either guise, she stands for the principle of freedom and transcendence.

ĀDITYA ("relating to *Aditi"), when used in the singular, an appellation of *Varuna, who, in *Vedic times, was venerated as the deity who maintained the cosmic order (*rita*).

ĀDITYAS, the sons of *Aditi. Originally six or seven, by the time of the *Shata-Patha-Brāhmana their number had been expanded to twelve, representing the twelve months of the year. They are all in some way related to the principle of light.

ĀDI-YĀGA ("primal sacrifice"), a synonym for *maithunā*, or *Tantric sexual intercourse.

ADORATION. See *ārādhana*.

ADRISHTA ("unseen"), fate or destiny, an invisible influence of which we can see only its effects. See also *karman*.

ADVAITA ("nonduality") characterizes the ultimate *Reality beyond all differentiation. Cf. *dvaita*.

ADVAITA VEDĀNTA ("nondual end of the *Vedas"), the metaphysics expounded in the *Upanishads and scriptures based on the *Upanishads*. Nondualism (*advaita*), the dominant philosophical tradition within *Hinduism, comprises many different schools, the most significant being *Shankara's absolute nondualism (*kevala-advaita-vāda*) and *Rāmānuja's qualified nondualism (*vishistha-advaita-vāda*).

*Yoga was originally panentheistic: the world emerged from and is contained in the *Divine but is not merely identical with it. The spiritual *path is a movement in *consciousness through progressive levels of the hierarchy of existence, until the original Consciousness (*cit*), or transcendental *Self, is realized. That Self experiences itself as an integral part (*amsha*) of the ultimate *Reality.

*Patanjali, who consolidated *Yoga as a philosophical system (*darshana*), appears to have favored a dualistic (*dvaita*) metaphysics that presumes an eternal chasm between *Consciousness (or Spirit) and matter. Reversing the position of the *Upanishads*, he contrasted the transcendental Self (*purusha*) with the transcendental ground of nature (*prakriti*).

The schools of *Postclassical Yoga reverted to a nondualist metaphysics, primarily that of *Shankara. See also Vedānta.

ADVAYA ("nondual"), a synonym of *advaita*, often found in the scriptures of Buddhist Tantrism.

ADVAYA-TĀRAKA-UPANISHAD ("Upanishad of the Nondual Deliverer"), one of the *Yoga-Upanishads of the common era. In nineteen short passages, this work propounds *tāraka yoga*, in which internally or externally perceived *light phenomena (known as photisms) play an important role. The "nondual deliverer" is the transcendental *Consciousness, which reveals itself to the *yogin in a "multitude of fires." See also *tāraka*.

AESTHETICS. It has sometimes been suggested that because of its spiritual orientation Indian thought is not true philosophy. On closer inspection, however, this opinion turns out to be a mere prejudice. Indian thought, though distinct in many ways from Western thought, shows a keen regard for the same major themes of philosophical inquiry that preoccupied the Greek philosophers and their descendants. Thus we find the Indian thinkers tackling significant issues such as the nature and means of knowledge (epistemology), the nature of rational thought (logic), and the nature of beauty (aesthetics), which are said to be hallmarks of mature philosophical consideration.

While some traditional Sanskrit authors considered style, figurative language, or suggestive content to be the essential element of poetry, most agreed that it rather is the flavor (*rasa*) of beauty. This concept was discussed in great detail in relation to poetry and drama in the common era (aesthetic philosophy probably has a much longer history in India, but any early writings are now lost). The greatest theorist in the field of Indian aesthetics was the philosopher-adept *Abhinava Gupta.

For a work of *art to evoke a feeling of beauty in the spectator, it must represent a unity under one of nine principal or permanent moods (also called *rasa* or "taste"), comprising the erotic, heroic, laughable, disgusting, terrible, pathetic, wondrous (*adbhuta*), and peaceful. To achieve this artistic unity, which alone can give rise to the feeling of beauty, the traditional Indian artists have since ancient times availed themselves of *Yoga practice, notably *concentration and visualization.

Nonetheless, however accomplished an artist may be in certain yogic techniques, his or her goal is not *liberation but the creation of beauty. From the yogic perspective, this is of course a limitation caused by the artist's unenlightened state. Thus, according to the *Tattva-Vaishāradī (1.2), a subcommentary on the *Yoga-Sūtra, even the most exquisite beauty (*atisundara*) comes to an end and therefore is a source of pain. Hence the *yogin* must endeavor to overcome all attachment to beauty.

AFFLICTION. See *klesha*, Suffering.

ĀGAMA ("come down"), testimonial or authoritative *knowledge, i.e., knowledge acquired through sensory perception or inferred by a trustworthy person; one of the three means of valid knowledge (*pramāna*) admitted in *Classical Yoga. The word is often translated as "tradition." See also *shruti*, *smriti*.

ĀGAMA, a work within a particular genre of sacred *Hindu literature belonging to *Shaivism. Some 200 such scriptures are known, though they have barely been studied. They are presented as revelations (*shruti*) of *Shiva. Their counterparts in *Vaishnavism are known as *Samhitās*, and in *Shaktism as *Tantras*. Traditionally, 28 Āgamas are recognized as forming the revealed canon of the *Shiva community of South India. These scriptures are equivalent to the four *Vedas of North Indian *Brāhmanism and are sometimes collectively referred to as the "fifth *Veda*." Like the *Tantras*, they purport to be for the spiritual aspirant of the present dark age (*kali-yuga*) who lacks the moral and mental capacity to follow more conventional *paths to *liberation. Regrettably, few of these texts have so far been published in book form, and fewer still have been translated into English.

ĀGĀMI-KARMAN ("present karma"). See *karman*.

AGARBHA-PRĀNĀYĀMA ("breath control without seed"), a synonym for *nirgarbha-prānāyāma*. See also *garbha*, *prānāyāma*; cf. *sagarbha-prānāyāma*.

AGASTYA (Tamil: Akattiyar), or Agasti; the name of several individuals. A seer (*rishi*) Agastya, composer of several of the hymns of the ancient *Rig-Veda*, was married to Lopamudra, the daughter of the ruler of the Videha tribe. The *Rig-Veda* (1.179.4) has preserved a conversation between the seer and his wife. He may have been the chief priest of the Vedic King Khela.

The name Agastya is also associated with works on grammar, medicine, gemology, and other sciences. Agastya is remembered to have been of small stature and in iconography is generally depicted as a dwarf. He is mentioned in a number of *Brāhmanas*, the *Mahābhārata* and the *Rāmāyana*, and several *Purānas*. The *Rāmāyana* (3.11.86) explains his name by his fabulous deed of stopping the mountains (*aga*) of the Vindhya range from pushing upward; indeed, legend has it that he humbled the proud mountain range by forcing it to bend over.

Agastya's hermitage (*ashrama) is said to have been in the extreme south of the Indian peninsula; according to legend, he was the first to establish a colony in the South. Agastya was a great adept (*siddha) who is to South India what *Matsyendra is to the North. His fame spread as far as Indonesia.

AGE. See kalpa, manvantara, yuga.

AGHORA ("Nonterrible"), an epithet of *Shiva, paradoxically referring to his terrifying aspect, which presumably is not so for the initiate worshiper.

AGHORASHIVA ACĀRYA (late 13th–early 14th cen. CE), the author of the Sarvajna-Uttara-Vritti ("Commentary on Ultimate Omniscience,") a commentary on the *Hatha-Ratna-Āvalī. He was patronized by King Prataparudra (1296–1323).

AGHORĪ, a *Tantra-based sect that evolved from the more widespread *Kāpālika ascetic order some time in the fourteenth century CE. Its followers, known as the Aghorī Panthīs, have always been held in low esteem because of their many eccentric practices, such as the use of human skulls as vessels, the frequenting of cemeteries, the eating of refuse, and not least cannibalism (until the end of the nineteenth century).

ĀGNEYĪ- or VAISHVĀNARĪ-DHĀRANĀ-MUDRĀ ("fiery concentration seal"), one of the five *concentration techniques described in the *Gheranda-Samhitā (3.61). The practitioner is asked to focus his *attention and *life force on the (digestive) "fire" (*agni) in the abdominal region for 150 minutes, thus stimulating the psychosomatic energy there. Accomplishment in this practice is said to make one immune against the heat of flames. See also dhāranā, mudrā, panca-dhāranā.

AGNI ("fire"), one of the five material elements (*bhūta) that compose the manifest *cosmos in its grossest dimension; also, digestive and psychosomatic heat. See also tattva, vahni.

AGNI, the god of fire, figured as a central deity (*deva) of the ancient *Vedic religion. He was closely associated with the Vedic sacrificial fire ritual. The symbolism of Agni is open to many interpretations, including his tentative equation with the "serpent power" (*kundalinī-shakti) in some contexts. See also jathara-agni.

AGNI-HOTRA ("fire oblation"), the daily fire sacrifice performed by pious Hindus, which involves the offering of milk into the fire. Since the time of the *Upanishads, *Yoga has been regarded as an internal fire sacrifice. See also yajna.

AGNI-SĀRA-DHAUTI ("cleansing by means of fire"), a synonym for *vahni-sāra-dhauti.

AGNI-YOGA ("fire Yoga"), the process whereby the "serpent power" (*kundalinī-shakti) is awakened through the joint action of *breath (or controlled psychosomatic energy) and *mind. A modern spiritual school by that name, founded by Russell Paul Schofield, uses visualization in combination with the *body's psychosomatic energy (*prāna) to dissolve undigested perceptual and emotional experiences that have created a blockage in the body-mind. This approach is also known as Actualization.

11

AHAM ("I"), the conditional *ego, the *ahamkāra. In Kashmiri *Shaivism, it designates the transcendental *Self, as *Shiva, and is also known as *ahamtā ("I-ness").

AHAM BRAHMA ASMI (aham brahmāsmi, "I am the Absolute"), one of the famous dicta of *Advaita Vedānta, introduced in the early *Upanishads and reiterated in medieval *Yoga scriptures that avow nondualism. It is more an ecstatic exclamation than a philosophical proclamation. In the condition of *enlightenment, the "I" is no longer the ego personality (*ahamkāra) but the transcendental Self (*ātman). See also brahman.

AHAM-IDAM ("I am this"), according to Kashmiri *Shaivism, the first level of distinction appearing in the *Absolute, as *Shiva, which is pure *aham. This level is characterized as a state of unity-in-difference in which the world is beginning to emerge as object from the ultimate subject, which is *Shiva. It is also known as *Sada-Shiva ("Ever-Shiva"). The next evolutionary level is *idam-aham ("this I am").

AHAMKĀRA ("I maker"), the *ego, or principle of individuation. In *Sāmkhya philosophy, it is regarded as one of the eight primary evolutes of nature and thus stands for a whole evolutionary category (*tattva). Often, however, it simply denotes the ego illusion, i.e., the sense of being a particular body-mind, of having certain properties ("my feelings," "my ideas," "my children," etc.), and of being an *actor originating *actions. All spiritual traditions are agreed that the ego sense must be transcended. Sometimes this is wrongly interpreted as a demand to be altruistic. Something much more profound is intended, namely, a radical shift in our sense of who we are: from self-identity, we are asked to move to Self-identity—from ahamkāra to *ātman. See also asmitā, jīva.

AHAMTĀ ("I-ness"), an expression of Kashmiri *Shaivism denoting the transcendental *Self, which, in the *Pratyābhijnā-Hridaya (20) is said to be constituted of the "essence of light and bliss" (prakāsha-ānanda-sāra).

AHAM-VIMARSHA ("I awareness"), the primary and principal creative activity (*kriyā) of the transcendental *Consciousness according to Kashmiri *Shaivism. The word *vimarsha generally has the meaning of "examination" or "discussion" but here refers to the primordial intelligence that witnesses all the processes of the objective *world. See also sākshin.

ĀHĀRA ("food" or "diet"). Dietary rules have formed an important part of *Yoga practice from the earliest times. Thus the *Chāndogya-Upanishad (7.26.2), which dates from the eighth century BCE, speaks of the close link between dietary *purity and purity of being. A favorite saying of modern *yogins is "You are what you eat."

The *Bhagavad-Gītā (17.8ff.) distinguishes foods according to the predominance of the qualities *sattva, *rajas, and *tamas in them:

Foods that promote life, lucidity (sattva), strength, *health, *happiness, and satisfaction (*prīti), and that are savory, rich in oil, firm, and heart[-gladdening] are agreeable to the sattva-natured [person].

Foods that are pungent, sour, salty, spicy, sharp, harsh, and burning are coveted by the rajas-natured [person]. They cause pain (*duhkha), grief (*shoka), and disease (*roga).

And [food] that is spoiled, tasteless, putrid, stale, leftover, and unclean is food agreeable to the *tamas*-natured [person].

The *Gheranda-Samhitā* (5.17ff.) makes a number of specific recommendations: The *yogin* should eat rice, barley, wheat, and various kinds of gram, in addition to fruits and vegetables native to India. In the beginning of *Yoga practice, one should avoid bitter, sour, salty, pungent, and scorched food, as well as curds, buttermilk, liquor, heavy vegetables, vegetable stems, gourds, berries, and a variety of other named fruits and plants; one should also avoid the company of women, travel, and open fires.

The *yogin* may consume fresh butter, ghee, milk, sugar, sugarcane, jaggery, ripe plantain, coconut, pomegranate, anise, grapes, cardamom, nutmeg, cloves, rose hips, dates, juice that is not sour, and a number of other named plants native to India. The food should be easily digestible, soft, and rich in oil. Food that is hard, polluted, putrid, stale, very cold, or very hot should be shunned. The *yogin* should eat more than once a day and avoid eating not at all or eating too frequently.

Specifically for the practice of *breath control, the *yogin* should take some milk or ghee twice a day, at noon and in the evening. The *Hatha-Ratna-Āvalī* (1.23) recommends milk and similar products at the outset of yogic discipline, but makes no rules for those who have become stabilized in their practice.

Not all yogic authorities, both ancient and modern, are in agreement over what constitutes a good diet. Without exception, however, they emphasize the importance of exercising restraint over the intake of food. This rule is known as *mita-āhāra. See also *anna-yoga*, *laghu-āhāra*, *upavāsa*.

ĀHĀRA-JAYA ("mastery over food"), disciplined eating; sometimes listed among the moral observances (*yama), which shows the great importance of this discipline. See also *anna-yoga*.

AHIMSĀ ("nonharming"), often translated as "nonviolence," though something more fundamental is intended by it. *Patanjali regards it as one of the five moral observances (*yama), that make up the "great vow" (*mahā-vrāta), which must be kept under all circumstances. Other authorities list *ahimsā* under the five restraints (*niyama). It is generally defined as the practice of abstaining from harming others physically, mentally, and vocally at all times. Mahatma *Gandhi, in advocating *ahimsā* as a viable moral and political practice, articulated an age-old tradition within *Hinduism, although his radical approach is not characteristic of all Hindu schools of thought. For instance, *Brāhmanism permits the slaughter of animals for sacrificial purposes. Also, the teachings of the *Bhagavad-Gītā* are set against the historical background of one of ancient India's fiercest wars. Here *Krishna admonishes Prince *Arjuna to participate in the *war rather than feel dejected about having to kill kinsmen and former teachers among the enemy. Because of its militaristic tenor, the *Bhagavad-Gītā* has often been interpreted as an allegory about the inner struggle of human beings. See also *vrāta*; cf. *himsā*.

AHIRBUDHNYA-SAMHITĀ, a *Pancarātra text from Kashmir, probably composed around the fifth century CE. The name Ahirbudhnya is an epithet of *Shiva and means "serpent of the deep" (from *ahi*, "serpent," and *budhnya*, "deep"). This *Samhitā, a fictitious dialogue between Shiva and the sage *Nārada, covers a wide range of subjects, from ritual to occultism, philosophy, and theology. It is of interest to the *Yoga researcher for its description of the lost Yoga text attributed to *Hiranyagarbha.

AIKYA ("union"), the highest stage of spiritual growth in *Vīra Shaivism. It refers to the realization of the singular (*eka) transcendental *Reality. See also shat-sthāla.

AIR. See prāna, vāta, vāyu.

AISHVARYA ("lordship"), one of the great magical attainments (*siddhi) by which the *yogin is said to gain mastery over the manifest and unmanifest aspects of the *cosmos, similar to the supremacy of the "Lord" (*īshvara). See also Parapsychology, vibhūti.

AJA ("unborn," from the root jan, "to be born"). Already in the ancient *Brihad-Āranyaka-Upanishad (4.4.20) the transcendental *Self is said to be unborn. This is a common *Vedāntic characterization of the *ātman and is found, for instance, numerous times in *Gaudapāda's *Māndūkya-Kārika.

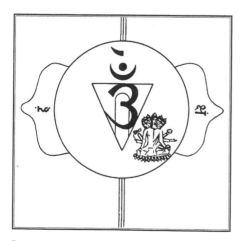

Ājnā-cakra, the psychoenergetic center situated in the middle of the head

When spelled ajā (with a feminine ending), the word means "goat," and it is used in this sense also in the *Brihad-Āranyaka-Upanishad (1.4.4) in a passage that describes the creation of everything in pairs (mithuna)—a reference to the inherently erotic nature of existence.

AJAPA-MANTRA, also known as ajapa-gāyatrī; the "unpronounced *mantra," i.e., the sound hamsa, which is continually produced by the *body as a result of the breathing process. The syllable ham is connected with inhalation, and sa with exhalation. According to the *Gheranda-Samhitā (5.84–85) and other medieval texts, this sound is automatically "recited" in the human body 21,600 times during a day. The same work (5.90) instructs that one should recite this potent sound (mantra) consciously and even double its *recitation in order to effect the state of exaltation (*unmanī). This idea is embedded in an esoteric teaching according to which the continuous sound hamsa-hamsa-hamsa can also be heard as so'ham-so'ham-so'ham, which means, "I am He, I am He, I am He," i.e., "I am the *Self." See also gāyatrī, hamsa, japa, mantra-yoga.

ĀJNĀ-CAKRA ("command wheel"), one of the seven major psychosomatic energy centers (*cakra) of the human *body, located in the middle of the head at the level of the eyebrows, also known as the "third eye." It derives its name from its being the receiver for the *guru's telepathic communications to the *student; hence it is also called guru-cakra. Graphically depicted as a gray or white two-petaled lotus, the ājnā-cakra contains a symbolic representation of the phallus (*linga)—as a symbol of masculine creativity, or *shiva—placed within a downward-pointing triangle, a symbol of the feminine principle, or *shakti. This center is connected with the sense of individuality (*ahamkāra), the lower mind (*manas), and the sacred syllable *om. Its presiding deities are Parama-Shiva ("Supreme *Shiva") and the Goddess Hākinī. It is the penultimate station in the ascent of the "serpent power" (*kundalinī-shakti) along the spinal axis. Its activation is said to lead to all kinds of psychic powers (*siddhi), notably *clairvoyance and the ability to communicate telepathically. See also bhrū-madhya.

AJNĀNA ("ignorance"), a synonym for *avidyā ("nescience"), signifying spiritual blindness, as a result of which we experience ourselves as individuated body-minds that know physical pain (*duhkha) and psychic torment and that are doomed to age and die. It is the opposite of spiritual wisdom (*jnāna, *vidyā), which is conducive to genuine self-knowledge and, ultimately, *Self-realization.

AKALA ("impartite"). This word is not yet found in the earliest *Upanishads, but from the time of the *Shvetāshvatara-Upanishad (6.5), which speaks of the *Divine as having no parts (kalā), it is frequently employed to describe the *Self. It is a synonym for the equally common nishkala. Cf. kalā.

AKARMAN ("inaction"). According to the *Bhagavad-Gītā (3.8), inactivity is impossible in the manifest world, because the very constituents of *nature, the *gunas, are forever in motion. Hence life cannot be maintained without a minimum of *action. Instead of abstention from action, this work proposes the ideal of action-transcendence (*naishkarmya-karman). Cf. karman, karma-yoga.

ĀKĀSHA "radiance"). Early on, this old Sanskrit word acquired the meaning of "space" or "ether" and served as a frequent comparison for the transcendental *Self, which is described as being brighter than a myriad of suns. Thus, in the ancient *Brihad-Āranyaka-Upanishad (2.1.17) the ākāsha is said to be located in the *heart, the secret seat of the *Self. In medieval works such as the *Advaya-Tāraka-Upanishad, the term has the specific meaning of "luminous [inner] space," which describes a set of mystical experiences in which *light phenomena play an important role. Five types of ākāsha are differentiated: (1) the guna-rahita-ākāsha ("ether-space devoid of qualities"); (2) the parama-ākāsha ("supreme ether-space"), which resembles palpable darkness lit up by the resplendent "deliverer" (*tāraka); (3) the mahā-ākāsha ("great ether-space"), which is bright like the conflagration at the end of time; (4) the tattva-ākāsha ("ether-space of verity"), which is effulgent beyond compare; and (5) the sūrya-ākāsha ("solar ether-space"), which is as brilliant as 100,000 suns. The *yogin is said to merge with these luminous realities, which are steppingstones to the transmental (*amanaska) state.

In later times, ākāsha came to be regarded as the finest of the five material elements (*bhūta) of the manifest *cosmos. In this sense, the concept is similar to Aristotle's "quintessence" and the "luminiferous ether" of nineteenth-century physics—a notion that was abandoned at the beginning of our century. See also kha, madhya-lakshya, tāraka-yoga, tattva, vyoman.

ĀKĀSHA-CAKRA ("ether wheel"), the ninth psychoenergetic center in the human *body, according to the *Siddha-Siddhānta-Paddhati (2.9). It is depicted as a lotus with sixteen petals facing upward; the middle of the pericarp has three peaks. This center may be the same as the *vyoma-cakra. See also cakra.

ĀKĀSHA-GAMANA ("walking in the ether"), a yogic power (*siddhi) that corresponds, if understood physically, to levitation or, if understood psychologically, to visualization involving the mind's journey through "other dimensions." In the latter sense, it is a precondition for the magical technique of entering the body of another being (*para-deha-pravesha), mentioned for instance in the *Yoga-Sūtra (3.38). See also khecaratva, mano-gati, Parapsychology.

ĀKĀSHĪ- or NABHO-DHĀRANĀ-MUDRĀ ("ethereal concentration seal"), one of the five *concentration techniques described in the *Gheranda-Samhitā (3.63). This practice consists in focusing one's *attention and life force (*prāna), through breath control, on the ether element for 150 minutes, thus stimulating the psychosomatic energy. This is said to be capable of "breaking open the door to *liberation." See also dhāranā, mudrā, pancadhāranā.

AKATTIYAR. See Agastya.

AKLISHTA ("nonafflicted"), one of two basic categories of mental activity (*vritti), namely, that which is conducive to *liberation, according to the *Yoga-Sūtra (1.5). See also klesha; cf. klishta.

AKRAMA ("nonsequential"), one of the characteristics of the ultimate *Reality, or *Self, according to Kashmiri *Shaivism. Whereas creation involves successive or sequential unfolding, called *krama, the transcendental *Being is beyond space and time and perfectly homogeneous or undivided (*akala). See also tattva.

AKRAMA-KRIYĀ ("nonsequential activity"). According to Kashmiri *Shaivism,

the ultimate *Reality, called *Shiva, is eternally creative, but this creativity is nonsequential. On the human level, this corresponds to what in some schools of thought is known as "action-transcendence" (*naishkarmya-karman).

AKSHARA ("immobile," "imperishable"; also "lettered" or "letter") the *Absolute; also, its symbol *om. Cf. kshara.

AKSHI-UPANISHAD (Akshyupanishad), one of the general Vedānta *Upanishads. Its curious name (akshi means "eye") indicates that it teaches visionary wisdom (cākshumatī-vidyā). The latter of its two parts deals with the seven stages of *Yoga (see sapta-bhūmi). Yoga is defined (2.3) as the "supraconscious, nonartificial obliteration (kshaya) of *consciousness."

AKULA, ("nonflock"), one of *Shiva's many epithets. See also Kaula school; cf. kula.

AKULA-ĀGAMA-TANTRA (Akulāgamatantra), a scripture belonging to the *Kaula tradition of *Matsyendra. Its first section deals with the sixfold path of *hatha-yoga. The third section explains the five "ingredients" of *Tantrism, the *ma-karas, as being a part of yogic practice, but condemns their literal enactment.

AKULA-VĪRA-TANTRA, a short work belonging to the *Kaula school; there appear to be two versions. The akula-vīra, or "akula hero," is the supreme *Reality.

ĀLAMBANA ("foundation"), the *object or stimulus of *consciousness acting as a prop for concentration (*dhāranā). See also bīja.

ĀLAMBUSĀ- or ĀLAMBUSHĀ-NĀDĪ ("plenteously misty channel"), one of the *body's principal conduits (*nādī), or pathways of life energy. It is generally thought to originate in the "bulb" (*kanda) in the lower abdomen, but its termination point is variously described as being in the *eyes, *ears, or mouth.

ĀLASYA ("sloth"), one of the obstacles (*antarāya) of *Yoga; explained in the *Yoga-Bhāshya (1.30) as inactivity resulting from bodily and mental heaviness. The *Shiva-Purāna (5.26.35) calls it one of the great enemies that must be conquered. In the *Mahābhārata (12.263.46) it is said to be one of the factors that prevent one from reaching *heaven. It can effectively be combated by *sīt-karī-prānāyāma, one of the chief types of *breath control employed in *hatha-yoga. See also styāna, tandrā.

AL-BĪRŪNĪ, a famous Persian traveler who visited India in the first half of the eleventh century. He composed the Kitāb Patanjal, a rather free Arabic rendering of the *Yoga-Sūtra, together with a lengthy commentary that could have been the *Tattva-Vaishāradī. His translation adds little to our knowledge of *Patanjali's Yoga; in fact, al-Bīrūnī seems to have misunderstood many of the more intricate technical matters.

ALCHEMY, the prescientific craft of using natural elements to produce seemingly supernatural results, notably physical *immortality. Whether in China, India, or Europe, the alchemists sought after the elixir of life, the philosopher's stone, that would outwit *nature's law of entropy. In India this elixir is known as *rasa ("taste" or "essence"), and alchemy is called rasa-āyana ("way of the elixir") or dhātu-vāda ("doctrine of the basic element"). From the reports of such seasoned travelers as

*al-Bīrūnī and Marco Polo, we learn that Indian *yogins have also practiced alchemy. Indeed, *Yoga is a form of alchemy, since it aims at the transmutation of human *consciousness and—in *Tantrism and *hatha-yoga—even at the *transubstantiation of the *body. At the center of the medieval *Siddha tradition lies the quest for a "divine body" (*divya-sharīra) endowed with a variety of paranormal abilities (*siddhi) and thoroughly enlightened. The *siddha's *enlightenment has permanently changed his body's chemistry.

ALCOHOL. See madya, surā.

ALINGA ("signless"), in *Classical Yoga, the highest (or deepest) level of the hierarchy of nature (*prakriti); the state of undifferentiated existence. The *Tattva-Vaishāradī (1.45) defines it as the equipoise of the three primary constituents (*guna) of nature. By contrast, in *Preclassical Yoga the term is sometimes used synonymously with *purusha, the transcendental *Self. See also Cosmos, tattva; cf. linga.

ALLĀMA PRABHUDEVA, a twelfth-century *adept and contemporary of *Basava remembered as the head of an order, Anubhava-Mandapa, of more than 300 enlightened beings, including about 60 women. He is mentioned in the *Hatha-Yoga-Pradīpikā (1.8) as one of the *teachers of *hatha-yoga. According to Gaurana's fourteenth-century Nava-Nātha-Caritra ("Life of the Nine Lords"), *Goraksha demonstrated to Allāma how no weapon could harm him. Then Allāma invited Goraksha to run his body through with a sword. To the latter's astonishment, the sword passed through Allāma's body as if it were made of space. It was then that Goraksha requested initiation from this great adept. Goraksha's meeting with Allāma is also described in the sixteenth-century *Prabhu-Linga-Līlā*. Allāma's date of death is traditionally given as 1196 CE.

ALOLUPTVA ("nonwavering"), according to the *Shvetāshvatara-Upanishad* (2.12), one of the characteristics of the first stage of yogic accomplishment, where the practitioner is firmly committed to the spiritual process. See also *anavasthitatva*.

ĀLOLYA denotes something like "dedication" or "enthusiasm," and in this sense is considered to be one of the signs (*cihna*) of *progress in *Yoga.

ALONENESS. See *kaivalya, kevalatā*.

ALPHABET. The transformative value of sound (*shabda*) is recognized in many spiritual traditions. But only a few traditions have developed full-fledged systems of alphabetic mysticism, notably the Hebrew Kabbalah, which some authorities deem to have been influenced by Eastern sources, and Indian *Tantrism. The Sanskrit alphabet comprises fifty letters (*varna*), which are used in the creation of sacred sounds (*mantra*) employed in meditative recitation (*japa*) or in the construction of geometric devices (*yantra* and *mandala*) serving the *yogin's *concentration.

According to the *Kaula school of Kashmir, the fifty letters of the *deva-nāgarī* alphabet correspond to the stages of creation or manifestation from the *Absolute down to the coarse (material) level of existence. Thus the first six vowels—*a, ā, i, ī, u,* and *ū*—are representative of the sequence in which the six primary powers (*anuttara, ānanda, icchā, īshana, unmesha,* and *ūrmi*) arise from the ultimate *Reality.

The consonants are symbolic of later phases of creation (*sarga*).

The letters are also called *mātrikās* ("little mothers") because they are thought to be not merely lifeless sounds but generative forces. In certain rituals the fifty letters are "placed" in various parts of the *body, particularly the psychoenergetic centers (*cakra*)—a practice known as *mātrikā-nyāsa*.

In *Tantric *kundalinī-yoga* the letters are pictured as being inscribed in the petals of the lotus flowers (*padma*) associated with the principal psychoenergetic centers (*cakra*) of the *body. The center at the crown of the *head, called *sahasrāra-cakra*, contains 1,000 petals, each with one letter of the alphabet. Since these centers are traditionally said to constitute the body of the "serpent power" (*kundalinī-shakti*), the *kundalinī* itself can be regarded as embodying—or being the psychocosmic force behind—the entire alphabet. Indeed, the *kundalinī* is considered to be the sonic Absolute (*shabda-brahman*).

The alphabet is picturesquely referred to as the "garland of letters" (*varna-mālā*). This alphabetic garland is represented in iconography as a necklace of skulls worn by the goddess *Kālī. The symbolism behind this is that, at the end of time (or in the moment of *enlightenment when the *world is transcended), the goddess withdraws or dissolves all human speech, including the letters of the alphabet. See also *vāc*.

ALTERED STATE OF CONSCIOUSNESS, a state of *consciousness that the experiencer feels to be qualitatively different from his or her ordinary mental functioning; a term coined by the psychologist Charles Tart, who wrote a pioneering work on the subject. The high value placed on the routine state of consciousness in our culture is a noteworthy historical oddity. Most premodern cultures valued such altered states as dreams, visions, trances, and ecstasies. By contrast, we tend to regard these states with perplexity and unease, seeing in them "abnormal" (i.e., deficient) manifestations of the psyche. The counterculture of the 1960s, mainly through the widespread exposure to "mind-altering" drugs such as LSD, has led to a softening of our attitude toward nonordinary states of awareness. This is most apparent in the growing New Age movement. Despite their popularization, however, altered states of consciousness are still only imperfectly understood. Most importantly, the condition of *enlightenment must be carefully distinguished from altered states, for it implies a transcendence of the *mind itself, even though this widely made claim is rejected by many psychologists. See also dhāranā, dhyāna, samādhi.

ĀLVĀRS. Southern *Vaishnavism remembers twelve ālvārs, who inspired the people with their devotional hymns expressing their burning love for the *Divine in the form of *Vishnu. Their name means "those who dive deep," that is, those who are deeply absorbed in the mystery of the *Divine. For the ālvārs, God was *Vishnu or Vishnu's various forms or incarnations, notably *Krishna and *Rāma.

The twelve included the untouchable *Tiruppan, the king *Kulasekhara, the *brahmin *Periy (also known as Vishnucitta), the chieftain *Tirumankaiy, the poet-saint *Āndāl, and the much-loved Namm-Ālvār ("Our ālvār"). These propagators of *bhakti-yoga lived in the period from 600 to 900 CE. Their devotional hymns were gathered in the Tamil compendium known as the Nalayirap-Pirapantam (Sanskrit: Nalayira-Prabandha). Most of the ca. 4,000 hymns are by *Tiruman-

kaiy and *Namm, the last of this group. Cf. Nāyanmārs.

AMĀ-KALĀ. This technical term of *Tantrism is composed of the word amā, denoting the night of the new moon or the sixteenth station (*tithi) of the moon, and the word *kalā, meaning "part." This is one of three aspects of the *kundalinī-shakti in its unmanifest state at the level of the highest psychoenergetic center, the *sahasrāra-cakra, of the *body. In this aspect, the "serpent power" is in a formless but subtle (*sūkshma) state and is associated with a reddish glow. It also is said to be in a half-coil. The amākulā is responsible for the transition from meditation (*dhyāna) to conscious ecstasy (*samprajnāta-samādhi). Cf. nirvāna-kalā, nirvāna-shakti.

AMANASKATĀ ("transmindedness") or amanaska ("transmental"), the sublime condition of *enlightenment in which the *mind (*manas) is transcended. It is also called "exaltation" (*unmanī).

AMANASKA-YOGA, a work on *hatha-yoga ascribed to Īshvara Vāmadeva. It consists of two chapters with a total of 208 stanzas and expounds what it calls *tāraka-yoga. This teaching is not identical with the photistic *Yoga of the *Advaya-Tāraka-Upanishad, however. Rather, it is a technique for the simultaneous stabilization of one's *gaze, *breathing, and *attention, founded in the *renunciation of everything.

AMĀNITVA ("humility"). According to the *Bhagavad-Gītā (13.7), this virtue is a manifestation of wisdom (*jnāna). Cf. abhimāna, darpa.

AMARA-NĀTHA-SAMVĀDA ("Dialogue with the Immortal Lord"), a twelfth-century Marathi text ascribed to *Goraksha.

AMARAUGHA-PRABHODHA ("Awakening to the Immortal Flood"), a work of seventy-four stanzas ascribed to *Goraksha. Many of its verses correspond to those of the *Hatha-Yoga-Pradīpikā. The title is composed of the words *amara* ("deathless" or "immortal") and *ogha* ("flood").

AMARAUGHA-SHĀSANA ("Instruction on the Immortal Flood"), a treatise on *Yoga ascribed to *Goraksha.

AMAROLĪ-MUDRĀ ("*amarolī* seal"). The word *amarolī* is difficult to translate; it denotes the "immortal (*amara*) nectar." This "seal" (*mudrā*) is one of the techniques that have brought *hatha-yoga* into disrepute with pollution-conscious *brahmins*. The *Yoga-Tattva-Upanishad* (128) describes it as the daily drinking of the *amarī*, or urine. The *Hatha-Yoga-Pradīpikā* (3.96ff.) contains a more detailed description of this practice: One should enjoy the middle flow of one's urine, discarding the first flow since it increases bile (*pitta*) and the last flow because it lacks essence. This is regarded as a variety of *vajrolī-mudrā*. The *Hatha-Ratna-Āvalī* (2.109) explains *amarolī* as the absorption of the "nectar" through the nose. See also *sahajolī-mudrā*.

AMĀTRA ("nonmeasure"), the transcendental aspect of the sacred syllable *om*, which cannot be heard or even perceived with the *mind. As *Shankara explains in his celebrated commentary on *Gaudapāda's *Māndūkya-Kārikā* (1.29), the *amātra* signifies the "Fourth" (*turīya*), that is, the *Absolute. See also *mātra*.

ĀMBHASĪ-DHĀRANĀ-MUDRĀ ("aqueous concentration seal"), one of the five *concentration techniques described in the *Gheranda-Samhitā* (3.72ff.) as follows:

The [*water] element is said to be like a conch, the moon, or white like the *kunda* flower, and auspicious. Its seed [syllable] is the letter *va*, [which is] its ambrosia, and *Vishnu is connected with it. One should concentrate the *mind and *breath for five *ghatikās* [ca. 150 minutes] thereon. This is the aqueous concentration that destroys all *evil, affliction, and *sorrow. Whoever know this seal will never meet with *death even in the deepest water. It should carefully be kept secret. By disclosing it, success is forfeited.

See also *panca-dhāranā*.

AMBROSIA. See *amarolī*, *amrita*, *soma*, *sudhā*.

ĀMNĀYA ("assemblage" or "group"). Writers within the prolific tradition of *Tantrism early on attempted to make sense of the vast variety of teachings by inventing a number of classificatory systems. One major grouping is into "streams" (*srota*), another is into "seats" (*pītha*), and a third and later grouping is into four, five, six, or even seven "assemblages." The arrangement into four groups appears to be the oldest and most common. These are based on the cardinal directions, though not in any strictly geographical sense, and they are also sometimes related to the four world ages (*yuga*).

The *Kula-Arnava-Tantra* (3.7ff.) subscribes to the following five *āmnāyas*, stating that they issued from the five faces of *Shiva: (1) *pūrva-* ("earlier," meaning east), (2) *pashcima-* ("last," meaning west), (3) *dakshina-* ("right," meaning south), (4) *uttara-* ("upper," meaning north), and (5) *ūrdhva-āmnāya* ("upward group"), which is said to be superior to the other four. All five groups lead to *liberation. The same *Tantra* (3.15–16, 19) declares:

He who [truly] knows one of the groups becomes undoubtedly liberated. What of someone who knows four groups? He directly becomes *Shiva.

Greater still than the knowledge of the four groups, dear one, is the upward group. Therefore one who desires perfection (*siddhi) should know it [fully].

O Goddess, know the ūrdhva-āmnaya as the direct means to liberation. The ūrdhva-āmnāyu, whose results exceed all other groups, is higher than the highest.

AMRITA ("immortal"), AMRITATVA ("immortality"). *Enlightenment is frequently equated with *immortality, for the transcendental *Self is deathless. In the literature of *hatha-yoga, however, the word amrita has a technical meaning. It refers to the nectar of immortality that trickles down from a secret center in the *head and is wasted by ordinary mortals because they do not know this secret. The intrinsic connection between this nectar and immortality is succinctly captured in the *Kaula-Jnāna-Nirnaya (14.94): "How can there be immortality (amaratva) without [the flowing of] the nectar?"

The nectar, variously called *soma, *sudhā, amara-vārunī, and pīyūsha, is of brilliant white-reddish color and is exquisitely bliss-inducing. According to the *Shiva-Samhitā (2.7f.), the nectar of immortality has two forms: one flows through the left conduit (the *idā-nādī) and nourishes the *body; the other flows along the central pathway (the *sushumnā-nādī) and creates the "moon" (*candra). The nectar's flow increases when the "serpent power" (*kundalinī-shakti) has ascended from the base center to the psychoenergetic center at the throat.

The *Hatha-Yoga-Pradīpikā (4.53) states that the whole *body should be flooded with this ambrosia, which produces a superior body endowed with enormous strength and vigor and free from *disease. This practice also prevents aging and bestows immortality as well as the eight magical powers (*ashta-siddhi). See also khecārī-mudrā, tālu.

AMRITA-BINDU-UPANISHAD (Amritabindūpanishad, "Upanishad of the Immortal Drop"), one of the *Yoga-Upanishads. Consisting of only twenty-two stanzas and based on *Vedānta metaphysics, it teaches a form of Yoga that combines renunciation with recitation (*japa) of the sacred syllable *om.

AMRITA-NĀDA-UPANISHAD (Amritanādopanishad, "Upanishad of the Immortal Sound"), one of the *Yoga-Upanishads. Consisting of thirty-eight stanzas, it expounds a *Vedānta-based sixfold *Yoga (*shad-anga-yoga). The text is prefixed with four verses dealing with a method for the recitation of the *pranava (i.e., *om) coupled with the *adoration of the God *Rudra. See also amrita, nāda.

AMRITA-NĀDĪ ("conduit of immortality"). According to the modern Indian sage and *jnānin *Ramana Maharshi and the contemporary American adept Da Avabhasa (a.k.a. Da Free John, Franklin Jones), the amrita-nādī is the esoteric structure that extends from the *head to the *heart to infinity. It is said to complete the circuit formed by the axial pathway (*sushumnā-nādī), which runs from the base of the spine to the crown of the head. See also amrita, nādī.

AMRITA-SIDDHI-YOGA ("Yoga of the Perfection/Attainment of Immortality"), a work on *hatha-yoga available only in manuscript form.

AMSHA ("part" or "fragment"). In the panentheistic teaching of the *Bhagavad-

Gītā and the *Bhāgavata tradition in general, the *cosmos and the embodied selves (**jīva-ātman*) are merely a fragment of the immeasurable body of the *Divine. Individual beings are the cells of the infinite organism that is the "Lord" (**bhagavat*). See also *Rāmānuja.

ANĀHATA-CAKRA ("wheel of the unstruck [sound]"), an esoteric center also known as the "lotus of the *heart" (*hrit-padma*), "heart center" (*hridaya-cakra*), "twelve-spoked center" (*dvādasha-ara-cakra*), and by many other synonyms. It has been recognized as a special locus of the sacred within the human *body since the time of the *Vedas*. The heart has since ancient times been viewed as the secret seat of the *Divine and the location where the immortal sound *om, which is not produced by anything, can be heard.

This psychoenergetic center is often depicted as a lotus having twelve petals of deep red color. Its seed syllable (**bīja-mantra*) is *yam*, which pertains to the *wind element. The center's presiding adept is Pinākin, the presiding *goddess is the yellow-colored, three-eyed Kākinī. The heart center is likened to the legendary wish-fulfilling tree. It is the abode of the "swan" (**hamsa*), i.e., the life force (**prāna*). Regular *contemplation of this esoteric structure yields a variety of paranormal abilities (**siddhi*), including immeasurable knowledge, *clairaudience, and *clairvoyance. See also *dahara*.

ĀNANDA ("bliss") can connote both joy and transcendental *bliss. The *Hatha-Yoga-Pradīpikā (4.75) distinguishes between bliss as a mental state (*citta-ānanda*) and as the unqualified innate delight (*sahaja-ānanda*) pertaining to the *Absolute. In *Classical Yoga, the term denotes one of the accompanying phenomena of conscious ecstasy (**samprajñāta-samādhi*).

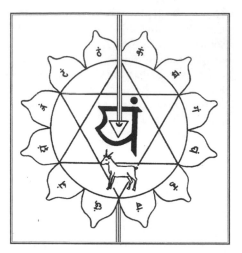

Anāhata-cakra, the psychoenergetic center located at the heart, considered to be the seat of the transcendental Consciousness

In Kashmiri *Shaivism, seven levels of blissful experience are distinguished: (1) *nija-ānanda* ("inborn bliss"), the experience of subjective *bliss as distinct from the objective *world; (2) *nirānanda*, the experience of bliss in the objective realm, resulting from the ascent of the life force (**prāna*) to the crown of the *head, the **dvādasha-anta*; (3) *para-ānanda* ("supreme bliss"), the realization of the *Self mixed with a successive grasping of objective contents, resulting from the descent of the life force from the head to the *heart, where it becomes **apāna*; (4) *brahma-ānanda* ("brahmic bliss"), in which the objective contents are grasped simultaneously, resulting from the conversion of the life force into *samāna at the heart; (5) *mahā-ānanda* ("great bliss"), which is devoid of all objective contents, resulting from the upward movement of the life force in the form of *udāna; (6) *cid-ānanda* ("conscious bliss"), the realization of the *Self as subject, object, and the means of knowledge, resulting from the conversion of the *udāna life force into the *vyāna current in the central conduit or *sushumnā-nādī; and (7) jagad-ānanda ("world bliss"), the realization of the *Self as perfectly identical with the *body and the *world. See also ānanda-maya-kosha, Happiness, mahā-sukha, sukha.

ĀNANDA BHAIRAVA, mentioned as a prominent *teacher of *hatha-yoga in the *Hatha-Yoga-Pradīpikā (1.5). See also Bhairava, Vijnāna-Bhairava.

ĀNANDA-MAYA-KOSHA ("sheath composed of bliss"), the highest or most subtle of the five "envelopes" (*kosha) covering the transcendental *Self. Its substance is bliss (*ānanda). It is sometimes identified with the Self as such.

ĀNANDA-SAMĀPATTI ("blissful coinciding [with the object of contemplation]"), according to the *Yoga-Bhāshya (1.17) and other commentaries on the *Yoga-Sūtra, a high-level conscious ecstasy (*samprajnāta-samādhi) consisting of the experience of pure *bliss. The bliss experienced in ānanda-samāpatti, or ānanda-samādhi, however, is conditional and temporary. In his *Tattva-Vaishāradī (1.17), *Vācaspati Mishra explains that the experience of bliss is generated when the *yogin's introverted *attention rests on one of the sense organs (*indriya), which contain a preponderance of the *sattva (luminosity) constituent of *nature. This experience is thus different from the "formless ecstasy" (*nirvikalpa-samādhi) of *Vedānta, which reveals the transcendental Being-Consciousness-Bliss (*sac-cid-ānanda). Here bliss is considered an essential aspect of the ultimate *Reality. See also ānanda, samādhi, samāpatti.

ĀNANDA-SAMUCCAYA, a thirteenth-century work on *hatha-yoga consisting of eight chapters, totaling 277 stanzas. Among other things, the text deals with the psychoenergetic centers (*cakra) and "channels" (*nādī) as well as the other esoteric structures of the *body.

ĀNANDA-SHAKTI ("power of bliss"), one of the characterizations of the divine, feminine energy of the *cosmos, also simply referred to as *shakti. *Abhinava Gupta and other authorities of *Tantrism distinguish this power from *Shiva's power of consciousness (*cit-shakti). See also ānanda.

ANANTA ("Infinite"), an epithet of *Vishnu, who is said in the *Mahābhārata (12.175.19) to be "difficult to be known even by *adepts owing to his infinity." Ananta, or Shesha, is the "thousand-headed" cosmic serpent of *Hindu mythology who serves as *Vishnu's couch. The name Shesha ("Remainer") is explained by the fact that Shesha remains after the destruction of the *cosmos. He is invoked by *Vyāsa at the beginning of his *Yoga-Bhāshya as the "Giver of *Yoga who is himself yoked in Yoga."

Ananta is also the name of the author of the late work Yoga-Sūtra-Artha-Candrikā ("Moonshine on the Meaning of the Yoga Aphorisms").

ANANTA-SAMĀPATTI ("coinciding with the infinite"), a precondition of the proper performance of posture (*āsana), according to the Yoga-Sūtra (2.47). The term presumably refers to the subjective experience of one's "widening out" in the state of deep relaxation (*shaithilya). Some of the Sanskrit commentators think that this is a reference to the serpent-king *Ananta. See also samāpatti.

ANĀTMAN ("non-Self"), a technical term denoting everything that is experienced as being different from the transcendental *Self (*ātman), i.e., the phenomenal world and the ego personality. In *Buddhism, anātman refers to the fact that nothing in nature has an eternal essence and that the human personality is an ever-changing composite of factors lacking a permanent identity.

ANATOMY. Conventional medical anatomy, based, as the word suggests, on dissection, is concerned with the material structures of the physical *body. Yogic anatomy, by contrast, is primarily concerned with the esoteric structures of the human body-mind, as it is experienced in such *altered states of consciousness as *meditation and *ecstasy. These esoteric structures include the distribution channels (*nādī) and vortices (*cakra) of the life force (*prāna). It also deals with the shock wave that rocks the body when its hidden psychospiritual power is tapped— the *kundalinī-shakti. Earlier generations of *Yoga researchers typically regarded the cakras and nādīs as fanciful representations of the nervous system. But the *yogins were well aware of the difference between their models of the body and the medical model of India's indigineous naturopathic system of health care, the *Āyur-Veda.

The fact that there is not one but many yogic models indicates that the *cakras and *nādīs are not altogether objective structures. Neither are they purely fictitious. A convenient way of looking at the different cakra models is that they are intended to be maps for the *yogin on his inward odyssey, during which he discovers the psychosomatic structures of his being, only to transcend them in the unqualified radiance of ultimate Being (*sat), or transcendental Consciousness (*cit). The purpose of yogic anatomy is thus to guide the yogin through and beyond the wonderland of

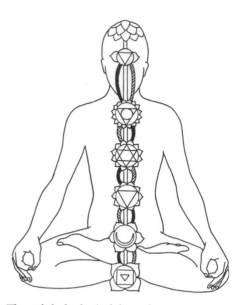

The subtle body (sūkshma-sharīra), with the seven principal psychoenergetic centers and the three major pathways

the inner world of the psyche, which is interlinked with the physical vehicle.

ĀNAVA-MALA, in *Shaivism, the blemishes or defects (*mala) attaching to the unenlighened psyche, known as *anu (hence the adjective ānava). The individual person is really *Shiva but because of spiritual ignorance (*avidyā) and other impurities is unaware of this truth. Specifically, ānava-mala is the defect by which one identifies with a limited human body-mind, thus creating an illusory *ego personality. Cf. kārma-mala, māyīya-mala.

ANAVASTHITATVA ("instability"), one of the obstacles (*antarāya) of *Yoga; occasionally also referred to as "mental unsteadiness" (citta-anavasthiti). According to the *Yoga-Sūtra (1.30), this is one of the distractions (*vikshepa). See also aloluptva.

ĀNAVA-UPĀYA (*ānavopāya*, "atomic means"), in *Shaivism, the approach to *Self-realization, or *enlightenment, through individual effort. The adjective "atomic" (*ānava*) is derived from the word *anu, signifying here the individuated psyche, which is deemed to be a "fragment" (*amsha*) of the Whole. Cf. *anupāya, upāya.*

ĀNDĀL (early 9th cen. CE), to this day venerated as one of the great poet-saints of South India; a worshiper of *Vishnu. Āndāl's poetry is reminiscent of the bridal mysticism of medieval Europe, though she tended to use far more explicit erotic imagery to express her *adoration of the *Divine. See also Ālvārs, Vaishnavism.

ANGA ("limb"), in addition to referring to the *body or, more specifically, to the male *genitals, also denotes the constituent practice categories of the yogic *path. The *Yoga-Rāja-Upanishad* (2) speaks of four basic categories that are common to all paths: posture (*āsana*), breath restriction (*prāna-samrodha*), meditation (*dhyāna*), and ecstasy (*samādhi*). The best-known tradition is the eightfold path, or *ashta-anga-yoga*, taught by *Patanjali. Another prominent approach is the sixfold path (*shad-anga-yoga*) taught, for instance, in the *Maitrāyanīya-Upanishad* (6.18). Also known are a sevenfold discipline (*sapta-sādhana*) and a fifteenfold path (*panca-dasha-anga-yoga*). In *Classical Yoga a distinction is made between "outer limbs" (*bahir-anga*) and "inner limbs" (*antar-anga*), whereby the latter comprise the higher mental practices.

ANGELS, in the Judeo-Christian tradition (inspired by Zoroastrianism), beings that stand midway between *God and humanity. As their Greek-derived name implies,

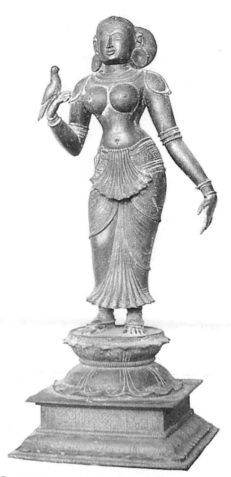

Āndāl with parrot in hand (Melakkarivalankulam, 16th century)

they are thought of as messengers. *Hinduism and the other Indian traditions likewise recognize the existence of beings on the subtle (*sūkshma*) planes, who are not merely the spirits of the departed but beings of light, power, and beauty who are yet lower in the celestial hierarchy than the *Divine itself. These beings are called *devas* or "bright ones," because they are perpetually drawn to the divine *Light. These are the many major and minor deities known to Indian humanity.

ANGER. See *krodha*.

ANGIRAS, one of the seven great seers (*saptarshi*) of the present world cycle (*manvantara*). Since *Vedic times, this name has been associated with *magic or sorcery and specifically with the *Atharva-Veda*.

ANGUSHTHA-MĀTRA-PURUSHA ("thumb-sized person"), the transcendental *Self, or *Consciousness, in its connection with the *body, according to the *Katha-Upanishad* (2.1.12). The same expression is found in the *Shvetāshvatara-Upanishad* (3.13), which adds that those who know this manikin become immortal (*amrita*).

ANIMAN ("atomization"), one of the great paranormal powers (*siddhi*) resulting, according to the *Yoga-Sūtra* (3.44f.), from the mastery over the *elements. It is the *adept's capacity to make himself infinitely small.

ANĪSHVARA ("lordless"). This term, which appears in a few passages of the *Mahābhārata* (notably 12.238.7 and 289.3), has given rise to scholarly debate. Some authorities have interpreted it in the sense of "atheist," but it is more likely to stand for the unliberated self, that is, the individuated psyche (*jīva*) who is not the "Lord" (*īshvara*).

ANJALI-MUDRĀ, the "seal" (*mudrā*) or gesture of placing the palms of the hands together, slightly cupped, in front of the *heart. This gesture is still used by modern *Hindus as a form of greeting. When greeting a spiritual personage, the palms are held at eye level, and when making reverent salutation to a *deity or the *Divine, they are held above the *head.

ANNA ("food"). See *āhāra*.

ANNA-MAYA-KOSHA ("sheath composed of food"), the lowest or coarsest of the five "envelopes" (*kosha*) covering the transcendental *Self, i.e., the physical *body, according to an ancient *Vedānta doctrine.

ANNA-YOGA ("Yoga of food"), contemporary term describing *Yoga as a spiritual discipline focusing on our relationship to food—its cultivation and consumption. See also *āhāra*.

ANOMIE. See *adharma*.

ANTAHKARANA ("inner instrument"), the psyche; a term found in *Sāmkhya, *Yoga, and *Vedānta texts. According to the *Sāmkhya-Kārikā* (32), it comprises the higher mind (*buddhi*), the "I maker" (*ahamkāra*), and the lower mind (*manas*). In *Classical Yoga the term *citta is used instead.

ANTA-KĀLA ("end time"), the time of a person's *death, one's final hour, which holds a particular obligation for the spiritual practitioner. From a materialistic point of view, death is simply the final and irrevocable cessation of the individual body-mind, followed by eternal oblivion. This view is denied by all spiritual traditions. Thus the ancient *Bhagavad-Gītā* (8.5f.) emphasizes the importance of dying well and how one's last thoughts or intentions determine one's postmortem existence. *Krishna admonishes:

And he who in the last hour, abandoning the *body, remembers Me alone, goes hence—he arrives at My state; there is no doubt of this.

Also, whatever state [a man] remembers when he abandons the body in the end, even to that [state] does he go, O Kaunteya [= *Arjuna], always forced to become that state.

Such esoteric knowledge dates back to the earliest *Upanishads. The *Bhāgavata-Purāna (5.8.1ff.) contains the popular story of Bharata that illustrates this age-old *ars moriendi*. Bharata was so intent on the young deer he had saved from the lion's clutches that he forgot to pursue his *Yoga practice and consequently was promptly reborn as a deer.

Expressing a classic yogic teaching, the *Shat-Cakra-Nirūpana (38) advises the *yogin to focus his *attention on the *ājnā-cakra (the brain core) at the moment of *death. See also *kāla*, *prayāna-kāla*.

ANTAR-ANGA ("inner limb"), a technical term in the *Yoga-Sūtra (3.7) denoting the last three constituents of the eightfold *path: concentration (*dhāranā), meditation (*dhyāna), and ecstasy (*samādhi). See also *anga*, *ashta-anga-yoga*; *panca-dasha-anga-yoga*, *sapta-sadhana*; cf. *bahir-anga*.

ANTARĀYA ("obstacle"). The *Yoga-Sūtra (1.30) lists the following impediments on the yogic *path: illness (*vyādhi), languor (*styāna), doubt (*samshaya), heedlessness (*pramāda), sloth (*ālasya), dissipation (*avirati), false vision (*bhrānti-darshana), nonattainment of the higher levels (*alabdha-bhūmikatva*) of the spiritual path, and instability (*anavasthitva) in a given level of attainment. These are also called "distractions" (*vikshepa) of *consciousness, and the *Yoga-Sūtra* (1.29) prescribes the practice of recitation (*japa) and contemplation (*bhāvanā) of the sacred syllable *om for their swift removal.

The *Linga-Purāna (1.9.1ff.) offers a slightly different list, which includes lack of *faith (*ashraddhā), suffering (*duhkha), and depression (*daurmanasya). This work states that such obstacles can be removed through constant practice and de-

votion to one's *teacher. The *Vedantic *Uddhāva-Gītā (10.33) additionally regards the paranormal powers (*siddhi) as obstacles for the person who seeks union with the "Lord" (*īshvara), calling them "time wasters." See also *upasarga*, *vighna*.

ANTAR-DHAUTI ("inner cleansing"), a practice comprising the following four techniques, according to the *Gheranda-Samhitā (1.12ff.): swallowing air and expelling it through the anus at will; completely filling the stomach with water (a risky practice); stimulating the "*fire" in the abdomen by repeatedly pushing the *navel back toward the spine, and washing one's prolapsed intestines (a dangerous practice if done without proper supervision).

ANTAR-DVĀDASHA-ANTA (*antardvādash-ānta*, "ending with the inner twelfth"), an esoteric concept of *Shaivism: the point where the life breath (*prāna) originates in the human *body, as opposed to *bāhya-dvādasha-anta ("ending with the outer twelfth"), the point where the life force ceases outside the body. According to an oral tradition from Kashmir, the inner space has three stages, beginning with the psychoenergetic center at the *heart, proceeding to the "throat well" (*kantha-kūpa), that is, the corresponding psychoenergetic center (*vishuddhi-cakra), and finally to the middle of the eyebrows (*bhrū-madhya). The distance between the *heart and the *throat, and between the throat and the eyebrows, is roughly twelve fingers wide, which explains the name. As *Kshemarāja's *Spanda-Nirnaya (3) explains, it is in this inner space that the *yogin must contemplate the *prāna-shakti* or power of life. The space between the inner and the outer *dvādasha-anta is sixteen *tuti or thirty-six fingers.

ANTAR-LAKSHYA ("inner sign"), a technical term belonging to the discipline of *tāraka-yoga and referring to one of three kinds of inner luminous experience (*lakshya). The *Advaya-Tāraka-Upanishad (13) describes it as the photistic experience of the *Absolute as the *light of awareness hidden in the cave of the higher mind (*buddhi). For the anonymous author of the *Mandala-Brāhmana-Upanishad (1.2.6), the object of this experience is the "serpent power" (*kundalinī-shakti), which is resplendent like myriads of lightning streaks, or it is the blue radiance that can be experienced in the middle of the eyes or in the *heart when one fixes the *mind thereon. Reference to this practice is also made in the *Siddha-Siddhānta-Paddhati (2.27). Cf. bahir-lakshya, madhya-lakshya.

ANTARYĀMIN ("inner controller"), the transcendental Self (*ātman) as it is effective in the human psyche (*jīva). This notion was first introduced by the *Brihad-Āranyaka-Upanishad (3.7.1ff.).

ANU ("atom"). The idea that physical objects are composed of minute indivisible parts dates back to the ancient Greek cosmologists. The notion was also current in India at that time and was very probably arrived at independently.

In Kashmiri *Shaivism, anu is a technical term referring to the individuated, "atomic" being (*jīva), or finite human personality, as opposed to the universal transcendental *Self. See also ānava, parama-anu.

ANUBHAVA ("experience"), personal experience, including the direct realization of the transcendental *Reality.

ANUBHŪTI ("experience"), a synonym for *anubhava used in the *Vedāntic technical expression aparoksha-anubhūti, meaning the unmediated experience, or realization, of the *Self.

ANU-GĪTĀ ("Subsequent Song"), part of the *Mahābhārata (14.16–51). Closely modeled after the *Bhagavad-Gītā, the Anu-Gītā purports to be a recapitulation of the teachings communicated by *Krishna to Prince *Arjuna at the eve of the Bharata *war. This second instruction occurs after the battles have been fought and the moral order (*dharma) has been restored.

ANUGRAHA ("favor"), divine *grace, frequently cited as the principal means of *Self-realization. In *Classical Yoga the "Lord" (*īshvara) is said to incline toward that *yogin who diligently strives for *perfection. See also kripā, prasāda; cf. Effort.

ANUMĀNA ("inference"), widely considered in *Hindu metaphysics as a valid means of knowledge (*pramāna). The *Yoga-Bhāshya (1.7) defines it as "the [mental] activity referring to that relation which is present in things pertaining to the same class as the thing-to-be-inferred (anumeya), which is absent from things pertaining to different classes, and which is chiefly [concerned with] the ascertainment of the genus." This is further developed in the *Tattva-Vaishāradī, where the logical structure of inference is examined.

ANUPĀYA ("without means"), in Kashmiri *Shaivism, the spontaneous realization of the *Self without any *effort. Cf. ānava-upaya, upaya.

ANUSVARA ("after-sound"), in grammar, the nasalized sound indicated by a dot above the Sanskrit letter m (or, in academic transliteration, by a dot below the letter *m*). The dot, or *bindu*, is connected with profound metaphysical associations, particularly in Kashmiri *Shaivism. See also *pranava*.

ANUTTARA ("unsurpassable"), ultimate *Reality, called *Shiva. In his *Parā-Trim-shikā-Vivarana* (1.1) *Abhinava Gupta states that the notion of *anuttara* is to the *Kaula school what the *heart is to the physical *body. He offers sixteen explanations for it.

ANUTTARA-CAKRA ("unsurpassable wheel"), *Shiva's manifestation as the *world, which, according to Kashmiri *Shaivism, flows out from the *heart through the "void" of the *eyes and toward the *objects of the senses. Shiva himself is said to be the wheel's lord (*cakra-īsha*, written as *cakresha*).

ANVAYA ("nexus"), a technical expression of *Classical Yoga. The *Yoga-Bhāshya* (3.44) explains it as referring to the primary constituents (*guna*) of *nature, which inhere in everything.

ANYATĀ-KHYĀTI ("vision of otherness"), in *Classical Yoga, the ecstatic "vision" of the distinction between the transcendental *Self and the *sattva*, which is the highest aspect of (insentient) *nature. It is synonymous with *viveka-khyāti*. See also *khyāti*.

AP ("waters"), a feminine plural word derived from the root *ap* ("to be active"). Water is one of the five material elements (*bhūta*) thought to compose the physical realm of *nature, including the human *body. It is specifically connected with the five bodily liquids: saliva, urine, semen, blood, and *perspiration. Water is sometimes said to govern the bodily region from the anus to the knees. Its symbol is

the crescent moon (*ardha-candra*) and its color is white, with *vam* being its seed syllable (*bīja-mantra*). See also *jala, tattva*.

APĀNA ("down-breath"), one of the principal currents of the life force (*prāna*), of which the *breath is its external manifestation. Together with the "forth-breath" (*prāna*), *apāna* is the great piston that powers the *body. According to various *Yoga-Upanishads*, it resides in the lower half of the body, from the *genitals to the knees or, alternatively, from the belly to the shanks or even the feet. This aspect of the universal life energy is responsible for the evacuation of waste matter and is connected with exhalation. When it is "mingled" with the *prāna* and the "*fire" at the *navel, it is instrumental in arousing the "serpent power" (*kundalinī-shakti*).

APARĀNTA-JNĀNA ("knowledge of one's end"), foreknowledge of one's *death through omens (*arishta*) and *dreams, etc.; one of the yogic powers (*siddhi*). It is important for the *yogin to die well, i.e., to die consciously so he can guide the death process and possibly effect *liberation during his last moments of bodily existence. There are numerous legends and anecdotes of *yogins* who correctly predicted the time of their death, in some cases years before it actually occurred. See also *jnāna*.

APARIGRAHA ("greedlessness"), one of the five moral disciplines (*yama*) in *Classical Yoga. When practiced to the point of perfection, it yields knowledge of the "wherefore" of one's birth, as the *Yoga-Sūtra* (2.39) states. The *Bhagavad-Gītā* (4.21) calls for the *abandonment of all possessions. This has given rise to schools of thought favoring radical world *renunciation. But other scriptural authorities, such as the *Bhāgavata-Purāna (3.28.4), espouse a minimalist interpretation of greedlessness, understanding it as "possessing [only] as much as is necessary."

APAROKSHA-ANUBHŪTI (*Aparokshānubhūti* "Unmediated Realization"), a short *Vedānta work attributed to *Shankara. See also *anubhūti*.

APAS ("water"), the singular form of *ap.

APAVĀDA ("refutation"), a key term of *Vedānta, also found in some works of *Postclassical Yoga, denoting the intellectual procedure whereby erroneous predications (*adhyāropa*) about the nature of reality can effectively be exposed as such. Thus it is a systematic attack on the consensus point of view of ordinary *consciousness, which, it is argued, fails to realize that *Reality is not finite and painful but infinite and blissful (*ānanda*.)

APAVARGA ("turning-off"), a synonym for *moksha*, *mukti*, *kaivalya*.

APPAR ("Father"), one of the epithets of the *Shaiva saint Tirunavukarasar (7th cen. CE). He is among the most venerated *Nayanmars and is remembered for reconverting apostatic Shaivites who had embraced *Jainism, notably King Mahendra Varman. Hagiography tells us that Appar himself, who was known by the name of Marulniki, was originally a Jaina. His conversion to *Shaivism was brought about by his miraculous cure from a painful stomach disease after entering the *Shiva temple at Virattanam in South India. In one of his many hymns Appar compares himself to a thief who steals unripe fruit when ripe fruit is close at hand. After his discovery of *Shiva within his own *heart, Appar went from temple to temple, performing menial tasks to sustain himself and to serve the *Divine, always proclaiming the glory of *God and the possibility of transcending all *fear. His success as a saintly minstrel caused the Jaina ruler Gunabhara (Mahendra Varman) to arrest and torture him for desertion and treason. When Appar miraculously survived all tortures, the king capitulated and declared himself the saint's disciple. He then demolished the Jaina monastery at his capital and built a Shiva temple in its place.

APPEARANCE. In philosophy, this concept offers a counterpoint to that of *reality. The question of the relationship between appearance and reality is a fundamental philosophical problem, which has been studied intensively by the Indian thinkers, especially since the time of the *Upanishads*. Various answers have been proffered, from *dualism to qualified nondualism (*Vishishta Advaita) to radical nondualism (*Kevala Advaita). Some schools consider the sensory world to be a distortion of the absolute Reality; others regard it as mere illusion (*māyā*). All metaphysical schools of India, however, are agreed that the objective *world presented to the *senses is, ontologically or at least spiritually, of a lesser status than the suprasensuous Reality, variously called *ātman*, *brahman*, or *tattva*. See also *ābhāsa*, Absolute, Divine, God.

APRABUDDHA ("unawakened"). Kashmiri *Shaivism distinguishes between individuals who are (1) completely oblivious of their spiritual nature (the *Self); (2) partially aware of their true nature, as is the case with practicing *yogins*; and (3) fully awakened or enlightened. The first are called *aprabuddha*, the second *prabuddha*, and the third *suprabuddha* ("well awakened"). See also *buddha*.

APRATIBUDDHA ("not fully awakened"), a synonym for *abuddha* in the terminology of *Preclassical Yoga.

APUNYA ("demerit" or "demeritorious"). Many *Hindu schools look upon demerit almost as a material substance that is accumulated in the body-mind, determining its *destiny. It is a part of the doctrine of *karma. Cf. *punya*.

ĀRĀDHANA ("adoration") synonymous with *īshvara-pūjana*; sometimes listed among the practices of self-restraint (*niyama*).

ĀRĀDHYA ("adorable" or "worshipful"). In the *Kula-Arnava-Tantra* (17.13), where it is treated as an epithet of the spiritual *teacher, the word's constituent syllables (*ā*, *rā*, and *dhya*) are explained as containing a reference to the *guru's transmission of the *Self's condition (*ātma-bhāva*), his transcendence of attachment (*rāga*) and aversion (*dvesha*), and his constant immersion into the state of meditation (*dhyāna*).

ĀRAMBHA-AVASTHĀ (*ārambhāvasthā*, "initial state"), the first of the four states (*avasthā*) of yogic accomplishment. According to the *Yoga-Tattva-Upanishad (64) it consists in the recitation of the sacred syllable *om, whereas the *Varāha-Upanishad (5.72) explains it as the giving up of external *actions and functioning inwardly instead. The *Hatha-Yoga-Pradīpikā (4.70f.), however, interprets it as that stage in which the "brahmic knot" (*brahma-granthi*) is pierced and *bliss arises out of the *void (in the *heart) and various mystical *sounds can be heard. For the anonymous author of the *Shiva-Samhitā (3.28), this stage is entered upon the *purification of the network of currents (*nādī*) in the *body.

ĀRANYAKA ("[Treatise] Pertaining to the Forest"), a type of ancient ritual work composed by and for forest anchorites. This genre of scriptures preceded the *Upanishads and ideologically stood midway between their esotericism and the sacrificial ritualism of the *Vedas and *Brāhmanas.

ARCĀ ("worship" or "adoration"), a synonym for *arcanā*.

ARCANĀ ("worship"), one of the elements of self-restraint (*niyama*); also one of the aspects of the *Yoga of devotion (*bhakti-yoga*). See also Worship.

ARCHAIC YOGA, also called Proto-Yoga, the body of beliefs and practices that can be reconstructed as a system of spiritual disciplines on the basis of the *Vedas, especially the *Rig-Veda, and the archaeological evidence of the *Indus-Sarasvati civilization. See also History, Yoga.

ARDHA-CANDRA ("half moon"; also called *ardha-indu* [*ardhendu*]), the graphic representation of the *ardha-mātra*.

ARDHA-MĀTRA ("half-measure"), the semicircular symbol placed above the syllable *om. It is sometimes likened to a flame flickering above a candle. See illustration at *om*.

ARDHANĀRĪSHVARA (*ardha*, "half"; *nārī*, "female"; and *īshvara*, "lord"), one the forms of *Shiva. Iconographically depicted as an androgynous figure, male on the right side and female on the left, Ardhanārīshvara represents the union of Shiva and *Shakti beyond all *duality. This image expresses a fundamental understanding of *Yoga.

ARISHTA ("omen"). Omens play an important role in *Yoga. The *yogin invests even seemingly irrelevant and arbitrary events with deeper significance. Nothing is thought to be due to chance. The universe (*vishva) is synchronistic and inherently meaningful, a belief captured in the idea that the *microcosm is a mirror of the *macrocosm. According to the *Yoga-Bhashya (3.22), an old commentary on the *Yoga-Sūtra, there are three kinds of omens: those generated by oneself, those involving others, and omens involving deities (*deva). Many scriptures furnish lists of omens relating to the *death of a *yogin, since this is an important spiritual transition and must be passed through with full *awareness. See also anta-kāla.

ĀRJAVA ("rectitude"), sometimes counted as one of the practices of moral observance (*yama). According to the *Bhagavad-Gītā (13.7), uprightness is a manifestation of knowledge or gnosis (*jnāna) and forms part of physical austerity (*tapas).

ARJUNA ("White" or "Bright"), the hero of the *Bhagavad-Gītā, which is essentially a dialogue between Arjuna and *Krishna. Like Hamlet, Prince Arjuna typifies the indecisive individual, suffering from *doubt.

ARMPIT. See kakshā.

ĀROGYA ("health"). According to the *Shvetāshvatara-Upanishad (2.13), *health is one of the initial signs of spiritual *progress. That this is a more comprehensive concept than the Western notion of health is evident, for instance, from the *Hatha-Yoga-Pradīpikā (2.2), which considers the following as manifestations of health: the ability to hold one's *breath as desired, increased activity of the gastric "*fire," and perception of the inner sound (*nāda). Cf. roga, vyādhi.

ARROGANCE. See abhimāna, darpa; cf. amānitva.

ART. In India the artist (shilpin) traditionally employed yogic *meditation for assisting the creative process. Any flaws in the artistic end product were attributed to laxity in *concentration and meditation. The textbooks not infrequently refer to the craftsman or artist as a *yogin or *sādhaka. Also, as a rule, these technical treatises contain prescriptions for the practice of *Yoga. Contemplation (*dhyāna) is thought to produce "vision" or "audition" (as in the case of Vālmīki, who inwardly heard the entire *Rāmāyana). Traditional (religious) Indian art was never concerned with the pursuit of beauty for its own sake. Rather, the artist aspired to communicate the infinite through his creative work and to uplift the person "participating" in his art. See also Aesthetics, Dance.

ARTHA ("object" or "thing"). In certain technical contexts, this word means "intended object" or "content of *consciousness." It also has the meaning of "purpose." A further meaning is "material welfare," as the lowest of the four human concerns (*purusha-artha) recognized in *Hindu ethics. See also parama-artha, vishaya.

ĀRŪDHA ("ascended"), an *adept who has risen to the top of the spiritual *path. According to the *Bhagavad-Gītā (6.3), this term applies to the *yogin whose means is quiescence (*shama). The same scripture

(6.4) states that the condition of *yoga-ārū-dha* is realized by that practitioner who has renounced all volition (*samkalpa*). Cf. *ārurukshu*.

ARULNANDI (13th cen. CE), one of the great teachers (*ācārya*) of South Indian *Shaivism; the author of the *Shiva-Jnāna-Siddhiyar*. See also Nayanmar.

ĀRURUKSHU ("desirous of ascending"), the spiritual aspirant whose discipline consists, according to the *Bhagavad-Gītā* (6.3), in the performance of action (*karman*) rather than the *renunciation of all activity. Cf. *ārūdha, siddha*.

ĀRYA ("noble"), an adjective applied to spiritual personages or teachings since *Vedic times. Those lacking spiritual nobility are said to be *anārya*. Interpreting the *Vedas*, Western scholars first turned *ārya* into a linguistic (Indo-European) category and then gave it a racial connotation with strong political overtones.

ARYAN INVASION THEORY. Because of its Eurocentric bias, nineteenth-century Western scholarship failed to appreciate the true age of the *Vedas*. In the absence of archaeological data, scholars relied exclusively on then-current linguistic models of the dispersion of Indo-European languages in the ancient world. This led them to the hypothesis that the Sanskrit-speaking *Vedic tribes originated outside India, entering the peninsula in the period from 1500 BCE to 1200 BCE as conquerors. These dates were arrived at from linguistic evidence found on Hittite clay tablets. Although this hypothesis was vehemently criticized by several eminent scholars, it quickly became "fact," largely because of the support it received from the renowned German Sanskritist Max Müller (1823–

1900). Disregarding all evidence to the contrary, the consensus of scholarly opinion also assumed that the *Rig-Veda* was composed after the "Aryans" had invaded northern India via the Hindukush mountains (mainly the Kyber pass, in present-day Afghanistan).

The standard chronology for the *Rig-Veda*, however, was thoroughly shaken by the discovery, in 1921, of the so-called Indus civilization (now renamed *Indus-Sarasvati civilization by a growing number of scholars). Researchers next sought to align the Aryan invasion theory with the chronology established for that early civilization. In particular, overinterpreting the archaeological evidence, they portrayed the invading Aryan tribes as the barbarous destroyers of the Indus cities. This obliged them to push back the date for the alleged invasion by half a millennium. But recent research has revealed the Aryan invasion theory to be a serious distortion of historical reality.

In light of the astonishing cultural continuity between the neolithic town of Mehrgarh (dating back to 6500 BCE), the *Indus-Sarasvati civilization, and the later *Hindu society and culture, a growing number of scholars now favor the view that the *Vedic tribes were native to India long before the decline of the Indus-Sarasvati civilization. In fact, there is good evidence to suggest that they were the builders and inhabitants of the towns along the Indus and Sarasvati rivers and their tributaries.

In keeping with this new understanding of ancient Indian *history, the chronology of the *Yoga tradition has been revised as well. Since the earliest expressions of yogic wisdom and practice can be found in the *Rig-Veda*, the development of Yoga is now thought to span 5,000 years or more.

ASAMPRAJÑĀTA-SAMĀDHI ("supraconscious ecstasy"), the technique leading to,
and the experience of, the state of unified
*consciousness beyond all cognitive con-
tent. In this superlative condition, subject
and *object become one. In Vedānta, this
is known as "formless ecstasy" (*nirvikalpa-samādhi). This realization presupposes the temporary deconstruction of the
ordinary consciousness (*citta). All that is
left is a residuum of subconscious tendencies (called *samskāra). If the state of supraconscious *ecstasy is maintained over a
prolonged period of time, these subconscious tendencies begin to neutralize one
another, leading to ultimate and irrevers-
ible *liberation, or *enlightenment. At
first, however, the supraconscious ecstasy
can be maintained only for brief intervals
because the powerful subconscious "activators" (samskāra) causing the ordinary
*waking state tend to reassert themselves.
However, the periods of restriction (*nirodha) of the contents of consciousness become increasingly longer until the subconscious deposits (*āshaya) are completely
eliminated. At this point the ultracon-
scious ecstasy is called "seedless" (*nir-
bīja). See also dharma-megha-samādhi, samādhi; cf. samprajñāta-samādhi.

ASAMSAKTI ("disconnection"), one of the
seven levels (*bhūmi) of wisdom (*jñāna).

ĀSANA ("seat"), originally, the surface on
which the *yogin is seated. That surface is
supposed to be firm, neither too high nor
too low, sufficiently big, level, clean, and
generally pleasant. The word is equally applied to the cover of the seat, which can
be made of grass, wood, cloth, or different
types of animal skin.
The most common meaning of the term
āsana, however, is "posture." This is considered as one of the regular "limbs"

(*anga) of the yogic *path. The *Yoga-
Sūtra (2.46) simply stipulates that posture
should be steady and comfortable. The latter qualification implies that it should be
practiced in a state of relaxation (*shaithilya). A common piece of advice is that one
should also sit up straight, with the trunk,
neck, and *head aligned, so that the life
force (*prāna) can freely ascend and de-
scend along the bodily axis. A variety of
postures are known and described in the
scriptures of *Yoga. Originally, they served
as stable poses for prolonged *meditation.
Later they were greatly elaborated and acquired a variety of therapeutic functions
leading to the sophisticated āsana technology of *hatha-yoga.
The scriptures of *Postclassical Yoga de-
clare that *Shiva propounded 840,000 different postures. This figure is thought to

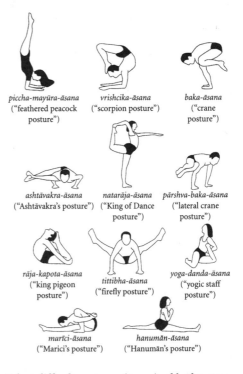

piccha-mayūra-āsana
("feathered peacock
posture")

vrishcika-āsana
("scorpion posture")

baka-āsana
("crane
posture")

ashtāvakra-āsana
("Ashtāvakra's posture")

natarāja-āsana
("King of Dance
posture")

pārshva-baka-āsana
("lateral crane
posture")

rāja-kapota-āsana
("king pigeon
posture")

tittibha-āsana
("firefly posture")

yoga-danda-āsana
("yogic staff
posture")

marīci-āsana
("Marici's posture")

hanumān-āsana
("Hanumān's posture")

Select difficult postures (āsana) of hatha-yoga

ASANGA

represent the total number of classes of living beings. Of this wide variety, only a limited number of "seats" (*pītha) are said to have been recommended by *Shiva for spiritual practitioners. Thus the *Goraksha-Paddhati (1.9) states that 84 postures are particularly suited, whereas the *Gheranda-Samhitā (2.2) claims that 32 are useful to human beings. Modern textbooks on *hatha-yoga describe as many as 200 such postures. The *Hatha-Ratna-Āvalī (3.8–19) names the 84 postures as follows, though it describes only 39 of them: (1) *siddha-, (2) *bhadra-, (3) *vajra-, (4) *simha-, (5) shilpa-simha-, (6) bandhakara-, (7) samputita-, (8) shuddha-, (9) *padma- (four varieties), (13) danda-pārshva-, (14) sahaja-, (15) bandha-, (16) pinda-, (17) eka-pāda-*mayūra- (six varieties), (18) bhairava-, (19) *kāma-dahana-, (20) pāni-pātra-, (21) kārmuka-, (22) *svastika-, (23) *go-mukha-, (24) *vīra-, (25) *māndūka-, (26) *markata-, (27) *matsyendra-, (28) pārshva-matsyendra-, (29) bandha-matsyendra-, (30) nirālambana-, (31) cāndra-, (32) kānthava-, (33) eka-pādaka-, (34) *phanīndra-, (35) *pashcimatāna-, (36) shayita-pashcimatāna-, (37) citra-karani-, (38) *yoga-mudrā-, (39) vidhūnana-, (40) pāda-pindana-, (41) hamsa- (misspelled himsā), (42) nābhī-tala-, (43) ākāsha-, (44) utpāda-tala-, (45) nābhī-lasita-pādaka-, (46) vrishcikā-, (47) cakra-, (48) utphālaka-, (49) *uttāna-kūrma-, (50) *kūrma-, (51) baddha-kūrma-, (52) kabandha-, (53) *goraksha-, (54) angushtha-mushtika-, (55) brahma-prāsādita-, (56) panca-cūli-, (57) *kukkuta-, (58) eka-pāda-kukkuta-, (59) ākārita-, (60) bandha-cūli-, (61) pārshva-kukkuta-, (62) ardha-nārīshvara-, (63) baka-, (64) candra-kānta-, (65) sudhā-sāra-, (66) vyāghra-, (67) rāja-, (68) indrāni-, (69) sharabha-, (70) ratna-, (71) citra-pītha-, (72) baddha-pakshī-īshvara-, (73) vicitra-, (74) nalina-, (75) kānta-, (76) shuddha-pakshi-, (77) sumandaka-, (78) caurangi-, (79) kraunca-, (80) dridha-, (81) khaga-, (82) brahma-, (83) nāga-pītha-, and (84) *shava-āsana.

According to the *Yoga-Sūtra (2.48), āsana desensitizes the *yogin to the effects of the "pairs of opposites" (*dvandva), such as heat and cold. Many scriptures of *Postclassical Yoga extoll posture as a means of conquering the worlds and as a preventive and curative panacea. Thus the *Hatha-Yoga-Pradīpikā (1.17) claims that the regular practice of posture induces *stability, *health, and bodily *lightness. Probably in reaction to the hypertrophy of this aspect of yogic practice in later times, the *Garuda-Purāna (227.44) makes this criticism: "The techniques of posture or 'seat' (sthāna) do not promote Yoga. Though called essentials, they all [merely] retard [one's *progress]."

See also nishadana.

ASANGA ("nonattachment"), one of the characteristics of the transcendental *Self, according to the *Brihad-Āranyaka-Upanishad (3.9.26). Since the *yogin seeks to emulate the absolute *Reality, nonattachment is also an important aspect of yogic practice. See also Abandonment, samnyāsa, tyāga, vairāgya; cf. sanga, sat-sanga.

ASANGA (4th cen. CE), the reputed founder of the *Yogācāra school of Mahāyāna *Buddhism. He propounded the teaching of *citta-mātra ("mind only"), which has many similarities with the philosophy of the *Yoga-Vāsishtha. This school of thought, which appears to have originated with the adept Maitreyanātha, is also known as Vijnānavāda. Even more important to the development of Indian Buddhism was Asanga's younger brother Vasubandhu, author of the famous Abhi-

dharma-Kosha. Both brothers were not only superb intellectuals but also great *yogins*.

ASAT ("nonbeing"). According to the traditions of *Yoga and *Sāmkhya, *being can arise only from being, which implies a rejection of the doctrine of creation ex nihilo, as espoused, for instance, in Christian theology. See also *abhāva*, *sat-kārya-vāda*; cf. *sat*.

ASCETICISM. *Yoga began to emerge as a distinct tradition around the middle of the first millennium BCE, with the early verse *Upanishads*, notably the *Katha-, *Shvetāshvatara-, and *Maitrāyanīya-Upanishads*, as well as the contemporaneous *Bhagavad-Gītā* (which considers itself to be an *Upanishad*). Yogic ideas and practices originated long before then, however, as is evidenced by the *Rig-Veda*. These proto-yogic elements were often loosely called *tapas* or asceticism. As *Yoga crystallized into a separate tradition, the concept of *tapas* also came to stand for a more articulated approach, stressing penance rather than the philosophically more consolidated and also more integrated orientation of the various branches and schools of Yoga. For several thousand years *tapas* has run parallel to the yogic stream of practice and nowadays is mostly evident in the form of fakirism practiced by many *sādhus*.

A practitioner of the ascetic tradition, called a *tapasvin*, relies on sheer willpower rather than grace (*prasāda*), coercion and self-discipline rather than submission and *self-transcendence. In his struggle for power, notably magical abilities (*siddhi*), the *tapasvin* seeks to win the support of the hidden forces of the universe—the *deities and spirits. In many respects, he continues the preyogic tradition

of *shamanism. See also Abandonment, *samnyāsa*, *tyāga*, *vairāgya*.

ĀSHĀ ("hope"). The *Chāndogya-Upanishad* (7.14.1) states that hope is more than memory (*smara*), for when stimulated by hope a person is able to memorize the sacred lore and perform the sacred rituals one has learned. The same work declares (7.14.2): "He who reveres (*upāste*) hope as *brahman*, through hope has all desires (*kāma*) fulfilled. . . . As far as hope reaches, so far he moves at will (*kāma-cāra*)." As the text continues, however, hope is not all-important. Only realization of the *Self has ultimate significance.

In some scriptures hope is portrayed as an obstacle on the path. Thus the *Bhagavad-Gītā* (16.12) speaks of the "demonic" (*āsura*) individual who is "bound by hundreds of cords of hope." In such contexts, hope refers to egoic exectations rather than genuine faith (*shraddhā*), which is always considered to be a constructive attitude.

ĀSHAYA ("resting place"), in *Classical Yoga, the subconscious "deposit," often called "action deposit" (*karma-āshaya*), which is the network of subliminal activators (*samskāra*) forming the structure of the subconscious or depth memory (*smriti*). This *action residuum is responsible for an individual's birth, span of life, and life experience. It must be transcended for *enlightenment to occur.

ĀSHCARYA ("wonder" or "marvel"). When we pause to consider life and the fact that there is something rather than nothing, we are filled with wonder. Similarly, we respond with wonderment when we ponder the existence of the transcendental *Self or *Reality. The *Bhagavad-Gītā* (2.29) contains the following verse, which describes people's relationship to the *Self: "One views Him as a marvel; another speaks of Him as a marvel; yet another hears of Him as a marvel. Yet, having heard, no one at all *knows* Him." In other words, the wonder that is the *Self must be realized through direct apprehension to be fully appreciated. Such appreciation necessarily transforms the person in a most profound way. Thus the *Katha-Upanishad* (1.27) speaks of the *adept who knows the Self and can teach about it from direct experience as wondrous, that is, beyond comprehension and awe-inspiring. See also *adbhūta*, *vismaya*.

ASHES. According to the *mythology of the *Purānas*, *Shiva burned the entire *universe, including all other deities, to ashes with an intense ray coming from his "third eye" in the middle of his *forehead, which is the *ājnā-cakra*. He then rubbed the ashes remaining after the conflagration on his *body as a sign of his mastery over the *world and his utter *renunciation. See also *bhasman*, *vibhūti*.

ĀSHRAMA (from *shrama*, "effort"), a hermitage where an *adept instructs *disciples who exert themselves in a sacred way of life. Also, a stage of life, of which the *Hindu social model distinguishes the following four: the stage of the student (*brahmacārin*), which is called *brahma-carya*; that of the householder (*grihastha*), *gārhasthya*; that of the forest dweller (*vāna-prastha*), *vānaprāsthya*; and that of the renouncer (*samnyāsin*), *samnyāsa*. See also *kutīra*.

ĀSHRAYA ("support" or "substratum"), in the *Yoga-Sūtra* (4.11), denotes the *consciousness underlying the subliminal activators (*samskāra*), whereas the term *ālam-bana* refers here to the object or stimulus presented to consciousness.

ASHTA-ANGA-YOGA (*ashtāngayoga*, "Yoga of eight limbs"), the *path of yogic maturation proposed by *Patanjali. It consists of the following eight practices: moral observance (*yama*), self-restraint (*niyama*), posture (*āsana*), breath control (*prānā-yāma*), sensory inhibition (*pratyāhāra*), concentration (*dhāranā*), meditation (*dhyāna*), and ecstasy (*samādhi*). See also *anga*; cf. *panca-dasha-anga-yoga*, *sapta sādhana*, *shad anga yoga*.

ASHTA-SIDDHI ("eight powers"), the classic set of eight paranormal powers (*siddhi*) ascribed to yogic *adepts. According to the *Yoga-Bhāshya* (3.45), these comprise the following abilities: miniaturization (*animan*), levitation (*laghiman*), expansion (*mahiman*), extension at will (*prāpti*), freedom of will (*prākāmya*), universal mastery (*vashitva*), lordship (*īshitritva*), and perfect wish fulfillment (*kāma-avasāyitva*). See also *vibhūti*.

ASHTA-VAKRĀ ("eight-curved"), a synonym for *kundalinī, according to the *Hatha-Ratna-Āvalī* (2.118).

ASHTĀVAKRA, a *Vedantic sage who figures prominently, in the *Ashtāvakra-Samhitā* (or -*Gītā*). According to legend, as recorded in the *Mahābhārata* (3.132–34), he acquired his name because of his eightfold physical deformity, caused by his father's curse. While still in his mother's womb, Ashtāvakra chided his father, Kahor, for committing errors in reciting the sacred *Rig-Veda. Kahor, a pious *brahmin, did not take kindly to his unborn son's criticism. Years later, Kahor was defeated in an intellectual debate at the royal court and was condemned to live out the rest of his life in the watery world of *Varuna. When Ashtāvakra, who was twelve years old at the time, learned of his father's misfortune, he went straight to the royal court to challenge Kahor's opponent in debate. At first he was refused entry because of his young age, but when the courtiers saw the boy's great scriptural learning, they admitted him. He promptly won the ensuing debate and thus rescued his father from Varuna. In return, Kahor asked his son to bathe in the Samangā River, which completely removed his deformity. But his name stayed the same.

Ashtāvakra's teaching, as found in the *Samhitā* bearing his name, is a pure form of *jnāna-yoga*, which is the pathway to the nondual *Reality.

ASHUDDHA ("impure"). See *ashuddhi*; cf. *shuddha*.

ASHUDDHI ("impurity"). According to the *Tattva-Vaishāradī* (1.2), impurity is of the nature of pleasure, pain, and delusion. Hence it must be overcome. Cf. *shuddhi*.

ASHVINĪ-MUDRĀ ("dawn horse seal") one of the twenty-five "*seals" (*mudrā*) described in the *Gheranda-Samhitā* (3.82); named after the Ashvins, the golden twin charioteers who, according to *Vedic mythology, pulled their sister Ushā's chariot at dawn. It is performed by repeatedly contracting the anal sphincter muscle. This is said to invigorate the *body, cure *diseases of the rectum, and awaken the "serpent power" (*kundalinī-shakti*). Cf. *mūla-bandha, yoni-mudrā.*

ASMITĀ ("I-am-ness"), the awareness of oneself as a discrete being. The *Yoga-Sūtra* (2.6) lists "I-am-ness" as one of the five causes of affliction (*klesha*) and defines it as the identification of the power of vision (i.e., the *mind) with the power of the visioner (i.e., the *Self). Furthermore, according to the *Yoga-Sūtra* (1.17),

this is one of the basic phenomena present in the state of conscious ecstasy (*samprajnāta-samādhi*). Some authorities describe an ecstatic state that is exclusively composed of the feeling of "I-am-ness," which they call *asmitā-samāpatti.*

ASMITĀ-MĀTRA ("mere I-am-ness"), in *Classical Yoga, the principle of primary individuation, which represents a distinct level in the hierarchy of being. It is the generic pool of all individualized consciousnesses (*nirmāna-citta*). See also *citta-mātra, mātra.*

ASMITĀ-SAMĀPATTI ("coincidence with I-am-ness"), in *Classical Yoga, an advanced form of conscious ecstasy (*samprajnāta-samādhi*), based on the mere feeling of being present as an entity; the most rarefied form of the ego identity. See also *sa-asmitā-samāpatti, samādhi*; cf. *nirasmitā-samāpatti.*

ASPARSHA-YOGA ("intangible Yoga"), an apophatic (negation-based) *Yoga based on the metaphysics of *nondualism, first announced by *Gaudapāda. *Shankara explains the term *asparsha* as that which is free from contact (*sparsha*) with everything and which is coessential with the *Absolute. Thus this *Yoga is not so much a *path as the practice of living from the *enlightened condition of nonduality. Cf. *sparsha-yoga.*

ASTEYA ("nonstealing"), one of the practices of moral observance (*yama*). According to the *Yoga-Sūtra* (2.37), when this virtue is practiced to perfection, it yields all sorts of gems (*ratna*), a statement best understood symbolically. The *Yoga-Bhāshya* (2.30) defines it as one's abstention from unauthorized appropriation of things belonging to another. In the *Shān-

dilya-Upanishad (1.1.7) it is explained as the noncoveting of another's property physically, mentally, and vocally.

ĀSTIKYA ("it-is-ness," from *asti*, "it is"), often regarded as one of the constituent practices of moral observance (**yama*) and also of self-restraint (**niyama*). The **Shān-dilya-Upanishad* (1.2.4) explains it as **faith in the knowledge of revelation (**sh-ruti*) and tradition (**smriti*).

ASTONISHMENT. See *camatkāra*; cf. *āsh-carya*.

ASTRAL TRAVEL. See *ākāsha-gamana*.

ASTROLOGY. The **adept, for whom the **universe is inherently meaningful, looks for **omens or portents, the better to understand the present moment and thereby act more in consonance with the flow of things. Thus some schools or authorities of **Yoga employ a variety of divination methods, including astrology, to determine the most auspicious moment in **time for an **initiation or other **ritual.

Indian astrology, called *jyotisha* in Sanskrit (which includes astronomy), originated at the time of the **Rig-Veda*, some 5,000 years ago. In **Hinduism it is regarded as one of the twelve auxiliary subjects. Indian astrology is based on the sidereal rather than the tropical zodiac and thus works with the actual position of the stars. The tropical zodiac, reckoned on the solar equinoxes and not the fixed stars, reflects a stellar pattern corresponding to 2,000 years ago. Thus a planet considered to be in the constellation of Aquarius is in fact positioned in the earlier constellation of Pisces.

Unlike the circular Western horoscopes, Indian horoscopes are rectangular (in South India) or diamond-shaped (in North India), emphasizing the twelve signs rather than the dynamic aspects between planets. Indian astrology works with the seven visible "planets" (including the Sun and the Moon) and the two lunar nodes (called *rahu* and *ketu* respectively). It also acknowledges twelve houses determined by the ascendant. The planets are assigned numerological values, associations with the five **elements, and fundamental qualities, as in Western astrology. Additionally, Indian astrology knows of twenty-seven lunar constellations (*nakshatra*), each of which is ruled by a planet. In contrast to Western astrology, where great attention is paid to the exact aspects between planets, Indian astrology reckons the aspects primarily on the basis of the houses in which the planets are placed. It emphasizes planetary combinations called *yoga*, of which long lists exist. Indian astrology has many unique features, showing a long history of experiential discovery. Its role in the practice of Indian medicine (**Ayur-Veda) and **Yoga has been considerable.

In the ancient world, the learned and wise turned to the stars not out of any theoretical fascination, as is the case with modern astronomy, but in order to obtain guidance for daily life. Hence for thousands of years, astronomy and astrology formed one and the same science. Their separation was made only with the ascendancy of rationalism in the modern era. Even such great astronomers as Kepler and Galileo were still deeply interested in the astrological aspects of their scientific discipline.

ASURA ("antigod"). In the **Vedic worldview, the *asuras* figure as the antagonists of the *suras* or **devas*, that is, the deities. In the Judeo-Christian tradition, the *asuras* might be described as fallen **angels. They are powerful beings, and in later

*Hinduism are considered demons. Curiously, the word *asura* originally denoted the supreme *Divine, a connotation it retained in the cognate *ahura* of Zoroastrianism. The post-Vedic literature furnishes all kinds of etymologies for *asura*, none of which is definitive.

The split into good and evil forces in the *subtle or invisible realms of existence is the archetype for a similar division on the human level. Thus the *Bhagavad-Gītā* (16.1ff.) distinguishes between divine (*daiva*) and demonic (*āsura*) beings and destinies in the *world. The latter are described as lacking understanding of action (*pravritti*) and renunciation (*nivritti*) and as being bereft of *purity, good conduct, and *truth, as well as suffering from insatiable *desire, hypocrisy, *pride, arrogance, and *delusion.

ĀSURI, the chief *disciple of *Kapila, the founder of the *Sāmkhya tradition. According to the *Suvarna-Saptati* ("Golden Seventy"), extant only in Paramārtha's sixth-century Chinese rendering, the sage Kapila appeared on the doorstep of the *brahmin* householder Āsuri to reveal to him the knowledge of Sāmkhya. However, Āsuri, who is described as an accomplished practitioner who had performed sacrifices for a thousand years, failed to respond. Kapila returned two more times, each time after an interval of a millennium. Finally Āsuri was ready to renounce his householder life and become the sage's disciple, adopting the lifestyle of a renouncer (*samnyāsin*). While Āsuri is remembered as one of the earliest Sāmkhya teachers, nothing substantial is known about him. The dialogue between him and Kapila found in the southern recension of the *Mahābhārata* is fictitious.

ĀSVĀDA ("taste"), in *Classical Yoga, the paranormal ability to taste "divine" (suprasensuous) delicacies. *Patanjali regards this as one of the flashes of illumination (*pratibhā*), a kind of supersense, which is considered to be an obstacle (*upasarga*) to *ecstasy.

ATATTVA, in *Shaivism, the *Divine in the form of *Shiva, who is not one of the principles or categories of existence, known as *tattva*.

ATHARVA-VEDA ("Knowledge of Atharvan"), one of the four *Vedic hymnodies. It received its name from the seer (*rishi*) Atharvan, who belonged to one of the greatest seer families of Vedic times. The name means "he who possesses fire," meaning a person skilled in the ritual of fire (*agni-hotra*). This *Veda*, probably compiled in the third millennium BCE, consists of some 6,000 magical incantations (in 730 hymns), though there are also hymns with a medical or healing intent and a number of fascinating philosophical riddles, as well as illuminating metaphysical passages that anticipate later *Sāmkhya and *Yoga ideas and practices, notably speculations about the *breath and breath control (*pranāyāma*). Of particular interest to Yoga researchers is the fifteenth book, known as the *Vrātya-Kānda*, which contains valuable information about the *Vrātya brotherhoods, in which early yogic practices were developed.

ATHEISM. In the context of Indian thought and culture, atheism can refer (a) to the materialism of the Cārvākas, who completely deny the existence of any higher or spiritual realities or entities, and (b) to traditions such as *Buddhism for which *Hinduism reserves the label *nāstika* ("not-is-ness"), meaning those that do not believe in the *Vedic revelation and the existence of a divine *Being. While the Buddhists do indeed reject the *Vedas as valid revelation, their founder's atheism is more properly described as a form of agnosticism, for the *Buddha refused to speculate about metaphysical questions. Some of his statements about *nirvāna, however, could be interpreted as an affirmation of an ultimate *Reality beyond the ever-changing world of *appearance. In fact, this interpretation seems to be favored by many of the philosophical schools of Mahāyāna and (Tibetan) Vajrayāna Buddhism. Moreover, all Buddhist schools affirm the existence of *deities, while the transcendental *buddhas of the Mahāyāna and Vajrayāna traditions are portrayed as creators of their own "fields," or universes.

ATIKRĀNTA-BHĀVANĪYA ("he who is intent on transcendence"). The *Yoga-Bhāshya (3.51) explains this high-level spiritual attainment as consisting in the intention to cause the "involution" (*pratiprasava) of the constituents (*guna) of *nature. The *adept who has reached this level of the spiritual process enjoys the sevenfold wisdom (*saptadha-prajnā). Cf. mādhu-bhūmika, prajnā-jyotis, prathama-kalpika.

ĀTITHYA ("hospitality"), sometimes regarded as one of the constituents of yogic self-restraint (*niyama). Since *Vedic times, guests (atithi) have been welcome in India as one might welcome a *deity, for they could well be deities in disguise. Hospitality is an aspect of generosity (*dāna). The word atithi means something like "wanderer," a person who does not stay in the same place (i.e., the host's home) very long.

ĀTIVĀHIKA-DEHA (lit. "superconductive body"), or simply ĀTIVĀHIKA, the migratory *body of the after-death state. According to the *Agni-Purāna (369.9), this body receives its nourishment from the funeral oblations. It is an intermediate vehicle for the ceased identity prior to the acquisition of the body peculiar to a deceased spirit (preta-deha) and, subsequently, an "enjoyment body" (bhoga-deha) in which the deceased reaps the auspicious or inauspicious fruits of his or her earthly deeds either in *heaven or in *hell. This body is also called *puryashtaka.

A different interpretation of the ātivāhika is found in the *Yoga-Vāsishtha (3.57.29) Here it is equated with the universal, omnipresent "body" of the singular *Reality. This is glorified as the true *body of human beings, the physical body being considered a mere illusion. See also Death, deha, pitri-yāna.

ĀTMA-DARSHANA ("Self-vision"), often used synonymously with *Self-realization or *enlightenment. In the *Yoga-Sūtra (2.41) this signifies the appearance of the transcendental *Self on the horizon of *consciousness in the highest mode of ecstasy (*samādhi). See also purusha-khyāti.

ĀTMA-JNĀNA ("Self-knowledge"), not mere self-understanding in the Socratic sense but the *ecstatic realization of the transcendental *Reality.

ĀTMA-KHYĀTI, a *Vedantic synonym for *purusha-khyāti in *Classical Yoga. See also khyāti.

ĀTMAN ("self" or "Self"). Since Sanskrit does not have capital letters, the context alone determines whether the empirical self, or ego personality (*jīva, jīva-ātman), or the transcendental *Self is intended. It is not always easy to make this distinction, however, as is clear from the following passage in the *Bhagavad-Gītā (6.5–6):

One should raise the *ātman* by the *ātman*; one should not let the *ātman* sink; for the *ātman* is indeed the *ātman's* friend, and the *ātman* is also the *ātman's* enemy.

The *ātman* is the friend of the *ātman* of him whose *ātman* is subdued by the *ātman*; but for [him who is] bereft of the *ātman*, the *ātman* is like an enemy in enmity.

The word *ātman*, though primarily a reflexive pronoun, has been used to denote the transcendental *Self since the time of the ancient *Upanishads*. As such it is a key concept of *Hindu metaphysics, notably *Vedānta and Vedānta-based schools of *Yoga. The Hindu sages and philosophers have mustered considerable ingenuity in determining and communicating the nature of the *ātman*. The problem is that the *Self is by definition not within reach of the *mind and the *senses. "The form of the Self cannot be seen by the eye," states the *Mahābhārata* (12.196.4), reiterating a point made already in the earliest *Upanishads*. As the archaic *Brihad-Āranyaka-Upanishad* (3.7.23) declares in a well-known passage, the *Self cannot be grasped because it is the grasper, the seer, of everything. In other words, the *Self reveals itself only to itself. No finite act of cognition is involved. Hence the *Shiva-Samhitā* (1.62) states: "Having abandoned the perception of false states [of *consciousness], the renouncer of all volition (*samkalpa) certainly beholds the Self in the Self by the Self."

ĀTMA-NIGRAHA ("self-control"), an important yogic virtue underlying all practices.

ĀTMA-NIVEDANA ("self-offering"), one of the aspects of the *Yoga of devotion (*bhakti-yoga). It means total surrender of the *ego and the unconditional worship of the *Divine as it is possible only in the state of ecstasy (*samādhi).

ĀTMA-PRATYĀBHIJÑĀ ("Self-recognition"), the state of *enlightenment in which the *adept recognizes his true nature as the ultimate *Self or *Reality in the form of *Shiva; the pivotal aspect of the *Pratyābhijñā school of Kashmiri *Shaivism.

ĀTMARĀMA. See Svātmarāma Yogīndra.

ATOMIZATION. See *animan*.

ATTACHMENT. See *rāga, sanga, sneha*.

ATTAINMENT. See *prāpti*.

ATTENTION (*avadhāna*), the focusing of the *mind or *consciousness upon a select *object, an intrapsychic process fundamental to all *Yoga. As the scriptures of *hatha-yoga point out again and again, it is closely associated with the flow of psychosomatic energy (*prāna) in the *body. In other words, attention and *breath are interconnected—a fact exploited by the *yogin. Attention permits consciousness to rest on ever more "subtle" (*sūkshma) aspects of existence. In the process of deepening *meditation or *contemplation, the mind is progressively emptied of contents, and ultimately there is no mental object left for attention to fasten on. In that moment, the *Self shines forth in its true nature and attention itself is totally transcended in the condition of supraconscious ecstasy (*asamprajnāta-samādhi).

ATYĀHĀRA ("overeating," from *ati* and *āhāra), according to the *Hatha-Yoga-Pradīpikā* (1.15), one of the six factors by which *Yoga is foiled. Cf. *mita-āhāra*.

AUM. See *om*.

AURA. In Western occultism, the aura is the subtle energy field surrounding the physical *body. It is simply the various layers of the subtle body (*sūkshma-sharīra*) insofar as they extend beyond the coarse body (*sthūla-sharīra*). The subtle layers of energy correspond to the various "sheaths" or "envelopes" (*kosha*) recognized in the *Yoga tradition. These are perfectly visible for the *yogin's* heightened vision or "divine eye" (*divya-cakshus*). The Sanskrit words for "aura" are *chāyā* ("shadow"), *prabhā-mandala* ("radiant circle"), and *dīpta-cakra* ("effulgent wheel"), the latter two referring to the energy field's luminosity.

The aura captured through Kirlian photography corresponds to what in Western occultism is known as the "etheric double" or "etheric aura." Properly, this still belongs to the physical *body or what in Sanskrit is known as the *anna-maya-kosha*. A more subtle auric field, which extends beyond the emanation of the physical aura, is the so-called astral body or emotional aura, corresponding to the *prāna-maya-kosha*. A still more subtle field, extending beyond the astral body, is the so-called mental aura or *mano-maya-kosha*. Beyond this, at a yet more subtle plane of existence, is the envelope of the higher mind, known as the *vijnāna-maya-kosha*. Finally, there is the so-called causal aura or causal body, known in *Hinduism as the *ānanda-maya-kosha*. Beyond all these sheaths, or bodies, is the transcendental *Self, which is unbounded and eternal.

AUROBINDO GHOSE (1872–1950), often referred to as Sri Aurobindo; one of modern India's most famous sages. Born into an Anglophile Bengali family, Aurobindo Ghose was educated in England and later entered the service of the maharaja of Baroda. During Curzon's vice-royalty, he became a leading figure in the Bengali nationalist movement. It was during his one-year imprisonment for political agitation that his spiritual transformation occurred. Upon his release he renounced politics and settled in the town of Pondicherry in South India. A prolific writer, he published numerous books on philosophy, art, education, and not least *Yoga, including *The Life Divine, The Synthesis of Yoga*, and *Essays on the Gita*. His work was continued by a Frenchwoman of Turkish-Egyptian descent, Mira Alfassa Richard, better known as "the Mother," in whom Sri Aurobindo saw the embodiment of the divine *shakti*.

Sri Aurobindo described his spiritual approach as "Integral Yoga" (*pūrna-yoga*). It has been hailed as the only new philosophical system to emerge from con-

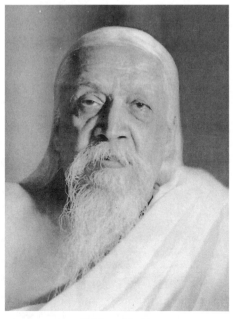

Sri **Aurobindo**

temporary India that is firmly founded in spiritual experience. Integral Yoga seeks to combine the quest for individual *liberation with the evolutionary destiny of humanity. This *Yoga purports to offer a viable spiritual *path for the present global crisis, which Sri Aurobindo understood as a transition from the mental to the supramental (or divinely inspired) consciousness.

AUSHADHI ("herb" or "herbal concoction"), certain drugs derived from plants and occasionally used by *yogins to procure *altered states of consciousness as well as paranormal powers (*siddhi). Herbs play an important role in Indian *alchemy. See also Parapsychology.

AUSPICIOUS POSTURE. See bhadra-āsana.

AUTOGENIC TRAINING. Invented by the German physician J. H. Schultz, Autogenic Training has been put forward as a kind of Western equivalent to *Yoga. It grew out of Schultz's extensive experimentation with *hypnosis during the period 1905–20. He understood his method as a "biological-rational technology," as opposed to the "mystical" approach of Yoga. He nonetheless expressed surprise at the subtleties of the yogic tradition, though remarking that it probably originated in a "cosmic hypochondria" leading to all sorts of mythologizing accretions.

AVADHŪTA ("cast off"), the spiritual *adept who has "shaken off" all worldly things and concerns. According to the *Mandala-Brāhmana-Upanishad (5.9), such a practitioner of radical *renunciation is accomplished in the practice of the highest type of supraconscious, supracognitive ecstasy (*nirvikalpa-samādhi). Also known as a "supreme swan" (*parama-hamsa),

the avadhūta is said to bring about the *liberation of 101 generations in his family. The *Mahānirvāna-Tantra (14.149) distinguishes two types of avadhūta: the perfect one, called "supreme swan," and the still imperfect one, known as "wanderer" (parivrāj). See also Baul sect, Crazy adept, samnyāsin.

AVADHŪTA-GĪTĀ, a late *Vedānta work that describes and extols the lifestyle of the *avadhūta who, in a blissful state of *Self-realization, bows to no social convention but utterly renounces everything.

AVASTHĀ ("state" or "condition"). *Yoga authorities distinguish several states or stages of maturity on the spiritual *path. Thus the *Hatha-Yoga-Pradīpikā (4.69) speaks of the initial state (*ārambha-avasthā), the active or "pot state" (*ghata-avasthā), the "accumulation state" (*paricāya-avasthā), and the "state of maturity" (*nishpatti-avasthā). These are more often styled "levels" (*bhūmi).

The word avasthā is also used to describe the four or five states of *consciousness according to the *Vedānta tradition. These are waking (*jāgrat), dreaming (*svapna), sleep (*sushupti), and the "fourth" (*turīya), which is the condition of *Self-realization. To these is sometimes added the state that transcends the "fourth" (*turīya-atīta), radical *enlightenment and absolute *transcendence.

Lastly, avasthā designates different states or stages of breath control (*prānāyāma).

AVATĀRA ("descent," from the root tri, "to cross over"), a manifestation, or incarnation, of the *Divine on earth—particularly of *Vishnu, of whom ten such descents, or incarnations, are generally mentioned. The *Bhāgavata-Purāna, however, also knows of sixteen, twenty-two, or twenty-three *avatāras*. The best known *avatāra* of these series are the God-men *Rāma and *Krishna. The divine incarnation for the present eon—the *kali-yuga* or dark age—is Kalki, or Kalkin, who is yet to come. Prophecy has it that he will appear riding a white horse and holding a blazing sword.

AVERSION. See *dvesha*.

AVIDYĀ ("nescience"), a synonym for *ajnāna*, generally denotes spiritual ignorance. In *Classical Yoga, *avidyā* is the principal among the five causes of affliction (*klesha*) that bind human beings to the endless cycle (*samsāra*) of *birth and *rebirth. The *Yoga-Sūtra* (2.5) defines it as seeing that which is eternal, pure, joyous, and of the *Self as that which is transient, impure, sorrowful, and not of the *Self. Nescience is not merely the absence of *knowledge but a positive misconception about *reality, just as a foe is not merely an absent friend but an enemy. Cf. *jnāna, vidyā*.

AVIRATI ("dissipation"), the squandering of one's energies on unworthy pursuits; one of the nine obstacles (*antarāya*) mentioned by *Patanjali.

AVISHESHA ("unparticularized"), a technical term of *Classical Yoga designating a distinct hierarchic level of nature (*prakriti*). According to the *Yoga-Bhāshya* (2.19), it is composed of six ontological categories (*tattva*), namely, the five potentials (*tanmātra*) and the principle of individuation (*asmitā-mātra*). See also Cosmos, *parvan*; cf. *vishesha*.

AVYAKTA ("unmanifest"), a term that belongs to the ancient vocabulary of the *Yoga and *Sāmkhya traditions, generally referring to the matrix of nature (*prakriti*), the source of the manifest forms, corresponding to the Greek notion of *archē*. *Patanjali employs the synonyms *alinga* and *pradhāna* instead. See also Cosmos, *parvan*; cf. *vyakta*.

AWAKENING. The idealist traditions of the world, including some schools of *Yoga, compare our ordinary *waking state to a *dream or hallucination: the *reality we experience has no objective existence but is a conjured image, a projection, that is based on the mistaken assumption that reality is external to our experiencing *consciousness. The split into an experiencing *subject (the ego consciousness) and an experienced objective *world is part of this dreamlike condition. Upon spiritual awakening, or *enlightenment, we understand that the duality (*dvaita*) between seer and seen is purely imaginary and that *Reality is singular. In this view, our ordinary state of *awareness is one of diminished consciousness; it is a semiconscious condition governed by habit patterns (*vāsanā*). This dream metaphor, however, is not used by *Patanjali, who believes that there is an ultimate, irrevocable chasm between the Self (*purusha*) and nature (*prakriti*). See also *bodha*.

AWARENESS. See *caitanya, cit, citi*, Consciousness.

ĀYUR-VEDA ("life science"), the native Indian system of *medicine. Although the original scripture by this title, traditionally considered to have been an appendix to the *Atharva-Veda*, is no longer extant, some of its medical lore has been preserved in the *Caraka-Samhitā*, the *Sushruta-Samhitā*, and other similar compilations. Āyur-Veda and *Yoga have influenced each other during their long history, starting in *Vedic times.

ĀYUR-VEDA-SŪTRA ("Aphorisms on the Life Science"), a sixteenth-century work attributed to Yogānanda Nātha. Its special interest for *Yoga researchers lies in the fact that it seeks to connect *Patanjali's eightfold *path with Indian *medicine.

· B ·

BABAJI. This Hindi honorific is bestowed upon an anonymous adept (*siddha) who is counted among the immortals. Also known as Kriya Babaji Nagaraja, he was introduced to Western spiritual seekers in *Autobiography of a Yogi* (1946) by Paramahansa *Yogānanda, who called him a great *avatāra. Various contemporary masters have referred to meetings with Babaji, who is particularly associated with *kriyā-yoga. According to this tradition, as kept alive by Yogi S. A. A. Ramaiah, Babaji was born into a priestly family on November 30, 203 CE in the South Indian village of Parangipettai, near the mouth of the Cauvery River. He was kidnapped at the age of five by a visiting trader from Baluchistan (in Pakistan), who sailed to Calcutta, where he sold the handsome boy. The owner, however, set him free, and the young child promptly joined a group of wandering ascetics. In this way he acquired great spiritual and scriptural knowledge. At the age of eleven he undertook a pilgrimage to the shrine of Katirgama in Sri Lanka, which was established by the South Indian *siddha *Boganāthar (Sanskrit: Bhoganātha).

Babaji became Boganāthar's *disciple and made swift progress on the path of *kriyā-yoga. At one point Boganāthar sent him to the famous adept *Agastyar. On the forty-eighth day of *prayer, *meditation, and *fasting, Agastyar revealed himself to the boy and then initiated him into the secrets of *breath control, called *vasi yogam* in the Tamil scriptures. Then he instructed Babaji to retire to Badrinath in the Himalayas, a few miles south of the Tibetan border. After eighteen months of practicing *kriyā-yoga* in the solitude of the high mountains, Babaji entered the state of *soruba-samādhi, which coincided with the *transubstantiation of his *body. He became one of the immortals.

Babaji is said to have initiated *Shankara, *Kabir, and *Lahiri Mahasaya, the teacher of Paramahamsa *Yogānanda's teacher.

BACK EXTENSION POSTURE. See *pashcima-tāna-āsana*.

BADDHA-PADMA-ĀSANA (*baddhapadmāsana*, "bound lotus posture"), performed by clasping the big toes with one's hands while seated in the lotus posture (*padmaāsana*) with one's arms crossed behind one's back; mentioned in the *Goraksha-Paddhati* (1.96), one of the older *hatha-yoga scriptures. It is often recommended especially for the *purification of the psychoenergetic pathways (*nādī-shodhana*).

BAHIR-ANGA ("outer limb"), in *Classical Yoga, one of the first five "limbs" (*anga) of the eightfold *path, which are contrasted with the three "inner limbs" (*antar-anga). See also *ashta-anga-yoga*.

BAHIR-LAKSHYA ("external sign"), one of the three kinds of photistic experience in *tāraka-yoga. The *Advaya-Tāraka-Upanishad (6) describes it as the perception of luminous "ether-space" (*vyoman) of blue, dark blue, red, and yellow color, at a distance of four, six, eight, ten, or twelve "breadths-of-thumb" (angula) in front of one's *nose. This is preceded by the manifestation of rays of golden *light that, as one becomes accomplished, are seen at the rim of the eyes or on the ground. See also lakshya.

BAHISH-KRITA-DHAUTI ("expelled cleansing"), one of the four types of internal cleansing (*antar-dhauti) used in *hatha-yoga. The *Gheranda-Samhitā (1.22) gives the following description: Perform the "crow seal" (*kākī-mudrā), then fill the abdomen with *air, hold it there for ninety minutes, and then force it down into the in-

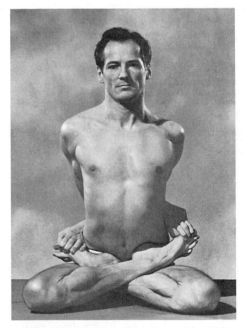

Baddha-padma-āsana, demonstrated by Theos Bernard

testines. Next, stand in navel-deep water, draw out the intestines, and wash them until they are completely clean; then pull them back up again. This procedure, which should not be done without supervision, is said to yield a "shining body" (deva-deha). See also dhauti.

BĀHYA-DVĀDASHA-ANTA ("ending with the outer twelfth"), the point reached by the exhaled *breath at a distance of twelve fingers from the tip of the *nose. See also dvādasha-anta; cf. antar-dvādasha-anta.

BALA ("power" or "strength"). Since ancient times, the practice of *Yoga has been said to lead to *power, both physical and psychic. This bears out the close historical association between Yoga and asceticism (*tapas). The *Yoga-Sūtra (3.46) lists bala as one of the marks of bodily perfection (*kāya-sampad). The *Bhagavad-Gītā (16.18), however, warns against the lust for power, which merely leads to repeated *rebirth. The word bala also signifies "strength" or "energy" as a positive requirement for *yogins. According to the *Mahābhārata (12.289.16), those who lack energy are bound to go astray.

BALANCE. See samatva.

BALI ("offering"), one of the "limbs" (*anga) of the *Yoga of sacred sound (*mantra-yoga). This practice, an aspect of most forms of ritual Yoga, consists in the offering of fruit and flowers to one's chosen deity (*ishta-devatā).

BANDHA ("bond" or "bondage") has a wide range of meanings in the Sanskrit literature and can stand for "tying" or "bridging" as well as "pledge" and "tendon." In *Yoga it first and foremost signifies the human condition of finite existence, that is, the state of *unenlightenment: our spiritual ignorance (*avidyā) is our bondage. It keeps us tied to the cycle of existence (*samsāra), from birth to *death to *rebirth to repeated death. In *Classical Yoga bandha denotes the "correlation" (*samyoga) between the transcendental *Self or *purusha and the finite *ego personality, or *consciousness. This relation is sometimes described as that between fire and wood. Moreover, according to the *Yoga-Sūtra (3.1), the term refers to the "binding" of consciousness to a particular *object or locus (*desha), which is the very essence of *concentration.

Finally, bandha stands for a particular class of techniques in *hatha-yoga that involve local stoppages of the flow of psychosomatic energy (*prāna). In this sense, the word is often translated as "lock" or "constriction." Three such locks are generally distinguished: the *mūla-bandha ("root lock"), the *uddīyāna-bandha

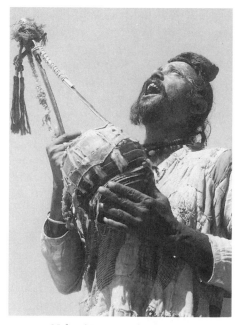

Nabani Das, a modern **Baul**

("upward lock"), and the *jālandhara-bandha ("Jālandhara's lock"). According to the *Yoga-Kundali-Upanishad (1.40), these should be practiced when *breath control is mastered properly. See also mudrā.

BAPTISM. See abhisheka.

BASAVA (12th cen. CE), the founder of the *Lingāyata or Vīra-Shaiva sect; a minister of King Bijjala Kalacuri. He rejected the authority of the *Vedas and the *brahmins and fervently opposed the customary practices of cremation, image worship, *pilgrimage, and *sacrifice. According to the Basava-Purāna (ca. 1370 CE), Basava was the son of a *brahmin and was married to the daughter of King Bijjala's chief minister, Baladeva. When Basava was appointed to Baladeva's position after the latter's death, he made large donations to the priests of his newly founded sect, who were known as the jangamas. When the king discovered that the state's treasury chest was rapidly being depleted, he tried to have Basava arrested, but this larger-than-life spiritual leader summoned his followers and defeated Bijjala in battle. They came to an agreement, and Basava was reinstated in his position. More unsavory is the story, told in both this and a *Jaina biography of Basava, that in due course he had the ruler murdered. When he learned that the king had indeed died, Basava himself dropped his *body and is said to have reached union with the *Divine.

BATH, BATHING. See snāna.

BAUL SECT. The Bengali word baul (Hindi: baur) can be derived from either the Sanskrit term vātula ("mad") or vyākula ("intent" or "perplexed"). Both make reference to the ecstatic intoxication and religious fervor for which the Bauls are renowned. This loosely organized sect originated in Bengal during the Indian middle ages. Its members are chiefly recruited from the lower strata of society. The Bauls are noted for their unconventional manners and customs. As *yogin*-bards they are famous for their songs, which typically revolve around the "man in the *heart," i.e., the transcendental *Self immanent in the human *body. See also *avadhūta*, Sahajiyā.

BEAUTY. See *kānti*.

BEE BREATHING. See *bhrāmarī*.

BEING (Sanskrit: *sat*), the ultimate *Reality, eternal and changeless (*akshara*). It is contrasted with becoming (*bhava*), which is equated with nonbeing or the unreal (*asat*).

BELLOWS BREATHING. See *bhastrikā*.

BHADRA-ĀSANA (*bhadrāsana*, "auspicious posture"), yogic posture (*āsana*) already mentioned in the fourth-century *Yoga-Bhāshya* (2.46), and described in the *Tat-*

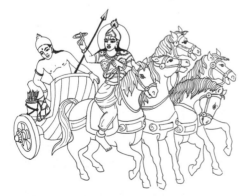

Lord Krishna and Prince Arjuna in the war chariot where the teachings of the *Bhagavad-Gītā* were imparted

tva-Vaishāradī (2.46) as follows: bringing the soles of both feet near each other at the scrotum, hollow the hands and place them above the feet in the shape of a tortoise. The *Gheranda-Samhitā* (II.9f.) states that one should place the heels crosswise under the scrotum, cross one's hands behind the back, and catch hold of the toes; while performing the "waterpipe lock" (*jālandhara-bandha*), one should fix one's gaze on the tip of the *nose. This, it is said, cures all kinds of *diseases. According to the *Hatha-Yoga-Pradīpikā* (1.53), this is also known as "Goraksha's posture" (*goraksha-āsana*). However, modern manuals of *hatha-yoga* tend to distinguish between the *bhadra-āsana* and the *goraksha-āsana*.

BHAGA ("dispenser"), an epithet of several *Vedic deities and the name of one of the *Ādityas. It also denotes the sun, good fortune, dignity, beauty, and love. Lastly, it refers to the female *genitals (*yoni*). See also *bhagavat*.

BHAGAVAD-GĪTĀ ("Lord's Song"), the most famous of all *Yoga scriptures; an episode in the *Mahābhārata* (6.13–40), into which it appears to have been neatly inserted prior to the common era. Like the epic as a whole, the *Gītā* ("song") belongs to what is called the "tradition" (*smriti*) literature of *Hinduism, but has for centuries in effect been treated as a part of the *Vedic canonical or *shruti* ("revelation") literature. According to its colophon, it wants to be understood as a secret teaching—an *Upanishad*. It was probably composed in the third or fourth century BCE, but earlier and also later dates have been suggested. It is possible that the *Gītā* as we know it, consisting of 700 stanzas, is not all of a piece, though scholarship has so far failed to reconstruct a satisfactory urtext.

The teachings of the *Gītā* stem from the *Pāncarātra tradition of the ancient *Bhāgavata sect. They bear a unique stamp, and especially the *Gītā's* emphatic *theism sets it off from other works of the same period. Its approach is markedly integrative, attempting to synthesize such diverse views as *Vedānta, *Sāmkhya, *Yoga, and orthodox *Brāhmanism, as well as the personal worship of *Krishna. Purporting to be both a moral (*dharma) teaching and mystical lore (*yoga-shāstra), the *Gītā* advocates a three-pronged *path to *liberation: *karma-yoga, *jnāna-yoga, and *bhakti-yoga. The first two approaches are expounded mainly in chapters 1–12, whereas the last six chapters are traditionally held to treat of the ideal and excellences of devotion (*bhakti). Though not rejecting the kind of world-negating *asceticism that characterizes many *Upanishads, the *Gītā* nevertheless places the ideal of disinterested action (*naishkarmya-karman) above that of the *renunciation of all *action. Yet devotion is put forward as especially worthy of pursuit, since it leads to a state of realization that is higher than mere "extinction in the world ground" (*brahma-nirvāna) insofar as it involves one's awakening in the divine person of Krishna, who is the all-encompassing suprapersonal (rather than impersonal) *Reality. See also *Anu-Gītā, Avadhūta-Gītā, Ganesha-Gītā, Īshvara-Gītā, Uddhāva-Gītā.*

BHAGAVAT ("blessed one"), an epithet generally applied to *Krishna but sometimes to other personal *deities of the *Hindu pantheon as well. It suggests that the ultimate *Reality is not an abstract condition but living *Being. When followed by words beginning with certain soft consonants, *bhagavat* is written *bhagavad*, as in *Bhagavad-Gītā, or *bhagavan*, as in *bhagavan-maya* ("intent on the Lord"). See also *bhaga, īshvara.*

BHĀGAVATA-PURĀNA or **SHRĪMAD-BHĀGAVATA**, a major *Purāna*, probably composed ca. 750 CE; the most important scripture of the *Bhāgavata sect. Its philosophical foundations are those of *Advaita Vedānta, mellowed by the conception and *worship of the *Divine in personal form as *Krishna. However, cultic *rituals do not play as significant a role in this work as they do in the *Samhitā literature of the *Pāncarātra tradition. The *Bhāgavata-Purāna* is replete with *Yoga and *Sāmkhya teachings. All the elements of the eightfold *path (*ashta-anga-yoga) are present, yet the overall focus is on *service and *devotion to the personal *God. Thus the path propounded in this *Purāna* is *bhakti-yoga, as contrasted with "Yoga," which presumably refers to the dualist approach of *Classical Yoga. Much space is given to instructions about visualizing the personal deity in *meditation.

Of particular interest is section 11.6–29, known as the *Uddhāva-Gītā. In imitation of the *Bhagavad-Gītā, this work expounds three types of *Yoga: *karma-yoga, *jnāna-yoga, and *bhakti-yoga. In one passage (9.20), *Vishnu declares that he is of nothing more fond than *devotion. Elsewhere (23.41), the *Uddhāva-Gītā* speaks out against the kind of body-oriented Yoga—meaning *hatha-yoga—that merely aims at the acquisition of paranormal powers (*siddhi), since, it is argued, the *body is after all mortal.

BHĀGAVATA SECT, a tradition based on the *worship of the "blessed one" (*bhagavat), i.e., *Vasudeva, who is *Vishnu and *Krishna. The antiquity of Bhāgavatism is well established, but its history is still rather obscure. The earliest available sources of this sect are the *Bhagavad-Gītā and the *Nārāyanīya* section of the *Mahābhārata (12.334–51). According to

*Shankara's learned commentary on the *Brahma-Sūtra* (2.2.42f.), a classic summary of *Vedānta metaphysics, the word *bhāgavata* applies to the followers of the religious tradition known as *Pāncarātra, though this distinction is not always so clear-cut. See also Vaishnavism.

BHAIRAVA, one of the terrifying forms of *Shiva; also the name of an *adept of "*hatha-yoga* mentioned in the *Hatha-Yoga-Pradīpikā* (1.6).

A certain Bhairava Ācārya is mentioned in Bāna's celebrated seventh-century *Harsha-Carita*, a historical novel featuring King Harshavardhana, of whose court the poet was a member. Bhairava Ācārya is portrayed as a saint from South India who had thousands of followers. Bāna furnishes the following vivid description of him: Seated on a tiger skin, he had long matted hair, into which rosary beads and shells were woven, and a thick beard. He wore crystal earrings (*kundala*) and an iron bracelet on one forearm, bound with a protective thread made from herbs. He also wore a loincloth (*kaupīna*) and a shawl (*yoga-pattaka*). See also Ānanda Bhairava, Ugra Bhairava, *Vijnāna-Bhairava*.

BHAIRAVA- or **BHAIRAVĪ-MUDRĀ,** a synonym for *khecārī-mudrā*.

BHAIRAVĪ, the feminine counterpart of *Bhairava, i.e., *Shakti.

BHAJANA ("worshiping"), a synonym for *kīrtana*.

BHAKTA ("devotee" or "worshiper"). Worship or devotion (*bhakti*) is a spiritual *practice by which the aspirant seeks to acknowledge his or her dependence on a higher power. The *Bhāgavata-Purāna*

(3.29.7ff.) distinguishes four types of devotee. The qualities of the first three are in consonance with the three primary qualities (*guna*) of *nature, whereas the fourth type is said to be *nirguna* or beyond nature's primary constituents. According to the *Bhagavad-Gītā* (9.23), even those who are completely dedicated to the worship of a deity (*deva*) other than *Krishna in reality worship Krishna, because he is the recipient of all *sacrifices. Because such worshipers do not know *Krishna to be the supreme *Being, however, they also do not attain final *liberation. There is always an exclusive element to such devotionalism, which is founded in *theism, but the ultimate virtue of the worshiper is to discover the *Divine in all beings and forms.

BHAKTI ("devotion" or "love," from the root *bhaj,* "to participate in"), loving attachment or devotion. From the beginning, the term was intimately connected with the theistic traditions of *Hinduism. It made its first appearance in the *Shvetāshvatara-Upanishad* (4.23), an early *Shaiva text, which demands devotion to the *Divine and one's *teacher.

Originally, however, the ideal of *bhakti* was mainly promoted among the worshipers of *Vishnu, who favored a strongly theistic philosophy. This orientation is best represented in the *Bhagavad-Gītā* (16.30), where *Krishna declares: "He who sees Me everywhere and who sees Me as all: to him I am not lost nor is he lost to Me."

The *Bhagavad-Gītā* (18.54f.) distinguishes two degrees of *liberation—one without devotion, the other with devotion:

Having become [identical with] the world ground (*brahman*) and being tranquil, he neither grieves nor craves. [Beholding] the same [*Reality] in all beings, he gains supreme *love for Me.

Through love (*bhakti*) he really knows Me; how great I am and who. Then, having really known Me, he forthwith enters into that [supreme state of My *Being].

These stanzas speak of what elsewhere is called the "higher love" (*para-bhakti*) of the person who, upon attaining *liberation, discovers that the ultimate *Reality is not impersonal but suprapersonal.

For the Marathi saint *Jnānadeva, whose *Jnāneshvarī is hailed as the finest commentary on the *Bhagavad-Gītā, devotion constitutes the fifth goal of humanity (*purusha-artha*). The *Bhāgavata-Purāna (6.9.47), again, insists that love and *knowledge are interdependent and that the one can be reached by means of the other. See also *bhakti-mārga, bhakti-yoga, guru-bhakti*.

BHAKTI-MĀRGA ("road of devotion"), the devotional religious movement that swept across the south of India in the seventh to ninth centuries and across the north in the fourteenth to seventeenth centuries CE. The modern Krishna Consciousness sect is a revival of those teachings. See Shrīla Prabhupāda.

BHAKTI-SŪTRA of *Nārada, a medieval *Vaishnava work probably composed after *Rāmānuja's time. In eighty-four aphorisms the sage Nārada explains in simple terms the essence of the devotional approach (*bhakti-yoga*) to the *Divine. He recommends contact (*sanga*) with the great *adepts and constant worship (*bhajana*) of *God, expressed in selfless *action, songs of praise, and listening to the scriptural expressions of his glory. *Liberation is gained through grace (*kripā*) alone. In aphorism 83 he mentions *Shāndilya, among other teachers of *bhakti.

BHAKTI-SŪTRA of *Shāndilya, in contrast to *Nārada's *Bhakti-Sūtra*, is more aca-

demic and polemical and has been more influential in philosophical circles. It consists of 100 aphorisms (*sūtra*) distributed over three chapters, and it probably precedes the *Bhāgavata-Purāna, which can be placed in the eighth century CE. The earliest extant commentary on Shāndilya's compilation is the *Bhāshya* ("Speech") of Svapneshvara, a Bengali *Vaishnava who may have lived between 1300 and 1400 CE. Another commentary is by the seventeenth-century scholar and spiritual practitioner *Nārāyana Tīrtha.

BHAKTIVEDANTA SWAMI, A. C. See Shrīla Prabhupāda.

BHAKTI-YOGA ("Yoga of devotion"), one of the principal branches of the *Yoga tradition of *Hinduism. It is often presented as complementing the approaches of *jnāna-yoga and *karma-yoga. Later *Vaishnava authorities of this type of Yoga mention the following nine "limbs" (*anga*): *shravana, or "listening" to the sacred scriptures; *kīrtana, or the "singing" of devotional songs in praise of *God; *smarana, or "remembering" the *Divine by meditating upon its form; *pāda-sevana, or "service at the feet" of the *Lord; *arcanā, or ritual worship; *vandana, or "prostration" before the image of God; *dāsya, or "slavish" devotion to the Lord; *sākhya, or "friendship" through which the Divine raises the humble *devotee to the status of a friend; and *ātma-nivedana, or "self-offering," through which the worshiper enters into the immortal body of God. These aspects, or stages, of *bhakti-yoga* are most lucidly expounded by Rūpa Gosvāmin in his work *Bhakti-Rasa-Amrita-Sindhu* ("Ocean of the Immortal Essence of Devotion").

According to the *Bhāgavata-Purāna (3.28.7), there are many *paths of *bhakti-

yoga, depending on the different inner constitution (*sva-bhava*) of practitioners. This scripture (3.29.14) also speaks of an *ātyantika* ("extreme") *bhakti-yoga* consisting in pure *devotion to the *Divine on the part of those who have resigned their will to the point where they do not even *desire to be uplifted to *Vishnu's paradise but have become utterly devoid of personal motivation apart from the desire to be *God's instrument. This is also known as "unqualified devotion" (*nirguna-bhakti*). See also *prapatti*.

BHANUKIN, an adept of *hatha-yoga* mentioned in the *Hatha-Yoga-Pradīpikā* (1.8).

BHARTRIHARI (7th cen. CE), poet and grammarian best known for his *Vairāgya-Shataka* ("Century of Dispassion") and *Shānti-Shataka* ("Century of Peace"). The former composition celebrates the ideal of *dispassion and depicts its author as still engaged in the struggle for *renunciation. The latter work, on the other hand, portrays him as having gained a certain spiritual vantage point. In this didactic poem (4.10) the author condemns false *yogins* who, through painful self-castigation, acquire *powers but lack genuine inner *peace. Bhartrihari was the first to propound the *Advaita Vedānta doctrine of *vivarta*, or illusory world emanation.

BHARTRIHARI (11th cen. CE), a king of Ujjain (western India) converted to *Nāthism, according to local tradition, by the great teacher *Goraksha himself. According to other traditions, it was *Jālandhari who initiated him. One of the subsects of the *Kānphata sect is named after him.

BHĀSHYA ("speech" or "discussion"), an original commentary on a primary scripture, such as a *Sūtra. See, for instance, *Yoga-Bhāshya*.

BHASMAN ("devouring"), that which has been devoured by fire, i.e., *ashes. As an outward sign of their inner *renunciation, *yogins* and *sādhus* mark a portion or all of their skin with ashes. The forehead (*lalāta*) mark made from ash dust is called *bhasma-lalātikā*. Some *ascetics live close to funeral pyres and use the ashes from the burning of corpses to express their symbolic *death in regard to all worldly things. The *Gheranda-Samhitā* (3.54) recommends smearing the *body with ashes for the practice of *shakti-cālana*. One of *Shiva's many epithets is Bhasmapriya, meaning "He who is fond of ashes."

Miraculous manifestations of ashes connected with the images of saints or produced at will by *yogins*, such as the contemporary miracle worker Satya Sai Baba, to strengthen their devotees' *faith are known as *vibhūti*.

BHASTRIKĀ or **BHASTRĀ** ("bellows"), one of the eight types of breath control (*prānāyāma*) described in the *Gheranda-Samhitā* (5.74f.) and other scriptures of *hatha-yoga*. It is explained as follows: as the bellows of the blacksmith move the air to and fro, so should the *breath be slowly moved through both nostrils. After twenty repetitions of this, the *yogin* should perform the "pot" (*kumbhaka*), that is, retention of the breath. It is clear from the description found in the *Hatha-Yoga-Pradīpikā* (2.59ff.) that inhalation should be done through the right nostril and exhalation through the left. In the *Yoga-Kundalī-Upanishad* (1.32ff.), however, a reverse procedure is stipulated. The principal purpose of *bhastrikā* is to awaken the "serpent power" (*kundalinī-shakti*). See also *shakti-cālana*.

BHĀSVATĪ ("Radiance") of *Hariharānanda Āranya, a twentieth-century Sanskrit commentary on the *Yoga-Sūtra*, offering many illuminating definitions.

BHAVA (from the root *bhū*, "to be") can mean such diverse things as "birth," "source," and "prosperity." In many contexts, however, the word denotes "existence" in the sense of *samsāra*. See also *sva-bhāva*; cf. Being.

BHĀVA (from the root *bhū*, "to be"), "being," "condition," "nature," "disposition," "feeling." The last-mentioned connotation is found primarily in works on *bhakti-yoga*, which distinguish five principal feelings, or moods: *shānta-bhāva*, the "tranquil mood" (of awe or humility); *dāsya-bhāva*, the "slavish mood" (of respect, subservience, or dedication); *vatsalya-bhāva*, the "calflike mood" (of tender filial or brotherly feelings); *sākhya-bhāva*, the "friendly mood" (of feelings of friendship); *mādhurya-bhāva*, the "sweet mood" (of delight between lovers). These should ultimately develop into *rasa*, the tasting of the pure *bliss of intimate love-participation in *God.

According to the *Sāmkhya-Kārikā* (23), there are eight fundamental conditions (*bhāva*) of the *mind: knowledge (*jnāna*), virtue (*dharma*), dispassion (*vairāgya*), lordship (*aishvarya*), ignorance (*ajnāna*), vice (*adharma*), lack of dispassion (*avairāgya*), and absence of lordship or potency (*anaishvarya*). Other *Sāmkhya texts mention fifty such *bhāvas*. It is possible that the mention of a sevenfold wisdom (*saptadha-prajnā*) in the *Yoga-Sūtra* (2.27) may be a reference to these mental states with the exception of knowledge, which is the means for transcending all others. *Vyāsa's *Yoga-Bhāshya* (2.27), however, offers a different, if not entirely convincing, explanation.

*Tantrism has a well-known classification of practitioners into three fundamental types: those with the "beastly disposition" (*pashu-bhāva*), the "heroic disposition" (*vīra-bhāva*), and the "divine disposition" (*divya-bhāva*). The word *pashu means "beast" or "creature" and generally refers to the individual who is fettered to the world of illusion (*māyā*). The predominant quality active in such a person is inertia (*tamas*). In some contexts, however, the word designates a full-fledged initiate of a certain level of spiritual attainment. The disposition of the hero (*vīra*), resulting from a preeminence of the quality of dynamism (*rajas*), is characteristic of the typical spiritual aspirant in the present dark age (*kali-yuga*). The divine disposition is due to a preponderance of the principle of lucidity (*sattva*), and it defines that rare individual who is naturally inclined toward *meditation, *equanimity, and remembering the *Divine.

BHĀVA GANESHA DĪKSHITA (prob. ca. 1550–1600 CE), the author of the *Yoga-Anushāsana-Sūtra-Vritti*, also titled *Pradīpikā*. He was a chief disciple of *Vijnāna Bhikshu.

BHĀVA-LINGA ("sign of being") refers to *Shiva as the *Reality beyond *space and *time. See also *linga*.

BHĀVANĀ ("cultivation"), a synonym for "meditation" (*dhyāna*). In *Tantrism the word is generally used in the sense of visualization.

BHĀVA-YOGA ("Yoga of being"), a yogic approach that does not include *mantra recitation, according to the *Shiva-Purāna* (7.2.37.9). Cf. *abhāva-yoga*.

BHAYA ("fear"), one of the defects (*dosha*) of the *ego personality that need to be overcome. That fear is a universal constant of human experience is recognized by all traditions of *Yoga, as is the possibility of transcending it. Upon full *Self-realization, all fear is extirpated. Cf. *abhaya*.

BHOGA ("enjoyment"), in *Classical Yoga, "world experience" as the antithesis of emancipation (*apavarga*). The *Yoga-Sūtra* (3.35) defines it as an idea based on the nondistinction between the *Self and the most translucent aspect of *nature, namely, the *sattva*. The *Bhagavad-Gītā* (5.22) speaks of the enjoyment that springs from contact with the sense objects as a womb of suffering (*duhkha*). See also *ābhoga*.

BHOJA (1018–60 CE), king of Dhārā; his personal name was Ranaranga Malla. A worshiper of *Shiva, Bhoja composed a much-acclaimed commentary on the *Yoga-Sūtra* entitled *Rāja-Mārtanda* and is also credited with the authorship of works on *Shaiva philosophy, grammar, *ethics, astronomy, and the art of war.

BHOJA-VRITTI. See *Rāja-Mārtanda*.

BHOKTRI ("enjoyer"), the *Self as the experiencing subject of mental states. According to *Sāmkhya metaphysics, the transcendental Self is the enjoyer of all things. Thus the *Maitrāyanīya-Upanishad* (6.10) asserts that the Self devours "*nature's food" (*prakritam annam*), its food being specifically the "elemental self" (*bhūta-ātman*). See also *bhoga, kartri*.

BHRAMA ("perplexity"), a wandering *mind in need of *discipline; one of the ten obstacles (*vighna*) of *Yoga.

BHRĀMARĪ ("bee"), one of the eight types of breath control (*prānāyāma*) of *hatha-yoga, described in the *Hatha-Yoga-Pradīpikā* (2.68) as follows: one should inhale while making the sound of a male bee, then exhale slowly (after having retained the air for some time) while making the sound of a female bee. According to the *Gheranda-Samhitā* (5.78ff.), this practice is performed somewhat differently and is connected with the perception of inner sounds. See also *nāda-yoga*.

BHRĀNTI ("delusion"), one of the ten obstacles (*vighna*) of *Yoga. According to the *Kaula-Jnāna-Nirnaya* (5.2), it is to be overcome through the persistent practice of meditation (*dhyāna*).

BHRĀNTI-DARSHANA ("false vision"), one of the obstructions (*antarāya*) mentioned by *Patanjali. The *Linga-Purāna* (1.9.7) explains it as erroneous knowledge relative to the spiritual goal, one's *teacher, the nature of *knowledge, *conduct, and the *Divine.

BHRIGU ("Bright"), one of the sons of the legendary *Manu, the ancestor of the human race. He is remembered as a *Vedic seer (*rishi*) who cursed *Agni, turning him into an omniverous deity. He is a member of the Vedic priestly family of the Bhrigus, who invented the fire *sacrifice. Bhrigu came to be associated with the tradition of *Vaishnavism. He often figures as a *teacher of *Yoga in medieval scriptures.

BHRŪ-CAKRA ("brow wheel"), better known as the *ājnā-cakra.

BHRŪ-MADHYA ("brow middle"), the place on the *forehead between the eyebrows (*bhrū*). *Yogins are often seen focusing their gaze (*drishti*) on this spot during *concentration. The *bhrū-madhya* is also the secret locus in the center of the *head, most frequently referred to as the *ajñā-cakra, a favorite anchor point for the aspirant's attention. This locus is also called tri-kunda, suci-hathā, govitha, shikhara, tri-shankhi-vajrī, and om-kārī, according to the *Hatha-Ratna-Āvalī (1.142). The *Tri-Shikhi-Brāhmana-Upanishad (2.132) regards the bhrū-madhya as one of the eighteen vital areas (*marman) of the *body and as the locus of the "fourth" (*turīya), i.e., the transcendental *Self. Cf. nāsa-agra.

BHŪ-CĀRA-SIDDHI or BHŪ-CĀRI-SIDDHI ("earth-moving power"), the paranormal ability (*siddhi) to levitate at will. According to the *Yoga-Tattva-Upanishad (59), this is one of the benefits of mastery in breath control (*prānāyāma). The *Shiva-Samhitā (5.88) also deems it achievable by means of *contemplation upon the vāna-linga in the *heart center. See also Levitation.

BHUJANGA-ĀSANA (bhujangāsana, "serpent posture," from bhuj and anga, lit. "crooked-limbed"), the posture (*āsana) popularly called "the Cobra." The *Gheranda-Samhitā (2.42f.) describes it thus: The body should touch the ground from the *navel down to the toes. Placing the palms on the ground, one should raise the *head and shoulders like a serpent. This is said to raise the body temperature and remove *diseases of all kinds, as well as awaken the "serpent power" (*kundalinī-shakti).

BHUJANGĪ ("serpent"), a synonym for *kundalinī.

BHUJANGINĪ-MUDRĀ ("serpent seal"), described in the *Gheranda-Samhitā (3.92f.) as follows: Extending the face a little forward, suck in air through the gullet. This is said to cure quickly all abdominal *diseases, especially indigestion. See also mudrā.

BHUKTI ("enjoyment"), a synonym for *bhoga.

BHŪMI ("earth") can stand for a variety of things. Thus it denotes (1) the ground on which the yogic practices are performed; (2) the earth element (*prithivī), (3) the planet Earth, and (4) a particular "stage" or "level" of practice.

The last-mentioned connotation deserves comment. *Yoga is a graduated endeavor, and the initiate is thought to progress to ever-higher levels of attainment until he or she reaches the final stage (prānta-bhūmi), which, according to the

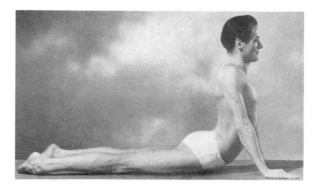

Bhujanga-āsana, demonstrated by Theos Bernard

Yoga-Sūtra (2.27), consists in the "sevenfold wisdom" (*saptadha-prajñā*). Since *progress depends on the individual's capacity and commitment, however, there can be no rigid objective scale, but only models that serve as signposts along the way. One such model is *Patanjali's classification of ecstasy (*samādhi*) into four principal types. Although one of *Patanjali's aphorisms (3.6) would seem to imply some kind of natural progression from one ecstatic level to the next, the great Yoga master nowhere actually states that a particular sequence must be followed. Sudden leaps to higher levels are in fact admitted by his commentator *Vyāsa, who in his *Yoga-Bhāshya* (3.6) remarks that "Yoga itself is the teacher." In the *Tattva-Vaishāradī* (1.17), *Vācaspati Mishra compares the *yogin* to an archer who first practices with a big target nearby and only later with a smaller target placed at a greater distance. Vācaspati suggests that at first *concentration should involve a "coarse" (*sthūla*) object and later, when the necessary skill has been developed, objects pertaining to the "subtle" (*sūkshma*) dimension of *nature.

Vācaspati also mentions four stages of the process of ecstatic involution: the *mādhu-mati-bhūmi* ("honeyed level"); the *mādhu-pratīka-bhūmi* ("honey-faced level"); the *vishoka-bhūmi* ("sorrowless level"); and the *samskāra-shesha-bhūmi* ("level consisting of a residuum of subconscious activators"). In the *Yoga-Bhāshya* (1.1), moreover, mention is made of five levels of mental activity (*citta-bhūmi*). See also *atikrānta-bhāvanīya*, *avasthā*, *mādhu-bhūmika*, *prajñā-jyotis*, *sapta-jnāna-bhūmi*.

BHŪTA (past participle of *bhū*, "to be, to become") has several connotations. It can signify a living being in general or an ele-

mental or disembodied spirit of a low order in particular. In many contexts, it denotes the five *elements (*panca-bhūta*) of which the material *cosmos is composed. These are, in ascending order: earth (*prithivī*), water (*ap*), fire (*agni*), air (*vāta*), and ether (*ākāsha*). See also *tattva*.

BHŪTA-ĀTMAN (*bhūtātman*, "elemental self"), the individuated *self. This concept first appears in the schools of *Preclassical Yoga but is also found in later *Yoga scriptures showing *Vedānta influence. According to the *Mahābhārata* (12.245.11), the elemental self resides in the *heart and is a fragment (*amsha*) of the supreme radiance, the transcendental *Self.

BHŪTA-JAYA (lit. "conquest of the elements"), one of the paranormal powers (*siddhi*). According to the *Yoga-Sūtra* (3.44), it results from the practice of ecstatic constraint (*samyama*) upon the various levels of a given *object.

BHŪTA-SHUDDHI ("purification of the elements"), often used synonymously with *kundalinī-yoga*, which attempts the gradual transformation of the *body into a "divine" or transubstantiated body (*divya-deha*) endowed with supernal faculties. As the "serpent power" (*kundalinī-shakti*) ascends from the base center to the crown of the *head, it is thought to successively "dissolve" the five elements (*bhūta*), interpreted as a process of gradual *purification. In practice, the ascent of the psychospiritual power leads to a progressive withdrawal of *consciousness from the body, leading to a state of insensitivity and coldness in the trunk and limbs. On the level of the *mind this spiritual *alchemy has a parallel effect inasmuch as consciousness becomes ever more unified, until the state of "formless ecstasy" (*nir-vikalpa-samādhi*) ensues. Now the *yogin's* awareness identity rests in the transcendental *Self, without any bodily awareness.

The process of *bhūta-shuddhi* also has a ritual counterpart whereby the material *elements are symbolically dissolved. The purpose of this *purification is to convert the *body into a temple ready to receive one's chosen deity (*ishta-devatā*). See also *shodhana, shuddhi*.

BHUVANA ("cosmos"). See Cosmos, *jagat, loka, samsāra, vishva*.

BĪJA ("seed"), the causes of affliction (*klesha*) that in *Classical Yoga are called the "seeds of the defects (*dosha*)," referring to the subconscious activators (*samskāra*). The term *bīja* can also mean the object or prop of *meditation, as in the compounds *sabīja- and *nirbīja-samādhi*. Finally, the word is short for *bīja-mantra*.

BĪJA-MANTRA ("seed word"), a central concept of *Tantrism. A *mantra of this category is monosyllabic and so called because it represents the quintessence of more complex *sound combinations. Such "shorthand" *mantras are characteristically meaningless and have a metalinguistic function. They are thought to represent, and be a part of, specific deities (*devatā*) who are invoked during the *Tantric rituals and with whom the initiate seeks to merge. These mystic phonemes are also associated with the seven (or more) psychoenergetic centers (*cakra*) of the *body.

BILE. See *pitta*.

BILESHAYA, a great *hatha-yoga* master mentioned in the *Hatha-Yoga-Pradīpikā* (1.5).

BIMBA ("reflection"), a technical term in the epistemology of *Classical Yoga as interpreted by *Vācaspati Mishra. It denotes the "reflection" of the transcendental *Self-awareness (*caitanya*) in the most lucid aspect of the *mind, i.e., the *sattva or *buddhi; also called the "shadow of *Consciousness" (*citi-chāyā*). See also *chāyā, pratibimba*.

BINDU ("drop" "dot") has many different technical connotations in *Yoga. It is occasionally used as a synonym for "seed" (*bīja*) or "source point." As such it is the origin of all manifestation, notably all sound (*nāda*). The *bindu* represents the inaudible, transcendental "sound" of the *Absolute, captured in the sacred syllable *om*. It is graphically depicted as the dot in the *ardha-mātra* symbol.

In *Tantrism and *hatha-yoga, *bindu* frequently denotes "semen." The loss of semen (*retas*) is considered to be one of the most potent *obstacles to spiritual development, and its preservation is regarded as imperative. The general recommendation is that in order to preserve the semen the *yogin* should abstain from sexual intercourse (*maithunā*). Even sexually active aspirants, however, are asked to circumvent seminal discharge. According to the *Hatha-Yoga-Pradīpikā* (4.28), the stabilization of the semen is effected by means of the stabilization of the *mind and the life force (*prāna*), for the movement of the *bindu* is closely connected with the circulation of the life energy in the form of the *breath. As the *Goraksha-Paddhati* (1.69) declares, so long as the *bindu* remains in the *body there is no need to fear *death.

A highly recommended practice for the prevention of seminal discharge is the *khecārī-mudrā*, which is said to be effective even during sexual embrace. When the semen has begun to flow down into the *genitals, it can be prevented from discharging by means of the *yoni-mudrā. When the semen has left the penis, it can be sucked back by means of the *vajrolī-mudrā.

The scriptures of *Yoga and *Tantrism obviously have a conception of semen that is quite distinct from the modern notion of seminal secretion. It comprises an esoteric dimension that is expressed in the doctrine of the two types of semen, male and female. The former is called shukla or *shukra (both words meaning "white"), and the latter is called *rajas (meaning literally "that which is brilliant"), mahā-("great")rajas, or shonita-bindu ("red semen"). Whereas the white or male bindu is situated in the "region of the moon" (*shashi-sthāna), that is, in the middle of the *head, the red or female bindu is to be found in the "genital region" (*yoni-sthāna). In the *Hatha-Ratna-Āvalī (2.89) the female secretion is also called bindu, and the practice of *vajrolī-mudrā is recommended for female initiates as well.

According to the *Goraksha-Paddhati (1.72), the union of these two bindus is most difficult to achieve. When accomplished, the *yogin attains to the supreme abode, or *liberation. As the *Yoga-Cūḍā-Mani-Upanishad (63) states, this union can be brought about through the activation of the "serpent power" (*kundalinī-shakti), a technique called *shakti-cālana. See also Sexuality.

BINDU-JAYA ("conquest of the semen"), also called bindu-siddhi ("power over the semen"). The *Hatha-Yoga-Pradīpikā (2.78) considers this to be one of the signs of *perfection in *hatha-yoga. See also khecārī-mudrā, vajrolī-mudrā, yoni-mudrā.

BINDUNĀTHA, mentioned in the *Hatha-Yoga-Pradīpikā (1.7) as an *adept of *hatha-yoga. Judging from his name, he was a master of the *bindu-siddhi. He may be identical with the author of the alchemical-medical work Rasa-Paddhati.

BIOFEEDBACK. Using technological instruments monitoring such bodily functions as heart rate, blood pressure, and brain wave patterns, this training method is sometimes touted as the modern equivalent to traditional *Yoga. Like Yoga, biofeedback training undoubtedly helps a person gain a degree of control over what are considered involuntary bodily functions. Unlike Yoga, however, it serves no spiritual purpose. While biofeedback training has proven successful in reducing or even eliminating chronic headaches and back pain, it does not end a person's existential *suffering through the realization of *enlightenment, nor does biofeedback training purport to do so. Yet this is the ultimate purpose of all yogic methods and techniques. In any case, the success of biofeedback training should be encouragement enough to look with new eyes at some of the claims made by *yogins. See also Autogenic training.

BIRD CATCHER SEAL. See pāshinī-mūdra.

BIRTH. See janman, jāti.

BLESSINGS (Sanskrit: āshī, mangala) have traditionally been taken very seriously as a form of spiritual *transmission, affording protection in life and promoting inner growth. Those aspiring to good fortune have always sought out the company of the virtuous (*sat-sanga) to benefit from their spiritual presence.

BLISS. The *Hindus conceive of degrees of bliss. The lowest degree is the relatively minor "bliss" of the *pleasure that can be derived from the stimulation of the *senses. Even the thrill of orgasm, which is the most intense pleasure known to many people, is only a shadow of the bliss experienced at the subtle (*sūkshma) levels of existence. Even the many degrees of bliss experienced by the *deities or higher beings amount to little, however, by comparison with the bliss of perfect freedom, inherent in the transcendental *Reality, as realized by the *enlightened adepts. See ānanda, mahā-sukha, sukha.

BOASTFULNESS. See katthana.

BODHA or BODHANA ("awakening" or "enlightenment"), a common synonym for *liberation (*moksha). See also Awakening.

BODHI ("awakening"), a synonym for bodha.

BODY. *Yoga, like all esoteric traditions of the world, envisions the human body as a complex hierarchic system of internesting "sheaths" (*kosha), each vibrating at a different frequency (or degree of subtlety). At the lowest level is the physical body, composed of the five material elements (*bhūta). At the highest level is the universal "body" of the transcendental *Reality, which is pure *Consciousness and unalloyed *Bliss. Between these two extremes are thought to exist a range of intermediary "vehicles" or bodily envelopes that are not normally accessible to our conscious *awareness, though their existence is inferable from their various activities. These subtle envelopes have been the subject of much introspective exploration by *yogins, who over many centuries have developed fascinating models of what has been called esoteric *anatomy. These seek to account for the phenomenology of *altered states of consciousness, notably mystical experiences. Their principal purpose, however, is not to furnish exhaustive descriptions or analyses but to serve as road maps for practitioners traveling on the spiritual *path.

One of the best-known yogic models of the subtle dimensions of bodily existence distinguishes seven major psychoenergetic centers (*cakra). These are thought to be aligned along the spinal axis and roughly correspond to the nerve plexuses in the physical or "gross" (*sthūla) body. These centers are connected by means of "conduits" or "channels" (*nādī) formed of life energy (*prāna). In fact, to the *yogin's clairvoyant sight, the person appears as a luminous bubble of energy made up of a dense network of psychoenergetic currents.

Recent studies in *parapsychology and bioelectricity have lent some credence to these models, though these findings remain controversial. Thus researchers using Kirlian photography have demonstrated the existence of a bioelectric field around living things, a field that disappears only gradually after *death. Researchers studying the meridians of acupuncture have also found positive proof for the existence of bioelectric currents and cakra-like vortices that cannot be explained by ordinary physiological principles. Mention must also be made of laboratory experiments on out-of-body experiences, which have yielded some evidence in favor of the traditional assumption that *consciousness can operate outside the body. Still, there is a need for much more substantive research in all these areas. Perhaps, as medicine outgrows its inherited nineteenth-century materialist paradigm, reputable researchers will be less fearful of entering investigations of this kind. Certainly, the esoteric models of the human body not only offer a far more exciting vision but are also inherently more plausible than the conventional physical model of modern medicine, for, however fanciful they may appear in their details, they do justice to the multidimensional nature of existence, as it is becoming obvious through the findings of contemporary physics. See also *deha*, Embodiment, *kāya*, *sharīra*, *tanu*.

BOGANĀTHAR (in Tamil), or BHOGANĀTHA (in Sanskrit); a South Indian adept (*siddha*) remembered as the *teacher of the legendary immortal master *Babaji. In the *Bogar-Jnāna-Sāgaram* ("Bogar's Ocean of Wisdom"), a poetic composition consisting of 557 verses, his teacher is said to have been Kalangi Nāthar, one of the nine *Nāthas. According to a modern account by Yogi S. A. A. Ramaiah, Boganāthar went to China and there became known as Lao Tzu, the author of the *Tao Te Ching*. He is also said to have visited South America, particularly Chile.

BOLDNESS. See *sāhasa*.

BONDAGE. See *bandha*; cf. Liberation.

BOOK LEARNING. See *grantha*, *shāstra*.

BOUND LOTUS POSTURE. See *baddha-padma-āsana*.

BOW POSTURE. See *dhanur-āsana*.

BRAHMA, the Creator in the classic triad of *Hinduism, the other two gods being *Vishnu and *Shiva. He is to be carefully distinguished from the *brahman*, the impersonal *Absolute beyond all distinctions. See also *brahma-loka*, *deva*, Prajāpati.

BRAHMA-ANDA (*brahmānda*, "brahmic egg"), the macrocosm. However, in the *Shiva-Samhitā* (1.91), for instance, the term signifies the microcosm, that is, the human *body. Cf. Microcosm, *pinda-anda*.

BRAHMA-BILA ("brahmic cave"). See *brahma-randhra*.

BRAHMA-CAKRA ("brahmic wheel"), a synonym for *mūlādhāra-cakra*. In the *Shvetashvatara-Upanishad* (1.6) this term is used to denote *God's lower nature, i.e., the finite manifest *world, or *prakriti*. See also *samsāra*.

BRAHMACARYA ("brahmic conduct"), the mode of life of the *Vedic student, *brahmacārin*. Brahmacarya essentially stands for the ideal of chastity. It is called "brahmic conduct" presumably because the *brahman* transcends all gender distinctions. The spiritual aspirant is asked to emulate that genderless condition so as to preserve and cultivate the great power inherent in the semen (*bindu*). Brahmacarya is one of the constituent practices of moral discipline (*yama*). According to the *Yoga-Sūtra* (2.38), the *yogin* who is firmly grounded in this virtue gains great vitality (*vīrya*). According to the *Bhagavad-Gītā* (17.14), it forms part of bodily asceticism (*tapas*). The *Kūrma-Purāna* (2.11.18) defines it as the abstinence from sexual intercourse (*maithunā*) in deed, *mind, and *speech at all times and in all circumstances. Similar definitions are found in many other works. The *Darshana-Upanishad* (1.13f.) also explains it as the mind's movement toward the state of the *brahman*.

The *Agni-Purāna* (372.9) understands *brahmacarya* as the *renunciation of the eight degrees of sexual activity: fantasizing (*smarana*); glorifying (*kīrtana*) the sex act or the opposite gender; dalliance (*keli*);

61

eyeing (*prekshana*) the opposite gender; talking in secret (*guhya-bhāshana*), i.e., love talk; longing (*samkalpa*); the resolution (*adhyavāsāya*) to break one's *vow of chastity; and *kriyā-nivritti*, the consummation of the sexual act. According to the *Linga-Purāna* (1.8.17), the above strict definition applies only to anchorites (*vaikhānasa*), forest dwellers (*vāna-prastha*), and widowers, whereas householders (*grihastha*) are allowed sexual intercourse with their wives but must practice chastity with regard to other women. See also *vajrolī-mudrā*.

BRAHMA-DVĀRA ("brahmic gate"). According to the *Shat-Cakra-Nirūpana* (3), the "brahmic gate" is situated at the mouth of the *citrinī-nādī* and is also called the "place of the knot" (*granthisthāna*), meaning the "brahmic knot" (*brahma-granthi*). This opening, at the base of the spinal column, is covered by the head of the hidden serpent, the *kundalinī-shakti*, and can be broken open by means of the "forceful Yoga" (*hathayoga*).

BRAHMA-GRANTHI ("brahmic knot"), the first of the "knots" in the human *body blocking the free flow of life force (*prāna*) along the central channel (*sushumnā-nādī*). It is located at the *mūlādhāra-cakra*, the lowest psychoenergetic center of the *body, though some traditional *Hindu authorities place it at the *heart. See also *granthi*.

BRAHMA-LOKA ("brahmic world"), the realm of the *saguna-brahman*, or the Lord (*īshvara*) or Creator, *Brahma, which is the highest level of cosmic existence. Beyond it is the unqualified *Absolute, which is called *nirguna-brahman*). See also Cosmos, *loka*.

BRAHMA-MUHŪRTA ("brahmic hour"), the time of sunrise, considered ideal for practicing *meditation and especially for rousing the "serpent power" (*kundalinī-shakti*). The brahmic hour is the last "hour" or watch of the traditional eight-*muhūrta* system. According to the sixteen-*muhūrta* system, it comprises the final three watches, lasting between 90 and 144 minutes. See also *muhūrta*.

BRAHMAN ("vast expanse," from the root *brih*, "to grow" or "to expand"), commonly translated as the "*Absolute." In the ancient *Vedas*, the term stands for *prayer or *meditation as a means of evoking the universal divine power, also called *brahman*. One hymn of the *Rig-Veda* (1.105.15) speaks of *Varuna, who knows the way, as "making the *brahman*." Elsewhere (10.50.4), *Indra is said to wax great by virtue of *brahman*, the creative word-power-prayer-meditation. For the Vedic seers, it was *Brahmanaspati, the Lord of *brahman*, who welded the upper and the lower worlds together like a blacksmith (10.72.2).

Not until the *Shata-Patha-Brāhmana* of the late third or early second millennium BCE did the word *brahman* acquire its well-known philosophical connotation as the supreme principle, the *Absolute, behind and above all the various deities (*devatā*), beings, and worlds. In this sense, the term is sometimes explained in fanciful folk etymology as that which grows (*brihati*) and causes everything to grow (*brihmyati*).

The earliest *Upanishads* are unique records of the intellectual struggle of the ancient sages to crystallize this philosophical concept, which was to become one of the anchor points of *Hindu metaphysics and theology. In the earliest references, *brahman* often still signifies the origin of the *cosmos, the primal entity that procreated the manifold world. Another, more sophisticated explanation understands the universe as being in essence identical with that *brahman*. As the *Chāndogya-Upanishad* (3.14) puts it: "All this *is* the *brahman*." This pantheistic conception was subsequently made more explicit in the *Brihad-Āranyaka-Upanishad*'s doctrine of the *brahman* that subsists in everything "as a razor is hidden in a razor case" (1.4.7). Next came the important notion of the identity of the *brahman* with the innermost self (or *Self) in human beings, called *ātman*. This identity forms the central theme of the *Upanishadic literature and *Vedānta philosophy. The Vedānta schools generally distinguish between a "lower" (*apara*) and a "higher" (*para*) aspect of the *Absolute, and often call the lower aspect the "sonic Absolute" (*shabda-brahman*). Cf. Brahma.

BRĀHMANA, or BRAHMIN; a person learned in the *Vedic lore; more generally, a member of the first of the four estates (*varna*) of traditional *Hindu society. The *brahmins* have traditionally been the custodians of the sacred *knowledge, though, as is evident from the *Upanishads, members of other estates—notably warriors (*kshatriya*)—also played a significant role in the development of *Vedānta and *Yoga. See also Brāhmanism.

BRĀHMANA, a work belonging to a particular genre of the sacred literature of *Hinduism, expounding the *Vedic sacrificial *ritual and *symbolism. The *Brāhmanas*, the oldest of which are now thought to date back possibly to the third millennium BCE, are exegetical works that seek to explain the archaic theological and ritual speculations of the four *Vedic "collec-

tions" (*samhitā*). They elaborated a kind of sacrificial mysticism that subsequently gave rise to some of the speculations in the *Upanishads. See also Brāhmanism, *yajna*.

BRAHMA-NĀDĪ ("brahmic conduit"), according to the *Shat-Cakra-Nirūpana* (2), a subtle channel situated inside the *citrinī-nādī*, which is located inside the *vajrā-nādī*, which is in turn to be found inside the central conduit (*sushumnā-nādī*) of the *body. In the *Siddha-Siddhānta-Paddhati* (2.27) the "brahmic channel" is said to be the proper object of the practice of the "inner sign" (*antar-lakshya*). See also *nādī*.

BRAHMA-NIRVĀNA ("extinction in the world ground"), a curious compound found in the *Bhagavad-Gītā* (2.72), where it stands for the condition of merging with the transcendental core of the world after *death. Here the word *brahman* appears to refer not to the *Absolute but to what elsewhere is called *brahma-loka*. The *Bhagavad-Gītā* (5.24–25) declares:

He who has inner joy, inner rejoicing (*ārāma*) and hence inner light, is a *yogin*. Having become the *brahman*, he approaches extinction in the *brahman*.

The seers whose defilements have dwindled, whose dualism (*dvaidha*) is destroyed, whose selves are controlled, and who delight in the good (*hita*) of all beings, reach extinction in the *brahman*.

This spiritual realization is imperfect because it lacks awareness of the radiating *love of *God, more specifically *Krishna. Cf. *nirvāna*.

BRĀHMANISM, the priestly culture of late *Vedic times, which centered on the esotericism of *sacrifice. It evolved into *Hinduism. See also *brāhmana*, Brāhmana.

BRAHMA-RANDHRA ("brahmic aperture"), the opening of the axial channel (*sushumnā-nādī*) at the crown of the *head, corresponding to the *sutura frontalis*. The *Siddha-Siddhānta-Paddhati* (2.8) calls it the "wheel of extinction" (*nirvāna-cakra*). See also *brahma-dvāra*.

BRAHMA-VID ("knower of the Absolute"), a *Self-realized *adept. See also *jīvanmukta, yoga-vid*.

BRAHMA-VIDYĀ ("knowledge of the *Absolute"), *Self-realization. See also *ātma-jnāna*, Awakening, Enlightenment.

BRAHMA-VIDYĀ-UPANISHAD (*Brahmavidyopanishad*), a medieval work belonging to the *Yoga-Upanishads* and consisting of 111 stanzas that deal with the "*Yoga of sound" (*nāda-yoga*) on the basis of the nondualist metaphysics of *Vedānta. Considerable space is given to speculations about the syllable *om and its three parts. Many *Tantra-type features are referred to, including the "serpent power" (*kundalinī-shakti*), though the text is highly conservative. Mention is made of a *hamsa-yoga*, and *breath control is said to be fivefold. The anonymous author recommends breath retention (*kumbhaka*) with mental *concentration on the navel (*nābhi-kānda*). He also subscribes to the ideal of radical *renunciation, enjoining the *adept who has realized the *Self to abandon absolutely everything. It is possible that after stanza 53 a new text begins, in which a person named Gautama is instructed once more in the secrets of the *hamsa* and related matters.

BRAHMA-VIHĀRA ("brahmic station"), a set of four practices well known not only to *Patanjali but also to authorities within *Buddhism. This technique consists of radiating the feelings of friendliness (*maitrī*), compassion (*karunā*), gladness (*muditā*), and equanimity (*upekshā*). According to the *Yoga-Sūtra (1.33), these are to be projected toward all beings and things, whether they are joyful or sorrowful, meritorious or demeritorious. This practice yields the pacification of *consciousness. As is evident from the *Yoga-Sūtra* (3.23), the four *brahma-vihāras* can also be made the theme of *ecstatic constraint (*samyama*), in which case the *yogin acquires the respective *powers of friendliness, and so on. *Vyāsa, however, thinks that *upekshā* is unsuitable for this.

BRAHMIN. See *brāhmana*.

BREATH, BREATHING. Early on, humanity appears to have discovered that by manipulating the breath, one can achieve *altered states of consciousness. This knowledge is reflected in the Indo-European languages, where the words for "breath" often also denote "spirit" or "psyche." Our modern civilization has all but forgotten this esoteric connection between *consciousness and the *breath. See also *prāna, pranāyāma, shvāsha*.

BREATH CONTROL. See *pranāyāma*.

BRIDGE. See *cakra-āsana*.

BRIHAD-ĀRANYAKA-UPANISHAD (*Brihadāranyakopanishad*, "Great Forest Upanishad"), probably the oldest text of this genre of *Hindu literature; its earliest portions may date back to 1500 BCE. This work contains the first clear enunciations of the doctrines of rebirth (*punar-janman*) and liberation (*moksha*).

BRIHAD - YOGI - YĀJNAVALKYA - SMRITI ("Great Codex of the Yogin Yājnavalkya"), a work dealing extensively with ritual worship, probably composed in the fourteenth or fifteenth century CE, though some researchers place it in the seventh century CE. Its unknown author, who is identified with the *Vedic sage *Yājnavalkya, stresses the practice of *meditation on the sacred syllable *om combined with breath control (*prānāyāma). The eight "limbs" (*anga) of *Classical Yoga are mentioned. This scripture must be distinguished from the *Yoga-Yājnavalkya, a shorter and probably earlier text.

BUDDHA ("awakened," past participle of the root budh, "to awaken"), a person who has achieved *enlightenment. Cf. abuddha, aprabuddha.

BUDDHA, GAUTAMA (ca. 563–483 BCE), the historical founder of *Buddhism; also called Siddhārtha Gautama and Shākyamuni Buddha. He is described in the Pali canon as a keen meditator, and the later Sanskrit scriptures of Mahāyāna *Buddhism often refer to him as a *yogin. For a period of time, Gautama studied under two well-known *teachers, and apparently quickly mastered the mystical state that each had put forward as the ultimate form of *enlightenment. One teacher, Arāda Kālāma, appears to have taught a kind of Upanishadic *Yoga culminating in the experience of the "sphere of no-thing-ness" (akimcānya-ayatana). This experience probably corresponds to the "formless ecstasy" (*nirvikalpa-samādhi) extolled as the highest goal in the *Upanishads. Udraka Rāmaputra, Gautama's other teacher, proclaimed the "sphere of neither consciousness nor unconsciousness" (naiva-samjnā-asamjnā-āyatana) as the most exalted spiritual state.

Unconvinced of the ultimacy of either realization, Gautama took to practicing the fiercest kind of asceticism (*tapas) for a period of six years. His efforts proved futile, however, and he adopted his famous "middle way" between ascetic discipline and the life of a *worldling. Remembering a spontaneous experience of *ecstasy that had suddenly overwhelmed him in his youth, Gautama began to simply sit in *meditation, resolving not to stir from his seat until he had broken through all conditional forms of *consciousness. After seven days of continuous meditation, he became an "awakened one" (buddha), reaching "extinction" (*nirvāna), that is, the cessation of all *desire. Soon afterward he began to communicate his newly won *enlightenment to others and to share with them his *wisdom about the "four noble truths": (1) life is suffering (*duhkha); (2) the *thirst for life is the cause of all suffering; (3) through the elimination of that innate craving, we can go beyond suffering; and (4) the means of eliminating

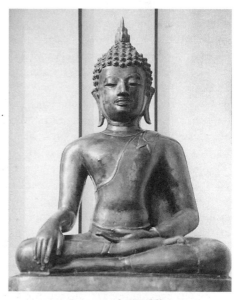

Gautama the **Buddha**

that thirst for life is the "noble eightfold path" to *liberation discovered by him.

The Buddha's eightfold *path comprises the following practices: (1) right vision (*samyag-drishti*), or the realization of the transience of conditioned existence and the understanding that there is indeed no continuous *ego or *self to which we could cling; (2) right resolve (*samyak-sam-kalpa*), or the threefold resolution to renounce what is ephemeral, to practice *benevolence, and to refrain from hurting any being; (3) right *speech (*samyag-vacā*), or the abstention from idle and false talk; (4) right conduct (*samyak-karmantā*), consisting mainly in abstention from killing, stealing, and illicit sexual intercourse; (5) right livelihood (*samyag-ājīva*), or the abstention from deceit, usury, treachery, and soothsaying in procuring one's sustenance; (6) right exertion (*samyag-vyāyāma*), or the prevention of future negative mental activity, the overcoming of present unwholesome feelings or thoughts, the cultivation of future wholesome states of *mind, and the maintenance of present positive psychomental activity; (7) right mindfulness (*samyak-smriti*), or the cultivation of awareness of the psychosomatic processes, i.e., the attentive observation of otherwise unconscious activities; and (8) right concentration (*samyak-samādhi*), or the practice of certain techniques for the internalization and ultimate transcendence of the individuated *consciousness. This practice comprises the meditative states from sensory inhibition (*pratyā-hāra*) to the various levels of ecstatic transcendence (*jhāna* in Pali, *dhyāna* in Sanskrit). But the goal of the eightfold path is *enlightenment, not any higher state of consciousness. The Buddha's teaching can be styled a pragmatic type of *Yoga, which in metaphysical matters favors agnosticism rather than *atheism, as often held.

The yogic nature of the Buddha's *path is further obvious from the use of such techniques as postures (*āsana*) and breath control (*prānāyāma*). The contribution of *Buddhism to the development of the *Yoga tradition has been considerable, just as the authorities of Yoga have contributed greatly to the unfolding of the Buddhist teachings.

BUDDHA ("Awakened One"), a *hatha-yoga* master mentioned in the *Hatha-Yoga-Pradīpikā* (1.6). He must not be confused with Gautama the *Buddha, the founder of *Buddhism.

BUDDHI (feminine form of *buddha*), one of the key concepts of the traditions of *Yoga and *Sāmkhya, as well as *Vedānta. Its first occurrence is in the *Katha-Upanishad* (3.3). In its primary technical meaning it signifies the first product, or evolute, of nature (*prakriti*). As such it is the most refined as well as the simplest form of existence and, by way of further *evolution, gives rise to all other categories (*tattva*) of existence, both material and psychic. The *buddhi*, which is similar to the *nous* in Neoplatonism, is also called *linga*, *linga-mātra*, and *sattva*.

A second, related connotation of the term *buddhi* is "wisdom faculty" or "higher mind" in contrast to the lower mind (*manas*). In a well-known simile first employed in the *Katha-Upanishad* (3.3), the *buddhi* is said to be the chariot driver, the chariot being the *body and the charioteer being the transcendental *Self. In this sense, the *buddhi* is the highest or deepest aspect of the human psyche—the birthplace of true *wisdom, or gnosis. Hence in some contexts the word denotes "wisdom." In *Classical Yoga, it simply stands for "cognition."

BUDDHI-INDRIYA (*buddhīndriya*, "cognitive sense"). See *indriya*.

BUDDHISM, the spiritual tradition founded by Gautama the *Buddha, can be understood as an elaborate yogic tradition that has developed its own schools of *Yoga. The Buddha's original doctrines, from what we know of them through the Pali canon, suggest an agnostic type of Yoga aimed at achieving the goal of "extinction" (*nirvāna*). The *Sūtras* of Mahāyāna Buddhism, which also claim to preserve the genuine teachings of the Buddha, balanced the pursuit of extinction with the positive ethical ideal of compassion (*karunā*), expressed in the *bodhisattva*'s vow to remain in the conditional realms until all other beings are freed from their *suffering by being liberated.

Later Buddhism saw several significant developments of a yogic nature, notably the Mahāyāna Buddhist *Yogācāra school of *Asanga (5th century CE) and the numerous schools of Buddhist *Tantrism, especially those of Tibet (known as the Vajrayāna), as well as the schools of Chinese Ch'an and Japanese *Zen Buddhism.

BUDDHI-YOGA, a compound met with repeatedly in the *Bhagavad-Gītā*. Thus, according to verse 2.49, it consists in one's taking refuge in the "wisdom-faculty" (*buddhi*) in order not to hanker after the fruit (*phala*) of one's deeds. In stanza 10.10, *buddhi-yoga* is said to be given by the *Lord to those who worship him with fondness. See also Wisdom.

BUDHYAMĀNA ("awakening one"), an important concept of *Preclassical Yoga, where it represents the twenty-fifth principle (*tattva*), the principle of conscious existence. When it "awakens"—that is, when it realizes its true nature as transcendental *Consciousness—it becomes the *Absolute (called *kevala*). Cf. *shad-vimsha*.

BULB. See *kanda*.

BULL POSTURE. See *vrisha-āsana*.

• C •

CAITANYA ("awareness" or "intelligence"), the individuated *mind; also, the transcendental *Consciousness, the very essence of the *Self. See also *cit*, *citi*; cf. *citta*.

CAITANYA (1486–1533 C.E.), or KRISHNA CAITANYA; the chief revivalist of *Krishna devotion in Eastern India. He probably wrote no more than eight devotional verses (called *Shiksha-Ashtaka* or "Eight [Stanzas] of Instruction"). His *bhakti school of *Vaishnavism is based on the teachings of the *Bhāgavata-Purāna*. He inaugurated the tradition of *go-svāmins* of which *Shrīla Prabhupāda (1896–1977) of the Krishna Consciousness movement was one of the last great leaders. Caitanya, a man of extraordinary charisma, was revered during his lifetime as an *incarnation of *Krishna. See also *bhakti-mārga*, *bhakti-yoga*.

CAKRA ("wheel," from the root *car*, "to move"; adopted into the English language as *chakra*), apart from its obvious secular

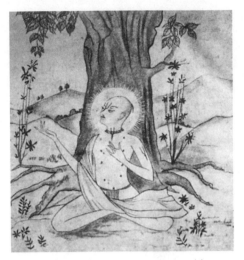

Caitanya (contemporary portrait)

meaning, has four principal esoteric connotations. First, it denotes the "wheel of becoming" (*bhava-cakra*) or "round of existence" (*samsāra*), that is, the phenomenal *cosmos. Second, it stands for the circle of initiates in the left-hand sexual ritual of *Tantrism where male and female participants sit in a circular arrangement around the *teacher. Third, it refers to a diagram similar to the *yantra used to determine the right kind of *mantra for a particular *student or situation; such diagrams are described, for instance, in the *Mantra-Yoga-Samhitā. Fourth, the word *cakra* denotes the psychoenergetic vortices forming the major "organs" of the *body composed of life energy (*prāna). These esoteric structures are also often referred to and graphically depicted as "lotuses" (*padma, kamala).

Most schools of *Yoga and *Tantrism propose six principal centers (*shat-cakra), with a seventh center being thought of as transcending bodily existence. These seven centers are, in descending order: (1) The *sahasrāra-cakra ("thousand-spoked

wheel"), at or above the crown of the *head; (2) The *ājnā-cakra ("command wheel"), in the center of the head, between and behind the *eyebrows; (3) the *vishuddha-cakra ("pure wheel"), at the throat; (4) the *anāhata-cakra ("wheel of the unstruck [sound]"), at the *heart; (5) the *manipura-cakra ("wheel of the jeweled city"), at the *navel; (6) the *svādhishthāna-cakra ("wheel of the self-base"), at the *genitals; and (7) the *mūlādhāra-cakra ("root-foundation wheel") at the anus.

Models involving nine, twelve, and more *cakras* are also known. Thus the *Kaula-Jnāna-Nirnaya (10), a medieval work, mentions eight centers, which remain unnamed however, and this scripture (3, 5) also speaks of "lotuses" with 100, 10 million, 15 million, 30 million, and even one billion petals. These belong to the secret centers that play an important role in higher Yoga practice. The *Kaula-Jnāna-Nirnaya (10) further claims that *contemplation upon these *cakras* leads to the conquest of *death and to the acquisition of paranormal powers (*siddhi).

A Kashmiri scroll examined by Fausta Nowotny (1958) lists the following twelve centers or lotuses, in descending order, with their respective location and number of petals: (1) the *bhramara-cakra* ("bee wheel"), at (or possibly above) the crown of the *head—number of petals not given; (2) the *sahasra-dala-cakra* ("thousand-petaled wheel"), at the crown of the head—1,000 petals; (3) the *pūrna-giri-pītha-cakra* ("wheel of the full mountain seat"), at the forehead—22 petals; (4) the *ājnā-cakra* ("command wheel"), at the "brow middle"—2 petals; (5) the *balavat-cakra* ("powerful wheel"), at the nose—3 petals; (6) the *vishuddha-cakra* ("pure wheel"), at the throat—16 petals; (7) the *anāhata-cakra* ("wheel of the unstruck [sound]"), at the *heart—12 petals; (8) the *manas-cakra* ("mind wheel"), at the center of the *navel—8 petals; (9) the *manipura-cakra* ("wheel of the jeweled city"), at the navel—10 petals; (10) the *kundalinī-cakra* ("wheel of the *kundalinī"), at the womb (*garbha)—number of petals not given; (11) the **svādhish-thāna-cakra* ("wheel of the self-base"), at the *penis—6 petals; and (12) the *ādhāra-cakra* ("base wheel"), at the anus—4 petals.

In Vajrayāna (Tibetan) *Buddhism, only five centers are singled out for special treatment, which are respectively located at the *forehead/crown, the *throat, the *heart, the *navel, and the *genital/anal region.

The most common explanation for these psychoenergetic centers proposed by noninitiates suggests a straightforward identification with the nerve plexuses known to medical physiology. This hypothesis contradicts the verbal and scriptural testimony of yogic authorities, however. A more moderate and credible opinion suggests a correlation between the cakras and the structures of the nervous system. According to some scholars, nota-

bly Agehananda Bharati (1965), such speculations make no sense because the *cakras* are merely "systematic fictions" or "heuristic devices" to aid the process of *meditation. While not denying the symbolic component of the *cakra* model, the transpersonal psychologist Ken Wilber (in John White, 1979) notes that the *cakras* are real insofar as they are associated with distinct sensations or states of *consciousness, just as they appear to be correlated with certain organs. See also *shat-cakra-bheda*.

CAKRA-ĀSANA (*cakrāsana*, "wheel posture"), a posture (**āsana*) mentioned in the **Vāraha-Upanishad* (5.17), where it is described as follows: Place the left thigh over the right ankle and the right thigh over the left ankle while holding the *body erect. This could be a description of what modern manuals know as the "mountain posture" (**parvata-āsana*), which is performed by assuming the "lotus posture" (**padma-āsana*) and then raising oneself until the body is balancing on the knees only, while both arms are stretched upward. In contemporary *Yoga practice, *cakra-āsana* signifies the complete backward bend or bridge.

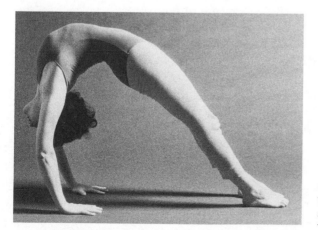

Cakra-āsana, the contemporary wheel or bridge posture, demonstrated by Kay Bird

CAKRĪ-KARMA ("stirring action"), a *cleansing practice of *hatha-yoga. The *Hatha-Ratna-Āvalī (1.28) describes it thus: Insert half a finger (sometimes stated to be the middle finger) into the rectum and move it around until the anal sphincter muscle is fully stretched. This practice is recommended for the curing of piles, *diseases of the spleen, and indigestion. This technique seems to be identical to the *mūla-shodhana described in other texts.

CAKSHUS ("eye"). See divya-cakshus, indriya, jnāna-cakshus.

CALMNESS. See upashama.

CAMATKĀRA ("astonishment," lit. "making the exclamation camat"), in Kashmiri *Shaivism, the moment of wonder (*vismaya) or astonishment when the *yogin experiences the blossoming forth of the ultimate *Consciousness of *Shiva, which transforms all his experiences of the *world. Cf. adbhūta.

CAMEL POSTURE. See ushtra-āsana.

CANDĪDĀS (Sanskrit: Candīdāsa, "Servant of [the goddess] Candī"; late 14th cen. CE), a leading Bengali *teacher of the *Sahajiyā movement. He achieved fame throughout Northern India for his numerous love songs, telling of the play between *Rādhā and her divine lover *Krishna and how to use the *body as a medium of prayerful *meditation. His compositions gave rise to a new school of *Vaishnava poetry. Of the thousands of poems attributed to him, about 200 are said to be authentic. See also bhakti-mārga.

CANDRA ("moon"), in *hatha-yoga and *Tantrism, an esoteric structure in the human *body from which oozes the "nectar of immortality" (*amrita, *soma). The "moon" showers its ambrosia continuously, but in the ordinary mortal this precious liquid is wasted. The *yogin, however, learns to check its flow and employ it in his quest for the *transubstantiation of the body. According to the *Yoga-Shikhā-Upanishad (5.33), a medieval text, the lunar orb is located at the "root of the palate" (*tālu-mūla), a location that the *Kaula-Jnāna-Nirnaya (5.16) cryptically refers to as the "navel" of the *head. The *Shiva-Samhitā (2.6) assigns the "moon" to a place at the top of "Mount *Meru," that is, at the upper terminal of the spine. This scripture also states that it has eight "portions" (*kalā), meaning that it is a half moon, though elsewhere (5.148) it speaks of it as having sixteen "portions," which amounts to a full moon. Furthermore, the *Shiva-Samhitā (5.146) announces that the "moon" becomes visible (presumably to the inner eye) through continuous *contemplation over a period of three days.

The "moon's" nectar is thought to ooze down into the trunk, where it is consumed by the "sun" (*sūrya) residing in the abdominal region. Bodily inversion techniques such as the *shoulder stand or the *headstand are designed to reverse the downward flow of the lunar nectar. The technique of *jālandhara-bandha, or throat lock, and the *khecārī-mudrā, in which the tongue is turned back against the *palate to block the cranial cavity, have the same purpose. This is analogous to the reversal of the "semen" (*bindu) attempted through such practices as the *vajrolī-mudrā.

The metaphor of sun and moon is a good example of the magical notion that the *macrocosm is mirrored in the *microcosm. The compound term *hatha-yoga is esoterically explained as the union (*yoga) of sun and moon, which refers to the two great microcosmic structures. Thus the *yogin attempts to make a true cosmos ("order") out of his inner environment by means of the integrative power of higher *consciousness.

The lunar excretion or *amrita has, even in some *Yoga texts, been prosaically identified as the saliva. Several modern interpreters have seen in it the cerebrospinal fluid. The preservation of this liquid is thought to promote *health and longevity. But, beyond this, the "moon" is, like the cakras, an important reference point for the yogic meditative journey. The *Shat-Cakra-Nirupana (41) refers to it as the "lunar orb" (candra-mandala), which is situated in the pericarp of the "thousand-petaled lotus (*sahasrara-cakra). The *Shiva-Purana (3.5.53) speaks of this region as being of the nature of supreme *Consciousness. Some scriptures call this location the indu- or soma-cakra, which is generally depicted as a lotus of sixteen moon-white petals. This is described as the seat of the higher mind (*buddhi).

CANDRA-GRAHANA ("lunar eclipse") occurs, according to the *Darshana-Upanishad (4.46), when the life force (*prana) reaches the abode of the "serpent power" (*kundalini-shakti) via the left channel (*ida-nadi).

CANGADEVA, a renowned *hatha-yogin who became a disciple of the young *Jnanadeva, who instructed him in sixty-five verses in the Marathi language. These came to be known as the Cangadeva-Pasasthi.

CARAKA-SAMHITA ("Caraka's Compendium"), a work attributed to Caraka, the court physician of King Kanishka (78–120 CE), though its present form dates probably from about 800 CE. One of the two

great texts of native Indian *medicine (*Ayur-Veda), it comprises eight sections dealing with subjects such as pharmacology, dietetics, pathology, anatomy, embryology, diagnosis, prognosis, toxicology, and general therapy. Its philosophical basis is *Preclassical Samkhya. See also Sushruta-Samhita.

CARPATA, one of the great preceptors of *hatha-yoga, credited with the authorship of the *Carpata-Shataka ("Carpata's Century [of Verses]"), the Ananta-Vakya ("Infinite Speech"), and the Carpata-Manjari ("Carpata's Flower Ornament"). One of his disciples was Sahila Varma (fl. ca. 920 CE), king of the Camba state (Punjab).

CARPATA-SHATAKA ("Carpata's Century [of Verses]"), an early work on *hatha-yoga ascribed to *Carpata, of which there appear to be several manuscripts.

CARPATI, mentioned in the *Hatha-Yoga-Pradipika (1.6) as a master of *hatha-yoga. It is not clear whether he is identical with the famous *Carpata.

CARYA ("conduct"), disciplined behavior intended to bring about inner *purification and the transformation of the *ego personality. This is one of four aspects of the spiritual *path discussed in the *Agamas and *Tantras, the other three being *jnana ("knowledge"), *kriya ("ritual"), and *Yoga ("unitive discipline").

CATURTHA ("fourth"), in *Vedanta, a technical term referring to the transcendental *Self beyond the three states (*avastha) of *waking, *dreaming, and *sleeping. It is also called turiya or turya, both words meaning "fourth." In *Classical Yoga, the word caturtha denotes that mode of breathing (*pranayama) that goes beyond inhalation and exhalation, namely, the total suspension of the *breath known as *kevala-kumbhaka.

CAURANGINĀTHA, also known as Caturanginātha; a younger contemporary of *Goraksha and apparently the son of King Devapala of Bengal. He is mentioned in the *Hatha-Yoga-Pradīpikā (1.5) as one of the early masters of *hatha-yoga. A posture (*āsana) named after him is referred to in the *Hatha-Ratna-Āvalī (3.19).

CAUSATION. See kārana, nava-kārana, sat-kārya-vāda.

CAUSATION, MORAL. See karman.

CAUSES OF AFFLICTION. See klesha.

CAVE. See guha.

CELĀ, the Hindi term for the Sanskrit *shishya.

CETAS ("mind" or "consciousness"), a synonym for *manas or *citta.

CHAKRA, the popular English spelling of *cakra.

CHĀNDOGYA-UPANISHAD (Chāndogyo-panishad), one of the oldest scriptures of the *Upanishadic genre, composed perhaps about the middle of the second millennium BCE. It contains, among other things, elaborate speculations about the sacred syllable *om (called *udgītha). The third chapter is essentially an exposition of the "honey doctrine" (*mādhu-vidyā) and the nature of the life force (*prāna). This scripture affords the historian of religion a valuable glimpse of the earliest formative phase of *Hindu metaphysics, when the *Vedic sacrificial ritual became internal-ized, thus paving the way for the development of *Yoga proper.

CHANGE. See parināma.

CHANNEL, SUBTLE. See hitā, nādī.

CHANTING. See bhajana, japa, kīrtana.

CHARITY. See dāna, dayā.

CHASTITY. See Abstinence, brahmacarya.

CHĀYĀ ("shadow" or "reflection") has a technical significance in *Classical Yoga. It stands for the "reflection" cast by the transcendental *Self, or *Consciousness, in the highest aspect of the mind, called *buddhi. This concept, which was first introduced by *Vācaspati Mishra in his *Tattva-Vaish-āradī (2.17), seeks to explain how *knowledge is possible given the fact that the mind (*manas, *citta) is an evolute of insentient nature (*prakriti).

In many works of *Postclassical Yoga the word signifies the *aura surrounding the physical *body and which, according to the *Vāraha-Upanishad (5.41), should always be perceived by the *yogin. See also bimba, pratibimba.

CHĀYĀ-PURUSHA ("shadow man"), the shadow cast by the *body, used by some *yogins for divining their own and other people's *destiny.

CIDGHANĀNANDA (prob. 18th cen. CE), the author of two works dealing with *diseases arising from faulty *Yoga practice, the *Mishraka and the *Sat-Karma-Sam-graha.

CIHNA ("sign"). Because *yogins experience the world as a psychophysical process, they believe that certain external signs are indicative of inner states or possibilities. Thus, according to the *Mārkandeya-Purāna (39.63), the first signs of *progress along the spiritual *path are as follows: enthusiasm (ālolya), *health, *gentleness, pleasant odor, scant urine and excrement, beauty (*kānti), clarity, and softness of voice. Similarly, the *Shiva-Samhitā (3.28f.) states that a sure sign of progress in the initial stage (*ārambha-avasthā) is the attainment of an "even body" (sama-kāya) that is handsome and emits a pleasant scent. Moreover, the *yogin on this level is said to enjoy a "strong (digestive) *fire," to eat well, and be happy, courageous, energetic, and strong, having well-formed limbs. In the *Yoga-Tattva-Upanishad (44ff.) four external signs are mentioned that result from the *purification of the psychoenergetic currents (*nādī): bodily *lightness, radiance (*dīpti), increase of the "abdominal fire" (*jāthara-agni), and bodily slimness. The *Yoga-Yājnavalkya (5.21f.) and the *Shāndilya-Upanishad (1.5.4), for instance, replace the last sign with the manifestation of the inner sound (*nāda).

The *Yoga scriptures also know of signs that occur immediately prior to, or that follow upon, *Self-realization. Thus the *Mahābhārata (12.294.20) has this stanza: "Like smokeless, seven-flamed [fire], like the radiant sun, like the lightning flash in space—thus the *Self is seen in the self." In a similar vein, the *Yoga-Shikhā-Upanishad (2.18f.) lists a number of signs that are styled the "gates" to the paranormal powers (*siddhi), namely, the experience in deep *meditation of *light resembling the flame of a lamp, the moon, a firefly, lightning, the constellations, and lastly the sun. See also pravritti, rūpa, tāraka-yoga.

CIN-MĀTRA ("pure awareness"; for euphony cit is here altered to cin), a common synonym for *ātman; the transcendental essence, which is supraconscious and mind-transcending. See also caitanya, cit, citi; cf. citta.

CIN-MUDRĀ ("seal of awareness"; for euphony cit is here altered to cin), one of the hand gestures (*mudrā) used in conjunction with certain postures (*āsana) or in sacred rituals. It is performed by bringing thumb and index finger together, while the remaining fingers are kept extended. See also yoga-mudrā.

CINTĀ ("thought"), often used in the sense of "pondering" or "*meditation"; e.g., in the *Maitrāyanīya-Upanishad (4.4) it is said that the *Absolute can be attained by means of asceticism (*tapas) and wisdom (*vidyā) or cintā. In other works such as the *Bhagavad-Gītā (16.11), however, the word means "concern" or "care."

CIRCUMAMBULATION. See pradakshina.

CIT ("awareness" or "consciousness"), a term widely employed in *Yoga and *Vedānta scriptures to denote the transcendental *Consciousness, or pure *Awareness. See also caitanya, cin-mātra, citi; cf. citta.

CITI ("awareness" or "intelligence"), a synonym for *cit. See also citi-shakti.

CITI-CHĀYĀ ("shadow of awareness"), a synonym for the mind (*citta). See chāyā, citi.

CITI-SHAKTI ("power of awareness"), a term found, e.g., in the *Yoga-Sūtra (4.34), where it refers to the transcendental *Self that continuously apperceives the contents of the *mind without itself being involved in the mental processes.

CITRINĪ-NĀDĪ ("shining channel") according to some *Tantric works, a subtle conduit within the central channel (*sushumnā-nādī). Within it lies the "brahmic channel" (*brahma-nādī), which is the actual pathway of the psychospiritual force known as the *kundalinī-shakti. See also nādī.

CIT-SHAKTI ("power of awareness"), a synonym for citi-shakti.

CITTA ("mind" or "consciousness"; past participle of the root cit, "to be conscious"), one of the key concepts of *Classical Yoga. Even though the term is not explicitly defined by *Patanjali, its meaning can be ascertained from its occurrences in his work. Thus the citta is a part of insentient nature (*prakriti), although it is not treated as a separate ontic category (*tattva). Instead, the word is used as an umbrella term for a variety of inner processes, primarily the capacity of *attention. It is in a sense the product of the transcendental *Consciousness (*citi) and the perceived object inasmuch as it is said to be "colored" by both. There exists a multitude of such consciousnesses, and in the *Yoga-Sūtra (4.15) Patanjali specifically rejects the idealist view of a single consciousness.

The citta is thought to be suffused with countless "subliminal activators" (*samskāra) combining into what are called the "traits" (*vāsanā). These are responsible for the production of the various psychomental phenomena, in particular the set of five "fluctuations" (*vritti). In the *Yoga-Sūtra (4.24) the citta is declared to be ultimately geared toward the *liberation of human beings. Upon the realization of the *Self, consciousness (which is really a material phenomenon) is dissolved because *Self-realization presupposes the "involution" (*pratiprasava) of the primary constituents or "qualities" (*guna) of nature. Like all other aspects of insentient nature (*prakriti), *consciousness undergoes continual change, and from the yogic viewpoint its most important modifications are the five kinds of "fluctuation" (vritti): accurate *cognition, erroneous *knowledge, *conceptualization, *sleep, and *memory. These must be stopped in order to actualize higher states of *awareness.

The Sanskrit commentators discuss at great length whether the citta corresponds to the size of the *body (which is the *Sāmkhya view) or whether it is really all-pervasive. They settle for the latter alternative and argue that it is only the mental "whirls" (*vritti) that can be said to contract and expand. *Vācaspati Mishra introduces the distinction between "causal consciousness" (kārana-citta) and "effected consciousness" (kārya-citta), arguing that the former is infinite, which presumably is intended to approximate *Patanjali's concept of "pure I-am-ness" (*asmitā-mātra).

To explain the cognitive processes the commentators resort to various metaphors. Thus the *Yoga-Bhāshya (1.4) compares *consciousness to a magnet that attracts *objects, and elsewhere (1.41) compares it to a crystal that reflects the color of the object near it. The *Tattva-Vaishāradī (1.7) also speaks of it as a mirror in which the "*light" of the *Self is reflected (see chāyā).

Outside the purview of *Classical Yoga, the term citta is generally employed in a less technically precise sense and mostly denotes "mind" in general. This tendency is present already in the commentaries on the *Yoga-Sūtra, where citta is often equated with *buddhi.

One of the most remarkable discoveries of the *yogins concerns the intimate relation that exists between *consciousness and the breath (*prāna). This discovery is especially emphasized in the literature of *Postclassical Yoga. For instance, the *Yoga-Shikhā-Upanishad (1.59) likens the *mind to a bird tied up by means of the cord of the life force (*prāna). Elsewhere (6.69) this work states that wherever the "wind" (i.e., the life force) abides in the *body, there too dwells consciousness. In the *Laghu-Yoga-Vāsishtha (5.9.73) the mind is defined as "the quivering of the life force" (prāna-parispanda). The general theorem is that by controlling the *breath, the mind can be conquered.

CITTA-BHŪMI ("level of consciousness"). See bhūmi.

CITTA-MĀTRA ("mere mind"). The notion of "mind only" is central to such idealist schools as Yogācāra *Buddhism and also the philosophy embedded in the *Yoga-Vāsistha. According to this doctrine, the world is nothing other than pure Mind, also called mano-mātra. *Patanjali, a staunch believer in realism, makes a point of refuting this teaching. In his *Yoga-Sūtra (4.16) he argues: "And the *object is not dependent on a single consciousness (eka-citta). This is unprovable. Besides, what could [such an imaginary object possibly] be?"

CITTAR, the Tamil word for *siddha.

CITTA-SHARĪRA ("mind body"). The *Yoga-Vāsishtha (3.22.15) makes a distinction between the "fleshly body" (māmsa-deha) and the "mind body" that neither dies nor is alive at any time, since it is the aspatial *Reality itself. See also Body, deha, linga-sharīra.

CIVAVĀKKIYAR (Sanskrit: Shivavākya; prob. 9th cen. CE), one of the great Tamil *adepts of Southern *Shaivism. His poetry, of which over 500 poems have survived, and the legends woven around his life show him to have been an outspoken rebel against the religious orthodoxy. He rejected the *Vedas and *Āgamas and condemned idol worship, the caste system, and the doctrine of *rebirth. His poetry, which is forceful and forthright, was left out of the *Shaiva canon. Kamil V. Zvelebil (1973), a renowned scholar of Tamil literature, considers Civavākkiyar "a greater poet than *Tirumūlar" (p. 81). His poetry is a clarion call reminding people to discover the great *God, *Shiva, who dwells within.

CLAIRAUDIENCE. See divya-shrotra, dūra-shravana, siddhi.

CLAIRVOYANCE. See divya-chakshus, dūra-darshana, siddhi.

CLASSICAL SĀMKHYA. See Sāmkhya.

CLASSICAL YOGA, the philosophical system that has evolved around *Patanjali's *Yoga-Sūtra and its extensive literature of commentary. This school of thought is generally referred to as the *yoga-darshana, or *rāja-yoga, which counts as one of the six classical systems of *Hindu philosophy. The other five are *Sāmkhya, *Vedānta (also known as Uttara-Mīmāmsā), *Pūrva-Mīmāmsā, *Nyāya, and *Vaisheshika.

*Patanjali was not the originator of *Yoga. He merely systematized existing knowledge and techniques. Traditionally, *Hiranyagarbha is credited with originating Yoga, though no actual scriptures have survived that could be identified as having been authored by this legendary *adept. Patanjali's aphorisms (*sūtra) on Yoga appear to have quickly eclipsed other similar compilations, which undoubtedly existed but are now lost.

The *Yoga-Sūtra provided an interpretation of *Yoga philosophy and practice that stimulated others to elaborate *Patanjali's metaphysical ideas. He taught a form of radical *dualism that remained quite controversial within the fold of *Hinduism. According to him, there are two eternal categories of existence—the transcendental *Self (*purusha) and the transcendental world ground (*prakriti). The former category comprises countless Selves that are omnipresent, omniscient, and passive spectators (*sākshin) of the spectacle of the *cosmos. The latter category, the world ground, comprises all the manifest and unmanifest dimensions and forms of *nature, which are inherently dynamic.

Whereas the Selves are innately conscious, or rather supraconscious, *nature is essentially unconscious or insentient. It has no purpose in itself but serves the countless Selves. They are either aware of their transcendental *freedom or they are entrapped in nature, believing themselves to be finite entities. This is possible because in its highest mode of existence, nature is transparent enough to "reflect" the "*light" of these Selves and thus create the illusion of sentience and intelligence in its evolutes. Thus the *mind (both as *manas and as *buddhi) is the product of this reflection (*chāyā) of *Consciousness in nature. The function of *Yoga is to oblige the *Self to awaken to its transcendental status through a progressive withdrawal from the forms of nature. This is accomplished through *Patanjali's eightfold *path (*ashta-anga-yoga), particularly the higher stages of meditation (*dhyāna) and ecstasy (*samādhi). The supreme goal is known as "aloneness" (*kaivalya), which is the perfect "isolation" of the Self.

This radical *dualism has provoked much criticism within and also outside *Hinduism, and it has definitely prevented Classical Yoga from becoming a more influential philosophical school. The tenor of Hinduism is nondualist, and this is reflected very well in the fact that the schools of *Postclassical Yoga are without exception informed by the metaphysics of *Advaita Vedānta rather than Classical Yoga. *Patanjali's system can almost be regarded as an interlude in a tradition that was from the outset nondualist, because the known schools of *Preclassical Yoga (with the exception of *Buddhism, if we wish to include it in this category) are all based on *Vedānta-type teachings.

CLEANSING PRACTICES. See dhauti, shauca, shodhana.

CLOTH, YOGIC. See dhoti.

COBRA POSTURE. See bhujanga-āsana.

COCK POSTURE. See kukkuta-āsana.

CODANĀ ("urging"), a yogic term found in the *Mahābhārata. In one passage (12.294.11) the *yogin is counseled to "impel" (codayet) himself by means of the ten or twelve codanās. This work further specifies that ten or twelve codanās are to be practiced in the first watch of the night and a further twelve in the middle of the night after having slept. Nīlakantha, the best-known commentator of the great epic, understands these as restraints of the *breath.

COGNITION. See buddhi, drishti, jnāna, prajnā, pratyaya.

COGNITION, ACCURATE. See pramāna.

COINCIDING, ECSTATIC. See samāpatti.

COLLECTEDNESS, MENTAL. See *samā-dhāna*.

COMPASSION. See *dayā, karunā*.

CONCEALED POSTURE. See *gupta-āsana*.

CONCENTRATION. Yogic concentration differs from ordinary efforts of focusing *attention by its duration, depth, and notably its purpose, which is to transcend the concentrated *mind itself. See also *dhāranā, mudrā, panca-dhāranā*.

CONCEPTUALIZATION. See *samkalpa, vikalpa*.

CONDUCT. See *ācāra, caryā*.

CONFUSION. See *moha, sammoha*.

CONSCIOUSNESS. The nature of consciousness has been a major philosophical concern in the long *history of *Yoga. Most yogic schools subscribe to the view that consciousness is transcendental, that is, not a product of the finite body-mind, much less a mere brain phenomenon. The transcendental nature of consciousness is thought to be philosophically self-evident and "verifiable" by means of the highest yogic condition—the supraconscious ecstasy (*asamprajnāta-samādhi* or *nirvikalpa-samādhi*). Consciousness is proposed as the ultimate identity of human beings. Hence it is also called the *Self (*ātman* or *purusha*), which is the *Spirit beyond *body, *mind, and *language.

According to the nondualist schools of *Yoga, that supreme Consciousness is utterly blissful (*ānanda*) and overwhelmingly real (*sat*). It cannot be known but it can be realized. *Self-realization is the alpha and omega of all approaches of Yoga. See also *cinta, cit, citi, citta, manas, prajnā*.

CONSECRATION. See *abhisheka*.

CONSTITUENT, BODILY. See *dhātu*.

CONSTRAINT, ECSTATIC. See *samyama*.

CONTEMPLATION. See *bhāvanā, dhyāna*.

CONTENTMENT. See *samtosha, tushti*.

CONTINUITY. See *santana*.

CONTRACTION. See *samkoca*.

CONVENTION. See *samketa*.

CONVICTION. See *mati*.

CORPSE POSTURE. See *mrita-āsana*.

CORRELATION. See *samyoga*.

COSMOS. The cosmological and cosmographical ideas of *Yoga are those current in the prescientific literature of *Hinduism, especially the *Purānas. Even though *Vyāsa, in his *Yoga-Bhāshya (3.26), outlines the essentials of the extraordinarily rich and imaginative cosmography of the *Hindus, these conceptions do not play a significant role in Yoga practice. However, they form a part of the general stock of knowledge of the educated sections of society.

According to *Vyāsa's cosmographical sketch, the universe is egg-shaped (see *brahma-anda*) and segmented into seven zones or regions (*loka*), which have their own subdivisions. The seven zones are, in descending order: (1) The *satya-loka* ("world of truth"), which is inhabited by four groups of *deities who live as long as there are world creations (*sarga*); (2) the *tapo-loka* ("world of asceticism"), which is inhabited by three groups of deities who live twice as long as the deities of the *jana-loka*; (3) the *jana-loka* ("world of people"), which is inhabited by four groups of deities who have mastered the *elements and the *senses; (4) the *mahar-prājāpatya-loka* ("*mahar* world of *Prajāpati), which is inhabited by five groups of deities who have mastered the elements and live for a thousand world cycles (*kalpa*); (5) the *mahā-indra-loka* (*mahendra-loka*, "world of the great Indra"), which is inhabited by six groups of deities who have acquired the major paranormal powers (*siddhi) and live for a full world cycle (*kalpa*); (6) the *antarīksha-loka* ("world of the midregion"), which extends from the summit of Mount *Meru, the mountain at the center of the world, to the pole star and which is populated by the planets and stars; and (7) the *bhū-loka* ("earth world"), which comprises (a) the earth (*bhūmi) with its seven continents, which have Mount Meru in their center and which are encircled by the seven seas and the *loka-aloka* mountains (the diameter of this curved disc being estimated at 500 million *yojanas* or ca. 4.5 billion miles); (b) the seven nether regions (*pātala); and (c) the seven hells (*nāraka).

Clearly, this and other similar models of the universe belong to the realm of *mythology. In *Tantrism and *hatha-yoga, such cosmographical concepts as *Meru and the seven worlds are descriptive of the microcosmic reality of the *body, as it is experienced during yogic *meditation. Thus, Mount Meru is the spinal axis or axial current (*sushumnā-nādī) of the life force (*prāna), while the seven worlds are the seven major psychoenergetic focal points (*cakra). See also *bhuvana, prakriti, sarga, tattva, vishva*.

COUCH (POSTURE). See *paryanka*.

COW. See *go*.

COW-MUZZLE POSTURE. See *go-mukha-āsana*.

CRAZY ADEPT. All major religious traditions of the world include the phenomenon of crazy wisdom—spiritual iconoclasm, whose representatives have been called crazy *adepts. For instance, in *Hinduism there is the figure of the *avadhūta, in Tibetan (Vajrayāna) *Buddhism the *lama myonpa*, and in Christianity the "fool for Christ's sake." These adepts seek to communicate spiritual truths by unconventional, even eccentric means. Their impromptu methods of instructing others are intended to shock, though their purpose is always benign: to reflect to the ordinary worldling the "madness" of his or her unenlightened existence, embroiled as it is in suffering and devoid of self-understanding.

The crazy adepts feel free to reject customary behavior and to be subversive, criticizing and poking fun at both the sacred and the secular establishment. They may dress in bizarre ways or even go about naked, ignoring the niceties of social contact, cursing and using obscene language, and employing stimulants and intoxicants, as well as *sexuality. They embody the esoteric principle of *Tantrism that *liberation (*mukti) is coessential with enjoyment (*bhukti) and that spiritual *Reality is not separate from the *world.

CREATION. See *sarga*, World ages.

CREATURE. See *pāshu*.

CRITICAL POSTURE. See *samkata-āsana*.

CROW SEAL. See *kākī-mudrā*.

CURLEW SEAT. See *kraunca-nishadana*.

78

· D ·

DAGDHA-SIDDHA ("burned adept"), a black magician. This term is used, for instance, in Dandin's seventh-century *Dasha-Kumāra-Carita* ("Life of Ten Princes") in regard to a practitioner of black *magic who had enslaved a married couple, sought to behead a princess, and was himself decapitated by Mantragupta, one of the ten princes referred to in the title. Dandin portrayed the black magician as a *Kāpālika-type ascetic, whose skin was covered with *ashes and who wore matted hair and ornaments made from human bone. See also *siddha*.

DAHARA ("minuscule," from the root *dabh*, "to be small"), the most subtle space within the *heart, or the "heart lotus" (*hrit-padma*), the connecting point between the body-mind and the transcendental *Self. The word also has overtones of radiance, since the associated root *dah* means "to burn" or "to be burned."

DAHARA-ĀKĀSHA (*daharākāsha*, "minuscule radiance-space"), one of the inner luminous spaces (*ākāsha*) on which the *yogin may *meditate in *tāraka-yoga*.

DAIVA ("divine," meaning "fate"), explained in the *Yoga-Vāsishtha* (2.9.4) as the inevitable consequence of one's auspicious or inauspicious deeds (*karman*). Elsewhere in this work (2.5.18), however, the existence of destiny is denied and reliance on it is firmly rejected. Instead the *virtue of self-exertion (*paurusha*) is recommended. Fate is sometimes listed as one of the obstacles (*vighna*) of *Yoga.

DAMA ("restraint"), occasionally regarded in the *Mahābhārata* (12.2ff.) as the highest *virtue. In the scriptures of *Postclassical Yoga, it is sometimes grouped with the moral disciplines (*yama*). The *Bhāgavata-Purāna* (11.19.36) understands it as *sense control (*indriya-samyama*).

DAMARU (from the root *dam*, "to resound"), a drum carried by some *yogins to exorcise demonic forces. Specifically, it refers to *Shiva's hourglass-shaped drum, which is the source of all the *vibrations or rhythms of the *cosmos.

DAMBHA ("ostentation") characterizes, according to the *Bhagavad-Gītā* (16.4), the person born to a demonic destiny. See also Pride.

DĀNA ("generosity" or "charity"). The *Tri-Shikhi-Brāhmana-Upanishad* (2.33) counts *dāna* among the ten practices of self-restraint (*niyama*), and the *Shāndilya-Upanishad* (1.2.5) explains it as giving with all sincerity wealth that has been acquired by righteous means. According to the *Bhagavad-Gītā* (17.20ff.), *dāna* is threefold, depending on the predominance of the three qualities (*guna*) of *nature. Thus it can be *sāttvika (when done in the right place and at the right time [*kāla*] as one's *duty without expecting any reward and for a worthy recipient), *rājasa (when a return favor is expected or when one hopes for *karmic merit), and *tāmasa (done without respect or with contempt at the wrong time in an inappropriate place for an unworthy recipient). The philosophy underlying the virtue of liberality is expressed in the *Mahanarayana-Upanishad* (523), which explains that all beings live from the donations of others. Curiously, the *Shiva-Samhitā (5.4) considers almsgiving to be one of the obstacles (*vighna) of *Yoga.

DANCE, since ancient times, a means of expressing religious or spiritual sentiments and aspirations, and of transcending *body and *mind. *Vaishnavism, for instance, celebrates the famous dance (*rasa-līlā) of the God-man *Krishna and the shepherdesses (*gopī). Through Krishna's *magic, each woman thought that she was the only one dancing with her beloved Lord—a striking simile of the spiritual aspirant's journey to the *Divine.

Dance has also been used as a metaphor for the rhythm of the *cosmos. This is beautifully captured in the iconographic image of *Shiva as "Lord of Dance" (nata-rāja), where the great god is seen dancing rapturously in a surround of flames, symbolizing the destruction of the universe. The dance itself represents Shiva's five primal activities—*creation, preservation, destruction, veiling, and salvific *grace.

Indian dance, like traditional Indian *art in general, can be looked upon as a form of *Yoga. It certainly requires considerable self-discipline and *concentration. Unlike European dancing, Hindu dance involves the entire *body: Every motion is charged with significance, and every pose and gesture is codified in great detail. Thus the classical texts mention thirteen positions of the *head, thirty-six of the *eyes, nine of the *neck, and hundreds of hand gestures (*mudrā).

Ecstatic dancing is known in the Tamil language as ananku ātulal. This phrase appears, for instance, several times in the *Tiruvāymoli, where *Nammālvār confesses (1.6.3f.):

There is none superior to the Lord, none even equal.
My tongue sings songs only to Him.

My limbs dance in ecstasy.
My limbs dance in ecstasy,
bowing to Him.

DANDA ("staff"), one of the traditional implements of an ascetic. It is carried by *sādhus and *samnyāsins and is an external representation of the central channel (*sushumnā-nādī) through which the "serpent power" (*kundalinī-shakti) ascends when properly awakened. See also tri-shūla.

DANDA-ĀSANA (dandāsana, "staff posture"), mentioned in the *Yoga-Bhāshya (2.46) and described by *Vācaspati Mishra as follows: One should sit down with the feet stretched out and close together.

DANDA-DHAUTI ("cleansing [by means of a] stalk"), one of the forms of "heart cleansing" (*hrid-dhauti). The *Gheranda-Samhitā (1.37f.) describes it thus: One should take a plantain stalk or a stalk of turmeric or cane and introduce it slowly into the gullet, then draw it out again. This is thought to expel all phlegm (*kapha), bile (*pitta), and other impurities from the mouth and chest. See also dhauti.

DANGEROUS POSTURE. See sankata-āsana.

DANTA-DHAUTI ("dental cleansing"), one of the four forms of cleansing (*dhauti) prescribed in *hatha-yoga. According to the *Gheranda-Samhitā (1.26), it consists of the following practices: cleansing of the teeth (*danta-mūla-dhauti), the tongue (*jihvā-dhauti), the ears (*karna-dhauti), and the frontal sinuses (*kapāla-randhra-dhauti).

DANTA-MŪLA-DHAUTI ("dental root cleaning"), is described in the *Gheranda-Sam-

hitā (1.27f.) as follows: Every day in the morning, rub the teeth with catechu powder or pure earth until all impurities are removed. See also *danta-dhauti*.

DARKNESS. See *tamas*.

DARPA ("arrogance"), universally condemned in the *Yoga scriptures as a character trait that blocks spiritual maturation. See also Pride; cf. *amānitva*.

DARSHANA ("vision" or "sight"), vision in both the literal and the metaphorical sense; viewpoint, as in the expression *yoga-darshana*. In the *Mahābhārata (12.232.21), visionary states are regarded as a by-product or sign (*cihna*) of *progress in *meditation. They are, however, also deemed obstacles (*upasarga*) in regard to ecstasy (*samādhi*). See also *ātma-darshana, bhrānti-darshana, siddha-darshana*.

DARSHANA-UPANISHAD (*Darshanopanishad*), one of the *Yoga-Upanishads*, consisting of 224 stanzas distributed over ten sections. Its teachings are expounded by *Dattātreya to his pupil Samkriti. The fundamental practices of Dattātreya's *Yoga are identical with those introduced in the *Yoga-Sūtra*. However, the text's metaphysical orientation is *nondualist. Much attention is given to the psychoenergetic currents (*nādī*) and their *purification, whereas the higher yogic practices are only sketchily described.

DATTĀTREYA, a historical teacher of *Postclassical Yoga who early on became deified. Dattātreya, whose name means "Datta, son of Atri," was a *crazy-wisdom adept who is mentioned in many *Purānas*. He taught an eight-limbed *path (*ashta-anga-yoga*), but his name is prom-

inently associated with the *avadhūta tradition. Mythology celebrates him as an incarnation (*avatāra*) of *Vishnu, but *Shiva worshipers also claim him as one of their great spiritual figures. Among other works, he is credited with the authorship of the *Avadhūta-Gītā*, the *Jīvan-Mukti-Gītā*, and the *Tri-Pura-Rahasya*, all of which are works espousing *Advaita Vedānta.

DAURMANASYA ("depression"), one of the symptoms accompanying the distractions (*vikshepa*) spoken of in the *Yoga-Sūtra (1.31). *Vyāsa, in his *Yoga-Bhāshya (1.31), explains the word as mental agitation resulting from the frustration of a *desire. According to the *Linga-Purāna (1.9.10), dejection is to be overcome by means of superior dispassion (*vairāgya*). Cf. *saumanasya*.

DAYĀ ("sympathy"), sometimes listed as one of the ten practices of moral discipline (*yama*). The *Yoga-Yājnavalkya (1.63) defines it as graciousness (*anugraha*) at all times toward all beings, in *mind, *speech, and *action. See also *karunā*.

DEAD POSE. See *shava-āsana*.

DEATH. Materialistic philosophies deny that any immaterial principle—such as a *soul or *spirit—survives the demise of the physical *body. This one-dimensional view of human nature is vehemently rejected by all schools of *Yoga, including the pragmatic tradition of *Buddhism. In fact, the authorities of Yoga are agreed that it is of acute importance *how* a person dies. Only complete control of the death process, as effected by full *awareness during and after the dropping of the body, guarantees a benign postmortem existence. The grand ideal is to "die," that is, to transcend the ego illusion, while yet alive, so that death comes as no surprise but is comparable to a simple change of clothes. The esoteric art of conscious dying is hinted at, for instance, in the ancient *Bhagavad-Gītā (8.10; 12f.):

That [practitioner who], at the time of going forth [i.e., death], directs with unmoving *mind the life force (*prāna) to the middle of the *eyebrows while being yoked by love (*bhakti) and by the power of *Yoga, comes to that supreme divine Spirit (*purusha). Controlling all the gates [of the body], confining the *mind in the *heart, fixing the life force in the *head, and established in yogic concentration (*dhāranā) while reciting *om, the [sacred] monosyllable [signifying] the *Absolute and remembering me [i.e., *Krishna]—he who [thus] departs, abandoning the *body, goes the supreme course [toward *liberation].

Such a person transcends the law of moral causation (*karma) and terminates the cycle of repeated births and deaths. This teaching is based on an even older account given in the *Brihad-Āranyaka-Upanishad (4.1f.). See also anta-kāla, āti-vāhika-deha, jīva, karman, mrityu, parānta-jnāna.

DEFECTS. See dosha, mala.

DEHA ("body," from the root dih, "to smear, anoint"). Two distinct and contrasting attitudes toward the *body and corporeality in general can be discerned in the spiritual traditions of India (and elsewhere). On the one hand, the body is characterized as an "ill-smelling . . . conglomerate of bone, skin, sinew, muscle, marrow, flesh, *semen, blood, mucus, tears, rheum, feces, urine, *wind, *bile, and *phlegm . . . which is afflicted with *desire, *anger, *greed, *delusion, *fear,

*despondency, *envy, separation from what is desirable, union with what is undesirable, *hunger, *thirst, senility, *death, *disease, *sorrow, and the like" (*Maitrāyanīya-Upanishad, 1.3). On the other hand, the *body is elevated to the status of "the temple of God" (deva-ālaya), as in the Maitreya-Upanishad (2.2). This second, world-affirmative viewpoint is already expressed in the archaic *Chāndogya-Upanishad (8.12.1): "This body is mortal, O Maghavan. It is subject to *death. Yet it is the resting place of the immortal, incorporeal Self (*ātman)."

In a similar vein, the *Yoga-Vāsishtha (5.66.32), almost two millennia later, declares the *body to be a most valuable instrument for discharging one's worldly duties. It is, as the text (4.23.189f.) affirms, a source of infinite trouble for the spiritually ignorant person, but a fountain of *happiness for the sage who, moreover, does not experience *death as a loss. The body serves him as a chariot and is conducive to his welfare and *liberation. Similarly, the *Mārkandeya-Purāna (39.61) states that the body should be carefully preserved, since it is the means of attaining virtue (*dharma), prosperity (*artha), sensual enjoyment (*kāma), and *liberation (*moksha). The *Uddhāva-Gītā (15.17) compares it to a well-constructed boat that is propelled forward by *Krishna as a favorable wind and that has one's *teacher as helmsman.

The preservation of the *body and the development of its latent powers (*siddhi) became the primary objective of such *Tantra-based schools as *hatha-yoga. Authorities of this type of *Yoga frequently compare the body to a pot (*ghata) that needs to be well baked in the fire of yogic disciplines. This comparison is curiously rejected, however, in the *Varāha-Upanishad (2.25). The *Yoga-Kundalī-Upanishad

(1.77) speaks of the transformation of the "material body" (*ādhibhautika-deha*) into the "divine body" (*ādhidaivika-deha*). The purest vehicle, however, is the "superconductive body" (**ātivāhika-deha*). As the **Yoga-Shikhā-Upanishad* (1.27) explains, the body is ordinarily insentient (**jada*) or "uncooked" (*apakva*) and it must be "energized" (*ranjayet*) by the **yogin*, so that it becomes "cooked" or "ripe" (*pakva*). In the **Uddhāva-Gītā* (10.29) such a ripe body is also called *yoga-maya-vapus*, or a "body fashioned through Yoga," and is said to be indestructible.

The **Yoga-Vāsishtha* (3.57.23) speaks of the "**yogin*'s body" (*yogi-deha*) as being invisible even to other *yogins*. Such a spiritualized body is attributed to many Yoga **adepts, and the idea has provided ample material for folklore and legend. See also *dridha-kāya, sharīra, vajra-deha*.

DEHIN ("embodied one"), the individuated **self, or human personality. See also *jīva, jīva-ātman, samsārin, sharīrin*.

DEITY. See *deva, devatā*, Divine, God.

DELUSION. See *bhrānti, moha*.

DEPRESSION. See *daurmanasya, vishāda*.

DESHA ("place"), a term denoting both the appropriate environment for yogic practice and special loci for **concentration, such as the psychoenergetic centers (**cakra*) and the sensitive places (**marma-sthāna*) of the **body.

Proper surroundings are deemed an essential precondition for success in yogic practice. *Desha* is counted among the constituent disciplines of the fifteen-limbed **Yoga (**panca-dasha-anga-yoga*). The most general stipulation is that the place should be clean and quiet. Some texts are considerably more specific. Thus the old **Shvetāshvatara-Upanishad* (2.10) asks that the ground be level, free from pebbles, gravel, and **fire, and that it be concealed, inoffensive to the **ear, pleasing to the **eye, and protected from the **wind. **Yogins* favor secluded spots such as mountains, caves, temples, and vacant houses. See also *samketa*.

DESIRE. See *icchā, ipsā, kama*.

DESIRE-BURNING POSTURE. See *kāma-dahana-āsana*.

DESIRE FOR LIBERATION. The self-transcending impulse, generally called **mumukshutva*, is the only motivational force that does not lead to **karmic embroilment.

DESPAIR. See *daurmanasya, vishāda*.

DESPONDENCY. See *daurmanasya, vishāda*.

DETERMINATION. See *nishcaya*.

DEVA ("god" or "divine," from the root *div*, "to shine") can stand for the personal **Divine, such as **Vishnu, **Shiva, **Indra, **Agni, **Brahma, **Rudra, or the goddesses **Kālī or **Durgā, or a lower deity comparable to the angelic beings in the Judeo-Christian tradition. In the latter sense, the *devas* or **devatās* are finite (and unenlightened) entities, though their life span far exceeds that of human beings (see Cosmos). Yet the **Hindu scriptures uniformly value human existence as higher than the existence of the inhabitants of the heavenly realms (**loka*), because human life affords a unique intensity of experience that can lead directly to spiritual **awakening, or **liberation. See also **Absolute, Angels, God, Reality.

DEVA-DATTA ("God-given"), one of the ten cardinal psychoenergetic currents (*nādī*) of the *body. According to the *Tri-Shikhi-Brāhmana-Upanishad* (2.82), it resides in the skin and bones and is responsible for *sleep. According to the *Siddha-Siddhānta-Paddhati* (1.68), however, its location is in the mouth, and it is responsible for the knitting of the *eyebrows. Most texts assign to it the function of yawning (*vijrimbhana*).

DEVA-MANDIRA ("abode of God"), temple. Temples are traditionally understood as replications of the *cosmos, which is a manifestation of the *Divine. Their geometry corresponds to the divine or celestial geometry. Conversely, the *world itself, or *nature, is regarded as a temple, and much of *Hindu worship occurs outdoors at riverbanks or confluences of rivers, under sacred trees, high up in the mountains, or on isolated islands. Hindu temples are not meeting places for a religious congregation, and no sermons are preached or confessions taken. They are treasured as the homes of *deities or emanations of deities, and pious folk visit them to pray, meditate, and offer incense, flowers, and other gifts to the image (*mūrti*) of the *gods or *goddesses whose presence they feel in the temples.

DEVATĀ ("deity"), a synonym for *deva often used to denote a presiding deity associated with a particular psychoenergetic center (*cakra*).

DEVA-YĀNA ("way of the gods"), the postmortem *destiny that leads one to the Absolute (*brahman*). See also *krama-mukti*; cf. *pitri-yāna*.

DEVĪ ("goddess"), the feminine aspect of the *Divine, often in the form of *Shiva's celestial spouse. See also *shakti*.

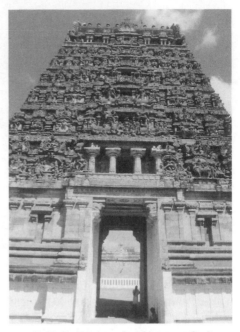

South Indian temple (***deva-mandira***)

DEVĪ-BHĀGAVATA-PURĀNA, or **SHRĪMAD-DEVĪ-BHĀGAVATA**; generally considered to be one of the secondary *Purānas*, though the *Shaktas venerate it as a major *Purāna*. It is dedicated to the worship of the Goddess (*Devī*) by means of *bhakti-yoga*. A central scripture of *Shaktism, it dates from the thirteenth century CE.

DEVĪ-GĪTĀ ("Song of the Goddess"), a *Shākta text forming chapters 29–40 of the seventh book of the *Devī-Bhāgavata-Purāna*. It expounds external *worship of the *Goddess and inner *meditation upon the *Divine transcending all forms.

DEVOTEE. See *bhakta*.

DEVOTION. See *bhakti, pranidhāna*.

DHAIRYA ("steadiness"), one of the factors promoting *Yoga, according to the

Hatha-Yoga-Pradīpikā (1.16). *Dhairya* is counted among the constituent practices of the "sevenfold discipline" (*sapta-sādhanā*). See also *dhriti*.

DHANAM-JAYA ("conquest of wealth"), one of the ten cardinal psychoenergetic currents (*nādī*) of the *body. Most *Yoga scriptures state that it pervades the entire body and does not leave it even after death, being responsible for the swelling of the corpse. It also sometimes thought to cause *phlegm (*shleshma*) and hiccups.

DHANUR-ĀSANA ("bow posture"), described in the *Gheranda-Samhita* (2.18) thus: Stretch the legs on the ground like a stick and catch hold of both feet with one's hands so as to make the *body resemble a bow (*dhanus*). The *Hatha-Yoga-Pradīpikā* (1.25) is a little more precise: Grasping the toes with one's hands, draw one foot up to the *ear as if one were drawing a bow.

DHĀRANĀ ("concentration," from the root *dhri*, "to hold" or "to retain"), sometimes called *samādhāna* ("collectedness"), one of the eight "limbs" (*anga*) of *Classical Yoga; also a component of other versions of the spiritual *path. The *Yoga-Sūtra* (3.1) defines it as the binding of consciousness (*citta*) to a single locus (*desha*). It is thus the practice of continuous *attention, which is of the essence of "one-pointedness" (*eka-agratā*). The *Amrita-Nāda-Upanishad* (15) understands it as the "compression" (*samkshepa*) of the *mind.

The practice of concentration, which precedes *meditation, is fundamental to the yogic process of introversion. It represents a gathering of one's psychic energy, which is accompanied by a high degree of sensory inhibition (*pratyāhāra*) and a slowing-down of thought. Yogic concentration can have a variety of mental objects (*artha*), ranging from the internalized image of a *deity to internalized sound (*nāda*), to a locus (*desha*) within the *body. Deepening concentration leads to meditation (*dhyāna*).

In some contexts, *dhāranā* denotes the retention of the *breath. See also *panca-dhāranā*.

DHARMA (from the root *dhri*, "to hold" or "to retain") is primarily employed in *Classical Yoga in the technical sense of "form" or "quality," which is contrasted with the concept of "form bearer" or

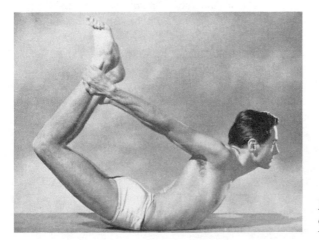

Dhanur-āsana, the bow posture, demonstrated by Theos Bernard

"substance" (*dharmin). *Patanjali, in the *Yoga-Sūtra (3.13f.), subscribes to *satkārya-vāda, that is, the view that change affects only the form of a thing, not its substance. Thus he distinguishes between three forms or states of a thing: its "quiescent" (shānta) or past aspect; its "uprisen" (udita) or present aspect, and its "indeterminable" (avyapadeshya) or future aspect. The word dharma can also simply stand for "thing" in general.

In the ethical field, dharma signifies "righteousness" or "virtue," that is, the moral order, as opposed to *adharma. In *Hinduism, morality is seen as the very foundation of the world. As such it is considered to be one of the four "human goals" (*purusha-artha). In the *Tattva-Vaishāradī (2.12), dharma is explained as that which leads to heaven (*svarga)—rather than to *liberation—and is said to stem from the inclination to perform desirable (kāmya) *actions. *Vācaspati Mishra, the author of this learned commentary on the *Yoga-Sūtra, even concedes that dharma can spring from righteous anger (*krodha), and he cites the legendary case of Dhruva, who took his father's slight as an incentive for performing austerities, which in the end raised him to a position above all others.

Historically, there has been a tension between the ideal of dharma and the ideal of *liberation, since the latter is deemed to be above good and evil, virtue and vice. Thus the *Mahābhārata (12.316.40) has this stanza: "Abandon dharma and adharma; abandon truth and falsehood. Having abandoned both truth and falsehood, abandon the [principle, i.e., the *mind] by which you abandon [everything]."

That the *yogin should eschew not only vice (*adharma) but also virtue (dharma) is, for instance, evident from the *Yoga-Sūtra (4.7), which makes a distinction between *karma that is black, karma that is white, and the karma of the *yogin, which is neither black nor white. The reason for the *yogin's extraordinary karmic status is his constant transcendence of the ego (*ahamkāra, *asmitā), which experiences itself as the performer of good or evil acts. See also rita.

DHARMA-MEGHA-SAMĀDHI ("ecstasy of the *dharma cloud"), the highest level of ecstasy (*samādhi) admitted in *Classical Yoga. It follows upon the "vision of discernment" (*viveka-khyāti) and is in turn the precursor to ultimate liberation (*kaivalya). This technical term also occurs in several *Vedānta works, including the Panca-Dashī (1.60), the Paingalā-Upanishad (3.2), and the Adhyātma-Upanishad (38). Its precise meaning is nowhere clearly defined, though many commentators understand the word dharma to denote "virtue" in this context. They may possibly have taken their cue from the Mahāyāna *Buddhist compound dharma-megha. But why should this elevated *ecstatic condition shower virtue upon the *yogin when it precisely signals the concluding phase in his transcendence of dharma and *adharma? In his *Yoga-Bhāshya-Vivarana (4.29), *Shankara interprets this high-level state somewhat more convincingly as "showering the supreme virtue called 'aloneness' (*kaivalya)." It is, however, more likely that in this context dharma means "constituent" and refers to the *gunas that, like a faint cloud, still stand between the *yogin and the ultimate condition of *liberation. The dharma-megha-samādhi is the highest form of "supraconscious ecstasy" (*asamprajnāta-samādhi). It is the final moment in the long and arduous yogic journey when the primary constituents of *nature resolve into their transcendental matrix. This "involution" (*pratiprasava) of the gunas coincides with *liberation or *Self-realization.

DHARMA-SHĀSTRA ("teaching of the law"), the body of precepts and interpretations of the notion of *dharma, which is at the core of the moral code of *Hinduism. This term also denotes a textbook (*shāstra) dealing with ethical matters.

DHARMA-SHĀSTRA of Manu, also known as the Mānava-Dharma-Shāstra or the *Manu-Smriti.

DHARMIN ("form bearer"), the unchanging substance, as opposed to the changeable form (*dharma). This is a key element of the theory of transformation (*parināma) adopted by *Patanjali in his *Yoga-Sūtra (3.13f.). See also dravya.

DHĀTU ("constituent") can refer to the three bodily humors: wind (*vāta), gall (*pitta), and phlegm (*shleshma or *kapha). It can also refer to the seven constituents that are listed, for instance, in the *Yoga-Bhāshya (3.29) as skin, blood, flesh, sinew, bone, marrow, and semen (*shukra). Some schools replace the skin with *rasa (thought to stream from the *heart and sustain the entire *body) and the marrow by fat. The *Tattva-Vaishāradī (1.30) mentions that the dhātus are so called because they "hold together" (dhārana) the physical frame. Sometimes dhātu denotes the principal constituent of the body, which is the "nectar of immortality" (*amrita). See also dosha, ojas.

DHĀTU-STRĪ-LAULYAKA ("longing for a base woman"), one of five obstacles (*vighna) mentioned in the *Yoga-Tattva-Upanishad (31).

DHAUTI ("washing" or "cleansing"), one of the "six acts" (*shat-karma) of *hatha-

yoga. According to the *Gheranda-Samhitā (1.13), it comprises the following four techniques: internal washing (*antar-dhauti); dental cleansing (*danta-dhauti); cleansing of the "heart" (*hrid-dhauti); and rectal cleansing (*mūla-shodhana). The *Hatha-Yoga-Pradīpikā (2.24f.) does not mention these subcategories but describes dhauti thus: One should slowly swallow a wet cloth four digits wide and fifteen spans long as instructed by one's *teacher, and then draw it out again. This technique is otherwise known as "cloth cleansing" (*vāso-dhauti). See also kapāla-randhra-dhauti.

DHĪ ("thought"), a key *Vedic notion referring to the illumination or visionary thought of the ancient seers (*rishi) through which they penetrated the veil of the material *world and caught glimpses of the unconditional *Reality.

DHOTĪ ("cloth"; Hindi word, derived from Sanskrit *dhauti), a long cloth worn by men, which is passed between the legs and tucked into the waist from behind.

DHRIK-STHITI ("steadiness of vision"), one of the practices of the fifteenfold *path (*panca-dasha-anga-yoga). It is defined in the *Tejo-Bindu-Upanishad (1.29) as that vision, consisting of *wisdom, which sees the world as the *Absolute and which must not be confused with mere gazing at the tip of the *nose. See also drishti.

DHRITI ("steadiness" or "steadfastness"), sometimes counted as one of the ten practices of moral discipline (*yama). The *Shāndilya-Upanishad (1.1.12) understands it as "mental stability" (cetah sthāpanam) at all times, especially in moments of personal loss. The *Uddhāva-Gītā (14.36) explains it as the "mastery over tongue and *genitals." The *Bhagavad-Gītā (18.33ff.) distinguishes three types of dhriti, depending on the preeminence of the three qualities (*guna) of *nature. Thus, sāttvika-dhriti is that steadiness by which one restrains the *mind, the *breath, and the *senses. Rājasa-dhriti is that steadiness by which one holds fast to virtue (*dharma), prosperity (*artha), and pleasure (*kāma) and also clings to their fruits. Finally, tāmasa-dhriti is characteristic of the deluded person who is attached to sleep (*svapna), fear (*bhaya), grief (*shoka), dejection (*vishāda), and intoxication (mada). See also dhairya.

DHŪPA ("incense"), sometimes listed as one of the "limbs" (*anga) of the devotional path of *Yoga. Incense is used to purify and render sacred the space (*desha) in which the yogic disciplines and *worship are to be conducted. The pleasant scent is thought to attract benign beings (*angels), who can be helpful to the *practitioner.

DHVANI ("sound"), a synonym for *shabda and *nāda.

DHYĀNA ("meditation" or "contemplation"), a fundamental technique common to all yogic *paths. The *Bhagavad-Gītā (12.12) places *meditation above intellectual *knowledge, and the *Shiva-Purāna (7.2.39.28) holds it to be superior to any *pilgrimage, austerity (*tapas), and sacrificial rite. As the Garuda-Purāna (222.10) declares: "Meditation is the highest *virtue. Meditation is the highest austerity. Meditation is the highest *purity. Therefore be fond of meditation."

In the eightfold path of *Classical Yoga, *meditation precedes *ecstasy (*samādhi). *Patanjali, in his *Yoga-Sūtra (3.2), defines it as the "one-directional flow" (*eka-tā-nata) of presented ideas (*pratyaya) relative to a single object of *concentration. As such, meditation is a natural continuation or deepening of concentration (*dhāranā). The Yoga-Sūtra (1.39) maintains that any *object whatsoever can be turned into a prop for the meditative process, though in the *Patanjali-Rahasya (1.39), for instance, the stipulation is made that it should not be a prohibited object such as a nude female.

*Meditation effects the arrest (*nirodha) of the five kinds of "fluctuation" (*vritti) of *consciousness mentioned by *Patanjali. The *Kūrma-Purāna (2.11.40), however, speaks of a meditation as a "continuum of fluctuations" (*vritti-samtati), with attention resting on a specific locus uninterrupted by other fluctuations. Meditation is marked by an advanced degree of sensory inhibition (*pratyāhāra). Hence the *Mahābhārata (13.294.16) describes the meditating *yogin thus: "He does not hear; he does not smell, neither does he taste nor see, nor experience touch; likewise, the *mind ceases to imagine. He desires nothing, and like a log he does not think. Then the sages call him 'yoked' (*yukta), 'one who has reached *nature' (prakritim āpannam)."

Many texts of *Postclassical Yoga distinguish between a "qualified" (*saguna) and an "unqualified" (*nirguna) meditation. Whereas the former has a concrete *object (such as one's chosen *deity), the latter has no immediate object but is a kind of absorption into oneself. These two categories are also respectively referred to as "formal" (mūrti) and "formless" (amūrti), or "partite" (sakala) and "impartite" (nishkala) meditation. The *Yoga-Yājnavalkya (9.9f.) gives as an example of the latter type of contemplation the persistent feeling of "I am the *Absolute."

Formal *meditation often contains a

strong element of visualization. This is especially true of *Tantrism and *hatha-yoga, where the *yogin is asked to construct elaborate inner environments calling for intense *concentration and imaginative capacity. Usually the object of such detailed visualization is the practitioner's "chosen deity" (*ishta-devatā). The *god or *goddess is so vividly imagined that he or she assumes overwhelming psychic reality for the practitioner. The *yogin can next attempt to identify with that deity in the unitive experience of *ecstasy until his own *ego identity is obliterated. The underlying idea is that most practitioners find it too difficult to engage the "formless" meditation of imageless absorption.

The *Gheranda-Samhitā (6.1ff.) makes a distinction between the following three types of meditation: "coarse meditation" (*sthūla-dhyāna), "light meditation" (*jyotir-dhyāna), and "subtle meditation" (*sūkshma-dhyāna). The first consists in the contemplation of a concrete form (such as one's chosen deity), and is said to be for beginners; the second consists in the contemplation of various *light phenomena, while the third is equivalent to absorption into the *Self during the performance of *shāmbhavī-mudrā.

Whatever approach one chooses, *meditation continues the potent transformative trend initiated by *concentration. If pursued with adequate rigor, that trend leads to the ultimate obliteration of the subconscious karmic "deposits" (*āshaya), i.e., the complete restructuring of one's personal identity—from *ego personality to transcendental Selfhood. Meditation is a steppingstone to ecstasy (*samādhi) and hence must be transcended at a certain point. Therefore it is not surprising that meditation is, as in the *Shiva-Samhitā (5.4), occasionally reckoned as one of the obstacles (*vighna) of *Yoga.

In some contexts, dhyāna is used in the sense of *samādhi. See also bhāvanā, nididhyāsana.

DHYĀNA-BINDU-UPANISHAD (Dhyānabindūpanishad), one of the *Yoga-Upanishads, consisting of 106 stanzas. This tract expounds the "*Yoga of meditation" (*dhyāna-yoga), which is understood to be the *path of meditative introversion by means of the sacred syllable *om, called the *pranava. A sixfold *path (*shad-anga-yoga) is put forward whose constituent practices are posture (*āsana), breath restraint (*prāna-samrodha), sense withdrawal (*pratyāhāra), concentration (*dhāranā), meditation (*dhyāna), and ecstasy (*samādhi).

The "serpent power" (*kundalinī-shakti) is used, though no detailed instructions about its arousal are given, and only the first four psychoenergetic centers (*cakra) of the *body are mentioned and roughly described. The "heart lotus" (*hrit-padma) is given prominence.

DHYĀNA-MUDRĀ ("seal of meditation"), one of the hand gestures (*mudrā) used in *Yoga, especially in conjunction with the various *meditation postures. It is performed by resting the open left hand, palm up, on one's folded legs and placing the right hand, also palm up, on top, with the tip of the thumbs touching.

The term dhyāna-mudrā is also used in the *Yoga-Mārtanda (159) to denote the balance (*samatva) of the *body during the practice of the "easy posture" (*sukha-āsana) when one is "inner-minded" even though the *eyes are open.

DHYĀNA-YOGA ("Yoga of meditation"), a common compound in the literature of *Yoga. It is frequently used as early as the *Mahābhārata, in which (12.188.1ff.) a

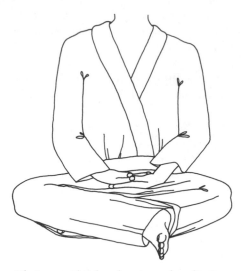

Dhyāna-mudrā, hand gesture of meditation

DHYEYA ("that which is to be contemplated"), the *object of *meditation. This can be any internalized object whatsoever, including the formless *Absolute itself. See also *ālambana, bīja, desha*.

DIET. See *āhāra, anna*.

DĪKSHĀ ("initiation") holds a central place in all branches and schools of the *Yoga tradition. According to the *Kula-Arnava-Tantra* (10.3), it is impossible to attain *enlightenment without initiation, a sentiment reflected in many other scriptures: "It is stated in the teaching of *Shiva that there can be no *liberation without initiation and that there can be no such [initiation] without a [qualified] preceptor (*ācārya*). Thus is the preceptorial lineage (*paramparā*)."

The great importance of *dīkshā* lies in that it consists essentially in the transference of *wisdom (*jnāna*) or power (*shakti*) from the *teacher to the *disciple. Through initiation the disciple comes to mysteriously participate in the teacher's state of being and even becomes a part of the teacher's line of transmission (*paramparā*). The *guru*'s lineage is a chain of spiritual empowerment that exceeds the world of space and time.

Both the word *dīkshā* and its underlying concept date back to the *Atharva-Veda*, which has the following pertinent stanza (11.5.3): "Initiation takes place in that the *teacher carries the pupil in himself as it were, as the mother [bears] the embryo in her *body. After the three-day ceremony the disciple is born."

Initiation is generally thought to have different degrees. Often a distinction is made between the following three types of initiation: (1) *mantra-dīkshā*, in which the *disciple is given an empowered *mantra* for *recitation and *meditation (also

fourfold *meditation is taught whose goal is "extinction" (*nirvāna*). It consists in making the *senses into a ball—the phrase is *pindī-kritya*—and sitting like a log while focusing the *mind on a single point. At the second stage, the mind is said to quiver like a lightning flash in a rain cloud. The mind is further described as tending to roam on the path of the *wind, which presumably means that it is inclined to follow the movement of the *breath, wherefore one should force it back on the path of *meditation. In the course of *meditation, we are told, different types of thoughts arise; these are referred to as *vicāra, *vitarka*, and *viveka*. While their precise meaning is not clear in this context, these terms have a parallel in the *Yoga-Sūtra*. The *Bhagavad-Gītā* (18.52) emphasizes that *dhyāna-yoga* must be cultivated in conjunction with dispassion (*vairāgya*).

DHYĀTRI ("meditator"), the meditating subject, as opposed to the object of *meditation or *contemplation *(dhyeya)*.

known as *ānavī-dīkshā); (2) *shakti-dīkshā*, in which the *teacher activates the disciple's "serpent power" (*kundalinī-shakti*) and which, according to the *Shiva-Purāna* (7.2.15.6), requires the teacher to enter the student's *body, a feat known as *para-deha-pravesha*; and (3) *Shiva-dīkshā*, the highest type of initiation, which is given by the teacher's mere touch or glance (*drishti*) and upon which the disciple is propelled into the state of ecstasy (*samādhi*). This is also known as *shāmbhavī-dīkshā*.

The process of transmission is frequently referred to as the "descent of power" (*shakti-pāta*). See also *abhisheka*.

DĪPA ("lamp" or "lantern"), one of the main implements for ritual *worship; sometimes listed as one of the "limbs" (*anga*) of the yogic *path.

DĪPTI ("radiance" or "luminosity"), a phenomenon associated with many yogic states. Thus it is listed in the *Yoga-Tattva-Upanishad* (45) as one of the signs (*cihna*) of the successful cleansing of the psychoenergetic conduits (*nādī*).

DĪRGHATAMAS ("Long Darkness"), a great seer (*rishi*) of the *Vedic age, born blind. He also figures prominently in the *Mahābhārata* and the *Purānas*.

DISCIPLE. See *shishya*.

DISCIPLESHIP, or *shishyatā*, is essential in all traditional forms of spirituality in which the secret and sacred *knowledge is primarily transmitted by word of mouth. See also *adhikāra, guru, shishya*.

DISCIPLINE. See *abhyāsa, yama, niyama*.

DISCRIMINATION, DISCERNMENT. See *tarka, vijnāna, viveka, viveka-khyāti*.

DISEASE. See *roga, vyādhi*.

DISPASSION. See *vairāgya, virāga*.

DISSIPATION. See *avirati*.

DISTRACTION. See *vikshepa*.

DIVINE. *Hinduism is well known for its astounding variety of metaphysical systems or theologies, which show considerable religious virtuosity and philosophical ingenuity. There are first of all the numerous popular deities (*deva, *devatā*), such as *Vishnu, *Shiva, *Krishna, *Rāma, *Durgā, and *Kālī. These are worshiped in rural India, and popular imagination views them as superhuman personalities who populate the heavenly realms (*svarga*) and who can be petitioned or even coerced through *prayer and magical incantations (*mantra*). The more literate sections of *Hindu society, however, believe that beyond this pantheon of deities abides a single ultimate *Being. In the monotheistic schools such as *Vaishnavism, this ultimate *Reality is conceived as suprapersonal. Thus *Vishnu is celebrated as the "supreme person" (*purusha-uttama*) beyond space-time. The pantheistic and panentheistic schools, again, envision the ultimate *Reality to be impersonal, without qualities (*nirguna*) and indescribable. They call it the *Absolute (*brahman*) or the transcendental *Self (*ātman*).

But then there are also philosophical schools such as *Classical Sāmkhya, *Mīmāmsā, and *Nyāya that make no reference to a single ultimate *Being but propose a pluralistic metaphysics of countless transcendental Selves (*purusha*). This is also the position of *Classical Yoga, which postulates a stringent dualism between nature (*prakriti*) and the conscious principle of existence called *purusha*. Like the *Nyāya school, it maintains that the "Lord" (*īshvara) is simply a special kind of transcendental *Self. Probably because of its dualist (or pluralistic) metaphysics and its attenuated concept of *God, Classical Yoga has never become widely influential as a philosophical school, although *Patanjali's systematization of the eightfold yogic *path has served many later authorities as a model. The schools of *Preclassical Yoga and *Postclassical Yoga subscribe without exception to the nondualist (*advaita) metaphysics developed in the *Vedānta tradition.

DIVYA ("divine"), the *Absolute, or ultimate *Reality; also, the suprasensuous realities and realms. Thus the term can simply stand for "sacred."

DIVYA-CAKSHUS ("divine eye"), also called *divya-drishti*, clairvoyance. It is among the paranormal abilities (*siddhi) attributed to *yogins and *sādhus. This is also called "far-sightedness" (*dūra-darshana*) in some texts, which is the modern Sanskrit word for "television" as well. See also *cakshus, kapāla-randhra-dhauti*.

DIVYA-DEHA or DIVYA-VAPUS ("divine body"), a lustrous *body acquired on the first stage of yogic accomplishment, or on the ninth level of the manifestation of the inner sound (*nāda), according to the *Hatha-Yoga-Pradīpikā (4.71). Sometimes this term denotes the *ātivāhika-deha*.

DIVYA-DESHA ("divine place"). In Southern *Shaivism, as encoded in the Tamil scriptures, 108 divine or sacred places are recognized, including the supreme *heaven known as Vaikuntha in Sanskrit or Tirunātu in Tamil, which is Lord *Vishnu's eternal abode. See also *tīrtha*.

DIVYA-PRABANDHAM or NĀLĀYIRA-DIVYA-PRABANDHAM ("Divine Collection"), a Tamil scripture of *Shaivism of 4,000 verses, which includes the famous *Tiruvāymoli of *Namm Ālvār. In South India, this collection has the same sacred status as the *Vedas have in the north.

DIVYA-SAMVID ("divine perception"), paranormal sensory activity, such as extremely acute sight or hearing, according to the *Yoga-Bhāshya (1.35). See also *samvid, siddhi*.

DIVYA-SHROTRA ("divine hearing"), clairaudience; a paranormal ability (*siddhi) mentioned, for instance, in the *Yoga-Sūtra (3.41), where it is explained as resulting from the practice of ecstatic "constraint" (*samyama) upon the relation between the *ears and space (*ākāsha).

DOLPHIN POSTURE. See *makara-āsana*.

DOSHA ("defect" or "blemish"), a common concept of *Hindu ethics. In the *Yoga tradition, it specifically refers to the five moral defects: lust (*kāma), anger (*krodha), greed (*lobha), fear (*bhaya), and sleep (*svapna or *nidrā). Sometimes this set is said to comprise passion (*rāga), delusion (*moha), attachment (*sneha), lust, and anger. Occasionally one of them is substituted for faulty breathing (*shvāsa or *nishvāsa). In the *Amrita-Nāda-Upanishad (27), again, seven such blemishes are cited: fear, anger, sloth (*ālasya), excessive sleep (*atisvapna), excessive waking (*atijāgara), overeating (*atyāhāra), and (excessive?) *fasting (anāhāra). The *Yoga-Tattva-Upanishad (12f.) furnishes a list of twenty blemishes that retard one's spiritual *progress: lust, anger, fear, delusion, greed, pride (*mada*), passion (*rajas), birth (*janman), death (*mrityu), meanness (*kārpanya), grief (*shoka), laziness (*tandrā), hunger (*kshudhā), thirst (*trishā), "thirst for life" (*trishnā), shame (*lajjā), anxiety (*bhaya), sorrow (*duhkha), dejection (*vishāda), and excitement (*harsha). The *Mahābhārata (12.290.56) suggests that there are even 100 such defects. It also states (12.205.18) that all these arise from spiritual nescience (*ujnānu) and are inborn (sahaja).

In the *Yoga-Sūtra (3.50) the term dosha is used only once, when *Patanjali speaks of the "seeds of the defects" (*dosha-bīja), meaning the subliminal "activators" (*samskāra) that generate all psychomental activity. Patanjali uses the technical term *klesha to refer to the "causes of suffering." In the medical scriptures of *Āyur-Veda, the term dosha stands for the three bodily humors, and this usage is occasionally adopted in the *Yoga texts as well. See also dhātu, mala.

DOUBT (Sanskrit: samshaya), universally regarded in the spiritual traditions as a great undermining force that saps the practitioner's *enthusiasm and will. It can be overcome by *faith.

DRASHTRI ("seer"), *Patanjali's term for the *Self in its role as *witness of the flux of psychomental phenomena. It is, as the *Yoga-Bhāshya (2.17) defines it, "the Self-conscious of the mind (*buddhi)." See also drishya, sākshin, samyoga.

DRAVYA ("substance"), defined in *Vyāsa's *Yoga-Bhāshya (3.44) as "a collection of distinct components that do not exist separately." Some scholars have argued that there is a discrepancy between the *Yoga master *Patanjali's explanation of

substance (called *dharmin in the *Yoga-Sūtra) and the grammarian Patanjali and that, therefore, the two authorities could not have been identical. This argument seems to be based on a misreading of the grammarian's work, however. Still, this does not mean that we must necessarily identify the two Patanjalis.

DREAMS. Dreaming (*svapna) is an *altered state of consciousness. In the nondualist schools of *Yoga, it is one of the states (*avasthā) that conceal the transcendental *Self. Yet, because dreams are often expressions of the deep structure of one's psychomental life, they can serve as divinatory signs (*arishta).

Moreover, the dream state can serve as a portal to higher states of *consciousness. Thus one of the distinct approaches of Vajrayāna (Tibetan) *Buddhism is the *Yoga of the dream state (milam in Tibetan), in which the *practitioner exercises control over his or her dreams so that they cease to manifest negative emotions but become an opportunity for generating merit through an increase of *awareness in the dream state. The perception of the illusory nature of dreams can then be transferred to the phenomena of the *waking state, which are similarly illusory. Cf. nidrā, sushupti.

DRIDHA-KĀYA, or DRIDHA-SHARĪRA ("firm body"); a *hatha-yoga term referring to the transformed body of the *adept. See also vajra-deha.

DRIDHATĀ ("firmness"), the second constituent of the sevenfold *path (*sapta-sādhana) expounded in the *Gheranda-Samhitā (1.10). It results from the practice of posture (*āsana). According to the *Hatha-Yoga-Pradīpikā (2.13), however, it is effected by rubbing into the *body one's perspiration (*sveda) produced in the course of exertions in *breath control.

DRISHI-MĀTRA ("pure seeing"), a technical expression of *Classical Yoga denoting the very essence of the *Self as the immutable and permanent apperceiving subject of the ongoing mental process. See also drashtri, purusha; cf. drishya.

DRISHTI ("view," "opinion," "gaze"). The *Mandala-Brāhmana-Upanishad (2.2.6) distinguishes three types of gaze during *meditation: the "new-moon glance" (amā-drishti), with the *eyes closed; the "first-phase-moon glance" (pratipad-drishti), with half-open eyes, and the "full-moon glance" (purnimā-drishti), with wide-open eyes. Some *postures or techniques of *breath control call for specific eye positions; the two best known are the gaze at the middle between the eyebrows (*bhrū-madhya) and the gaze at the tip of the nose (*nāsa-agra). See also dhrik-sthiti.

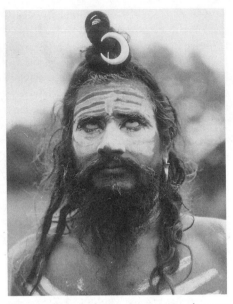

Bhrū-madhya-drishti, yogic concentrative gaze at the middle of the eyebrows

DRISHYA ("that which is to be seen"), the *object. In *Classical Yoga, this is a comprehensive term for nature (*prakriti). The *Yoga-Sūtra (2.18) defines it as having the character of brightness, activity, and inertia, which refers to the three types of primary constituents (*guna) of nature. Cf. drashtri, sākshin.

DRUM. See damaru.

DUALITY. See dvaita.

DUHKHA originally meant "having a bad axle hole," but early on came to signify "sorrow," "suffering," or "pain." According to the spiritual traditions of India, existence is inherently sorrowful. This doctrine has frequently led Western critics to summarily portray Indian philosophy as profoundly pessimistic. This typification is demonstrably misleading, however, since the avowed goal of Indian spirituality is the perfect transcendence of sorrow or pain. Indeed, most schools of Indian spirituality describe the ultimate *Reality as utterly blissful (*ānanda). Sorrow, then, pertains only to the ego-ensconced individual, not to the *Self. What more optimistic orientation could there be?

According to *Patanjali's *Yoga-Sūtra (2.17), the "correlation" (*samyoga) between the immutable *Self and *nature (or the body-mind), is the cause of the experience of suffering. When that correlation is severed, suffering ceases. Already in the *Bhagavad-Gītā (6.23) *Yoga is defined as the "disunion of the union with suffering" (duhkha-samyoga-viyoga). Cf. sukha.

DULLNESS. See jādya.

DURGĀ ("Difficult to Reach"), the cardinal *goddess of *Hinduism. The *Purānas celebrate her as the divine spouse of *Shiva, but her historical roots reach back into archaic agricultural religion. Riding on a lion and carrying different weapons, this goddess is a veritable symbol of destruction. Yet to her *devotees she is a benign, loving force because she removes all *obstructions and, ultimately, obliterates the *ego illusion. See also Kālī.

DURVASAS ("Ill-Clad"), a mighty but irascible sage whose fierce *asceticism had brought him many extraordinary powers (*siddhi). Even *Krishna was unable to dispel the sage's curse after Krishna had refused to accept an offering of flowers. Durvāsas's exploits are told in the *Purānas.

DUTY. See dharma.

DVĀDASHA-ANTA (dvādashānta, "ending with the twelfth"), an esoteric psychoenergetic center (*cakra) that, according to some schools of *Shaiva Yoga, is said to be situated twelve digits above the *head. It is commonly equated with the *sahasrāra-cakra. The expression can also refer to a point in space twelve digits from the tip of the *nose, which is as far as the life force (*prāna) is thought to extend into *space during exhalation. This point in space is employed in *tāraka-yoga to visualize certain *light phenomena. Some texts distinguish between ūrdhva-dvādasha-anta, referring to the *sahasrāra-cakra; antar-dvādasha-anta, referring to the center of the *body); and bāhya-dvādasha-anta, denoting a locus outside the body. See also ākāsha.

DVĀDASHA-ARA-CAKRA (dvādashāra-cakra, "twelve-spoked wheel"), a psychoenergetic center in the center of the *body known to *Postclassical Yoga. In some contexts, it denotes the *heart lotus

(*hrit-padma), while in others it refers to the "wheel of channels" (*nādī-cakra).

DVĀDASHA-STHĀNA ("twelve stations"), in Kashmiri *Shaivism, the twelve loci traversed by the ascending "serpent power" (*kundalinī-shakti). In the commentaries on the *Vijñāna-Bhairava (30), these are named as follows: (1) janma-agra ("birth point"), or the sexual organs; (2) mūla ("root"), or the perineum, which is the seat of the *kundalinī; (3) *kanda ("bulb"), or the source of the countless subtle "conduits" (*nādī); (4) *nābhi ("navel"); (5) *hrid ("heart"); (6) *kantha ("throat"); (7) *tālu ("palate"); (8) *bhrū-madhya ("brow middle"); (9) *lalata ("forehead"); (10) *brahma-randhra ("brahmic fissure"); (11) *shakti ("power"), or the conscious energy beyond the *body; and (12) vyāpinī, or the divine energy manifesting when the *kundalinī has completed its ascent.

DVAITA ("duality"). In the schools of *Preclassical and *Postclassical Yoga, which are founded in the metaphysics of *Advaita Vedānta, the experience of duality (or the schism between *subject and *object) is the result of spiritual nescience (*avidyā).

DVANDVA ("pair"), a common designation for such pairs of opposites, or polarities, as heat and cold, *light and darkness, or *pleasure and *pain. These bewilder all beings, as the *Bhagavad-Gītā (7.27) admits. According to *Patanjali's *Yoga-Sūtra (2.48), the *yogin becomes immunized against these dualities through the practice of posture (*āsana), which includes an element of sensory inhibition (*pratyāhāra).

DVĀRA ("gate"). The *Bhagavad-Gītā (16.21) speaks of lust (*kāma), anger (*krodha), and greed (*lobha) as the three gates of *hell. More commonly, however, the word dvāra stands for the bodily apertures. Already in the ancient *Atharva-Veda (10.2.31) the *body is likened to a citadel with nine gates. The *Katha-Upanishad (5.1) speaks of eleven apertures, presumably the two *eyes, two *ears, two nostrils, the mouth, the genital opening, the anus, the *navel, and the sagittal suture (*vidriti), through which the psyche (*jīva) exits in the moment of *death. Occasionally ten such gates are differentiated. The *Amrita-Nāda-Upanishad (26), again, lists seven gates, but these are esoteric loci in the body, such as the "heart gate" (hrid-dvāra); the "wind gate" (*vāyu-dvāra), which probably refers to the *vishuddha-cakra at the *throat; and four unidentified gates located in the *head.

DVESHA ("hatred" or "aversion"), in *Classical Yoga, one of the five "causes of affliction" (*klesha); defined in the *Yoga-Sūtra (2.8) as one's dwelling upon what is painful (*duhkha). However, that hatred can also have a positive spiritual effect is borne out by the story of Shishupāla, the king of Codi, who was released from the grip of the world by virtue of his abiding hatred for *Vishnu over a period of three lifetimes. As the *Uddhāva-Gītā (4.22) explains:

> On whatever the individual concentrates the *mind fully and intelligently either through attachment (*sneha) or even through hatred—with that he becomes coessential.
>
> Or again: That [*Absolute] sees no distinctions, therefore one should unite [with the *Divine] through the bond of enmity or *friendship, *fear or *attachment or desire (*kāma).

These ideas express the position of *samrambha-yoga, one of the most astonishing developments within *Hindu spirituality. See also rāga.

· E ·

EAGLE POSTURE. See garuda-āsana.

EARRINGS. See kundala, mudrā

EARS. In many esoteric traditions the ears, which are associated with the ether-space (*ākāsha), have great significance. Thus in India elongated earlobes, as seen on many Buddha statues, are taken as a sign of *renunciation. The *yogins of the *Kānphata sect bore holes into the cartilege of the ears and insert large rings (*kundala) into them in order to stimulate a particular subtle channel (*nādī), which is thought to make them more receptive to hearing the inner sound (*nāda).

EASY POSTURE. See sukha-āsana.

ECLIPSE. See grahana.

ECSTASY, as this Greek-derived word suggests, is a "standing outside" of oneself. It is a nonordinary or *altered state of consciousness that involves a significant shift in one's sense of identity. The experience entails at least a partial *transcendence of the *ego, accompanied by blissfulness (*ānanda). Because the term ecstasy connotes emotional rapture and mental exaltation, characteristics that do not apply to the typical yogic state of mind-transcending consciousness, Mircea Eliade (1969) and others have proposed to render the term *samādhi as "enstasy" or "enstasis." "Enstasy" means literally a "standing within" oneself and, ultimately, within one's authentic being, i.e., the transcendental *Self (*ātman, *purusha).

But this distinction cannot always be made in such a clear-cut way. Some yogic *samādhis—especially in the *bhakti tradition—resemble more ecstasy as commonly understood than *enstasy. The general thrust of the yogic states of consciousness, however, is toward the calming of the *body and *mind so that there is no emotional or intellectual excitation but simply a blossoming of pure Awareness (*cit).

EFFORT. In some yogic schools the question is raised about the relationship between personal effort (*prayatna, *yatna) and grace (*anugraha, *kripā, *prasāda). The answers range from complete reliance on self-effort to complete reliance on divine intervention. In most cases, however, a middle *path is recommended, whereby a practitioner earns the favor of the *Divine by his or her consistent application to the spiritual process. In Southern *Shaivism, a distinction is made between the *path of the monkey and the path of the cat. On the former path, the *practitioner makes the effort of clinging to the *Divine, as a young monkey clings to its parent. On the latter path, however, the Divine carries the devotee (*bhakta) as a mother cat carries a kitten. See also paurusha.

EGO. In religious or spiritual contexts, the ego refers to the psychological principle of individuation, whereby a person experiences himself or herself as an individual apart from all other beings. This egoic existence is thought to lie at the root of all human *experience of suffering (*duh-

kha), and thus the ego is considered to be the principal stumbling block on the spiritual *path.

Two broad approaches to this problem can be distinguished. The first approach seeks to extirpate the ego together with all typically human forms of self-expression. Here the goal is to realize the transcendental *Reality apart from the *world. This involves the pursuit of extreme inwardness and a radical withdrawal from the world and from participation in human culture. This is the ideal of *abandonment.

The second, more integral orientation also seeks *Self-realization through ego-transcendence, but it is basically world affirmative. The underlying argument is that if there is only one *Reality it must necessarily include the *world, which means that the world and therefore the human personality must be viewed as valid manifestations of that ultimate Reality. Hence *self-transcendence does not imply ego denial as in the former approach. Rather the ego personality is used as an instrument for *action in the world, while at the same time it is continually transcended through acts of conscious *self-surrender. This ideal is best expressed in the approach of *karma-yoga. See also aham, ahamkāra, aham-vritti, asmitā, jīva.

EKA ("one"), the singular *Reality, or transcendental *Self, beyond the multiplicity experienced by the *unenlightened, ego-bound individual. See also advaita, advaya, aikya.

EKĀGRATĀ ("one-pointedness," from eka "one, single," and agra-tā, "pointedness"), the single-mindedness, or focused *attention, that is the very essence of yogic *concentration. Through the *practice of one-pointedness, the *mind is prevented from attaching itself to one *object after another. In the *Mahābhārata* (12.242.4), *ekāgrya* (a synonym for *ekāgratā*), is praised thus: "The "singleness" (*ekāgrya*) of the *senses and the *mind is the highest [form of] austerity (*tapas*)."

It is *attention's natural tendency to wander. The reason for this constant movement is the vibratory (*spanda*) nature of existence itself. Everything is in continuous flux (*parināma*). The *yogin attempts to slow down this perpetual motion of *nature within the *microcosm of his own *consciousness to the point where his true identity, the pure Consciousness (*cit*), becomes obvious to him. See also *ekatānatā*; cf. *sarva-arthatā*.

EKANĀTHA (ca. 1533–99 CE), a celebrated Marathi *adept who edited the famous *Jñāneshvarī and also wrote many original works of his own, notably his commentaries on the *Bhagavad-Gītā and on the eleventh canticle of the *Bhāgavata-Purāna, as well as his numerous didactic poems (*abhanga*). Ekanātha's approach to *Self-realization combines devotion (*bhakti*), gnosis (*jñāna*), renunciation (*samnyāsa*), and meditation (*dhyāna*). See also Jñānadeva, Nāmadeva.

EKĀNTA-VĀSA ("dwelling in solitude"), sometimes counted among the practices of self-restraint (*niyama*). Like silence (*mauna*), periodic or long-term solitude is a powerful means for achieving self-sufficiency and self-control (*ātma-nigraha*).

EKATĀNATĀ ("single extension"), the continuation of *ekāgratā on the level of *meditation (*dhyāna*). It is the continuous flow of "presented ideas" (*pratyaya*) with regard to the same *object of meditation.

ELEMENTS. The five material elements (*bhūta*)—earth, water, fire, air, and ether—are the final products of the process of cosmic *evolution. They form the "coarse" (*sthūla*) dimension or outermost layer of existence. See also *ādhibhūta*, *tanmātra*, *tattva*.

ELEPHANT SEAL. See *mātanginī-mudrā*.

ELEPHANT TECHNIQUE. See *gaja-karanī*.

ELEVATION, ECSTATIC. See *prasamkhyāna*.

EMBODIMENT. For many spiritual traditions, embodiment is the problem to be solved, in that embodiment implies the *experience of being a specific *body and *mind—an individual, or *ego. Only those traditions, such as Mahāyāna *Buddhism, that do not oppose the ultimate *Reality (*nirvāna*) against conditional existence (*samsāra*) have developed a more body positive and world positive *ethics. For them, embodiment is a unique spiritual opportunity, in terms of both personal *liberation and the exercise of compassion (*karunā*) toward all *beings.

EMISSION, DIVINE. See *visarga*.

EMOTION. See Feeling.

ENERGY. See *bala*, *shakti*, *vīrya*.

ENJOYMENT. See *bhoga*, *bhukti*.

ENLIGHTENMENT is that condition of the body-mind in which it is perfectly synchronized with the transcendental *Reality. It is identical with *Self-realization. See also *ātma-jñāna*, Awakening, *bodha*, Liberation, *purusha-jñāna*.

ENSTASY. See Ecstasy, *samādhi*.

ENTHUSIASM, in the form of consistent dedication to the spiritual process, is a basic requirement on the *path to *Self-realization. This must be more than emotional excitement, which tends to be fleeting and unsuited for a long-term commitment to the difficult task of *self-transcendence. Enthusiasm must, rather, be a measure of one's understanding (*jnāna), or *wisdom, and be borne by a strong faith (*shraddhā) in the reality of the spiritual process. See also ālolya.

ENVIRONMENT. See desha.

ENVY. See mātsarya.

EPIC YOGA, the collective designation for the different *Yoga schools and teachings represented in the *Mahābhārata. This designation is sometimes used interchangeably with *Preclassical Yoga, which, strictly speaking, is a more comprehensive concept. See also History of Yoga.

EPISTEMOLOGY. See pramāna.

EQUANIMITY. See sama-darshana, sa-matva.

EQUILIBRIUM. See sama-rasatva.

EROTICISM. See kāma, maithunā, Sexuality.

ERROR. See viparyaya; cf. pramāna.

ETHER. See ākāsha, kha, Space, vyoman.

ETHICS (Sanskrit: *dharma-shāstra), the science of the moral law (*dharma). It is concerned with formulating guidelines for deciding between *good and *evil, right and wrong. See also Morality.

EVEN POSITION. See sama-samsthāna.

EVEN VISION. See sama-darshana, sama-drishti; see also Same-mindedness.

EVIL. See adharma, pāpa; cf. Good, Morality, punya.

EVOLUTION, the unfolding of forms by stages. Many spiritual traditions postulate a hierarchical series of developmental stages in *nature. In *Hinduism it was particularly the schools of *Sāmkhya and *Yoga that created comprehensive evolutionary models intended to map out the principal categories (*tattva) of the manifest and unmanifest *cosmos. The purpose of these models is, however, not so much to offer cosmological theories as to serve the involutionary journey of the spiritual aspirant.

Both *Yoga and *Sāmkhya subscribe to a doctrine called *sat-kārya-vāda, which states that the effect (*kārya) is preexistent (sat) in the cause. What this means is that all evolving categories of existence are potentially present in earlier categories. Thus, out of the single transcendental matrix (*pranidhāna) of *nature evolves the category of the *buddhi, or *mahat, the unified prephysical and prepsychic field from which in turn emerge the distinct categories of physical and psychic existence. A common illustration of this evolutionary principle is that of an urn (the effect) that was fashioned out of clay (the cause). We can also think of a marble sculpture that preexists in a block of marble and is given shape through the artist's vision and skill.

In the tradition of *Advaita Vedānta, which has largely adopted the *Sāmkhya account of this cosmogenetic process but which also denies ultimacy to the *world of multiple forms, these transformations from one category into another are considered to be illusory. They are the product of the hypnotizing agency of spiritual nescience (*avidyā). Hence this teaching is known as "phantom development" or *vivarta. By contrast, Sāmkhya and *Yoga subscribe to a realist philosophy. Their position is known as *parināma-vāda* or the "doctrine of [real] development." See also *parināma, prakriti, sarga*.

EXALTATION. See *unmanī*.

EXCITEMENT. See *harsha*.

EXISTENCE. See *bhāva*, Cosmos. Cf. Being.

EXPERIENCE. See *ābhoga, anubhava, anubhūti*.

EXTINCTION. See *nirvāna*.

EYE OF WISDOM. See *jnāna-cakshus*.

EYEBROWS. See *bhrū, bhrū-cakra, bhrūmadhya*.

EYES. Being one of the most intricate organs of the *body, the human eye is given special significance in many esoteric traditions. It is the most important sense organ (*indriya*) and traditionally is said to be not merely a passive receptor of incoming light but an active transmitter of *energy that establishes actual contact with the perceived object (*vishaya*). Thus the eye is the medium for projecting the *yogin's will upon another being, by way of the "third eye" or *ājnā-cakra.

It is with his third eye that *Shiva burned Kāma, the deity of *desire, to *ashes. The third eye is the eye of *fire. When closed, it suggests inner vision or higher *perception. Shiva's other two eyes represent the *sun and *moon respectively. Because of his three eyes, Shiva is also known as Tri-Netra, Tri-Aksha (written Tryaksha), or Tri-Nayana, all meaning "Three-Eyed."

Some researchers have equated the third eye with the small pine-cone-shaped pineal gland located in the midbrain, which is light sensitive. The physiological function of this gland is ill understood. See also Gaze.

· F ·

FAITH, as opposed to mere belief, is a deep-felt trusting attitude toward existence. As such it is fundamental to all spiritual traditions. Maturation on the yogic *path is unthinkable without faith, especially faith in one's teacher (*guru*), who is thought to testify to the reality of the spiritual dimension of life. In the *Bhagavad-Gītā* (7.3), *Krishna emphasizes the importance of faith (*shraddhā*) in this manner: "The faith of every [person] is in accordance with his essence (*sattva*), O Bharata [i.e., *Arjuna]. A person (*puru-sha*) is of the form of faith. Whatever his faith, that verily is he." See also *pratīti*.

FASTING, (*upavāsa; anāhāra*) plays a significant role in many religious and spiritual traditions. It is employed as a means of purifying *body and *mind in preparation for higher practices of *self-transcendence, notably *concentration, *meditation, and *ecstasy. Occasionally, fasting is regarded as a defect (*dosha*). See also *laghu-āhāra, mita-āhāra*; cf. *atyāhāra*.

FATE. See *daiva, karma*.

FEAR. See *bhaya*.

FEARLESSNESS. See *abhaya*.

FEELING. It is sometimes thought that the *Yoga tradition, and *Hinduism in general, pays little attention to feelings or emotions. In fact, however, the *Hindu authorities have catalogued the entire range of feelings or sentiments known to modern psychology. Indeed, the Yoga scriptures refer to affective experiences to be had at the higher levels of ecstasy (*samādhi*) for which there are no straightforward equivalents in psychology. The ecstatic "coincidence with bliss" (*ānanda-samāpatti*) is a case in point. The *Taittirīya-Upanishad* (2.7) affirms that the "[ultimate *Being] verily is but feeling (*rasa*)."

Perhaps what has given rise to the above mistaken impression is the tendency of Indian philosophers to think more holistically. Thus in *Yoga the affects are generally treated together with the motivations, anticipating certain contemporary affecto-motivational theories. This psychological holism is epitomized, for instance, in the *klesha doctrine of the *Yoga-Sūtra*, which identifies the five principal factors governing a person's life: spiritual nescience (*avidyā*), which is not merely the absence of right *knowledge but a positive misreading of reality; "I-am-ness" (*asmitā*); the "will to survive" (*abhinivesha*); attachment (*rāga*); and aversion (*dvesha*). Attachment and aversion form part of a motivational continuum. The life of the ordinary, unenlightened individual revolves around the pursuit of *pleasure and the avoidance of *pain. Within this motivational framework, a plenitude of emotions occurs.

The yogic process consists initially in the transmutation of negative emotions into positive feelings such as compassion (*karunā*), friendliness (*maitrī*), and love (*bhakti*). This is accomplished through adherence to the principles of moral discipline (*yama*) and self-restraint (*niyama*). However, *Yoga does not stop at the humanistic objective of creating a benign and functional personality. It endeavors to transcend the body-mind and hence also the affective dimension. At the same time, however, it must be emphasized that in most schools the ultimate accomplishment of *Self-realization, or *enlightenment, does not signal the termination of the *yogin's emotional life. Rather as a fully liberated being, an *adept, he is now able to engage life spontaneously and to freely animate all kinds of emotions without getting bound by them. This is especially evident in the case of the *crazy adepts, who, because their identity rests in the *Self and not in the *ego, are able to activate the entire range of human emotion to instruct others. Although the condition of *Self-realization is said to be beyond *good and *evil, the Self-realized adept is essentially a benign being.

FEET. Because it is through the feet that *yogins and other saintly folk connect their own psychospiritual energy to the energy of the *earth, the feet or footwear (*pāduka*) of holy men and women have tradiionally been objects of reverence.

FETTER. See *pāsha*; see also Bondage.

FICKLENESS. See *laulya*, *loluptva*; cf. *dhairya*.

FIRE. See *agni*, Elements, *jāthara-agni*, *vahni*, *vaishvānara*.

FIRMNESS. See *dridhatā*.

FISH POSTURE. See *matsya-āsana*.

FOOD. See *āhāra, anna, anna-yoga*.

FOOT BENCH POSTURE. See *pāda-pītha-āsana*.

FORCE. See *bala, shakti*.

FOREHEAD. See *lalāta*.

FORM. See *mūrti, rūpa*.

FORTUNATE POSTURE. See *svastika-āsana*.

FOUNDATION. See *ādhāra, ālambana, pradhāna*.

FOURTH, a *Vedānta designation for the transcendental *Reality. See also *caturtha, turīya, turya*.

FRAGMENT, DIVINE. See *amsha*.

FREEDOM. All spiritual traditions are in agreement that the ordinary human condition is one of *bondage and that freedom resides in our authentic identity, which is variously called *Self or *Spirit. Conditional existence is governed by the iron law of cause and effect. According to *Hinduism, this is so even in the moral dimension, where our *actions and *volitions determine our future through the mechanism of *karma and *rebirth. So long as we identify with the limited *body and *mind that is called the human personality, we cannot be free. Freedom reigns beyond the *ego. Thus the spiritual traditions of India all offer means of transcending the self in favor of the universal Self (*ātman, *purusha). The Self is coessential with radical freedom and is often equated with *immortality. Upon *Self-realization, or *enlightenment, the limiting conditions of the body-mind and its environment are no longer experienced as curtailing our essential freedom. The *adept is thus able to act with utter spontaneity (*sahaja) in the world, and to experience its ordinary *pleasures and *pains, without in the least feeling diminished by it in his being. See also Liberation.

FRIENDLINESS. See *maitrī*.

FROG POSTURE. See *manduka-āsana*.

· G ·

GAHINĪNĀTHA (12th cen. CE), the *teacher of *Nivrittinātha. He lived in Maharashtra.

GAJA-KARANĪ ("elephant technique"), also called *gaja-karinī* in the *Hatha-Ratna-Āvalī* (1.25), is described in the *Hatha-Yoga-Pradīpikā* (2.38) as follows: Draw up the *apāna life force to the *throat and then vomit the contents of the stomach. This practice is said to bring the network of psychoenergetic currents (*nādī*) gradually under control. This technique is not listed among the "six practices" (*shat-karma*), though it obviously belongs to this set, and resembles *vamana-dhauti*.

GĀNDHĀRĀ- or GĀNDHĀRĪ-NĀDĪ ("*gāndhārā* channel"), one of the fourteen principal conduits (*nādī) of the life force (*prāna) circulating in the *body. It commences at the "bulb" (*kanda) and extends to the left eye or, as the *Darshana-Upanishad (4.22) insists, to the right eye. The *Siddha-Siddhānta-Paddhati (1.67) gives both ears as its termination point. Its position is generally given as being behind the *idā-nādī, but according to the *Var-āha-Upanishad (5.26), it runs between the central channel (*sushumnā-nādī) and the *sarasvatī-nādī.

GANDHI, MOHANDAS KARANCHAND (1869–1948), known as Mahatma ("Great Soul") Gandhi, Indian nationalist and spiritual leader. A lawyer by profession, while living in India he developed satyā-graha (lit. "devotion to truth"), a means of applying political pressure through nonviolent passive resistance. Returning to his homeland in 1914, he played an instrumental role in achieving India's political independence. He was an exemplary practitioner of *karma-yoga.

GANESHA-GĪTĀ ("Ganesha's Song"), part of what some scholars call the "pseudo-Gītā literature." It celebrates the elephant-headed, pot-bellied god Ganesha ("Lord of the Hosts"), who is widely invoked as the remover of *obstacles, as the supreme Godhead. It prescribes a *Tantric type of *Yoga for his *worship. The text consists of 414 stanzas distributed over eleven chapters that form a part of the latter portion of the Ganesha-Purāna. Most of the verses are identical with those of the *Bhagavad-Gītā, though the author omits principal verses focusing on the worship of *Krishna. This compilation, composed some time between 900 and 1300 CE, has a commentary by Nīlakantha (ca. 1700 CE), which contains many references to Yoga.

GARBHA ("womb" or "seed"). See agar-bha-prānāyama, sagarbha-prānāyāma, nir-garbha-prānāyāma.

GARIMAN ("heaviness"), the power to make oneself physically heavy at will; one of the classic paranormal powers (*siddhi) ascribed to accomplished *yogins.

GARUDA, or GARUTMAN; described in the *Vedas as *Vishnu's mount, half eagle, half human. Traditionally, Garuda represents the sacred *Vedic utterances by which the spiritual aspirant can rise to the highest realms of *existence. According to the ancient *Shata-Patha-Brāhmana (6.7.2.6), Garuda is a personification of courage. Symbolically, this mythological being represents the *life force without which neither the priests nor the *yogins can accomplish the exacting task of the *ritual of

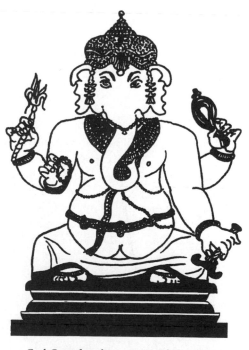

God **Ganesha**, the remover of obstacles

*concentration and *meditation. Vedic lore remembers him as the mighty being who succeeded in stealing the ambrosia (*soma) bestowing immortality.

GARUDA-ĀSANA (garudāsana, "eagle posture"), described in the *Gheranda-Samhitā (2.37) as follows: Pressing the thighs against the ground, one should keep the *body steady by placing the hands on one's knees. Modern textbooks explain this posture (*āsana) differently: One should stand upright on one leg, wrapping the other leg around the outstretched one. The arms are raised together in front of the body till they are parallel to the ground. Then one should bend them at the elbows and wrap one forearm around the other.

GATE, BODILY. See dvāra.

GATE OF HELL. See nāraka-dvāra.

GAUDA ABHINANDA (Kashmir, early 10th cen. CE), the author of the *Laghu-Yoga-Vāsishtha. He is also credited with the authorship of the *Yoga-Vāsishtha-Sāra, and some scholars even think that he composed the longer *Yoga-Vāsishtha as well, but this seems unlikely.

GAUDAPĀDA, the author of the *Māndūkya-Kārikā, an early exposition of the metaphysics of *Advaita Vedānta. Often accused of having been a crypto-Buddhist, Gaudapāda's own testimony (4.99) is that his view is by no means identical with that of the *Buddha. According to tradition, he was the teacher of Govinda, *Shankara's preceptor. Gaudapāda's Kārikā is of interest to *Yoga researchers because it introduces the "intangible Yoga" (*asparsha-yoga).

GĀYATRĪ ("hymnal," from the root gai, "to sing" or "chant"), the most famous

तत् सवितुर् वरेण्यं
भर्गो देवस्य धीमहि
धियो यो नः प्रचोदयात् ॥

Gāyatrī-mantra

*mantra of *Hinduism, which has been recited daily since ancient *Vedic times. The word also refers to the specific meter in which this mantra is composed. According to the *Rig-Veda (3.62.10), it runs as follows: tat savitur varenyam bhargo devasya dhīmahi dhiyo yo nah pracodayāt, "Let us contemplate that beautiful splendor of the divine Savitri [the solar God], that he may inspire our visions." This mantra is often prefixed with bhūr bhuvar svar, referring to the three realms; *Earth, midregion (or astral plane), and *heaven. The *recitation of this *mantra was early on assimilated into the *Yoga tradition. See also ajapa-mantra.

GAZE. See drishti.

GENEROSITY. See dāna.

GENITAL CONTROL. See upastha-nigraha.

GENITALS. See anga, linga, medhra, upastha, yoni.

GESTURE. See mudrā.

GHANTĀ or GHANTIKĀ ("bell" or "alligator"), an esoteric structure of the *body, mentioned in some texts as being situated at the *throat. In most contexts it would seem to correspond to the uvula. See also tālu-cakra.

GHATA-AVASTHĀ (gatāvasthā, "state of the pot"), the second of the four stages (*avasthā) mentioned in some *hatha-yoga texts. It is defined in the *Shiva-Samhitā (3.56) as that stage in which the inbreath (*prāna), the outbreath (*apāna), the mystic sound (*nāda), the "seed" (*bindu), the individuated self (*jīva) and the transcendental *Self are all united. According to the *Hatha-Yoga-Pradīpikā (4.73), this coincides with the piercing of the "knot of *Vishnu" (*vishnu-granthi).

GHATASTHA-YOGA ("pot-based Yoga"), the designation given to *hatha-yoga in the *Gheranda-Samhitā (1.9). The "pot" (ghata) is the *body, which has to be matured in the *fire of *Yoga.

GHATIKĀ, a period of twenty-four minutes. See also muhūrta.

GHERANDA-SAMHITĀ ("Gheranda's Compendium"), a late seventeenth-century manual on *hatha-yoga consisting of 351 stanzas distributed over seven chapters. It counts among the three classic scriptures of this school of *Yoga, and the techniques outlined in this tract form the basis of much of contemporary Yoga practice. The teachings are presented in the form of a dialogue between the sage Gheranda, about whom nothing is known, and his disciple Canda Kāpāli. This *Vaishnava work is modeled on the *Hatha-Yoga-Pradīpikā, and some verses correspond verbatim to that manual.

Gheranda teaches a sevenfold discipline (*sapta-sādhana) and describes no fewer than thirty-two postures (*āsana) and twenty-five "seals" (*mudrā). The most original part of his work is the extensive treatment of the various purification techniques (*shodhana). He also proposes an interesting classification of the phenomenon of *ecstasy (*samādhi). There are a number of commentaries on this text.

GHODACOLIN, mentioned in the *Hatha-Yoga-Pradīpikā (1.8) as a teacher of *hatha-yoga.

GHŪRNI ("swaying") in Kashmiri *Shaivism, the realization of the ever-present ultimate *Being; the high-energy state of all-pervasiveness in which the *adept experiences himself or herself as absolutely one with everything.

GIRDLE, YOGIC. See yoga-kaksha.

GĪTĀ ("Song"). See Avadhūta-Gītā, Bhagavad-Gītā, Ganesha-Gītā, Īshvara-Gītā, Uddhāva-Gītā.

GĪTĀ-GOVINDA ("Song of Govinda"), an artful composition by the twelfth-century poet Jayadeva. It celebrates the love play between the God-man *Krishna and his favorite shepherdess, *Rādhā; in its strong erotic overtones it resembles the most daring medieval Christian writings on bridal mysticism. It is an allegory of the love (*bhakti) between the *Divine and the human psyche striving for union with the ultimate Lover.

GITANANDA GIRI, SWAMI (1906–1993). The son of a Sindhi father and an Irish mother, he went to England at the age of sixteen and spent most of his professional life as a physician in the West, holding many posts with the World Health Organization. Upon returning to India in 1968, he founded the Ananda Ashram in Pondicherry, Tamil Nadu, which now has seventy-five centers around the world. Apart from training thousands of Western Yoga students, he was also a leading cultural figure in South India. The Kambliswamy Yoga and Cultural Arts Program launched by him has provided training in Yoga and classical dance and music for over 20,000

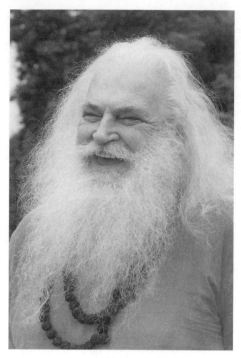

Swami **Gitananda** Giri

village children. Swami Gitananda Giri also wrote twenty-five books and published the monthly magazine *Yoga Life* for a quarter of a century.

GLADNESS. See *mudita, saumanasya*.

GO ("cow"), in the *Rig-Veda*, denotes both "bull" (when in the masculine case) and "cow" (when in the feminine case), the *Vedic people's most prized material possession. The word also stood for "cow's milk," sacred "speech," the "earth," and a "ray" of light. Additionally, when used in the plural, it could signify the stars. Much later, in the literature of *hatha-yoga*, the term acquired an esoteric meaning, referring to the *tongue. "Milking" the tongue is an important preparatory practice for the *khecarī-mudrā*. See also Govinda.

GOD. See Absolute, Being, *deva*, Divine, *īsh, īshvara*, Reality.

GODDESS. See *devī, shakti*.

GO-MUKHA-ĀSANA (*gomukhāsana*, "cow-muzzle posture"), described in the *Gheranda-Samhitā* (2.16) as follows: Place one's feet on the ground with the heels crossed beneath the buttocks. The *body should be kept steady so as to resemble a cow's muzzle. In many other texts we find this description: Place the right ankle next to the left buttock and the other ankle similarly next to the right buttock. Modern manuals add that one should reach over one's shoulders with one arm and clasp one's hands.

GOOD. See *dharma, punya*; cf. *adharma, pāpa*.

GOPA ("shepherd"), a male devotee of *Krishna. See also *gopī*.

GOPĪ ("shepherdess"). Medieval works such as the *Bhagavata-Purāna* and the *Gītā-Govinda* point to the great love between the God-man *Krishna and the love-sick shepherdesses of Vrindavāna (Brindavan) as an example of the intensity of passion necessary in the *Yoga of devotion (*bhakti-yoga*). The *gopīs* had become so distracted by Krishna that they promptly forgot about their husbands and families whenever they heard his magical flute play. See also *gopa*.

GOPĪCANDRA, an eleventh-century king of Bengal whose sensational abdication and conversion to the *Nātha cult is remembered in numerous legends and poems. This event is most articulately presented in the cyclic Hindi poem *Manikcandra Rājar Gan* ("The Song of King Manik Candra").

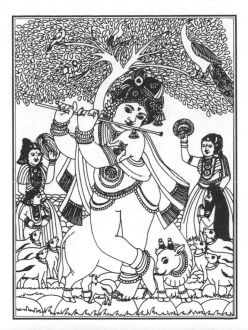

Lord Krishna enchanting the shepherdesses (*gopī*) with his flute playing

GORAKH, Hindi for *Goraksha.

GORAKH-BODH ("Illumination of Gorakh"), an archaic Hindi text, possibly dating from the twelfth century CE. It consists of a presumably fictitious dialogue between *Goraksha and his teacher *Matsyendra. Its thirty-three verses deal with such diverse topics as the life of the *avadhūta*, the concept of the void (*shūnya*), the mystic sound (*nāda*), the six esoteric bodily centers (*cakra*), the "unrecited recitation" (*ajapa-japa*), which is the *ajapa-mantra*, and the doctrine of spontaneity (*sahaja*).

GORAKH-UPANISHAD, an old text of the *Nātha sect. It is composed in mixed Hindusthani and Rajasthani and speaks of the lifestyle of the *avadhūta*, the doctrine of *kula* and *akula*, and the eight "limbs" (*anga*) of *Yoga.

GORAKSHA or **GORAKSHANĀTHA** (Hindi: Gorakhnāth; prob. 9th or 10th cen. CE), the best-known and certainly one of the greatest masters of *hatha-yoga*; appears to have been a native of the Punjab. He is acclaimed by some as the first writer of Hindi or Punjabi prose and is credited with the authorship of numerous works, including the *Goraksha-Samhitā*, the *Amaraugha-Prabodha*, the *Jnātā-Amrita-Shāstra*, and the *Siddha Siddhānta-Paddhati*. Folklore gives varying accounts of Goraksha's origins, but according to traditions in Assam, he belonged to the weaver caste. Most sources are agreed that he renounced the world at an early age and traveled widely as a miracle worker and *teacher. In many parts of Northern India he still commands respect and veneration as a perfected adept (*siddha*) and even as a *deity. He was made the patron saint of Gorkha and was deified early on, his principal shrine being in Gorakhpur. Although the Tibetan sources speak of him as a *Buddhist magician, the works ascribed to him and his school have a distinct leaning toward *Shaivism. Goraksha's place of death is unknown. The several accounts of his spiritual lineage unanimously position him after *Ādinātha (who must be identified with *Shiva) and *Matsyendra.

According to some authorities, *goraksha* and *matsyendra* are appellations given to initiates of a certain level of spiritual attainment. While this may be correct, there is no reason to doubt the historicity of either personage. The title *goraksha* means literally "cow protector," and it may refer to someone who has achieved control over the tongue—both in the sense of mastery of *speech and mastery of the technique of *khecarī-mudrā*, which involves the "swallowing" of the tongue.

Goraksha was one of the luminaries of the *Nātha sect, though his name is

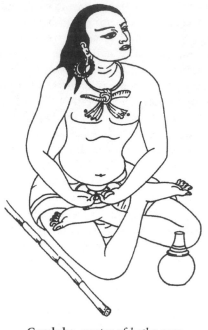

Goraksha, master of *hatha-yoga*

GORAKSHA-ĀSANA (*gorakshāsana*, "Goraksha's posture"), described in the **Gheranda-Samhitā* (2.24f.) thus: Place the upturned feet between the knees and the thighs, covering carefully the heels with both outstretched hands, while contracting the throat (**kantha-samkoca*) and fixing the gaze (**drishti*) upon the tip of the **nose. In the **Hatha-Yoga-Pradīpikā* (1.54), however, this posture is identified with the **bhadra-āsana.

GORAKSHA-BHUJANGA ("Goraksha's Serpent"), a relatively late **hatha-yoga* tract consisting of nine stanzas in praise of **Goraksha, written by Lakshmidhāra.

GORAKSHA-PADDHATI ("Goraksha's Tracks"), also known as the **Goraksha-Samhitā* ("Goraksha's Compendium"); one of the many works ascribed to **Goraksha. A good many of its 202 stanzas are found in other texts of **hatha-yoga*, and its probable date is the twelfth or thirteenth century CE. It expounds a sixfold **path (**shad-anga-yoga*) and provides detailed descriptions of the main concepts of esoteric **anatomy. It also contains instructions for the arousal of the "serpent power" (**kundalinī-shakti*). Great emphasis is placed on the recitation of the **pranava*, i.e., the sacred monosyllable **om.

GORAKSHA-SAMHITĀ ("Goraksha's Compendium"), another name for the **Goraksha-Paddhati*; also the title of a work on **alchemy ascribed to **Goraksha.

GORAKSHA-SHATAKA ("Goraksha's Century [of Verses]"), a tract comprising 101 stanzas; apparently a fragment of the **Goraksha-Paddhati.

GORAKSHA - SIDDHĀNTA - SAMGRAHA ("Collection of Goraksha's Doctrines"),

equally associated with the **Kānphata sect, which he is traditionally said to have founded. The probable historical relationship between Goraksha and **Matsyendra has been embroidered in numerous legends that depict both teachers as highly accomplished thaumaturgists. Goraksha appears to have modified his **guru's more **Tantric teachings without, however, abandoning that tradition. There is some truth in Mohan Singh's (1937) observation that the teachings of Goraksha are to be searched for not in the **hatha-yoga* scriptures but in the **Samnyāsa-Upanishads* that extol the ideal of **renunciation. Nevertheless, even if Goraksha cannot be considered as the originator of **hatha-yoga* as we know it from such works as the **Hatha-Yoga-Pradīpikā* and other earlier texts, there can be no doubt that he was instrumental in the development of this branch of **Yoga.

an eighteenth-century work that, as the title suggests, draws on earlier *hatha-yoga scriptures, some fifty in all.

GORAKSHA-VACANA-SAMGRAHA ("Collection of Goraksha's Sayings"), an anonymous work of 164 stanzas with a short appendix of eight verses, perhaps authored in the eighteenth century. It opens with the statement that *Reality transcends both dualism (*dvaita) and nondualism (*advaita). It teaches a sixfold *path entailing the awakening of the "serpent power" (*kundalini-shakti) primarily through the *recitation of the sacred syllable *om combined with *breath control and the ten seals (*mudrā) of *hatha-yoga. Several verses (150ff.) describe the marks of a radical renouncer (*avadhūta).

GORAKSHA-VIJAYA ("Goraksha's Victory"), a work on the legendary exploits of master *Goraksha that to this day is sung in ballad form throughout Northern India.

GOVINDA ("Cow Finder"), one of the epithets of *Krishna. In Sanskrit, the word *go ("cow") also stands for sacred treasure, the philosopher's stone, a usage already known to the ancient seers of the *Rig-Veda.

GRACE. See anugraha, kripā, prasāda.

GRACIOUSNESS. See mādhurya.

GRAHA ("grasper"), planet. The planets were traditionally thought to shape or "seize" the *destiny of human beings and whole nations. In addition to the two lights—sun and moon—Hindu *astrology recognizes seven "planets": Mercury, Venus, Mars, Jupiter, Saturn, and the two lunar nodes (known as Rāhu and Ketu respectively). The word graha is applied especially to Rāhu, who seizes and eclipses the sun and the moon.

GRAHANA ("grasping"), in *Classical Yoga, the process of cognition, especially sensory perception. See also grahītri, grāhya, pramāna.

GRAHĪTRI ("grasper"), the cognizing or perceiving subject. See also grahana, grāhya, pramāna.

GRĀHYA ("to be grasped"), the *object of cognition or perception. See also grahana, grahītri, pramāna, vishaya.

GRANTHA ("that which is knotted" or "that which is held together by a knot"), the typical palm leaf manuscript on which India's sacred and other texts have been written for countless generations. In the broader sense, grantha means "book."

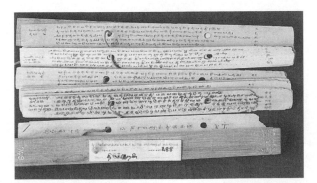

Grantha (palm leaf manuscript) of the Tirukkural

109

Spiritual traditions generally deem mere book learning barren in comparison to firsthand experience. Even though the *Yoga tradition has developed an extensive literature expounding sophisticated doctrines, it has never lost sight of the importance of personal commitment and actual practice. The *Mahābhārata (12.293.25) epitomizes this orientation: "He who does not know the meaning of a book carries only a burden; but he who knows the reality behind a book's meaning, for him the teaching of that book is not in vain." Some schools of *Yoga, however, are positively antispeculative and decry all forms of learning. This approach is found, for instance, among the followers of the *Sahajiyā movement. See also *pandita, shāstra*.

GRANTHI ("knot"). Early on the ancient *Chāndogya-Upanishad (7.26.2) speaks of the "knots" from which those who know the traditional teachings (*smriti) are released. The *Katha-Upanishad (6.15), again, states that "when all the knots of the *heart here [in the *body] are cut, then a mortal becomes immortal." In this usage, "knot" generally stands for "*desire" or, perhaps, "*doubt," which must be removed before *Self-realization can occur.

Later traditions know of three knots, collectively referred to as the *tri-granthi* ("triple knot"): "Brahma's knot" (*brahma-granthi*), "Vishnu's knot" (*vishnu-granthi*), and "Rudra's knot" (*rudra-granthi*). They are thought to be located at the *heart, the *throat, and the spot between the *eyebrows respectively, though according to some authorities their respective locations are the base center (*mūlādhāra-cakra), the heart lotus (*hrit-padma*), and the "command center" (*ājnā-cakra) in the *head.

These knots are blockages in the axial current (*sushumnā-nādī) and prevent the "serpent power" (*kundalinī-shakti) from ascending to the crown center (*sahasrāra-cakra). The *Yoga-Shikhā-Upanishad (1.113–14) compares their being pierced by the *kundalinī to the piercing of the joints of a bamboo stick by means of a heated iron rod. This process is also known as *vedhaka-traya-yoga* ("threefold piercing Yoga") and *shat-cakra-bheda*.

GRASANA ("swallowing"), the astronomical phenomenon of the eclipse; also, the eclipse of the internal *sun and *moon.

GREAT (adjective). See *mahā*.

GREAT (noun). See *mahat*.

GREED. See *lobha*.

GRIEF. See *shoka*.

GRIHASTHA or GRIHIN ("householder"). That *Yoga is not exclusively for ascetics who retire to the forest or mountain cave is borne out, for instance, by the *Shiva-Samhitā (5.186), which promises success to the householder who follows the methods outlined in that text. This is the great ideal of the Yoga of action (*karma-yoga), first announced in the *Bhagavad-Gītā. Cf. *samnyāsin*.

GUHĀ ("cave"). In the *Upanishads, the *Self (*ātman) is said to lie hidden in the cave of the *heart. This idea goes back to early *Vedic times. See also *hrid-ākāsha*.

GUHYA ("hidden" or "secret"), the status of the *Self hidden in the *heart. Thus in the *Katha-Upanishad (1.2.12), the *Divine is said to be concealed (*gūdha*), "stationed in the cave" (*guhā-hita*). Only the sage who leaves behind excitement (*harsha) and grief (*shoka) can behold it. See also Mystery, Secret.

GUHYĀVĀSI SIDDHA, a seventh-century *adept of Central India who spread the teachings of *Shaiva Siddhānta; also, one of the many epithets of *Shiva as a cave-dwelling (guha-āvāsin) ascetic.

GUILT. See kilbisha.

GUNA ("strand" or "quality"). This word has a great many connotations. Its two most common and connected usages are "quality" and "constituent." In this sense, the term belongs to the technical vocabulary of the *Yoga and *Sāmkhya traditions, where it refers to the well-known triad of forces—*sattva, *rajas, and *tamas—that are thought to be the principal building blocks of *nature. The origin of the guna doctrine is obscure, though the Dutch scholar J. A. B. van Buitenen (1957) has speculated that it may be linked with the archaic *Atharva-Veda (10.8.43), which speaks of the lotus flower with nine *gates, meaning the human *body, covered with three "strands." Van Buitenen has shown that in its earliest conception this doctrine sought to explain the psychocosmological *evolution of the higher *mind (called *buddhi) into the lower mind (*manas), the senses (*indriya), and the material elements (*bhūta).

*Patanjali, in his *Yoga-Sūtra (2.15), pictures these three types of fundamental force—comparable perhaps to the energy quanta of modern physics—as being in continual conflict with each other. As a result of this inherent tension between them, they create the different levels (*parvan) of existence. The declared goal of Patanjali's *Classical Yoga is to bring about the "involution" (*pratiprasava) of the gunas, that is, their resorption into the transcendental matrix of nature (*prakriti), at least on the personal, microcosmic level.

According to the *Bhagavad-Gītā (13.21), the gunas are "born of nature" (prakriti-ja), and they bind the individuated or embodying self (*dehin) to a particular body (*deha). In the *Mahābhārata (12.301.15), *nature is said to unfold the gunas a hundredfold or a thousandfold through its *desire and free will and for the sake of cosmic *play. *Patanjali, on the other hand, appears to think of the gunas as three types of force or energy whose existence can be deduced from the behavior patterns (*shīla) of nature. From the *Yoga-Bhashya (2.18), the oldest extant commentary on Patanjali's aphorisms, we learn that (1) although the gunas are distinct, (2) they are nonetheless interdependent and (3) in combination create the phenomenal *cosmos, wherefore (4) everything must be regarded as a "synergization" of these three factors. It was not until *Vijnāna Bhikshu's voluminous *Yoga-Vārttika (2.18), composed in the sixteenth century CE, that the gunas were conceived as substances existing in infinite numbers and producing the multiple phenomena of the material and the immaterial universe.

The characteristics (*shīla) of the gunas are often described. Thus *Patanjali (*Yoga-Sūtra, 2.18) mentions their respective disposition toward brightness (*prakāsha), activity (*kriyā), and inertia (*sthiti). Other authorities are more explicit but generally emphasize the psychological aspects. See also nirguna, saguna, tattva.

GUNA-ATĪTA (gunātīta, "transcending the qualities"), the condition of radical *freedom from *nature; also, the person thus free. As the *Bhagavad-Gītā (14.22ff.) puts it, such a person neither rejects nor pines for the manifestations of the three *gunas but remains the same (*sama) in *pleasure and *sorrow, honor and disgrace, etc. In other words, the liberated being is thought to be beyond the qualities of nature, or *nirguna.

GUPTA-ĀSANA (guptāsana, "concealed posture"), described in the *Gheranda-Samhitā (2.2) thus: Conceal the feet between one's knees and thighs and then place the buttocks on one's feet. See also siddha-āsana.

GURU ("weighty one"). In contrast to most of the hybrid forms of *Yoga taught in the Western world, traditional Yoga is characterized by an intense teacher-disciple relationship that is thought to extend even beyond this lifetime. The guru, whose counsel or judgment is "weighty," is the pivot of the entire initiatory structure of Yoga. The following stanzas from the *Shiva-Samhitā (3.11; 13f.) illustrate the superlative importance of the guru's role in practically all schools.

[Only] the *knowledge imparted through the guru's mouth is productive [of *liberation]; otherwise it is fruitless, weak, and the cause of much affliction.
There is no doubt that the guru is one's father; the guru is one's mother; the guru is *God. Therefore he should be served by all in deed, *speech, and thought.
By the guru's favor (*prasāda) everything auspicious for oneself is obtained.

Similarly, the *Hatha-Yoga-Pradīpikā (4.9) declares that without the compassion (*karunā) of a true teacher (*sad-guru), the *sahaja state is difficult to attain. As the *Shiva-Purāna (7.2.15.38) states, if a *preceptor is merely "nominal," so is the *liberation that he bestows on the disciple (*shishya). The *Yoga-Kundalī-Upanishad

(3.17) compares the guru to a helmsman who assists the pupil in crossing the ocean of phenomenal existence in the boat built from his knowledge. The *Advaya-Tāraka-Upanishad (14ff.) has these verses:

The [true] teacher is well versed in the *Veda, a devotee of *Vishnu, free from envy, pure, a knower of *Yoga and intent on Yoga, and always having the nature of Yoga.
He who is equipped with *devotion to the teacher, who is especially a knower of the *Self, possessing such characteristics [as are mentioned above], is designated as a guru.
The syllable gu [signifies] darkness; the syllable ru [signifies] the destroyer of that [darkness]. By reason of [his power] to destroy darkness, he is called guru.
The guru alone is the supreme *Absolute. The guru alone is the supreme way. The guru alone is the supreme knowledge. The guru alone is the supreme resort.
The guru alone is the supreme limit. The guru alone is supreme wealth. Because he is the teacher of that [nondual *Reality], he is a guru greater than [any other] guru.

The significance of such a guru stems from his having realized the *Self. This realization represents a change in his very state of being that spontaneously communicates itself to others, even to the natural environment. The *Self-realized adept is always transmitting his native condition of *liberation, which is the true condition of all beings and things. Thus he constantly initiates others into the same realization, though they may be slow in experiencing this consciously.

Because of their flawless identification with the transcendental *Reality, such enlightened masters were traditionally approached with the utmost reverence. They were even regarded as embodiments (*vi-graha*) of the *Divine. In practice, however, only a small number of teachers alive at any given time are Self-realized. As the *Kula-Arnava-Tantra* (13.106ff.) counsels:

O *Devī, there are many *gurus* on Earth who give what is other than the *Self, but hard to find in all the worlds is the *guru* who reveals the *Self.

Many are the *gurus* who rob the *disciple of his wealth, but rare is the *guru* who removes the disciple's afflictions.

He is the [true] *guru* by whose very contact there flows the supreme bliss (**ānanda*). The intelligent man should choose such a one as his *guru* and none other.

The fact that so few *gurus* enjoy full *enlightenment has undeniably led to the occasional exploitation of credulous students. Many preceptors expected not only unquestioned *obedience but also constant *service, possibly even a hefty remuneration for this or that initiation (**dīkshā*). For instance, the *Shiva-Sam-hitā* (5.33) stipulates that one should make over all one's property and livestock to the teacher in exchange for *initiation. Already the *Maitrāyanīya-Upanishad* (7.8ff.) warns against false teachers who merely deceive the naive.

On the other side we have warnings against abandoning one's *guru*, which is thought to have dire *karmic consequences. For example, the *Saura-Purāna* (68.11), a medieval encyclopedic compilation, contains this curselike threat:

May he who deserts his teacher meet with *death. May he who discontinues [the recitation of] the *mantra* [given to him by the teacher] become poverty-stricken. May he who deserts both [teacher and *mantra*] be cast into *hell, even if he be a perfected [*adept].

One of the most heinous of *sins was to violate the preceptor's marital bed, for which the only expiation, according to the *Mahābhārata* (12.159.46f.), was *death by embracing a heated female statue of iron, or by self-castration. This capital punishment was presumably felt necessary because of the *guru-kula* system, where the disciple became part of the teacher's household (*kula*).

Particularly in medieval times, with the rise of the elaborate and often dangerous psychotechnology of *Tantrism, the guidance of a *guru* was considered absolutely essential. Perhaps partly in order to counterbalance the excessive authority traditionally granted to the *guru* and the strong trend toward the deification of spiritual teachers, some *Hindu schools began to emphasize that the real teacher is none other than the transcendental *Self. Thus the *Uddhāva-Gītā* (2.20) states: "The *Self is the teacher of [all] selves, especially of humans, because it guides one to the highest good (*shreya*) by means of *perception and *inference."

The practice of *guru-yoga* as the foundation for spiritual *transmission is alive even today. The importation of *Yoga and other similar esoteric traditions into the West has raised a number of questions, not least that of the appropriateness of spiritual discipleship and the legitimacy of spiritual authority. See also *ācārya*, Crazy adept, *upādhyāya*.

GURU-BHAKTI ("devotion to the teacher"), a requirement on all yogic *paths except (at least in theory) in the most radical schools of *sahaja-yoga*. It is sometimes listed as one of the nine constituent practices of self-restraint (**ni-yama*). The *guru* serves the *disciple as a concrete image of the ultimate *Reality, that is, his or her own higher *Self. By constantly thinking about the *guru, the disciple tunes into and indeed participates in the *guru's extraordinary state of being, which is thought to effect a gradual transformation in the disciple. The underlying idea, known in all spiritual traditions, is that one becomes what one makes the focus of one's *attention. The *Yoga-Shikhā-Upanishad (5.53) states: "There is no one greater in the three worlds [i.e., in the total universe] than the guru. It is he who grants divine knowledge (divya-jnāna) and who should be worshiped with supreme devotion (*bhakti)."

That devotion is a form of loving *attachment. Instead of being attached to ordinary things, the disciple channels all his or her emotive energies toward the *guru. This is expressed through constant service (*sevā), *meditation upon the guru, and complete obedience (shushrūshā). This process can be understood in terms of the transference phenomenon known to psychiatry, and therefore it is important that the guru should carefully monitor the disciple's spiritual maturation and ensure that he or she does not become neurotically dependent on the teacher but is truly set free. See also guru-pūjā.

GURU-CAKRA ("teacher's wheel"), a synonym for *ājnā-cakra, because it is at this psychoenergetic center in the *head that the *guru telepathically contacts the *disciple.

GURU-GĪTĀ ("Song to the Teacher"), a popular *Hindu work of 352 stanzas that forms part of the Sanatkumāra-Samhitā in the second section of the Skanda-Purāna. It is presented as a dialogue between Maheshvara (i.e., *Shiva) and his divine spouse, Pārvatī.

GURU-PŪJĀ, or GURU-PŪJANA ("worship of the teacher"); the mental or bodily worship of one's *guru, either in person or in the form of an image (*mūrti). See also guru-bhakti.

GURU-PŪRNIMĀ, a celebration in honor of one's *teacher, held annually on the full moon (pūrnimā) in July.

GURU-SEVĀ ("service for the teacher"), which is listed in the *Shiva-Samhitā (3.35) as one of the means to success in *Yoga, is fundamental to most schools of Yoga. It is a form of *guru-bhakti and a concrete way of cultivating *self-transcendence. See also ācārya-sevana, sevā.

GURU-SHUSHRŪSHĀ ("obedience to the teacher"), occasionally counted among the rules of self-restraint (*niyama), as for instance in the *Linga-Purāna (1.89.25). The word shushrūshā is the desiderative form of the root shru ("to hear") and means the "desire to listen" to the *teacher. See also Obedience.

GURU-YOGA, the spiritual discipline of submitting to the *guru's will in all matters. This practice is sometimes made into a distinct spiritual *path, involving the ceremonial worship of the *teacher or sacred articles belonging to the teacher, notably his or her sandals (*pādukā).

· H ·

HAIR plays an important role in many sacred traditions. Some *yogins* shave all their head hair as a sign of utmost *renunciation; others allow their hair to grow unchecked. Still others, imitating *Shiva, gather their long hair into locks, besmear it with mud and *ashes, or hide it under a turban. Esoteric reasons are given for all such practices. Long-haired *ascetics were already known in early *Vedic times as *keshins*. The lock of golden hair on *Krishna's left breast is known as *shrivatsa* or "fortunate beloved." It symbolizes the source of the manifest *world.

HALA-ĀSANA (*halāsana*, "plow posture"), as described in modern manuals of *hatha-yoga*, is performed by lowering one's legs from the shoulder stand (*sarvaanga-āsana*) or head stand (*shirshaāsana*) to the ground.

HAMSA, usually translated as "swan" but refers more precisely to the wild goose (*Anser indicus*), whose high flight has inspired the ancient Indians to make it the symbol of the sun and, later, of the luminous transcendental *Self (*ātman*) as well as a certain type of renouncer (*samnyāsin*) who has realized that Self.

In the scriptures of *hatha-yoga*, the word *hamsa* frequently stands for the individual self (*jīva*), especially in its aspect as the life force (*prāna*) and its external aspect, the *breath. Thus already the *Shvetāshvatara-Upanishad* (1.6) states that the *hamsa* flutters about in the *brahma-cakra*, which here means the lower nature of *God, that is, the *world. Elsewhere (3.18) this text declares that although the *hamsa* is embodied in the

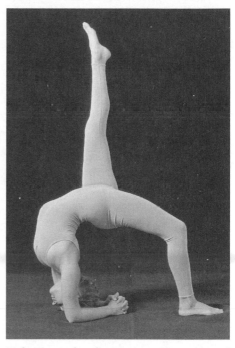

Hala-āsana, the plow posture, demonstrated by Amy Cooper. This difficult variation is often called *cakra-āsana* in contemporary manuals.

"nine-gated city" (i.e., the *body), it hovers to and fro outside the body. This may be the source of the later notion that it leaves the body (in the form of the breath) to a distance of thirty-six digits via the left and the right path (i.e., the nostrils).

In the *Yoga-Upanishads* speculations about the *hamsa* abound. For instance, according to the *Hamsa-Upanishad* (5), the *hamsa* is said to pervade all bodies as fire pervades wood or oil pervades sesame seed. The *Kaula-Jnāna-Nirnaya* (17.23), again, states that the *hamsa* is in the shape of a coil extending from the *feet to the top of the *head and is also known as *vāma, which can mean "beautiful," "crooked," and "left." In other words, it is identical with the "serpent power" (*kundalinī-shakti), the hidden spiritual energy of the *body. The *Pashupāta-Brāhmana-Upanishad (1.25), however, states that the hamsa circulates between the left arm and the right hip, whereas the *Yoga-Shikhā-Upanishad (6.35) teaches that it moves up and down within the central channel (*sushumnā-nādī) of the body.

The word hamsa is often explained as the *sound produced by the *breath, the ejection of *prāna causing the sound ha and its reentry into the *body the sound sa. This spontaneous sound is widely known as the *ajapa-mantra, ajapa-gāyatrī, or hamsa-mantra. The body is thought to recite this mantric sound automatically 21,600 times a day. The *Yoga-Shikhā-Upanishad (6.54) counsels that this sound should be recited in reverse, namely as so'ham, "I am He." This is the "wedge" (kīlaka) spoken of in the *Hamsa-Upanishad (10), by which the door to *liberation can be forced open.

HAMSA, an *incarnation of *Vishnu during the golden age, or krita-yuga. According to the *Mahābhārata epic, he instructed great sages such as *Sanaka, *Sanānanda, *Sanātana, and Sanatkumāra in *Yoga. His spiritual advice to the Sādhya-devas is contained in the so-called Hamsa-Gītā, a tract found in the twelfth book of the *Mahābhārata (chapter 288).

HAMSA-UPANISHAD ("Swan Upanishad"), one of the *Yoga-Upanishads, consisting of twenty-one short sections expounding in a very condensed fashion the theory and practice of the *hamsa. The text is in the form of a conversation between Sage *Sanatkumāra and his pupil

Gautama. The teaching propounded here is a form of *kundalinī-yoga. The text mentions eight functions of the *hamsa but actually describes twelve. These are related to the "lotus of the heart" (*hrit-padma). It also gives a description of the ten levels of manifestation of the inner sound (*nāda).

HAMSA-YOGA ("Yoga of the swan"), an expression found, for instance, in the *Nāda-Bindu-Upanishad (5) where it stands for the *recitation of the sacred syllable *om.

HĀNA ("cessation"), in *Classical Yoga, the discontinuation of the "causes of affliction" (*klesha).

HAND VESSEL POSTURE. See pāni-pātra-āsana.

HANŪMAT (in the nominative case, HANŪMĀN), the erudite and clever ruler of the monkey race, according to the *Rāmāyāna. He was instrumental in the recovery of Sītā, King *Rāma's beloved wife, who had been abducted by the demon Ravana ruling over Sri Lanka. In the *Purānas, Hanūmat is typically hailed as a son of *Shiva, and is remembered as a faithful servant of Rāma, an *incarnation of *Vishnu. The *Mahābhārata acknowledges Hanūmat as the monkey perched on *Arjuna's banner.

HAPPINESS. The pursuit of happiness is intrinsic to human life. Ordinarily, it takes the form of one's search for pleasurable (*sukha) experiences and one's simultaneous avoidance of painful (*duhkha) experiences. But from a spiritual point of view, neither sensual nor emotional nor intellectual *pleasure can ultimately satisfy a person. Only the recovery of one's true identity, as the transcendental *Self, guarantees the end of our incessant thirst (*trishnā) for ever new pleasurable experiences. In other words, we tend to look for happiness in the wrong places—either in external things or in internal states—whereas the nature of the Self is inherent *bliss (*ānanda). At least this is the teaching of most nondualist schools of *Yoga, though this idea is also implicit in dualist conceptions of the Self, as in *Classical Yoga. For why would anyone want to realize the Self, or the *Absolute, if that realization were connected with *pain or even a mediocre experience? The universal testimony of the *adepts is that recovering one's true identity is the most rewarding of all possible human aspirations (*purusha-artha). See also Joy.

HARA ("Robber" or "Remover"), an epithet of *Shiva as the destructive aspect of the *Divine. In modern terms, he is the principle of entropy.

HARI ("He who is tawny"), one of *Vishnu's or *Krishna's many names.

HARIHARĀNANDA ĀRANYA (1869–1947), a Bengali *adept who wrote, among other works, the *Yoga-Kārikā and the *Bhāsvatī commentary on the *Yoga-Sūtra. He was the founder of the Kapila Matha in Bihar, one of the last remaining schools in the tradition of *sāmkhya-yoga.

HARSHA ("excitement"), widely regarded as an undesirable emotional state; sometimes grouped with the defects (*dosha) preventing *progess on the yogic *path.

HASTI-JIHVĀ ("elephant tongue"), one of the fourteen principal channels (*nādī) of the life force (*prāna) of the *body. It is generally stated to be located to the rear of the central channel (*sushumnā-nādī) and to extend to the right *eye. According to the *Darshana-Upanishad (4.14), however, it is situated behind the *idā-nādī and extends to the big toe of the right foot. The *Yoga-Yājnavalkya (4.44) insists that it is connected to the toes of the left foot, while the *Siddha-Siddhānta-Paddhati (1.67) has it proceed to the *ears.

HASTI-NISHADANA ("elephant seat"), a sitting posture (*āsana) mentioned but not further described in the *Yoga-Bhāshya (2.46). See also nishadana.

HATHA-PĀKA ("forceful cooking"), a term used in *Kshemarāja's Pratyabhijnā-Hridaya-Sūtra (11) to denote the intense process by which the spiritual aspirant is brought to maturity. This is an excellent characterization of *sādhanā.

HATHA-RATNA-ĀVALĪ ("String of Jewels on Hatha[-Yoga]"), a work of 397 verses expanding in masterly fashion on the information contained in the *Hatha-Yoga-Pradīpikā. It appears to have at least one commentary (by *Aghorashiva Acārya). Its author, Shrīnivāsa Bhatta (mid-17th cen. CE), whose *teacher was a certain Ātmārāma, also wrote works on *Vedānta, *Nyāya, and *Tantra.

HATHA-SANKETA-CANDRIKĀ ("Moonlight on the Conventions of Hatha[-Yoga]"), an eighteenth-century work by Sundara Deva, son of Vishvanātha Deva, belonging to the Kashyapa clan (gotra) of Benares. The author quotes profusely from other works, and his text runs to some three thousand stanzas. Interestingly, this text contains no references to the *Gheranda-Samhitā.

HATHA-TATTVA-KAUMUDĪ ("Moonlight on the Principles of *Hatha[-Yoga]"), a work by Sundara Deva, who also authored the *Hatha-Sanketa-Candrikā. One known manuscript comprises 121 folios.

HATHA-YOGA ("forceful Yoga"), also called hatha-vidyā ("science of hatha"); the type of *Yoga specific to the *Kānphata sect, though this designation is also applied in general to the vast body of doctrines and practices geared toward *Self-realization by means of perfecting the *body. As such hatha-yoga is an important aspect of the pan-Indian movement of *Tantrism. The historical roots of this eclectic Yoga are varied. On the one side, it is anchored in the Tantric *Siddha cult with its *kāya-sādhana ("body cultivation"); on the other side, it was inspired by *alchemy (rasāyana). It also received vital stimuli from *Shaivism, *Shaktism (in the form of the *kundalinī doctrine), *Advaita Vedānta, and even Vajrayāna (Tantric) *Buddhism. There also appears to be a strong link with the "practice of the (inner) sound" (*nāda-anusamdhāna), as described in the *Samnyāsa-Upanishads, esoteric Vedānta works dealing with *renunciation.

The most popular teacher of hatha-yoga, who is widely celebrated as its inventor, is *Goraksha (9th or 10th cen. CE), a member of the *Nātha tradition, in which *body cultivation played a crucial role. Many Western scholars consider hatha-yoga to be the product of a period of cultural decline, and even in India it came under attack early in its development. For instance, it is clearly rejected in the *Laghu-Yoga-Vāsishtha (5.6.86, 92), which maintains that it merely leads to *pain. The most formidable critic of hatha-yoga was *Vijnāna Bhiksu, a sixteenth-century savant and *Yoga practitioner. Some of his criticisms, especially against the magical undercurrents present in this yogic approach, are undoubtedly justified. Yet we must guard ourselves against a wholesale condemnation of this tradition, which clearly has spawned some outstanding *adepts. The label "decadent Yoga" (J. H. Woods, 1966) lacks credence. Occasional excesses and aberrations notwithstanding, its body-positive orientation exemplifies the integral spirit of *Tantrism at its best. Like all *Tantric schools, it purports to be a teaching for the difficult conditions of the present dark age (*kali-yuga).

That hatha-yoga must also not be dismissed as an "easy" way is hinted at in the word hatha itself, which means "force" or "forceful." In the *Jīvan-Mukti-Viveka (1, p. 156) it is explicitly contrasted with what its author, *Vidyāranya, calls "gentle Yoga" (*mridu-yoga). He characterized the two approaches thus: One can lead an animal into its stall either by enticing it with some fresh grass or by whipping it. The first way is better; the second merely causes the animal to panic. Similarly, equanimity (*samatva) toward friend and foe is the easy method of subduing the *mind. The other, difficult method is that of breath control (*prānāyāma) and sensory inhibition (*pratyāhāra). This shows the kind of bias against hatha-yoga that is common among followers of the *Vedānta tradition, which tends toward world negation and denial of the *body.

The word hatha also has a deeper, esoteric significance. Thus its two component syllables, ha and tha, are frequently explained as standing for the microcosmic sun (*sūrya) and moon (*candra) respectively, while *yoga* is the union (*aikya*) between these two psychoenergetic principles.

Hatha-yoga is often contrasted with *raja-yoga*, the "royal" eightfold path of *Patanjali, also known as *Classical Yoga. This distinction is relatively recent, however, and perhaps was first introduced by *Vijnāna Bhiksu. From the beginning, *hatha-yoga* included the higher yogic stages of *concentration, *meditation, and *ecstasy. Yet in the *Gheranda-Samhitā (1.1), the *Hatha-Yoga-Pradīpikā, and the *Shiva-Samhitā (5.181)—the three most widely used manuals—*hatha-yoga* is presented as a "stairway" to *raja-yoga*. The *Hatha-Yoga-Pradīpikā (4.104) proffers the following metaphor: Reality (*tattva*) is the seed, *hatha-yoga* the soil, and indifference (*udāsīnya*) the water that together promote the growth of the legendary wish-fulfilling tree (*kalpa-vriksha*), which is the sublime condition of *unmanī, or the ecstatic transcendence of the *mind.

But *hatha-yoga* does not seek mere transcendental experiences. Its objective is to transform the human *body to make it a worthy vehicle for *Self-realization. *Embodiment is understood as a genuine advantage, and *enlightenment is thought to have definite bodily repercussions. As the *Shiva-Samhitā (2.49) affirms: "When the *body, obtained through *karma, becomes the means of extinction (*nirvāna), then the burden (*vahana*) of the body is fruitful, not otherwise." Or, in the words of the *Gheranda-Samhitā (1.8): "Like an unbaked urn left in water, the [bodily] vessel is ever [so soon] decayed. Baked well in the fire of Yoga, the vessel becomes purified [and enduring]." In the *Yoga-Shikhā-Upanishad (1.161ff.), we find these stanzas:

He whose body (*pinda*) is unborn and deathless is liberated in life (*jīvan-mukta*). Cattle, cocks, worms, and the like verily meet with their *death.

How can they attain *liberation by shedding the body, O Padmaja? The life force [of the *yogin] does not extend outward [but is focused in the axial channel, or *sushumnā-nādī]. How then can the shedding of the body [occur]?

The liberation that is attainable by shedding the body—is that liberation not worthless? Just as rock salt [is dissolved] in water, so Absoluteness (*brahmatva*) extends to the body [of the enlightened being].

When he reaches the [condition of] non-otherness (*ananyatā*), he is said to be liberated. [But others continue to] distinguish different bodies and organs.

The *Absolute has attained embodiment (*dehatva*), even as water becomes a bubble.

Thus the *hatha-yogin strives after *liberation by means of the creation of a "yogic body" (*yoga-deha*) immune to *disease and free from the limitations that characterize the ordinary flesh *body. The yogic body is said to be endowed with "supersenses" (*atīndriya*) and powers far beyond the capabilities of the normal person. According to the *Yoga-Shikhā-Upanishad (1.134), *hatha-yoga* removes the "dullness," or *impurity, resulting from the defects (*dosha*). This is mentioned as the second level of yogic attainment, the first being the obliteration of all diseases (*roga*). The third level is reached when the inner moon (*candra*) showers forth the "nectar of immortality" (*amrita), where-upon the body becomes youthful and the *yogin acquires a variety of paranormal powers (*siddhi).

The *body of the enlightened *adept is really the universal Body, and hence it is said that he can assume any form or shape at will. This transubstantiated body is also styled *ātivāhika-deha or "superconductive body." It is an omnipresent, luminous vehicle. This is explained in the *Yoga-Bīja (53ff.) thus:

The [*yogin's] body is like the *ether, even purer than the ether. His body is more subtle than the subtlest, coarser than any coarse [object], more insensitive [to pain, etc.] than the [most] insensitive.

The [body of] the lord of *yogins conforms to his will. It is self-sufficient, autonomous, and immortal. He entertains himself with play wheresoever in the three realms [i.e., on earth, in the "midregion," and in the celestial worlds].

The *yogin is possessed of unthinkable powers. He who has conquered the *senses can, by his own will, assume various shapes and make them vanish again.

The *adepts of hatha-yoga are thus not only *enlightened masters but also magical theurgists, considered on a par with the world creator (see Prajāpati).

Hatha-yoga's philosophy of the *body is most elaborately discussed in five of the six chapters of the *Siddha-Siddhānta-Paddhati, an early work ascribed to *Goraksha. This body-oriented approach has led to a plethora of inventions in yogic technology, notably in the areas of cleansing practices (*shodhana, *dhauti), postures (*āsana), and breath control (*prānāyāma). Generally, *hatha-yogins accept the eightfold *path

outlined by *Patanjali, though they have greatly developed some of its aspects. The *Gheranda-Samhitā, however, puts forward a sevenfold discipline (*saptasādhana). In the *Yoga-Tattva-Upanishad (24ff.), again, hatha-yoga is presented as having the following twenty "limbs" (*anga), of which the first eight coincide with those of the eightfold path: moral discipline (*yama); self-restraint (*niyama); posture (*āsana); breath control (*prāna-samyama); sense withdrawal (*pratyāhāra); concentration (*dhāranā); meditation (*dhyāna); ecstasy (*samādhi); the "great seal" (*mahā-mudrā); the "great lock" (*mahābandha); the "great piercer" (*mahāvedha); the "space-walking seal" (*khecarī-mudrā); the "water-retention lock" (*jālandhara-bandha); the "upward lock" (*uddīyāna-bandha); the "root lock" (*mūla-bandha); the "practice of the prolate *pranava" (dīrghapranava-samdhāna); listening to (i.e., study of) the teachings (*siddhāntashravana); the "vajrolī seal" (*vajrolīmudrā); the "amarolī seal" (*amarolīmudrā); and the "sahajolī seal" (*sahajolī-mudrā).

The "locks" (*bandha) and "seals" (*mudrā) are all designed to control and regulate the flow of life force (*prāna) in the *body. Mastery of the life force is fundamental to all schools of hatha-yoga. Hence *breath control (*prānāyāma) is given such prominence in the scriptures. In the *Amaraugha-Prabodha (4) hatha-yoga is virtually defined as that *Yoga which involves the regulation of the *breath. The underlying idea is that control of the breath implies control of the *mind, for the two are intimately connected.

The *hatha-yogin's primary objective is to intercept the oscillating current of the life force within his own *body. Normally, the life force circulates along the left and right channels (*nādī), maintaining the bodily activities and producing all the phenomena of ordinary *consciousness, be it awake or asleep. The *hatha-yogin seeks to focus this innate bodily force and prevent it from dissipating. He endeavors to redirect it along the central axis of the body, called *sushumnā-nādī. This is thought to arouse the body's dormant psychospiritual energy, which is known as the "serpent power" (*kundalinī-shakti), and to guide it progressively from the basal center (*mūlādhāra-cakra) to the "thousand-spoked wheel" (*sahasrāra-cakra) at the top of the *head. The crown center is considered to be the seat of the transcendental god *Shiva. The union of the feminine principle, or *goddess energy, in the form of the *kundalinī-shakti with Shiva, the masculine principle, yields the temporary state of nondual *Self-realization, or *nirvikalpa-samādhi.

This ecstatic realization is held to be more complete than the *samādhi that results from mere *meditation, as in the *Vedānta tradition, for example, because it includes the *body. In hatha-yoga and *Tantrism in general, *enlightenment is a matter of the illumination of the whole body. This approach is epitomized in the Tantric saying that *liberation (*mukti) and enjoyment (*bhukti) are perfectly compatible.

The literature of hatha-yoga is fairly extensive and barely researched. Very few texts have been edited or translated. Especially we are still in the dark about the earliest *history of this tradition. The two most popular manuals are the *Hatha-Yoga-Pradīpikā and the *Ghe-

randa-Samhitā. Other works include the *Amanaska-Yoga, *Amaranātha-Samvāda, *Amaraugha-Prabodha, *Ānanda-Samuccaya, *Brihad-Yogi-Yājnavalkya, *Carpata-Shataka, *Gorakh-Bodha, *Gorakh-Upanishad, *Goraksha-Bhujanga, *Goraksha-Paddhati, *Goraksha-Shataka, *Goraksha-Siddhānta-Samgraha, *Goraksha-Vacana-Samgraha, *Goraksha-Vijaya, *Hatha-Ratna-Āvalī, *Hatha-Samketa-Candrikā, *Hatha-Tattva-Kaumudī, *Jnana-Amrita, *Jyotsnā, *Nava-Shakti-Shatka, *Sat-Karma-Samgraha, *Shiva-Samhitā, *Shiva-Svarodaya, *Shiva-Yoga-Pradīpikā, *Yoga-Bīja, *Yoga-Kārnikā, *Yoga-Mārtanda, *Yoga-Shāstra, *Yoga-Vishaya, and *Yoga-Yajnavalkya. Possibly one of the oldest texts is the *Siddha-Siddhānta-Paddhati. In addition to these works there are also twenty-one *Yoga-Upanishads.

HATHA-YOGA-PRADĪPIKĀ ("Light on the Forceful Yoga"), the most widely used manual on *hatha-yoga. It was authored by Svātmārāma Yogin (mid-14th cen. CE). This work seeks to integrate the physical disciplines with the higher spiritual goals and practices of *rāja-yoga. Its great popularity can be gauged from the numerous Sanskrit commentaries written on it, notably those by Umāpati, Mahādeva, Rāmānanda Tīrtha, and Vrajabhūshana. The best-known commentary is the *Jyotsnā of Brahmānanda. The Hatha-Yoga-Pradīpikā comprises four chapters totaling 389 couplets, though the numbering varies from edition to edition. Some manuscripts have an additional chapter of twenty-four stanzas, but this supplement seems to belong to a later period.

Significantly, Svātmārāma does not systematize the yogic *path, but he furnishes many fundamental definitions of core techniques. He describes as many as six-

श्री:

हठयोगप्रदीपिका

ज्योत्स्नायुता

प्रथमोपदेश:

श्रीआदिनाथाय नमोऽस्तु तस्मै येनोपदिष्टा हठयोगविद्या ।
विभ्राजते प्रोन्नतराजयोगमारोढुमिच्छोरधिरोहिणीव ॥ १ ॥

श्रीगणेशाय नम: ॥

गुरुं नत्वा शिवं साक्षात्ब्रह्मानन्देन तन्यते ।
हठप्रदीपिकाज्योत्स्ना योगमार्गप्रकाशिका ॥
इदानीतनानां सुबोधार्थमस्या: सुविश्राय गोरक्षसिद्धान्तहार्दम् ।
मया मेरुशास्त्रिममुख्यामियोगात् स्फुटं कथ्यतेऽत्यन्तगूढोऽपि भाव: ॥

मुमुक्षुजनहिताथें राजयोगद्वारा कैवल्यफलां हठप्रदीपिकां विधित्सु:
परमकारुणिक: स्वात्मारामयोगीन्द्रस्तत्स्मरुह्यनिवृत्त्ये हठयोगप्रवर्तक:श्रीमदादिनाथ-
नमस्कारलक्षणं मङ्गलं तावदाचरति—श्रीआदिनाथायेत्यादिना । तस्मै श्रीआदि-
नाथाय नमोऽस्त्वित्यन्वय:। आदिश्चासौ नाथश्च आदिनाथ: सर्वेश्वर: । शिव
इत्यर्थ: । श्रीमानादिनाथ: तस्मै श्रीमदादिनाथाय । श्रीशब्द आदित्यस्य स:

Opening page of the printed Sanskrit text of the *Hatha-Yoga-Pradīpikā* with the *Jyotsnā* commentary

teen postures (*āsana), most of them variations of the cross-legged sitting posture. For those who suffer from disorders of the bodily humors (*dosha), he prescribes the "six acts" (*shat-karma). These purificatory practices are to be engaged prior to *breath control. Svātmārāma distinguishes eight types of breath control, which he calls "retentions" (*kumbhaka). These are thought to arouse the "serpent power" (*kundalinī-shakti). This esoteric process is also aided by the ten "seals" (*mudrā), which include the three "locks" (*bandha) of the *throat, the abdomen, and the anus. However, the text also contains descriptions of the *amarolī-mudrā and *sahajolī-mudrā. A prominent feature of Svātmārāma's teaching is "worship through sound" (*nāda-upāsana) by means of which the condition of mental absorption (*laya) is achieved.

HATHA-YOGIN (masc.), or HATHA-YOGINĪ (fem.); a practitioner of the "forceful Yoga" (*hatha-yoga). In the *Hatha-Yoga-Pradīpikā (4.79), the hatha-yogin is sharply contrasted with the *rāja-yogin: "[There are those who are] only performers of *hatha[-yoga], without knowledge of *rāja-yoga. These practitioners I deem deprived of the fruit of [their] efforts." This distinction is, however, not meant to apply to all hatha-yogins.

HATRED. See dvesha, samrambha-yoga.

HAVIS, is a sacrificial oblation consisting of grain milk, butter, or *soma, which is poured into the *fire.

HEAD (Sanskrit: shīrsha, shiras, kapāla, or mūrdha) a frequent locus of *concentration. The *Bhagavad-Gītā (8.12) states that the life force (*prāna) should be driven up into the head. The *Yoga-Sūtra (3.32) speaks of a "light in the head" (mūrdha-jyotis), upon which the *yogin should focus his *attention for the practice of ecstatic "constraint" (*samyama) that yields the vision of the *adepts (*siddha-darshana). The head is also the location of several important psychoenergetic centers (*cakra): the *dvādasha-anta-, *sahasrāra-, *ājnā-, and *tālu-cakra. See also Body, Heart.

HEADSTAND. See shīrsha-āsana, viparīta-karanī, sarva-anga-āsana.

HEALTH (*ārogya), which is understood as the harmonious interaction of the three bodily humors (*dosha), is deemed desirable on all spiritual *paths, presumably because *illness has an adverse influence on one's *attention. However, it is a precondition rather than the goal of *Yoga, even *hatha-yoga. Cf. roga, vyādhi.

HEART. In the spiritual traditions of India, as elsewhere, the "heart" refers not so much to the physical organ as to a psycho-spiritual structure corresponding to the heart muscle on the material plane. This spiritual heart is celebrated by *yogins and mystics as the seat of the transcendental *Self. It is called *hrid, *hridaya, or *hrit-padma ("heart lotus"). It is often referred to as the secret "cave" (*guhā) in which the *yogin must restrain his *mind. In some schools, notably Kashmiri *Shaivism, the word hridaya applies also to the ultimate *Reality. See also anāhata-cakra, Body, Head, marman.

HEAVEN. See svarga.

HEEDLESSNESS. See pramāda.

HELL. See nāraka.

HERBS. See aushadhi.

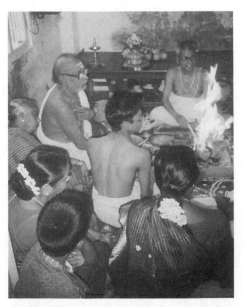

Hindu religious ceremony involving recitation from the sacred texts

HERMITAGE. See āshrama, kutira, matha.

HERO. See vīra.

HEROIC POSTURE. See vīra-āsana.

HIMSĀ ("harm" or "violence"). According to Vyāsa's *Yoga-Bhāshya (2.34), there are eighty-one types of violence depending on whether harm is done, caused to be done, or approved; whether its source is *greed, *anger, or *delusion; whether that impulse is mild, moderate, or vehement (each of which degree has again three forms of intensity). The general principle is that the very intention to harm another being is wrong and is harmful to the intender. Violence breeds violence. The ideal held high in *Yoga is thus nonviolence, or *ahimsā.

HINDU, a member or an aspect of *Hinduism.

HINDUISM, the dominant culture of India, which, in theory at least, is based on the sacred tradition of the brahmins (*brāhmana). The designation is rather problematical, since "Hindu" describes an amorphous mass of ideas, practices, institutions, and attitudes. What they have in common, however, is a shared *history reaching back to the time of the *Rig-Veda and the indigenous *Indus-Sarasvati civilization. The *wisdom and lore contained in the four *Vedic hymn "collections" (samhitā), which are collectively known as the *Veda, form the bedrock of later Hinduism.

The following eight periods can usefully be distinguished in the evolution of Hinduism: (1) The *Vedic Age (ca. ?4000–2000 BCE), epitomized by the teachings of the *Rig-Veda and the other three ancient hymnodies. (2) The Brahmanical Age (ca. 2000–1500 BCE), marked by the composition of the *Brāhmana* ritual literature. (3) The Upanishadic Age (ca. 1500–500 BCE), marked by the teachings embedded in the early *Upanishads*, the first full-fledged mystical communications on Indian soil of which we have knowledge. In the concluding phase of this era, *Buddhism and *Jainism emerged, challenging and stimulating Hinduism. (4) The Epic Age (ca. 500 BCE–200 CE), so called because of the composition and influence of the *Mahābhārata* epic, which contains the famous *Bhagavad-Gītā*, the earliest and perhaps most beautiful work on *Yoga. (5) The Classical Age (200–800 CE), characterized by the crystallization of the earlier traditions into philosophical schools and the triumph of *Advaita Vedānta. This is the period of the composition of the *Yoga-Sūtra*, the textbook of *Classical Yoga. (6) The Tantric Age (800–1500 CE), marked by the creation of a new cultural style representing a synthesis of a variety of approaches and embodied in the vast literature of the *Tantras*. This period also saw the emergence of *hatha-yoga*. (7) The Sectarian Age (1500–1700 CE), captured in the great popularity of the *bhakti* movement, which was the culmination of the monotheistic aspirations of the two great sectarian cultures of Hinduism, *Vaishnavism and *Shaivism. (8) The Modern Age (from 1700 CE), marked by the collapse of the Mughal empire and the establishment of British rule in India and, then, in 1947, India's independence. In the late nineteenth century Hinduism entered a great renaissance, which brought its teachings to many Western countries.

The conglomeration of religious cultures known as Hinduism claims today nearly 700 million adherents worldwide. It is important to know that not all Hindu schools of thought acknowledge the Vedic revelation (*shruti*). For instance, the *Tantras* purport to be a teaching for the present dark age (*kali-yuga*) in which the religious doctrines and practices of the *Veda* are no longer useful. Similarly, in South India millions of adherents of *Shaivism have replaced the four *Vedas* with the *Tirukkural*, a poetic compilation mostly dealing with ethical matters and dating approximately from the sixth century CE.

HIRANYAGARBHA ("Golden Germ"), hailed in the *Yogi-Yājnavalkya-Smriti* (as cited in the *Tattva-Vaishāradī* 1.1) as the original propounder of *Yoga. The same claim is made in the *Mahābhārata* (12.337.60). Most scholars assume that Hiranyagarbha is an entirely mythological figure. In the archaic *Rig-Veda* (10.121), he stands for the supreme lord of all beings who upholds *heaven and earth. In subsequent times, *hiranya-garbha*— "golden germ" or "golden womb"—came to designate the "first-born" entity in the evolutionary series, as taught in *Vedānta but also in some schools of *Preclassical Yoga. According to the *Mahābhārata* (12.291.17f.), *hiranya-garbha* is none other than the higher *mind, that is, the *buddhi* of the *Sāmkhya tradition or the *mahān* of the *Yoga tradition. Other synonyms are *virinca* ("extended"), *vishva-ātman* ("all-self"), *vicitra-rūpa* ("multiform"), *eka-akshara* ("single immutable" or "monosyllable"), and, in *Classical Yoga, *linga-mātra* ("pure sign").

Despite these psychocosmological connotations, however, it is likely that there was a sage called Hiranyagarbha, for a person by that name is remembered as having authored a textbook on *Yoga (*yoga-shāstra*). Thus, according to the *Ahirbudhnya-Samhitā* (12.31ff.), a work belonging to the *Pāncarātra-Vaishnava tradition,

Hiranyagarbha composed two "collections on Yoga" (*yoga-samhitā*). The *Ahirbudh-nya-Samhitā* even supplies an apparent and rather sketchy list of their contents, which appear to echo certain notions found in the *Yoga-Sūtra*.

HISTORY OF YOGA. The history of *Yoga is barely known, because of the paucity of available chronological materials. The following six phases in the unfolding of Yoga can be distinguished: (1) *Archaic or Proto-Yoga of the ancient period, which can be reconstructed from the archaeological evidence of the *Indus-Sarasvati civilization (ca. 3000–1800 BCE) and also from the descriptions in the hymns of the four *Vedic collections. (2) *Preclassical Yoga, which started with the earliest *Upanishads (ca. 1500 BCE.) expounding a form of sacrificial *mysticism based on the internalization of the *brahmanical ritual. These efforts led to the development of a rich contemplative technology involving early yogic concepts and practices based on the *Vedānta metaphysics of nondualism. (3) *Epic Yoga (ca. 500 BCE–200 CE), which evolved in the era of the middle *Upanishads and the *Mahābhārata epic. Here we witness a proliferation of schools and doctrines that for the most part continue to espouse nondualism. Yogic teachings developed in close association with *Sāmkhya ideas. Because many of these developments are recorded in the *Mahābhārata, this phase of *Preclassical Yoga can also be called *Epic Yoga. (4) *Classical Yoga (starting at the latest ca. 200 CE), which has its source in the *Yoga-Sūtra of *Patanjali and was developed over several centuries through an extensive literature of commentary. Its metaphysical foundations are no longer those of *Vedānta, but it avows a strictly dualistic interpretation

of *reality. (5) *Postclassical Yoga (ca. 200–1900 CE), which continued the nondualist teachings of *Preclassical Yoga, ignoring for the most part the dualistic philosophy of *Patanjali but making occasional use of his delineation of the eightfold path (*ashta-anga-yoga) and his fine definitions. This is the period of the *Yoga-Upanishads and the scriptures of *Tantrism and *hatha-yoga. (6) Modern Yoga (starting ca. 1900 CE), which is epitomized in the *Integral Yoga of Sri *Aurobindo and the many Western schools of *hatha-yoga. Other classificatory systems are possible.

HITĀ ("salutary"), the *good (also called shubhā); also, an early synonym for *nādī. According to the *Brihad-Āranyaka-Upanishad (2.1.19), there are 72,000 "salutary" rays or channels of the life force (*prāna) that extend from the *heart to the pericardium (puritāt). According to the Prashna-Upanishad (3.6), however, these 72,000 hitās branch off from the 101 *nādīs.

HITĀ-ICCĀ (hiteccā, "desire for the good"), the wish to promote the welfare of others—an important moral value since ancient *Vedic times. See also loka-sam-graha.

HOMA ("offering"), a ritual sacrificial oblation, sometimes counted among the practices of self-restraint (*niyama). See also yajna.

HOSPITALITY. See atithya.

HOTRA ("sacrifice"), the *Vedic sacrificial ceremony; also, the offering made by the priest (*hotri) in that ceremony.

HOTRI ("sacrificer"), the chief priest in the *Vedic sacrificial ceremony (*hotra). The term is also applied to sacrificial priests in general. They were the *yogins of the Vedic mainstream.

HOUSEHOLDER. See grihastha.

HRĪ ("modesty"), occasionally regarded as one of the practices of self-restraint (*niyama); sometimes counted among the constituents of moral discipline (*yama).

HRID ("heart"), the physical *heart or chest cavity; also, the spiritual organ so called, as well as the transcendental *Self.

HRID-ĀKĀSHA ("heart ether"), the esoteric, radiant space of the *heart, where the transcendental *Self can be experienced. See also guhā, hrit-padma.

HRIDAYA ("heart"), a synonym for *hrid. The three syllables of this word—hri, da, and ya—are explained in the *Brihad-Āranyaka-Upanishad (5.3.1) as conveying the ideas of bringing a gift, receiving a gift, and going to heaven. See also Heart.

HRIDAYA-GRANTHI ("heart knot"), sometimes used as a synonym for *vishnu-granthi. See also granthi.

HRID-DHAUTI ("heart cleansing"), a *purification technique of *hatha-yoga, described in the *Gheranda-Samhitā (1.36ff.). It consists of three practices: *danda-dhauti ("cleansing by means of a stick"), *vamana-dhauti ("cleansing by vomiting"), and *vāso-dhauti ("cleansing by means of a piece of cloth"). See also dhauti.

HRISHĪKESHA ("He whose hair bristles"), an epithet of *Krishna, who is ever in a sublime state of *ecstasy, the *bliss of which makes his *hair stand on end.

HRIT-PADMA ("heart lotus"), also called hridaya-pundarika or *anāhata-cakra; the *heart in the spiritual sense. According to the *Goraksha-Paddhati (2.68), it is "radiant like lightning." It is described as having eight or twelve petals.

HUMILITY. See amānitva; cf. Pride.

HUMMING SOUND. See pranava.

HUMORS. See dhatu.

HUNGER. See kshudhā.

HUTA or HUTI ("sacrifice"), a synonym for *yajna.

HYPNOSIS. Some *Yoga researchers, notably Sigurd Lindquist (1932), have argued that many of the yogic practices, including the postures (*āsana) but especially the higher meditative and *ecstatic states, are based on self-hypnosis. This explanation is, however, reductionistic and not borne out by a careful study of the yogic technology and literature. Besides, the yogic authorities themselves carefully distinguish between hypnosis and higher spiritual phenomena. As a case of hypnosis, the *Mahābhārata (13.40f.), for instance, relates the story of Devasharman, who asked his disciple Vipula to protect his wife Ruci from the charms of *Indra while he, Devasharman, was on a *pilgrimage. Vipula promptly gazed into Ruci's *eyes and transferred his *mind into her *body, rendering her immobile. When Indra, enamored with her *beauty, arrived at the hermitage, Ruci was unable to respond to him, because Vipula had "bound all her *senses by the bonds of Yoga."

The condition of ecstasy (*samādhi), though it is preceded by sensory inhibition (*pratyāhāra*), does not amount to a diminished state of *consciousness. This is emphasized throughout the spiritual literature of *Hinduism as well as *Buddhism and *Jainism. See also Autogenic Training, Psychology.

· I ·

I. See *ahamkāra*, Ego, *jīva*.

ICCHĀ ("will," "wish," or "desire"). See *kāma*, *shubha-icchā*.

ICCHĀ-RŪPA ("will form"), the magical ability to assume any shape whatsoever. Hindu legends are filled with stories of *yogins* who are able to drop their *body at will and take possession of another body. Thus the traditional biography of *Shankara, the famous expounder of *Advaita Vedānta, recounts how he animated the corpse of a recently deceased king in order to learn the bedroom arts, that he might win a doctrinal contest against an opponent, Mandana Mishra, which he did. See also *kāma-avasāya-vitva*, *para-deha-pravesha*.

ICCHĀ-SHAKTI ("willpower"), not ordinary willpower but, according to some schools of *Shaivism, the first of the three aspects of the divine power, the other two being *jnāna-shakti* and *kriyā-shakti*. The *icchā-shakti* is the impulse toward manifestation within the unmanifest principle of power (*shakti*). According to some schools, the supreme power (*parā-shakti*) first gives rise to the power of consciousness (*cit-shakti*) and the power of bliss (*ānanda-shakti*).

IDAM-AHAM ("This I am"), in Kashmiri *Shaivism, the second level of differentiation in the process of *world emanation

out of the *Absolute. See also *aham*, *aham-idam*.

IDĀ-NĀDĪ ("channel of comfort"), one of the three primary ducts or currents (*nādī*) of the life force (*prāna*) circulating in the human *body, according to esoteric *anatomy. It is situated to the left of the axial channel called *sushumnā-nādī*, which runs vertically from the psychoenergetic center (*cakra*) at the base of the spine to the crown of the *head. The *idā-nādī* is generally thought to commence at the "bulb" (*kanda*) and to extend to the left nostril. It coils around the central channel and is associated with the cooling energy of the internal moon (*candra*). The *Shiva-Samhitā* (2.25) curiously states that the *idā* terminates at the right nostril, but this medieval *hatha-yoga text gives divergent positions for most other esoteric structures, perhaps in order to deliberately mislead the uninitiated.

The word *idā* dates back to the *Rig-Veda* (1.40.4), where it denotes "libation" or "oblation." It is also the name of the female deity of *devotion. The word is connected with the feminine noun *id*, one of whose meanings is "comfort." Thus the technical term *idā-nādī* could be interpreted to mean "the comforting channel"— comforting because it cools the *body during the heat of the day. The *idā* current of the life force corresponds on the physical level to the parasympathetic nervous system. It must, however, not be confused with it. According to the *Hatha-Ratna-Āvalī (2.144), it is also known as candrā, shashī, vālī, gangā, and vāma. Cf. pingalā-nādī.

IDEA. See buddhi, pratyaya.

IDEALISM, PHILOSOPHICAL. This label can be applied to all those many schools of *Hindu thought that espouse the existence of an ultimate *Reality considered to be more real than the *world of phenomena. Various versions of this philosophical position can be distinguished, from the moderate nondualism (*advaita) of the early *Upanishads to the radical idealism of the *Māndūkya-Kārikā and the *Yoga-Vā-sishtha.

IDENTITY, PSYCHIC. See ātman, Self.

IDLENESS. See akarman, ālasya.

IGNORANCE. See avidyā, ajnāna.

ĪHĀ ("exertion" or "desire"), a synonym for *yatna.

IJYĀ ("sacrifice"), the offering of oblations as part of a more ritualistic *Yoga practice; sometimes counted as one of the constituent practices of self-restraint (*niyama). See also bali, Sacrifice.

ILL. See adharma, pāpa; cf. dharma, punya.

ILLNESS. See roga, vyādhi; cf. Health.

ILLUMINATION. See bodha, Enlightenment.

ILLUSION. See māyā, moha.

IMAGE. See mūrti.

IMAGINATION. The imaginative powers of the *mind play an important role in *Yoga theory and practice. It is through the imagination that we experience the *world and, according to some schools of thought, even create our particular experienced environment. Hence the *yogin is charged with carefully controlling his imaginative powers, so that he can come to realize the transcendental *Reality beyond all *illusion. See also bhāvanā, kalpanā, samkalpa.

I MAKER. See ahamkāra, Ego.

IMMORTALITY is often equated with the condition of *liberation, or *enlightenment, in which case it signifies immortality of the Spirit, or transcendental *Self. Traditions such as *hatha-yoga and *alchemy, however, aspire to bodily immortality, though here the *body is understood to be radically transformed. See also amrita.

IMPERFECTION. See dosha.

IMPURITY. See dosha, mala; cf. Purity.

INACTION. See akarman.

INATTENTION. See pramāda.

INCARNATION. See avatāra.

INCENSE. See dhūpa.

INDIVIDUALITY. See ahamkāra, Ego, jīva.

INDRA ("Ruler"), the principal *deity and ruler of the *Vedic pantheon during the most ancient period of *Hinduism. He has often been characterized as a rain god, or god of thunder and lightning. It is clear from certain hymns of the *Rig-Veda, however, that the Vedic people also saw in him a spiritual power, granting flashes of inner illumination. His name is also related to *indu* ("juice"), meaning the ambrosial fluid or *soma, as well as the esoteric moon (*candra) that is thought to ooze the precious nectar in the human *body. See also *deva*, God.

INDRIYA ("pertaining to *Indra"), the sense organs, which are the most powerful influence in the life of the ordinary mortal. As the *Agni-Purāna* (373.20) puts it succinctly: "The senses are all that which [leads to] *heaven or *hell. [A person goes] to heaven or hell, [depending on whether the senses are] restrained or active." The *Bhagavad-Gītā* (2.62f.) offers the following analysis of the play of *attention:

When a man thinks of *objects, contact with them occurs. From that contact springs desire (*kāma), and from desire anger (*krodha) is bred.
From anger comes bewilderment (*sammoha), from bewilderment [springs] disorder of the *memory, and from disorder of the memory [comes] the destruction of wisdom (*buddhi). On the destruction of *wisdom [a person] is lost.

The *Bhagavad-Gītā* (2.64f.) then recommends the following attitude:

Although moving with the senses among *objects, [the person with] a well-governed self, disjoined from passion (*rāga) and aversion (*dvesha), under the control of the *Self, approaches serenity (*prasāda).
[On reaching] serenity, there arises for him the obliteration of all *suffering. For the clear-minded, the wisdom faculty (*buddhi) is at once firmly grounded.

According to the *Sāmkhya tradition, which is widely accepted on this point by other schools, there are eleven sensory instruments. These can be arranged into three groups: (1) the cognitive senses (*jnāna-* or *buddhi-indriya*), composed of *eyes (*cakshus*), *ears (*shrotra*), *nose (*ghrāna*), *tongue (*rasa*), and skin (*tvac*); (2) the conative senses (*karma-indriya*, written *karmendriya*), composed of voice (*vāc*), hands (*pani*), *feet (*pāda*), anus (*pāyu*), and *genitals (*upastha*); and (3) the lower mind (*manas*). Although these designations suggest physical organs, the *indriyas* are rather their intrinsic capacities.

In the *Mahābhārata* (12.195.9) the five (cognitive) senses are compared to lamps set on high trees that illumine things and produce *knowledge. They entice *attention to focus on external reality rather than the *Self. Hence the *yogin is constantly counseled to practice sensory restraint (*indriya-jaya). In the *Katha-Upanishad* (3.3f.) the *body is likened to a chariot and the senses to unruly horses that need to be checked. Another popular metaphor for the process of sensory inhibition (*pratyāhāra) is that of a tortoise withdrawing its limbs. See also *bhūta*, *buddhi*, Cosmos, Evolution, *tanmātra*.

INDRIYA-JAYA ("conquest of the senses"), the capacity to control the outflowing of *attention through the sensory pathways. According to the *Yoga-Sūtra* (2.41), such mastery is one of the benefits of cultivating perfect purity (*shauca). *Patanjali also speaks of the "obedience" (*vashyatā*) of the senses as a result of the constant practice of sense withdrawal (*pratyāhāra).

INDRIYA-NIGRAHA ("sense restraint"), sometimes counted among the practices of moral discipline (*yama). It is equivalent to *pratyāhāra.

INDU-CAKRA ("wheel of the nectar"), also called *shodasha-cakra;* an esoteric psychoenergetic center (*cakra) located in the *head above the *manas-cakra. It is generally thought to have sixteen petals of moon-white color, and to be the seat of the higher mind (*buddhi). See also Indra.

INDUS-SARASVATI CIVILIZATION, more commonly known as the Indus or Harappan civilization, was discovered in the early 1920s. It existed first along the Indus River in the Punjab (now Pakistan) and, after a great natural catastrophe occurring around 1900 BCE, shifted eastward to the Ganges River. In its Indus phase, it extended for over 1,000 miles from north to south. Its origins are obscure. The large, well-organized cities of Harappa and Mohenjo Daro, which have been excavated, appear to date from the middle of the third millennium BCE, though they show a remarkable cultural continuity with the town of Mehrgarh in Afghanistan, dated back to 6500 BCE.

As revealed by satellite photography, most of the settlements can be found in the long-dry bed of the Sarasvati River, which is hailed in the *Rig-Veda as the mightiest river of India. The new geological and archaeological evidence seriously challenges the long-standing model of the *Aryan invasion, which hitherto has been used to explain the collapse of the big cities of the Indus. Scholars now increasingly believe that the Vedic Aryans came to India long before the advent of the urban culture of the Indus and that they were in fact its creators.

Since the pictographic Indus script has not yet been deciphered, it is difficult to get a clear idea of the religious world of this great civilization. However, the archaelogical evidence suggests that the Indus-Sarasvati people were, like the later *Hin-

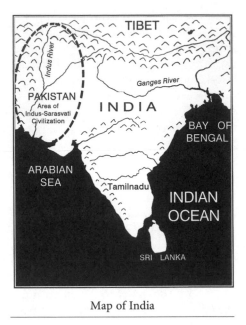

Map of India

dus, very pollution conscious and engaged in a variety of rituals of *purification. Particularly remarkable is the absence of weapons in the more than sixty excavated sites. This could point to a strict morality of nonharming (*ahimsā), which would be extraordinary for that historical period. Apart from architectural clues, there are above all the over 2,000 terra-cotta (steatite) seals featuring inscriptions and artistic motifs that convey some idea of the mythological and religious notions current in that civilization.

One seal, dubbed the *pashupati* seal, in particular has attracted the attention of *Yoga researchers. It shows a horned deity seated cross-legged in the fashion of the later *yogins, surrounded by animals. The figure has been identified as *Shiva in his role as *Pashupati, or Lord of Beasts.

Other evidence, suggesting an early Goddess cult and fertility beliefs, indicates a remarkable continuity between the

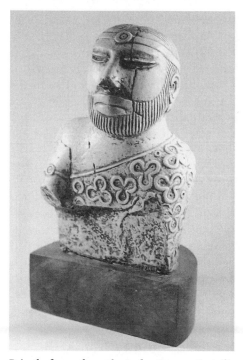

Priestly figure from the **Indus-Sarasvati** civilization

Indus-Sarasvati civilization and later *Hinduism.

If we regard the Indus-Sarasvati civilization as essentially Vedic in character, it is entirely plausible to assume that some of the constituent elements of *Yoga should have derived from that civilization. Yoga has many roots, however, and certainly its emergence as a full-fledged tradition did not occur until about 500 BCE. See also Archaic Yoga, Preclassical Yoga.

INFERENCE. See *anumāna.*

INFINITE. See Ananta.

INITIATION. See *abhisheka, dīkshā.*

INNER INSTRUMENT. See *antahkarana.*

INSTABILITY. See *anavasthitatva.*

INTEGRAL YOGA. See *pūrna-yoga.*

INTELLECT. See *buddhi, manas,* Mind.

INTERCOURSE, SEXUAL. See *maithunā,* Sexuality.

INTUITION, called "inborn knowledge" (*sahaja-jnāna*) or "inner knowledge" (*antar-jnāna*) in Sanskrit. At the highest level, it is the immediate certainty of one's essential nature, which is the *Self. See also Consciousness, Knowledge.

ĪPSĀ ("desire"), a synonym for *kāma.*

ĪRSHYĀ ("jealousy"), a synonym for *mātsarya.*

ĪSH, ĪSHA, ĪSHANA ("ruler"). The theistic schools of *Hinduism often describe the *Divine as the ruler of the *world and the individual body-mind. One of the most beautiful expressions of this idea is found in the *Īsha-Upanishad,* a work predating the common era. See also *īshvara.*

ĪSHITRITVA, or ĪSHITVA ("lordship"); one of the classic paranormal powers (*siddhi*) granting the accomplished *adept sovereignty over *nature. According to the *Yoga-Bhāshya* (3.45), this power allows the adept to create, rearrange, or even destroy the material elements (*bhūta*).

ISHTA-DEVATĀ ("chosen deity"). Since it is difficult to relate to the transcendental *Reality in abstract terms, many *Hindu practitioners choose to worship the *Divine in the form of one of the many deities (*deva*) known in *Hinduism, such as *Vishnu, *Krishna, *Shiva, or *Kālī. These are thought to be actual spiritual forces, not merely products of the religious imagination. They can be invoked and approached for grace (*prasāda*). According to the *Yoga-Sūtra* (2.44), the *yogin* can come into contact with his chosen deity especially by immersing himself into the study (*svādhyāya*) of the sacred lore.

ĪSHVARA ("foremost ruler," "lord"), a word found already in the ancient *Brihad-Āranyaka-Upanishad* (1.4.8, e.g.). In the *Vedānta-inspired schools of *Yoga it refers to the transcendental *Self as it governs the *cosmos and the individuated being. This is epitomized in the following stanza from the *Bhagavad-Gītā* (18.61): "The Lord abides in the *heart region of all beings, O *Arjuna, whirling all beings by [His] power (*māyā*), [as if they were] mounted on a machine (*yantra*)."

In the *Epic Yoga schools of the *Mahābhārata*, the *īshvara* is also referred to as the "twenty-fifth principle," since he transcends the twenty-four principles or evolutionary categories (*tattva*) of *nature. In *Classical Yoga, the *īshvara* is defined as a special *Self (*purusha*). This specialness consists in that the Lord was at no time embroiled in the *play of nature, whereas all other Selves will, at one time, have been or become caught up in the illusion of being embodied and thus bound to the mechanisms of nature. Specifically, the *īshvara* is said to be untouched by the "causes of affliction" (*klesha*), action (*karman*), action's fruition (*vipāka*), and the subconscious deposits (*āshaya*). The Lord's *freedom is eternal.

This view has led to theological difficulties, since *Patanjali also regarded the *īshvara* as the first teacher. How can an utterly transcendental *Self possibly intervene in the spatiotemporal world? In his *Yoga-Bhāshya* (1.24) *Vyāsa tries to deal with this issue. He explains the *īshvara's* teaching role in terms of the Lord's assumption of a perfect medium, which Vyāsa calls *sattva* ("beingness"). *Vācaspati Mishra compares this to the role played by an actor who nevertheless is aware that he is not identical with the character of his role. He also emphasizes that this is possible because the Lord's *sattva* is devoid of any trace of *rajas and *tamas. Vyāsa also explains that the Lord appropriated such a perfect *sattva* vehicle for the "gratification of beings" (*bhūta-anugraha*). Both exegetes further insist that the proof for this belief is to be found in the sacred scriptures, which are manifestations of that perfect *sattva*. See also *anugraha, bhagavat, prasāda*.

ĪSHVARA-GĪTĀ ("Song of the [divine] Ruler"), one of the imitations of the *Bhagavad-Gītā*. A part of the *Kūrma-Purāna* (2.1–11), it consists of eleven chapters with a total of 497 stanzas, presented as a conversation between *Shiva and a group of sages. This scripture (2.40) defines *Yoga as "one-mindedness" (*eka-cittatā*) and emphasizes the interrelation between *Yoga and wisdom (*jnāna*). Thus we find the following stanza (2.3), for instance: "*Wisdom springs from Yoga [practice]; Yoga derives from wisdom. For him who is dedicated to Yoga and wisdom, nothing is unattainable." It is through the favor (*prasāda*) of *Shiva that extinction (*nirvāna*) is reached. The spiritual *path is the eightfold Yoga (*ashta-anga-yoga*) taught by *Patanjali.

ĪSHVARA KRISHNA (prob. 4th cen. CE), the author of the *Sāmkhya-Kārikā*, which is to *Classical Samkhya what the *Yoga-Sūtra* is to *Classical Yoga.

ISHVARA-PRANIDHĀNA ("devotion to the Lord"), one of the constituents of self-restraint (*niyama*). The *Yoga-Bhāshya* (1.23) explains this practice as a special kind of love (*bhakti*) or intention (*abhidhyāna*) by which the Lord (*īshvara*) becomes inclined to favor the *yogin*. Elsewhere (2.1, 32) in this commentary, it is explained as the offering up of all *actions to the supreme *teacher, that is, the *īsh-vara, and as the renunciation (*samnyāsa*) of the fruit (*phala*) of one's actions.

ISHVARA-PŪJANA ("worship of the Lord"), sometimes counted among the practices of self-restraint (*niyama*). The *Darshana-Upanishad* (2.8) explains it as a *heart devoid of passion (*rāga*), speech not tainted by untruth, and *action free from harm (*himsā*).

· J ·

JĀDYA ("dullness"). According to the *Yoga-Shikhā-Upanishad* (1.134), the ordinary *body suffers from "dullness," or *impurity, which can be removed through the practice of *hatha-yoga. The *hatha-yogin seeks to draw the life force (*prāna*) up into the central channel (*sushumnā-nādī*), which is said to render his body lustrous. This practice also gives him the paranormal ability (*siddhi*) to move in space (*khecara*). See also *khecarī-mudrā.

JAGAT ("world"). See Cosmos, *vishva*.

JAIGĪSHAVYA, a prominent *teacher of *Epic Yoga whose views on *Sāmkhya and *Yoga are quoted several times in the *Yoga-Bhāshya (e.g., 3.18). In the *Matsya-Purāna* (180.59) he is said to have attained the state of "aloneness" (*kaivalya*) after kindling the "fire of *Yoga" by means of *meditation. His didactic conversation with Asita Devala is recorded in the *Mahābhārata (12.222.4ff.). He is also credited with the authorship of the *Dhāranā-Shāstra* ("Textbook on Concentration"), a late work more akin to *Tantrism than *Yoga.

JĀGRAT ("waking"), one of the five states (*avasthā*) of *consciousness; the ordinary *waking state, marked by a sharp awareness that has a narrow focus. By contrast, the condition of *ecstasy is characterized by suprawakefulness that has no focus because the limiting *ego is absent in it. Whereas the former type of *consciousness is inherently dis-eased, the latter is experienced as whole and indescribably blissful (*ānanda*).

JAINISM, the spiritual tradition founded by Vardhamāna Mahāvīra, an older contemporary of Gautama the *Buddha. The historical roots of Jainism, however, reach back into a hoary past. Thus the Jaina scriptures speak of a lineage of twenty-four "ford makers" (*tīrthankāra*), or *adept teachers, of whom Mahāvīra was the last. The spirituality of Jainism has preserved many archaic features, and it tends toward ascetic rigor. It has greatly influenced the development of the ethical aspects of *Yoga, especially the virtue of "nonharming" (*ahimsā*) and the teachings on moral causation (*karma*). Later Jaina writers articulated ideas and practices that are rather similar to *Hindu Yoga. Thus the renowned scholar Haribhadra (ca. 750 CE) made use of some of the codifications of *Patanjali. Among his over 1,400 works are several treatises on Yoga, notably his *Yoga-Bindu* ("Seed of Yoga") and *Yoga-Drishti-Samuccaya* ("Collection of Yoga Views"). Hemacandra, in his seventh-century *Yoga-Shāstra* ("Yoga Teaching"), also availed himself of some of the formulations found in Patanjali's *Yoga-Sūtra*.

JALA ("water"), one of the five material elements (*bhūta*). The *Yoga-Shikhā-Upanishad* (5.50) mentions that *concentration on water bestows the paranormal power (*siddhi*) of never being overcome by that element. See also *ap*.

JĀLA can mean "watery" but also "net" or "web," and in the latter sense is sometimes used as a synonym for "illusion" (*māyā*).

JĀLANDHARA. See *Jālandhari*.

JĀLANDHARA-BANDHA ("Jālandhara's lock"), an important practice of *hatha-yoga* consisting in the "contraction of the *throat" (*kantha-samkocana*), which is achieved by placing the chin on the chest, usually after inhalation. In the *Gheranda-Samhitā* (3.13) this technique is praised as a "great seal" (*mahā-mudrā*). It is practiced in conjunction with a variety of postures (*āsana*) and "seals" (*mudrā*). According to the *Goraksha-Paddhati* (1.79), this *bandha* "binds" the network of channels (*sirā*) and prevents the ambrosial liquid (*amrita*) from flowing into the trunk. It is also thought to cure *diseases of the throat.

JĀLANDHARA-PĪTHA ("Jālandhara's seat"), a synonym for *vishuddha-cakra*.

JĀLANDHARI ("Net Bearer," from *jāla*, "net," and *dhara*, "carrying"), a famous

master of *hatha-yoga* and, prior to his *renunciation of the *world, allegedly ruler of Hastinapur in Northern India. He is said to have initiated King *Bhartrihari into *Yoga. According to some traditions, he was also called Hadipā (Hadipāda), who is known to have initiated King *Gopīcandra of Bengal.

JALA-VASTI ("water syringe"), one of two forms of *vasti*. The *Gheranda-Samhitā* (1.46f.) describes it as follows: One should immerse oneself in *water up to the *navel and while performing the "raised posture" (*utkata-āsana*) should contract and dilate the anal sphincter muscle. This is thought to cure urinary disorders, digestive troubles, and "cruel wind" (*krūra-vāyu*), or diseases related to the wind *element. Cf. *shushka-vasti*.

JAMADAGNI, was one of the seven seers (*rishi*) of the *Vedic era. The *Hindu tradition remembers him as the son of Ricīka and as the father of Parashu-Rāma, an *incarnation of *Vishnu preceding both *Rāma and *Krishna. Several stories of doubtful historicity are told about him in the *Mahābhārata*. According to one ac-

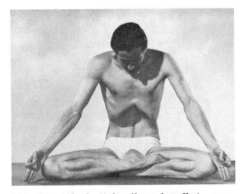

The throat lock (*jālandhara-bandha*), combined with the upward lock (*uddīyana-bandha*), demonstrated by Theos Bernard

count, he had his wife, Renukā, put to *death for having lustful thoughts about him. The homicide was committed by Par-ashu-Rāma, but only after having been as-sured of her prompt *rebirth in a com-pletely virtuous state. The story has a deep symbolic meaning, as Renukā's name also denotes *semen, which must be controlled in order to achieve *virtue and *tapas. Ja-madagni is said to have been murdered by King Kārtavīrya.

JANAKA, an early king of Videha who was not only fabulously wealthy but also wise. He is mentioned in the *Brihad-Āranyaka-Upanishad (4.1ff.) as a disciple of the illus-trious sage *Yājnavalkya. Many later sages and others took the same name in honor of this sagacious ruler.

JANA-SANGA ("contact with people"). So-cializing is, according to the *Hatha-Yoga-Pradīpikā (1.15), one of the factors by which *Yoga is foiled. See also *sanga.*

JANMAN ("birth"). In *Hinduism, a per-son's birth into the *world is merely one phase in a beginningless series of births, lives, and *deaths, which is known as *samsāra, the round of existence. This process of ever-renewed *embodiment at different levels of *manifestation, whether material or *subtle, is dependent on the cosmic moral law or *karma. However, because we can choose *good over *evil, or right over wrong, a person can improve his or her individual *destiny. More im-portantly, a person can break entirely out of the cycle of births and deaths and re-cover his or her essential being, the *Self, which is unborn (*aja) and continuously conscious. See also *jāta.*

JAPA ("recitation"), defined in the *Yoga-Yājnavalkya (2.12) as the "repetition (*ab-*hyāsa) of *mantras in accordance with the rules." This extremely old practice, be-longing to the earliest developments of *Yoga, probably grew out of the medita-tive recitation of the sacred *Vedic texts, which required the utmost *concentration from the priest, since each holy word had to be accurately pronounced lest it should adversely influence the outcome of the sacrificial ritual (*yajna).

The *Yoga-Sūtra (1.28) recommends the recitation of the sacred syllable *om for the removal of all obstacles (*antarāya). This recitation should naturally lead over into the contemplation (*bhāvanā) of the inner significance of this *mantra. Mind-less repetition of words has no desirable effect. *Japa,* like all other practices of *Yoga, is to be performed with great atten-tiveness and dedication. According to the *Mahābhārata (12.190), a person who fails to be intent on the meaning of the words he recites is destined to go to *hell.

Japa can be practiced verbally or men-tally. In the former case, a *mantra* can be whispered (*upāmshu*) or voiced (*ucca,* elsewhere called *vācika*). According to the *Yoga-Yājnavalkya (2.15f.), whispered rec-itation is a thousand times better than voiced *japa,* whereas mental (*mānasa*) rec-itation is a thousand times better than whispered *japa.* *Meditation, however, is stated to be a thousand times better than even mental *japa.* The *Linga-Purāna (1.85.106) makes the point that recitation in one's home is good, but recitation in a cow pen is a hundred times better and on a riverbank a thousand times better. Fur-thermore, the text notes, in the presence of *Shiva, recitation is infinitely effica-cious. See also *hamsa.*

JAPAKA ("reciter"), a practitioner of *japa,* a *japa-yogin.*

JĀTA ("birthed"), the class of being in which a person is born. See also *janman*, *jāti*; cf. *aja*.

JĀTI ("birth"), the social rank or status of a person's *birth, especially his or her caste. See also *janman*, *jāta*.

JĀTHARA-AGNI ("belly fire"), the digestive heat in the stomach area; on the esoteric level, the inner sun (*sūrya*) that devours the divine nectar (*amrita*) dripping from the inner moon (*candra*) in the *head. Some techniques of *hatha-yoga, such as *vahni-sāra-dhauti, *shushka-vasti, and *viparīta-kāranī, are specifically designed to stimulate that abdominal "fire." Indeed, the anonymous author of the *Yoga-Tattva-Upanishad (45) values increased digestive heat as a sign (*cihna*) of the successful cleansing of the channels (*nādī*) through which the *life force circulates. See also *agni*, *vaishvānara*.

JEALOUSY. See *irshyā*, *mātsarya*.

JIHVĀ-BANDHA ("tongue lock"). See *mahā-bandha*.

JIHVĀ(-MŪLA)-DHAUTI ("cleansing of the tongue's [body]"), also called *jihvā-shodhana* ("purification of the tongue"); part of what is known as "dental cleansing" (*danta-dhauti*). The *Gheranda-Samhitā* (1.29f.) describes it as follows: One should rub and clean the tongue by means of the index, middle, and ring fingers, then massage it with butter and milk and thereafter slowly pull it out with the help of an iron tool. This should be done daily with diligence at sunrise and again at sunset. Gradually the tongue's tendon (here called *lambikā*) becomes elongated, which is said to remove aging, *disease, and even *death. See also *khecarī-mudrā*, *lambikā-yoga*.

JĪTA-INDRIYA (*jītendriya*, "he whose senses are conquered"), a master of *Yoga. See also *indriya*.

JĪVA ("life" or "alive") roughly corresponds to what is called the psyche or, as the *Mahābhārata* (12.180.30) puts it, "the mental fire." This is the individuated self (*jīva-ātman*) as opposed to the transcendental Self (*parama-ātman*). The *Laghu-Yoga-Vāsishtha* (5.10.18) calls it the mind (*citta*) that does not know *Reality and hence is afflicted with *suffering. According to the schools of *Vedānta, the numerous individuated selves are the product of an *illusion. Their multiplicity, which stems from spiritual nescience (*avidyā*, *ajnāna*), is not ultimately true. Upon *enlightenment, the seeming diversity of existence melts away, and there is only the singular transcendental *Self (*ātman*).

In the *Goraksha-Paddhati* (2.35) the *jīva* is compared to a bull who is "triply bound" and "roars a mighty roar." The phrase "triply bound" suggests the individual's experience of confinement by the three primary constituents (*guna*) of *nature. The *Shiva-Purāna* (1.16.99f.) defines the *jīva* as "that which decays from the moment of *birth" and as "that which is born enmeshed and entwined." For the same reason, the *Gheranda-Samhitā* (3.50) styles it an "animal" (*pashu*) so long as the spiritual force, or *kundalinī-shakti, is still dormant and not yet awakened. The *Kaula-Jnāna-Nirnaya* (6.7) states that the individual is called *jīva* while it abides in the *body, whereas it is the supreme *Shiva upon release from the bodily fetters. In the moment of *death, the *jīva* is generally thought to escape through the crown of the *head (in the case of *yogins) or through other bodily orifices (in the case of those who are spiritually unprepared).

The close relationship between the *jīva* and the life force (*prāna*) as *breath has been carefully studied in *hatha-yoga. Thus in the *Goraksha-Paddhati (1.38ff.) we find this important verse:

Even as a ball struck by a club flies up, so the psyche (*jīva*) struck by *prāna and *apāna does not stand still. Under the influence of *prāna* and *apāna*, the psyche rushes up and down through the left and right paths [i.e., through the *idā- and *pingalā-nādī], and because of this moving to and fro cannot be seen.

Even as a hawk tied to a rope can be brought back again when it has flown off, so the psyche bound by [*nature's] strands (*guna) is pulled about by *prāna* and *apāna*.

It leaves [the body] with the sound *ha* and it enters with the sound *sa*, both sounds being continually recited [and forming the *hamsa-mantra].

The *Yoga-Vāsishtha (appendix to 6.50.2ff.) has this fascinating division of *jīvas* into seven types depending on their spiritual maturity and power: (1) the *svapna-jāgara* ("dream waking"): one whose *dreams are the waking world of others; (2) the *samkalpa-jāgara* ("imagination waking"): one whose imagination is so powerful that it creates a waking world for others; (3) the *kevala-jāgara* ("sole waking"): one who experiences the waking state for the first time; a "new soul"; (4) the *cīra-jāgara* ("long waking"): one who has experienced the *waking state for many lifetimes; an "old soul"; (5) the *ghana-jāgara* ("solidified waking"): one whose repeated evil *actions have reduced him to a state of relative unconsciousness; (6) the *jāgrat-svapna* ("waking dream"): one for whom the *world perceived in the *waking state is but a *dream; and (7) the *kshīna-jāgara* ("dwindled waking"): one for whom the waking world has ceased to

exist as an apparently independent *creation because he has realized the transcendental *Self.

Elsewhere (3.94.2ff.) this scripture proposes a twelvefold classification of *jīvas* on the basis of the interplay of the primary constituents (*guna) of *nature. All such schemas serve the principal purpose of driving home the point that the *waking state, which is so highly valued in our modern civilization, does by no means express the ultimate human potential. Rather it reflects a particular degree of awareness that is characterized by a certain level of moral and spiritual maturity. See also Actor, *dehin*, *hamsa*; cf. *ātman*.

JĪVA-ĀTMAN (*jīvātman*, "living self"), the individuated *consciousness or psyche (*jīva). According to *Vedānta and the *Vedānta-based schools of *Preclassical and *Postclassical Yoga, *liberation consists in the merging of the individuated self with the transcendental or supreme *Self (*parama-ātman).

JĪVAN-MUKTA ("living liberated"), the *adept who is *liberated, or *enlightened, while still embodied. This is the grand ideal of those spiritual schools of *Hinduism that subscribe to *nondualism, or the teaching that upon *Self-realization the distinction between transcendence and immanence collapses: The *world is seen to arise in and as the *Divine. Hence *liberation is not an otherworldly alternative that implies disembodiment. The *Bhagavad-Gītā (2.56f.) proffers this description of a *jīvan-mukta:

[He whose] *mind is unagitated in suffering (*duhkha), devoid of longing during pleasure (*sukha), and free from passion (*rāga), fear (*bhaya), and anger (*krodha)—he is called a sage (*muni) steadied in the vision [of the *Self].

He who is unattached toward everything, who does not rejoice at whatever auspicious [events] happen to him, nor hates whatever inauspicious [events occur]—his wisdom (*prajnā) is well established.

Thus the jīvan-mukta's continual immersion in the *Self expresses itself in his stoic attitude toward existence, which allows him to recognize the same (*sama) in all things. His *equanimity also has more positive, outgoing characteristics, however. He is, above all, a compassionate being. This is made clear in the following stanzas from the *Bhagavad-Gītā (12.13ff.), where *Krishna instructs Prince *Arjuna:

[He who feels] no *hatred toward any being, [who is] friendly and compassionate . . . [that] *yogin who is ever content, self-controlled, of firm resolve, with *mind and wisdom (*buddhi) offered up in Me, who is My *devotee—he is dear to Me.

He from whom the *world does not shrink and who does not shrink from the world and who is free from exultation, *anger, *fear, and agitation, is dear to Me.

In the *Yoga-Vāsishtha (5.77.7ff.), authored over a millennium after the above Gītā verses were composed, we find these memorable stanzas:

He does not concern himself with the future, nor does he abide [exclusively] in the present, nor does he recall [i.e., live in] the past, but he acts out of the *Whole.
*Sleeping, he is awake. Awake, he is like one asleep. Performing all [necessary] *actions, he "does" nothing whatsoever inwardly.
Inwardly always renouncing everything, without inner *desires and performing externally what has to be done, he remains [completely] balanced (*sama).

Remaining perfectly happy and experiencing *enjoyment in all that is expected [of him], he performs all *actions while abandoning the misconception of doership.
[He behaves] as a boy among boys; an elder among elders; a *sage among sages; a youth among youths, and as a sympathizer among the well-behaved afflicted.
[He is] wise, gracious, charming, suffused with his *enlightenment, free from pressure (kheda) and distress, an affectionate friend.
Neither by embarking on the performance of *action nor by abstention, nor by [such concepts as] *bondage or *emancipation, underworld or *heaven [can he be perturbed].
[For,] when the objective *world is perceived as the unitary [*Reality], then the *mind fears neither bondage nor emancipation.

Some schools claim that the jīvan-mukta is capable of shape-shifting and that therefore he enjoys *immortality. However, for most authorities his physical *body is by no means incorruptible, but *death does not affect his existential status as a free being in the least.

JĪVAN-MUKTI ("living liberation"), the condition of a *jīvan-mukta. Cf. videha-mukti.

JĪVAN-MUKTI-VIVEKA ("Discernment about Living Liberation"), a remarkable *Vedānta text by Vidyāranya Tīrtha, a fourteenth-century scholar and spiritual practitioner. This comprehensive work offers a detailed discussion of the yogic *path from a Vedantic point of view. Vidyāranya cites a great many scriptures, and his work contains illuminating commentaries particularly on the *Yoga-Vāsishtha and the *Yoga-Sūtra.

JNĀNA ("wisdom" or "knowledge"), a word that is applied in both sacred and secular contexts. It can stand for learning, or conceptual *knowledge, and also for higher, intuitive insight and *wisdom, or gnosis. Occasionally jnāna is even equated with the ultimate *Reality itself.

The *Bhagavad-Gītā (18.20ff.) distinguishes three types of jnāna depending on the predominance of one or the other of the three primary constituents (*guna) of *nature: (1) sāttvika-jnāna, by which one sees the one immutable *Reality in all things; (2) rājasa-jnāna, by which one sees but the composite nature of things, not their underlying unity; and (3) tāmasa-jnāna, by which one irrationally clings to a single thing as if it were the whole, without concern for *Reality.

The *Yoga-Vāsishtha (3.118.5ff.), composed about 1100 CE, mentions seven stages or levels (*bhūmi) of *wisdom: (1) shubha-icchā, or the impulse toward what is spiritually auspicious; (2) vicāranā, the profound consideration of spiritual teachings; (3) tanu-mānasī, the refinement of one's thinking; (4) sattā-āpatti, the acquisition of a pure being; (5) asamsakti, nonattachment; (6) pada-artha-bhāva, the recognition of what truly matters, which is *enlightenment; and (7) turya-ga, the *intuition of the "Fourth" (*turya). These stages of jnāna lead to final and irrevocable *liberation. Thus, as is stated in the *Bhagavad-Gītā (4.36), wisdom is a raft (plava) by means of which one can cross the "crooked stream of life." As another stanza (4.38) has it, wisdom is the "greatest purifier on earth."

Sometimes jnāna is contrasted with *yoga (in the sense of specific practices).

Thus the *Tri-Shikhi-Brāhmana-Upanishad (2.19) declares: "Wisdom is brought about by *Yoga. Yoga is developed by wisdom." See also prajnā, sapta-jnāna-bhūmi, vijnāna; cf. ajnāna, avidyā.

JNĀNA-AMRITA ("Immortal Nectar of Wisdom"), a medieval work on *hatha-yoga ascribed to *Goraksha.

JNĀNA-BANDHU ("friend of knowledge"), an intellectual who studies spiritual matters but fails to convert his interest into living practice. See also grantha, shāstra.

JNĀNA-BHŪMI ("level of wisdom"). See jnāna, bhūmi, sapta-jnāna-bhūmi.

JNĀNA-CAKSHUS, or JNĀNA-NETRA ("eye of wisdom"). Although the transcendental *Self is invisible to the human *eye, the metaphor of vision has almost universally been employed to describe *Self-realization. The *Bhagavad-Gītā (15.10), for instance, states that the Self can be seen through the eye of *wisdom. According to another stanza (13.34), this inner eye helps one distinguish between the "field" (*kshetra) and the "field knower" (*kshetra-jna), that is, between *nature and the Self. See also manas-cakra.

JNĀNADEVA, or JNĀNESHVARA (late 13th cen. CE); Maharashtra's greatest mystical and poetic genius. He died at the age of twenty-one, apparently by voluntarily dropping his mortal coil while in the state of *ecstasy. His *Jnāneshvarī, a comprehensive verse commentary on the *Bhagavad-Gītā, is the first philosophical work in the Marathi language. He also authored the Amrita-Anubhava ("Experience of Immortality") and a number of shorter tracts. His spiritual roots lie in the *Nātha tradition on the one side, and the *bhakti

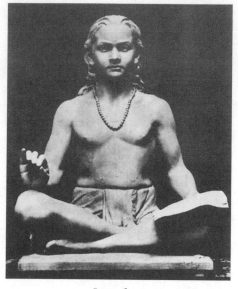

Jnānadeva

of *Yoga. His works extol the virtue and liberating power of *devotion.

JNĀNA-INDRIYA (jñānendriya, "cognitive sense"). See indriya.

JNĀNA-KĀRIKĀ ("Wisdom Activity"), a text of the *Kaula school consisting of 137 verses (kārikā) distributed over three chapters. The last chapter describes the proper *environment for the *kaula-yogin, including such settings as cave, cremation ground, the confluence of rivers, and crossroads, all interpreted symbolically as locations within the *body.

JNĀNA-MĀRGA ("path of wisdom"), the nondualistic approach of the *Upanishads; also, a synonym for *jñāna-yoga. See also Path.

movement on the other. In the Jnāneshvarī (18.1751ff.) he gives his spiritual lineage as follows: *Shiva, *Shakti, *Matsyendra, *Goraksha, *Gahinī, and *Nivritti (his elder brother).

Jnānadeva's philosophy revolves around the notion that the manifest *world is a "sport" (vilāsa) of the *Absolute, an expression of the supreme *love of the singular *Reality. He refutes the dualism of *Classical Sāmkhya, the *idealism of later *Buddhism, and especially *Shankara's theory of nescience (*avidyā) as the ultimate cause of the world's existence. Jnānadeva regards *bhakti, instilled with *wisdom, as the alpha and omega of spiritual life. His philosophical position is known as sphūrti-vāda, or the doctrine of spontaneous manifestation. Although he was initiated into *hatha-yoga by his brother, it is clear from some passages in his Jnāneshvarī (e.g. 18.1138) that he was critical of the techniques and *rituals of this branch

JNĀNA-MUDRĀ ("wisdom seal"), one of the hand gestures (*mudrā) used during *meditation, performed by touching the thumb to the index finger so they form a circle, while the remaining three fingers are extended. In the *Brahma-Vidyā-Upanishad (64) the jñāna-mudrā is interpreted symbolically as consisting in the recollection of the *hamsa-mantra in the state of *ecstasy.

In Kashmiri *Shaivism the term refers to the inner spiritual union between *Shiva and *Shakti. A similar interpretation prevails in Buddhist *Tantrism. See also abhaya-mudrā, cin-mudrā, dhyāna-mudrā, vishnu-mudrā.

JNĀNAPRAKĀSHA, (16th cen. CE), a South Indian *adept and the author of a commentary on the *Shiva-Jnāna-Siddhi. He is also credited with the authorship of several other works, including the *Shiva-Yoga-Sāra and the *Shiva-Yoga-Ratna. He understands *yoga not in the sense of "union" but as a means of realizing one's identity (*sayujya*) with *Shiva, or "Shiva-hood" (*shivatva*). His *path is that of gnosis (*jnāna*) through *meditation and *ecstasy, though he also values *breath control.

JNĀNA-SHAKTI ("power of wisdom"), one of three aspects of the *Divine, whereby the ultimate *Reality is not insentient but supraconscious and the matrix for all levels of manifest awareness or intelligence. See also *icchā-shakti*, *kriyā-shakti*.

JNĀNA-YOGA ("Yoga of wisdom"), one of the principal branches of *Yoga, the others being *bhakti-yoga* and *karma-yoga*. It is virtually identical with the spiritual *path of *Vedānta, which places a premium on gnosis. Specifically, *jnāna-yoga* consists in the constant exercise of discriminating *Reality from unreality, the *Self from the "non-Self" (*anātman*).

The compound *jnāna-yoga* is first employed in the *Bhagavad-Gītā* (3.3), where *Krishna tells his pupil *Arjuna, "Of yore I proclaimed a twofold way of life in this *world, O guileless one—the Yoga of *wisdom for the *sāmkhyas* and the Yoga of action (*karma-yoga*) for the *yogins*." Here the *sāmkhyas* are not so much the followers of any particular school of *Sāmkhya as what could be called contemplatives. Accordingly, the principal technique of *jnāna-yoga* is *meditation. It is in the simplified inner *environment of meditation that *discrimination between the Real and the unreal can be pursued most effectively. *Krishna equates *jnāna-yoga* with *buddhi-yoga*, for it is the *buddhi* or "wisdom faculty" that makes such discernment possible.

In the fifteenth-century *Vedānta-Sāra* ("Essence of *Vedānta") of Sadānanda, the *path of *jnāna-yoga* is stated to consist of four principal means: (1) discrimination (*viveka*) between the permanent and the transient, the Real and the unreal; (2) renunciation (*tyāga*) of the enjoyment of the fruit (*phala*) of one's *actions; (3) the "six accomplishments" (*shat-sampatti*) consisting of tranquillity (*shama*), sense restraint (*dama*), abstention (*uparati*) from *actions that are not relevant to the maintenance of the body-mind or to the pursuit of *enlightenment, endurance (*titikshā*), mental "collectedness" (*samādhāna*), and faith (*shraddhā*); and (4) the urge toward *liberation (*mumukshutva*).

Some works, such as *Shankara's brilliant commentary on the *Brahma-Sūtra* (1.1.4), speak of a sevenfold *path of *jnāna-yoga*. It consists of the above-mentioned practices with the exception of mental collectedness, and includes listening (*shravana*) to the sacred lore, pondering (*manana*) the truth of the scriptures, and *meditation (*nididhyāsana*). See also *jnāna-mārga*.

JNĀNA-YOGIN (masc.), or JNĀNA-YOGINĪ (fem.); a practitioner of *jnāna-yoga*. See also *jnānin*.

JNĀNESHVARĪ ("Goddess of Wisdom," from the words *jnāna* and *īshvarī* or "goddess"), also called *Bhāva-Artha-Dīpikā* ("Light on the Meaning of Being"); the major work of *Jnānadeva. He is said to have delivered its 9,000 verses extempore at the age of fifteen in 1290 CE.

JNĀNIN ("knower"), a synonym for *jnāna-yogin*. The *Tri-Pura-Rahasya* (19.16ff.) distinguishes between three types of practitioners of this *Yoga. The first type suffers from the fault of *pride. The second suffers from the *illusion of doership, that is, from the assumption of being an ego personality engaged in acts rather than the

*Self beyond *ego and *action. The third and most common type suffers from the "monster" of *desire, i.e., from motivations that run counter to the primal impulse toward *self-transcendence. Depending on the practitioner's *efforts and personality type, *jnāna-yoga* can manifest differently in different individuals. However, the unknown author of the *Tri-Pura-Rahasya* (19.71) is quick to point out that these differences do not mean that *wisdom itself is manifold. Rather, *jnāna* admits of no distinction; it is coessential with *Reality.

In some contexts the word *jnānin* stands for the individual who ponders the great teachings of the scriptures but cannot really be considered a spiritual practitioner (see *jnāna-bandhu*). The *Yoga-Shikhā-Upanishad* (1.48f.), again, contrasts the *jnānin* with the *yogin*, arguing that whereas the former does not rid himself of future *births, the latter learns to master his *body and hence is assured of *liberation.

JNĀTA-AMRITA-SHĀSTRA (*Jnātāmritashāstra*, "Teaching on the Immortal Knower"), a rare work attributed to *Goraksha, consisting of 227 verses.

JNĀTRI ("knower"), the knowing subject, as opposed to the known object (*jneya*) and the process of knowledge (*jnāna*). In some schools, this term is used to denote the transcendental *Self.

JOY. See *ānanda*, Bliss, Happiness, *sukha*.

JYOTIR-DHYĀNA ("light meditation") also called *tejo-dhyāna*; one of three kinds of *meditation described in the *Gheranda-Samhitā* (6.1). It involves *concentration on the esoteric center at the base of the spine, where the individual psyche (*jīva-ātman*) is said to be located in the form of *light. An alternative process is concentration on the "*fire" of the *pranava (i.e., *om), visualized at the spot between the *eyebrows.

JYOTIS ("light"). Since ancient times the transcendental *Reality has been described as unimaginably luminous. The *Bhaga-vad-Gītā* (13.17) calls that Reality "light of lights beyond darkness." Most *Hindu scriptures make reference to the *light aspect of the *Self. The *Shiva-Samhitā* (5.23) epitomizes this trend: "He who sees that brilliance unobstructed even for an instant is released from all *sin and reaches the highest estate." See also *tār-aka-yoga*.

JYOTSNĀ ("Moonlight"), the principal commentary on the *Hatha-Yoga-Pradī-pikā*. Its author, Brahmānanda, offers many valuable explanations of the ideas and practices of *hatha-yoga.

· K ·

KABĪR (1440–1518 CE), one of the great medieval *Hindu saints. He was brought up by a Muslim weaver in Benares (Varanasi) but converted to *Hinduism through the influence of Rāmānanda (1440–1470 CE). He was also greatly influenced by the female *adept *Lallā, by *Nāmadeva, and not least the teachings of Sufism. Kabīr, at heart a *bhakta, was critical of the forced approach of *hatha-yoga. Although he did

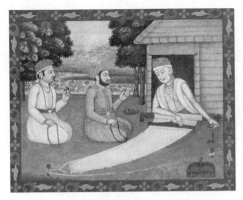

Kabīr, the weaver-mystic

not deny that by manipulating the life force (*prāna) one could experience exquisite *bliss, he saw little value in this because, as he noted, such artificially produced states are exceedingly temporary. He also opposed the caste system and excessive image *worship.

KAIVALYA ("aloneness"), the state of unconditional existence of the *Self. In *Classical Yoga the term refers more precisely to what the *Yoga-Sūtra (2.25) styles the "aloneness of seeing (*drishi)," which refers to the Self's innate capacity for unbroken apperception of the contents of consciousness (*citta). In an alternative definition, the *Yoga-Sūtra (4.34) explains this as the "involution" (*pratiprasava) of the primary constituents (*guna) of *nature, which have lost all purpose for the Self that has recovered its transcendental autonomy. According to yet another of *Patanjali's aphorisms (3.55), kaivalya is said to be established when the *sattva (the highest ontological aspect of *nature) and the *Self are of comparable *purity. The *Hatha-Yoga-Pradīpikā (4.62) defines kaivalya as that which remains after the lower *mind has been "dissolved" through yogic practice. The *Mandala-Brāhmana-Upanishad (2.3.1) speaks of the "*light of alone-

ness" (kaivalya-jyotis), which is motionless and full, "resembling a flame in a windless place." The *Jīvan-Mukti-Viveka (chapter 2) explains it as "the condition of the isolated (kevala) Self, that is, freedom from the *body, etc.," which is "obtainable through gnosis (*jnāna) alone."

In the Yatīndra-Mata-Dīpikā (8.16f.), a seventeenth-century *Vedānta work, kaivalya is contrasted with *moksha, or *liberation, as follows:

The seekers after liberation are of two kinds: the followers of kaivalya and the followers of moksha. [That which is] named kaivalya, [as reached] through *jnāna-yoga, is of the nature of realization as distinct from *nature. They say this realization is a realization without the Lord (*bhagavat). . . .

The followers of moksha are of two kinds: the *bhaktas and the *prapannas [for whom the *Lord is the ultimate *Reality].

Thus, according to this interpretation, kaivalya is founded in a dualistic metaphysics, whereas the metaphysical underpinning of the ideal of *moksha is distinctly theistic. Historically speaking, however, kaivalya originated in the schools of *Epic Yoga, which were panentheistic, and the term continued to be used as a synonym for moksha in many of the schools of *Postclassical Yoga.

KĀKACANDĪ ĪSHVARA, mentioned in the *Hatha-Yoga-Pradīpikā (1.7) as an *adept of *hatha-yoga. He is credited with the authorship of a *Tantra scripture on *alchemy bearing his name.

KĀKA-MATA ("crow doctrine"), referred to in the *Yoga-Shikhā-Upanishad (1.144) and explained in *Upanishad Brahmayogin's commentary on this text as the doctrine that Maheshvara (i.e., *Shiva) is the "master of illusion" (*māyin*), i.e. the source of the illusion (*māyā*) that is called the *world.

KĀKĪ-MUDRĀ ("crow seal"), mentioned in the *Gheranda-Samhitā* (1.22) in connection with the "expelled washing" (*bahish-krita-dhauti*). According to stanzas 3.86f., it is performed by shaping the mouth like a crow's beak and then sucking in the *air. This work also states that by practicing this technique one becomes free of *disease "like a crow."

KAKSHĀ ("armpit"). The *Vijnāna-Bhairava* (79), a principal text of Kashmiri *Shaivism, mentions the curious practice of focusing *attention on the armpit while raising the arms in an arc above the head, an action that is thought to yield inner *peace.

KĀLA ("time" or "death"). The principal reason why conditional existence (*bhava*) is experienced as filled with suffering (*duhkha*) is that it is temporal. Time is seen as the great enemy of all creatures. As the *Yoga-Vāsishtha* (1.23.4) puts it, "There is nothing here in this universe that all-voracious time does not devour, like the submarine fire [swallows] the overflowing ocean." The author of the *Yoga-Vāsistha* (6.7.34) compares time to a potter who, continually turning his wheel, produces innumerable pots only to smash them whenever he fancies to do so. The *Mahābhārata* (11.2.8, 24) has these two stanzas:

Time pulls along all creatures, even the *gods. There is none dear to time, none hateful.
Time "cooks" [all] beings. Time destroys [all] creatures. [When all else is] asleep, time is awake. Time is hard to overcome.

Yet the transcendence of *time is precisely the objective of all spiritual traditions. Hence the *yogin seeks to "cheat" time and *death by realizing the transcendental *Reality, which is immortal. The perfected *adept is also called *kāla-atīta*, "he who has transcended time." This attitude is epitomized in a verse from the *Hatha-Yoga-Pradīpikā* (4.108): "The *yogin* yoked through *ecstasy . . . is not devoured by time." The same work (4.17) discloses that the *sun and *moon create time in the form of day and night, whereas the central channel (*sushumnā-nādī*) consumes time. This means that when the life force (*prāna*) enters the axial channel, the *mind stands still and all perception of *space and time ceases.

Probably under the influence of later *Buddhism, *Patanjali and his commentators speculated about the nature of *time. According to *Classical Yoga, time consists of a series of moments (*kshana*). This idea of the discontinuous nature of time corresponds with modern quantum-physical notions. The time intervals cannot be perceived in themselves. According to the *Yoga-Sūtra* (3.52), however, the *yogin can focus on the reality of time while in the *ecstatic condition, which yields "discernment-born wisdom" (*viveka-ja-jnāna*). The commentaries compare these minute intervals of time to the atoms (*parama-anu*) of matter. These *kshanas* are considered to be real, whereas temporal duration is merely a "mental construct" (*buddhi-samāhāra*).

The term *kāla* is also used in the scriptures of *Yoga to denote the appropriate time for *practice. Thus the *Gheranda-Samhitā* (5.8ff.) stipulates that one should not commence practice when the weather is either too hot or too cold, or during the rainy season. The two ideal seasons, therefore, are spring (*vasanta*) and autumn (*sha-*

144

rad). The *Mārkandeya-Purāna (39.47) adds to this that one should also abstain from practicing Yoga when it is windy or where other extremes (*dvandva) prevail. The *Mahābhārata (12.294.9) additionally mentions three occasions when Yoga practice should be interrupted: during urination, defecation, and eating. This puritanical prescription is not upheld by other, more body-positive schools, however. A favorable time for Yoga practice, particularly *meditation, is sunrise, known as "Brahma's hour" (*brahma-muhūrta). Some scriptures also recommend the time of sunset and just before and after midnight. See also anta-kāla, Cosmos, ghatikā, kalpa, muhūrta, prayāna-kāla, World ages.

KALĀ ("part" or "segment"), one of the categories (*tattva) of existence distin-

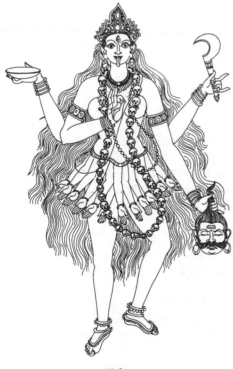

Kālī

guished in Kashmiri *Shaivism, where it stands for secondary or partial creatorship. In *Tantrism and *hatha-yoga, it also refers to the potentiality of *sound, often mentioned together with *nāda and *bindu. In the Parā-Trishikā-Vivarana of *Abhinava Gupta, the Sanskrit letters from a to ah are called the sixteen kalās. The sixteenth is known as visarga-kalā, which is unchanging.

Kalā signifies the sixteenth part of anything, especially the *moon. Thus a number of medieval works on *Yoga mention the lunar "part" in the "thousand-spoked wheel" (*sahasrāra-cakra). In the *Shat-Cakra-Nirūpana (46), it is called amā-kalā, amā being one of the many synonyms for *candra, the esoteric moon from which drips the "nectar of immortality" (*amrita). This work (47) also mentions a *nirvāna-kalā ("part of extinction"), which is to be found within this amā-kalā. Such concepts are best understood as attempts to explain specific experiences in *meditation and *ecstasy. The experience of the amā-kalā is associated with supraconscious ecstasy (*asamprajnāta-samādhi).

KĀLĀMUKHA sect, a *Tantric cult (ca. 1000 CE) generally regarded as a branch of the *Lakulīsha tradition. Since none of the scriptures of this cult, whose members were fond of learning, have survived, it is difficult to get a clear picture of its metaphysics and spiritual practice. This well-organized sect has frequently and apparently unjustly been accused of indulging in eccentric and obscene *rituals similar to those of the *Kāpālikas. The sect got its name "black face" (kālāmukha) from the fact that its adherents wore a striking black mark on their *foreheads, indicating their *renunciation of the *world.

KĀLĪ, the "black" goddess, portrayed with bulging *eyes and protruding *tongue, represents the destructive aspect of the *Divine. She destroys the illusion of the *ego and, for her devotees, removes all obstacles and limitations in the way of *Self-realization. See also *deva, mahā-vidyā*.

KALI-YUGA ("*kali* age"), the present dark age of spiritual decline. It is traditionally said to have started with the *death of *Krishna in 3002 BCE. This idea is fundamental to *Tantrism, which purports to be a new gospel for the dark age. The word *kali*, often incorrectly translated as "dark," derives from the losing throw of the dice, dice playing being a favorite activity of the ancient Indians. See also *kalpa, yuga*.

KALKI, or KALKIN; the prophesied tenth incarnation (*avatāra*) of *Vishnu. He is said to come at the end of the present dark age (*kali-yuga*), riding a white stallion and brandishing a sword blazing like a comet. According to *Vaishnava theology, he will establish the next golden age.

KALPA ("usage" or "rule"). *Hindu cosmology knows of world cycles of immense duration. A *kalpa* represents one full day in the life of the Creator, *Brahma. It translates into 4.32 billion human years, or 12 million divine years, or 1,000 "great ages" (*mahā-yuga*), a total that comes surprisingly close to modern computations for our solar system. Brahma is thought to live for 36,000 *kalpas*. Each *kalpa* has a "day" and a "night." During the night phase the *cosmos is temporarily dissolved. This dissolution is known as an "absorption" (*pralaya*). Since the creation of the present universe almost 2 billion years are reckoned to have elapsed. See also World ages.

KALPANĀ ("fashioning"), a synonym for *samkalpa*. See also Imagination.

KĀMA ("desire"), *pleasure in general and the sexual urge, or sensuality, in particular. In the sense of a pleasurable experience, *kāma* is considered to be one of the legitimate goals of human aspiration (*purusha-artha*). Yet from the point of view of the highest human potential, which is liberation (*moksha*), it is typically viewed as unworthy of one's pursuit. In fact, together with anger (*krodha*) and greed (*lobha*), *kāma* is widely deemed to be one of the three "gates of *hell."

KĀMA-AVASĀYITVA (*kāmāvasāyitva*, "desire dwelling"), the paranormal power (*siddhi*) of perfect wish-fulfillment. A *yogin endowed with this ability realizes all his *desires. The *Yoga-Bhāshya* (3.45) wisely observes that this does not mean that the *adept can overthrow the natural order of the *universe, as instituted by the Lord (*īshvara*). This cautionary objection is seldom heeded in the popular *Yoga literature, however, which abounds in stories of *yogins and ascetics who do not hesitate to set the world topsy-turvy in order to force the *gods to do their bidding.

KĀMA-DAHANA-ĀSANA (*kāmadahan-āsana*, "desire-burning posture") described in the *Hatha-Ratna-Āvalī* (3.48) as follows: While seated in the *bhadra-āsana*, arrange the *feet in the opposite manner. Thus it is a variation of the *bhadra-āsana*.

KAMALA-ĀSANA (*kamalāsana*, "lotus posture"), a synonym for *padma-āsana*.

KĀMA-RŪPA ("desire form"), the geographic region of Assam, a stronghold of *Tantrism; also, an esoteric structure of the human *body. In the latter sense, it refers to the secret locus at the perineum (*yoni*). It forms a part of the basal center (*mūlādhāra-cakra) and is represented as a deep red triangle (trikona), also called "triple city" (tripura, traipura). According to the *Shat-Cakra-Nirūpana (8), it has the brightness of ten million suns. It is here that the lower opening of the central channel (*sushumnā-nādī) is found. It is the seat of the "serpent power" (*kundalinī-shakti).

Additionally, kāma-rūpa (sometimes kāma rūpatva) is the paranormal power (*siddhi) to assume any shape at will. See also icchā-rūpa.

KAMPA or KAMPANA ("tremor" or "trembling"), a curious yogic phenomenon associated with the arousal of the "serpent power" (*kundalinī-shakti). According to the *Yoga-Yājnavalkya (6.26) and a number of other *hatha-yoga scriptures, trembling occurs during the second stage of breath control (*prānāyāma). The *Kaula-Jnāna-Nirnaya (14.16) speaks of two degrees, (1) general trembling and (2) violent shaking of the limbs, accompanied by the hearing of inner *sounds. The *Mārkandeya-Purāna (39.56) recommends as a remedy that one should fix the *mind on the image of a mountain (a symbol of *steadiness).

KANĀDA. See Vaisheshika.

KANDA ("bulb": sometimes spelled kānda), the point of origin of the network of channels (*nādī) along or through which the life force (*prāna) circulates in the *body. Some schools specify its location as being at the base of the spine, corresponding to the position of the perineum (*yoni), others as being in the "middle of the body" (*deha-madhya). It is unanimously said to be egg-shaped, though the *Hatha-Yoga-Pradī-pikā (3.113) describes it as having the ap-

pearance of a "rolled cloth." Its size is often given as nine digits long and four digits wide, and it is generally stated to be soft and white. It is also known as kanda-yoni ("bulb source") and kanda-sthāna ("bulb place"). The *Yoga-Kundalī-Upanishad (1.49) mentions a kanda near the ankles, by which this text probably means a sensitive area (*marman).

KĀNERIN, mentioned in the *Hatha-Yoga-Pradīpikā (1.7) as a master of *hatha-yoga.

KĀNIPĀ, a pupil of *Jālandhari; the reputed founder of the *Aghorī sect.

KĀNPHATA SECT. The Hindi word kān-phata means "ear splitting," which refers to the custom of slitting the cartilages of both *ears to accommodate large earrings (called darshan or kundal in Hindi). This originally ascetic order is said to have been founded by *Goraksha, who is also credited with inventing *hatha-yoga. Today the sect comprises men and women, some of whom are married. Their social status is generally low, and they engage in *occultism, dream interpretation, and psychic healing.

During the late sixteenth century CE, the order experienced the destruction of many of its temples at the hands of the Sikhs (see *Sikhism). There are still numerous Kān-phata monasteries (*matha) found scattered throughout India. Each belongs to one of the original twelve subdivisions of the order. Two levels of initiation (*dīkshā) are generally recognized: First there is a probationership of up to six months during which the student lives in confinement to test his or her resolution. This is followed by the candidate's formal acceptance as a *disciple, at which time he or she receives a *mantra and the *yogin's garb. In the second stage of initiation, the disciple's *ears are pierced, which is thought to stimulate a particular current (*nāḍī) of the *life force associated with the acquisition of magical power.

There is no question that the Kānphatas were instrumental in the development of *hatha-yoga. They produced a fairly extensive literature on this type of *Yoga, though today few of its members are literate. Undoubtedly many texts are lost forever. See also Nātha sect, Siddha cult, Tantrism.

KANTHA-BANDHA ("throat lock"), a synonym for *jālandhara-bandha; also occasionally called kantha-mudrā ("throat seal") and kantha-samkoca ("throat contraction").

KANTHA-CAKRA ("throat wheel"), a synonym for *vishuddhi-cakra.

KANTHADI, mentioned in the *Hatha-Yoga-Pradīpikā (1.6) as an *adept of *hatha-yoga.

KĀNTI ("beauty"). Physical beauty is sometimes considered one of the signs (*cihna) of successful *Yoga practice. It is the result of enhanced *prāna activity in the *body.

KAPĀLA ("skull"), one of the implements used by certain types of *yogins, notably the members of the *Kāpālika sect, who use human skulls for dinner plates. The skull cup symbolizes the *world, which the *yogin has mastered. Its esoteric significance is the union (yoga) between *Shiva and *Shakti.

KAPĀLA-BHĀTI ("skull brightening"; also called mastaka-bhāti in some texts), one of the "six acts" (*shat-karma). The *Gheranda-Samhitā (1.55) describes it as consist-ing of three practices, which are said to remove phlegm (*kapha). They are the "left process" (*vāma-krama), the "inversion" (*vyutkrama), and the "process [of the sound] shīt" (*shīt-krama). According to the *Hatha-Yoga-Pradīpikā (2.35), kapāla-bhāti simply consists in rapid breathing similar to the "bellows" (*bhastrikā), which is recommended as a means of curing disorders (such as corpulence) resulting from a surplus of *phlegm. See also sīt-karī.

KAPĀLA-KUHARA ("cranial cavern"), the cavity in the skull into which the back-turned tongue is inserted in the practice of the *khecarī-mudrā.

KAPĀLA-RANDHRA-DHAUTI ("cleansing of the skull opening"), a part of dental cleansing (*danta-dhauti) in *hatha-yoga. The *Gheranda-Samhitā (1.34f.) describes it thus: One should rub with the thumb of the right hand the depression in the *forehead near the bridge of the *nose. It further states that this practice, which should be done daily in the morning, after meals, and in the evening, induces "divine sight" (divya-drishti), or clairvoyance. See also divya-cakshus.

KĀPĀLIKA, mentioned in the *Hatha-Yoga-Pradīpikā (1.8) as a master of *hatha-yoga. His historicity is uncertain.

KĀPĀLIKA SECT, a *Shaiva sect, also known as Soma-Siddhānta, that may have originated in the south of India in the first centuries CE. It belongs to the more eccentric manifestations of *Hindu spirituality. The name "Kāpālika" means "skull bearer" and is explained by the curious practice of carrying a human skull (*kapāla), which serves as a food bowl. The Kāpālikas' other distinguishing mark is a club (*khatvanga*). This sect can be considered as belonging to *Tantrism, as its practitioners consume *meat and *wine and engage in sexual rites (*maithunā*). No scriptures of this religious school are extant.

KAPĀLIN, mentioned in the *Hatha-Yoga-Pradīpikā* (1.7) as a master of *hatha-yoga*.

KAPHA ("phlegm"; also called *shleshma*), one of the three humors (*dhātu*) recognized by native Hindu medicine (*Āyur-Veda), many of whose principles came to be adopted in *Yoga. Phlegm is described as heavy, cold, oily, sweet. Cf. *pitta, vāta*.

KAPILA, traditionally believed to be the founder of the *Sāmkhya tradition, though in later texts, such as some of the *Purānas*, he is hailed as a great *yogin*. It is likely that there were several historical personages by that name. The word *kapila* appears already in the *Rig-Veda (10.27.16), where it stands for the color reddish brown. It is in the *Shvetāshvatara-Upanishad* (5.2) that the seer (*rishi*) Kapila is mentioned.

Kapila, the Sāmkhya authority, is widely celebrated as the author of the *Sāmkhya-Sūtra*, but this work appears to be relatively recent, dating perhaps from ca. 1400 CE. Kapila's actual teaching can no longer be reconstructed, though it was in all likelihood a panentheistic doctrine revolving around the concepts of Self (*purusha*) and nature (*prakriti*). The southern recension of the *Mahābhārata includes a probably fictitious dialogue between Kapila and his chief disciple, Asuri.

KĀRANA ("cause"), as opposed to "effect" (*kārya*). See also *karma, kartri, nava-kārana, sat-kārya-vāda*.

KARMAN ("action"; also written *karma*, in the nominative case), *action in general.

The *Bhagavad-Gītā* (18.23ff.) distinguishes three fundamental types of acts, depending on the *actor's inner disposition: (1) *sāttvika-karman*, actions that are prescribed by tradition and performed without *attachment by a person who does not hanker after the "fruit" (*phala*); (2) *rājasa-karman*, performed out of ego sense (*ahamkāra*) and in order to experience *pleasure; and (3) *tāmasa-karman*, performed by a deluded or confused individual who has no concern for the moral and spiritual consequences of his or her deeds.

A further meaning of *karman* is "ritual act." But more specifically, *karman* (generally anglicized as *karma*) refers to the moral force of one's intentions, thoughts, and behavior. In this sense, *karma* often corresponds to *fate, as determined by the quality of one's being in past lives and the present *life. The underlying idea is that even the moral dimension of existence is causally determined. As the *Shiva-Samhitā* (2.39) puts it: "Whatever is experienced in the *world—all that is springs from *karma*. All creatures have experiences in accordance with [their] *karma*." The *Gheranda-Samhitā* (1.6f.) has these two stanzas:

Through good and bad deeds the pot (*ghata*) [*i.e.*, the *body] of living beings is produced; from the body, *karma* arises. Thus [the circle] revolves like a waterwheel (*ghati-yantra*).

As the waterwheel moves up and down powered by the bullocks, so the psyche (*jīva*) passes [repeatedly] through life and *death, powered by *karma*.

The doctrine of *karma* is intimately connected with the idea of rebirth (*punar-janman*). Both teachings were first disclosed in the earliest *Upanishads but appear to have been already an integral part of the ancient *Vedic heritage.

Generally, karma is thought to be of three kinds: (1) sancita-karma, the total accumulated stock of karmic deposits (*āshaya) awaiting fruition; (2) prārabhda-karma, which has come to fruition in this life (e.g., our bodily constitution); and (3) vartamāna- or āgāmi-karma, karma acquired during the present lifetime and that will bear fruit in the future. The *Yoga-Sūtra (3.22) distinguishes between moral retribution that is acute (sa-upakrama, written sopakrama) and deferred (nirupakrama). *Vyāsa, in his *Yoga-Bhāshya (3.22), imaginatively likens the former type to a wet cloth that is spread out to dry quickly, and the latter type to wet cloth rolled into a ball, which dries slowly.

All karma, whether "good" or "bad," is considered to be binding. Karma is the mechanism by which conditional existence maintains itself. Notwithstanding the sweeping influence of karma, India's philosophers and sages, with few exceptions, have not succumbed to fatalism. On the contrary, their thinking has revolved around the question of how this nexus of moral causation can be escaped. All spiritual *paths start from the assumption that the law of moral retribution, which is comparable to what modern physics calls a natural law, can be transcended. Thus in his *Yoga-Sūtra (4.7), *Patanjali states that karma is fourfold, a statement explained in the *Yoga-Bhāshya as follows: Karma can be "black," "black and white," "white," and "neither white nor black."

In order to outwit the iron law of karma, one has to transcend the very *consciousness that generates mental and physical *actions and their consequences. In other words, one must go beyond the *ego personality, the *illusion that one is an agent (*kartri). This philosophy is beautifully epitomized in the teaching of *karma-yoga in the *Bhagavad-Gītā. Realizing that *life is synonymous with activity, *Krishna taught that mere abstention from action does not lead to *liberation, or *enlightenment. Hence he recommended the path of "action transcendence" (*naishkarmya-karman). Only acts done without postulating a subjective center—the *ego—are nonbinding. By constantly cultivating a self-transcending disposition, the vicious circle of karmic existence can be intercepted. Thus future karma is prevented, whereas past karma is simply allowed to play itself out as it will. Spiritual practice is thought to be capable of diffusing otherwise severe physical karma. For instance, karma that would ordinarily cause a car accident may be neutralized in a dream experience of that predestined accident, and so on.

KARMA-INDRIYA (karmendriya, "action organ"). See indriya.

KĀRMA-MALA. See mala.

KARMA-YOGA ("Yoga of [self-transcending] action") was first communicated under this name well over 2,000 years ago in the *Bhagavad-Gītā, though it undoubtedly existed prior to that scripture. The Gītā introduced this *path as one of the two "ways of life" (*nishthā) taught by *Krishna, the other being *sāmkhya-yoga. Karma-yoga encourages an active life, though from an ingenious perspective: All work must not only be appropriate, which for the most part means allotted to one by one's position in *life, but must also be performed in the spirit of an inner sacrifice (*yajna). Only then are one's *actions not karmically binding.

Karma-yoga, according to the Matsya-Purāna (52.5f.), is a thousand times better than *jnāna-yoga, which here means the path of *meditation and *renunciation. In the *Uddhāva-Gītā (15.7), however, karma-yoga is introduced as the first step toward *jnāna-yoga. It is intended for those who are not "disgusted" with *actions and who still entertain all kinds of *desires. Karma-yoga is sometimes also called *kriyā-yoga.

The *Manu-Smriti (2.2) understands karma-yoga as ritual activity, which is the older meaning of the term.

KARMIN ("worker"), a synonym for karma-yogin, the spiritual practitioner who follows the *path of *karma-yoga.

KARNA-DHAUTI ("ear cleansing"), one of the practices of *danta-dhauti. According to the *Gheranda-Samhitā (1.33), it should be done with the index and ring fingers. Regular daily practice leads to the perception of inner sounds (*nāda).

KĀRPANYA ("meanness"), sometimes listed as one of the defects (*dosha) on the spiritual *path.

KARTRI ("actor" or "agent"), one link in the "action nexus" (karma-samgraha), the other two being the object (kārya), and the causal process (*kārana) itself. The *Bhagavad-Gītā (18.26ff.) distinguishes three types of agents: (1) the sāttvika-kartri, who is free from *attachment, steadfast, dedicated, unchanged by success or failure, and who does not utter "I"; (2) the rājasa-kartri, who hankers after the fruit (*phala) of his *actions, is passionate, greedy, impure, subject to elation and depression, or of a violent nature; and (3) the tāmasa-kartri, who is undisciplined, vulgar, obstinate, deceitful, base, slothful, despondent, and procrastinating. See also Actor, guna, karma.

KARUNĀ ("compassion") is mentioned, e.g., in the *Yoga-Sūtra (1.33) as a positive emotion to be projected in *meditation. *Patanjali probably borrowed this term from *Buddhism. In certain schools of *Shaivism and also in *Rāmānuja's school of *Vaishnavism, karunā stands for divine *grace. See also dayā.

KĀSHYAPA or KASHYAPA; the name of several ancient sages. Spelled with a long a, the name refers particularly to one of the great seers (*rishi) of *Vedic times, who is also known as Kanva and traditionally is said to have descended directly from *Brahma. He is first mentioned in the *Atharva-Veda (e.g., 1.14.4) as a sage knowledgeable in *magic. A different Kashyapa figures prominently in the *Mahābhārata and many of the *Purānas as a wise preceptor of *Vedānta. One of these Kashyapas was a renowned teacher of *medicine and the author of a medieval tract on *Āyur-Veda, entitled Kāshyapa-Samhitā.

KATHA-UPANISHAD (Kathopanishad), probably the oldest verse *Upanishad, which, in its earliest portions, dates back to the fifth century BCE. It is also the first Upanishad to contain explicit *Yoga and *Sāmkhya ideas. These are grafted onto an ancient narrative in which the student Naciketas is initiated into the higher mysteries by the god of death (*Yama). The second chapter, which appears to be a self-contained unit, expounds a type of *Epic Yoga consisting in the "firm binding of the *senses." In one verse (2.12) the compound *adhyātma-yoga occurs, the goal of which is the realization of the transcendental Self (*purusha). The general tenor of this work is panentheistic.

KATTHANA ("boastfulness"), one of the five obstacles (*vighna) of *Yoga according to the *Yoga-Tattva-Upanishad (3). See also abhimāna; cf. mauna.

KAULA ("pertaining to the *kula," short for *kaula-mārga, "path relating to the *kula"), a spiritual approach extolled in the *Kula-Arnava-Tantra (2.13–14; 20–21):

Just as the footprints of all creatures are lost in an elephant's footprints, so the [philosophical] viewpoints of all people are [absorbed] in the kula [teaching].

Just as iron is never comparable with gold, so the kula teaching should never be likened to any other [teaching].

Riding on the vehicle of the kula teaching, the most excellent person goes across the island [of this world] to *heaven and [then] obtains the jewel of *liberation.

In all other [philosophical] viewpoints, people attain to liberation through prolonged *practice. In the kaula [school], however, [they are liberated] instantly.

Fundamental to the practice of the *Kaula school is the divinization of the *body through stimulating the flow of the "nectar of immortality" (*amrita). In the *Kaula-Jnāna-Nirnaya (14.94) this ambrosial liquid is stated to be the "true condition of the kaula."

The term kaula also applies to a practitioner of the spiritual *path of the *Kaula school. According to the *Akula-Vīra-Tantra (version B, 43), there are two classes of kaulas: the kritaka ("artificial")-kaulas, who know the "serpent power" (*kundalinī-shakti) and who seek to manipulate it to gain *enlightenment, and the *sahaja ("spontaneous")-kaulas, who have achieved identity with *Shiva and abide perpetually in the state of *samarasa. See also Adept, kaula-yogin, kaula-yoginī, Spontaneity.

KAULA-ĀGAMA (kaulāgama), a synonym for *kula-āgama.

KAULA-JNĀNA-NIRNAYA ("Ascertainment of Kaula Knowledge"), an ancient *Tantric work ascribed to *Matsyendra; the oldest known source about the *kaula-mārga taught by him. According to the colophon, this work comprises 1,000 verses, but all the available manuscripts, dating back to the mid-eleventh century CE, appear to be incomplete. The first chapter, most of which is missing, deals with the process of cosmic *creation. The second chapter discusses macrocosmic and microcosmic dissolution (*laya, *pralaya). The third chapter outlines the different bodily locations (*sthāna) for *meditation and also speaks of the true nature of the phallus (*linga) and how it is to be worshiped. This is followed by a lengthy treatment of the paranormal powers (*siddhi) accruing from spiritual *practice. The next three chapters deal with the hidden bodily centers (*cakra) and various esoteric processes, including the *khecarī-mudrā. The eighth chapter introduces rituals of *worship of the different kinds of female power (*shakti). The next chapter is a list of *teachers of this particular school. The tenth chapter discloses the seed mantras (*bīja-mantras) for the various *cakras. Then come chapters dealing with dietary and behavioral considerations. The thirteenth chapter is dedicated to a discussion of the means of *liberation, especially the esoteric teaching of the *hamsa. The remaining eleven chapters deal with all kinds of esoteric processes for initiates.

KAULA-MĀRGA ("kaula path"), a synonym for *kula-āgama. See also Kaula school.

KAULA SCHOOL. The beginnings of this school within the broad movement of *Tantrism may reach back to the fifth century CE. Traditionally, *Matsyendra is venerated as its founder, though it appears that he merely founded the *yoginī-kaula* branch in Assam. Be that as it may, by the time *Abhinava Gupta wrote his learned works on Kashmiri *Shaivism in the tenth century CE, the Kaula tradition was well established, looking back on a long history.

In consonance with the *Siddha tradition, the *kaulas* believe that *enlightenment is a bodily event and that the *body's structures, if rightly manipulated, would yield *Self-realization. The central mechanism of this process is the "serpent power" (*kundalinī-shakti*), also known as the *kula* or *kula-shakti*. The body-positive orientation of the *kaulas* included the employment of *sexual rites (*maithunā*), a feature of many *Tantric schools.

The literature of the Kaula school, which was probably very comprehensive, is poorly preserved and very little researched. The most popular work is undoubtedly the *Kula-Arnava-Tantra*. Another treatise, less well known but for the historian more significant, is the *Kaula-Jnāna-Nirnaya*.

KAULA-YOGIN (masc.), or KAULA-YOGINĪ, (fem.); a practitioner of the *kaula-mārga*. See also *kaula*.

KAULIKA ("relating to *kula*"), is a synonym for *kaula*.

KAUPĪNA is the loincloth worn by many *yogins* and *sādhus*.

KAUSHALA ("skill"). In the *Bhagavad-Gītā* (2.50) *Yoga is defined as "skill in action." See also *buddhi-yoga*, *karma-yoga*.

KĀYA ("body"), a synonym for *deha* and *sharīra*.

KĀYA-KALPA ("body fashioning"), an *Āyur-Veda treatment for rejuvenating the *body, calling for seclusion, *meditation, and the application of various herbal concoctions. Tapasviji Maharaj, a renowned *Hindu saint who supposedly lived for over 180 years, underwent this treatment several times and attributed his long *life to it.

KĀYA-SAMPAT ("perfection of the body"), mentioned in the *Yoga-Sūtra* (1.45) as resulting from the total "conquest of the elements" (*bhūta-jaya*) and consisting in beauty, gracefulness, strength, and "adamantine robustness" (*vajra-samhana-natva*). See also Body, *kāya-siddhi*.

KĀYA-SHUDDHI ("body purification"). See Purification, Purity.

KĀYA-SIDDHI ("perfection of the body"), one of the results of asceticism (*tapas*), according to the *Yoga-Sūtra* (2.43). As the *Yoga-Bhāshya* (2.43) explains, such perfection is demonstrated in the acquisition of the eight major paranormal powers (*siddhi*), as well as by such paranormal abilities as clairvoyance (*dūra-darshana*) and clairaudience (*dūra-shravana*). See also Body, *kāya-sampat*.

KESHIDVĀJA, a teacher of *Epic Yoga. In the *Agni-Purāna* (379.25) he defines *Yoga as the union (*samyoga*) of the *mind with the *Absolute (*brahman*).

KESHIN ("long-haired"), a *Vedic type of ecstatic sage to whom a whole hymn is dedicated in the *Rig-Veda* (10.136). Some scholars have seen in the *keshin* a forerunner of the later *yogin*. He appears to represent a mystical culture distinct from the sacrificial *ritualism of the Vedic "seers" (*rishi).

KEVALA ("alone"), the *Self. According to the *Yoga-Tattva-Upanishad (12f.), this term refers to the psyche (*jīva) "devoid of the twenty defects (*dosha)."

KEVALA ADVAITA, the *Vedānta teaching of radical nondualism propounded, for instance, by *Shankara. It postulates that *Reality is singular and that all multiplicity is simply a cognitive error. Cf. Vishishta Advaita.

KEVALATĀ or KEVALATVA ("aloneness"), a synonym for *kaivalya employed in *Vedānta.

KEVALĪ-BHĀVA ("condition of aloneness"), a synonym for *kaivalya used in the *Yoga-Vāsishtha (3.4.53). This concept is found already in the *Mahābhārata (12.306.77), where it is stated that he who has "become alone" (kevalī-bhūta) sees the twenty-sixth principle (i.e., the *Self). This appears to be the conceptual source of the later notion of kaivalya in *Classical Yoga.

KEVALA- or KEVALĪ-KUMBHAKA ("absolute retention"), one of the forms of breath control (*prāṇāyāma) in *hatha-yoga. The *Hatha-Yoga-Pradīpikā (2.73) defines it as the retention of the *breath without inhalation and exhalation. This work (2.72) also stipulates that one should practice *sahita-kumbhaka so long as one is not accomplished in kevala-kumbhaka. The *Gheranda-Samhitā (5.89) explains it thus: "When the breath is confined to the pot (ghata) [i.e., the *body], this is kevala-kumbhaka." This text (5.92f.) further specifies that one should start by retaining the

*breath between one and sixty-four times. This should be done every three hours or, if this is not possible, five times a day (in the early morning, at noon, twilight, midnight, and in the fourth quarter of the night), or three times (morning, noon, and evening). One should also try to increase the duration of each retention daily.

KEVALIN ("that which is alone"), the transcendental *Self. The term is used, e.g., in the *Yoga-Bhāshya (1.24), which states that there are numerous kevalins who have severed the three "fetters" (bandhana), perhaps referring to the bonds of the three types of primary constituent (*guna) of *nature. The kevalins are the liberated *adepts who have perfectly recovered their transcendental Selfhood. This term has the same meaning in *Jainism, which may in fact be the source from which this concept was borrowed by *Yoga authorities. See also eka.

KHA ("hole" or "space/ether"), a synonym for *ākāsha. See also duhkha, sukha.

KHANDA, mentioned in the *Hatha-Yoga-Pradīpikā (1.8) as an *adept of *hatha-yoga.

KHECARĪ-MUDRĀ ("space-walking seal"; khecarī [fem.] is derived from *kha and the root car, "to move"), one of the principal "seals" (*mudrā) of *Tantrism and *hatha-yoga. Already hinted at in the *Maitrayanīya-Upanishad (6.20), this technique has immense importance in *hatha-yoga, where it is used in conjunction with *breath control. In the *Gheranda-Samhitā (3.25ff.) we find the following description: One should cut the *tongue's fraenum and move the tongue constantly, milking it with butter and pulling it out by means of an iron implement. When the tongue has been elongated to the point where it can reach the spot between the *eyes, one is fit for the khecarī-mudrā. In this technique, the tongue is turned back and slowly inserted into the "skull cavity" (*kapāla-kuhara). This produces all kinds of sensations, including a whole range of tastes—from salty to bitter to sweet—as the ambrosial liquid (*amrita) begins to flow abundantly. One's gaze (*drishti) should be fixed on the middle of the *forehead. This *mudrā is said to prevent fainting (*mūrchā), *hunger, *thirst, lassitude (*ālasya), *disease, aging, and even *death. It is also stated to create a "divine body" (deva-deha). Such a transubstantiated, beautiful *body is beyond the vicissitudes of the *elements and specifically of snakebite.

The *Hatha-Yoga-Pradīpikā (3.34) advises that one should cut the fraenum only a hair's breadth at a time and rub the *tongue with powdered rock salt (and yellow myrobalan). This procedure should be done every seven days, until the fraenum is completely severed after about six months. This scripture (3.41) also explains that both the tongue and the *mind must move into the "space" (*kha) for this *mudrā to be effective.

Stanza 3.42 makes the further point that by this technique the *semen is prevented from falling even when one is embracing a passionate woman. The *yogin who is skilled in this practice is claimed (3.44) to conquer *death within fifteen days. Another verse (4.49) states that the khecarī-mudrā should be practiced until the "Yoga sleep" (*yoga-nidrā) sets in.

The *Shāndilya-Upanishad (1.7.15) defines khecarī-mudrā as the state in which the *breath and *mind have come to rest upon the "inner sign" (*antar-lakshya).

The anonymous author of the *Yoga-Kundalī-Upanishad (2.44), which devotes a long section to the "science of the khecarī" (khecarī-vidyā), observes that while performing this technique one should also block the nostrils with a small plug made out of gold, silver, or iron wrapped with a thread soaked in milk. This work also makes the anatomically doubtful claim that some *yogins can extend their *tongues to the crown of the *head, though some practitioners have succeeded in elongating their tongue by two inches and more. See also lambikā-yoga.

KHECARATVA ("space-walking"), variously understood as either *levitation or an *out-of-body experience, which books on *occultism call "astral travel." This paranormal ability (*siddhi) is also called khe-gati. See also ākāsha-gamana, laghava.

KHYĀTI ("vision"). See anyatā-khyāti, ātma-khyāti, viveka-khyāti.

KILBISHA ("guilt"), a synonym for *dosha. Guilt is a transgression of the laws of life, a violation of the *life force. Hence since ancient times the discipline of breath control (*prānāyāma) has been recommended as a means for expiating guilt and thus restoring the moral order. See also klesha, pāpa.

KIND SPEECH. Many of India's spiritual traditions consider kind speech an important *virtue, presumably because it represents an aspect of nonharming (*ahimsā). Thus the *Shiva-Samhitā (3.18) states that success in *Yoga escapes those who are given to harsh speech (nishtura-bhāshā). See also vāc.

KĪRTANA ("chanting"). Singing songs of praise in the ritual *worship of one's chosen deity (*ishta-devatā) is one of the "limbs" (*anga) of *bhakti-yoga. This practice tends to lead more often to an emotionally charged *ecstasy, with tears of *joy, rather than the quietistic *ecstasy aspired to in other schools of *Yoga.

KLESHA ("trouble" or "affliction"), a word found already in the *Mahābhārata, where it is generally used in the sense of "toil" or "struggle." At least one passage (12.204.16), however, suggests a more technical use of the term: "As seeds roasted in fire do not sprout again, so the *Self (*ātman) is not bound again by the kleshas [once they have been] burnt by means of wisdom (*jnāna)." Here the term stands for what has been called the "causes of affliction." Presumably reiterating an earlier tradition, *Patanjali distinguishes five such causes: nescience (*avidyā), "I-am-ness" (*asmitā), attachment (*rāga), aversion (*dvesha), and the will to live (*abhinivesha). These factors, which can be compared to the drives of an earlier generation of psychologists, provide the cognitive and motivational framework for the ordinary individual enmeshed in conditional existence (*samsāra) and ignorant of the transcendental *Self. As the *Yoga-Sūtra (2.12) states, these kleshas are the root of the *karmic "deposit" (*āshaya) in the subconscious. Their effects are not only felt in one's present life but also determine the quality of one's future *rebirths.

According to the *Yoga-Sūtra (2.4), the kleshas exist in various states. They can be (1) dormant (prasupta), i.e., exist in the form of subliminal "activators" (*samskāra) ready to manifest as psychomental activity; (2) attenuated (tanu), i.e., temporarily prevented from taking effect by way of *concentration or other yogic techniques; (3) intercepted (vicchinna), which is the case when one kind of klesha blocks the operation of another; or (4) aroused (udāra), i.e., fully active. According to *Patanjali, it is the purpose of *kriyā-yoga to achieve the attenuation (tanū-karana) of these kleshas. Ultimately, the kleshas are completely obliterated through the realization of the "cloud of dharma" ecstasy (*dharma-megha-samādhi).

In the *Yoga-Bhāshya (1.8) the following alternative designations are furnished: *tamas ("darkness"); *moha ("delusion"); mahā-moha ("great delusion"); tāmisra ("the dark"); and andhatāmisra ("the pitch-dark"). Another name for klesha is *viparyaya ("error"). See also aklishta, dosha, duhkha, klishta.

KLISHTA ("afflicted"), the past participle of the root klish, from which the noun *klesha is derived. *Patanjali looks upon the five types of mental activity (*vritti) as being either "afflicted" or "nonafflicted" (*aklishta). The *Yoga-Bhāshya (1.5) explains the former as "caused by the *kleshas," but the *Mani-Prabhā (1.5) offers the more convincing interpretation of "resulting in *bondage."

KNOTS. See granthi.

KNOWLEDGE. In Western thought, knowledge is simply information about the *world. It is not attributed with any metaphysical function. However, the Indian sages early on distinguished between knowledge as information, or knowledge of the differentiated phenomenal world, and knowledge as *wisdom, which reveals the *Self and is therefore liberating. The second kind of knowledge is rated higher than pragmatic knowledge, because it not merely satisfies the curious *mind but also leads to perfect *happiness through *Self-realization. See also abhijnā, jnāna, prajnā, vidyā, pramāna; cf. ajnāna, avidyā, viparyaya.

KRAMA, one of the leading schools of *Shaivism, especially prominent in Kashmir. It considers the ultimate *Reality to be process (*krama*): the transcendental *Consciousness (*samvid*) emanates out of itself the multiplex universe, while itself remaining eternally the same. This school's beginnings are connected with the name of Shivānanda (8th cen. CE), a native of Kashmir.

KRAMA-MUKTI ("gradual liberation"), one of two *paths taught in the early *Upanishads. It is also called *deva-yāna because it leads virtuous folk to the realms of the *gods before delivering them from the bonds of conditional existence (*samsāra*) altogether. Those who are capable of radical *renunciation in the moment are instantly liberated, which is the second path of *sadyo-mukti* (from *sadyas*, "immediate"). See also *pitri-yāna*.

KORANTAKA, is mentioned in the *Hatha-Yoga-Pradīpikā (1.6) as a master of *hatha-yoga.

KOSHA ("sheath" or "casing"). All major spiritual traditions of the *world sanction the belief that the physical *body is not the only vehicle in which *consciousness can express itself or in which the Spirit, or Self (*ātman*), manifests itself. Thus most schools of *Postclassical Yoga and *Vedānta accept the doctrine of the five sheaths (*panca-kosha*), which was first introduced in the ancient *Taittirīya-Upanishad (2.7). This scripture speaks of the five envelopes that occlude the pure *light of the transcendental *Self: (1) the "sheath composed of food" (*anna-maya-kosha*); (2) the "sheath composed of life force" (*prāna-maya-kosha*); (3) the "sheath composed of *mind" (*mano-maya-kosha*); (4) the "sheath composed of awareness" (*vijnāna-maya-kosha*); and (5) the "sheath

composed of *bliss" (*ānanda-maya-kosha*). The last-mentioned envelope is equated in the *Taittirīya-Upanishad with the transcendental *Reality itself, though later schools consider it still to be a fine veil around the *Self.

This model is not accepted in *Classical Yoga; yet here too the existence of a supraphysical *body is postulated, which is composed of more subtle (*sūkshma*) matter-energy than the material body. While the *Yoga-Sūtra does not mention such a body directly, it is implied, e.g., in the notion that there are highly evolved masters of *Yoga who have merged with the very ground of *nature. This merging (*prakriti-laya*) is of exceedingly long duration and is a condition of quasi-liberation. Also, the deities (*deva*) exist in some form or another, and the "Lord" (*īshvara*) himself is held to have assumed a highly refined supramaterial condition, called *sattva, in order to instruct the ancient sages. Furthermore, techniques such as "space-walking" (*khecarī-gati*), or *astral projection, imply the existence of a subtle body.

In one passage in the *Yoga-Bhāshya (4.10), however, *Vyāsa distinctly argues that consciousness (*citta*) is all-pervasive and that therefore there can be no question of a subtle or "superconductive" (*ātivāhika*) *body. This all-pervasive *citta* contracts and expands only in its manifestation as mental activity (*vritti*). Possibly the differences in opinion are the result of taking the concept of *body too literally. We can conceive of a universal field of *consciousness that, seen hierarchically, is yet delimited from another universal field of different quality, such as the highly attenuated *sattva field that certainly *Vyāsa assumes for the *īshvara in his teaching mode. It is possible to speak of such a field as a body.

KRAUNCA-NISHADANA ("curlew seat"), a *posture mentioned in the *Yoga-Bhāshya (2.46). The *Tattva-Vaishāradī (2.46) unhelpfully observes that for its performance one should study the typical posture of a curlew.

KRI-KARA ("kri maker"; sometimes spelled kri-kala), one of the five secondary forms of the life force (*prāna) circulating in the *body. It is responsible for causing hunger (*kshudhā) or sneezing.

KRIPĀ ("grace"), a synonym for *anu-graha, *prasāda. See also Grace; cf. Effort.

KRISHNA ("Puller"), the incarnate *God worshiped in the *Vaishnava tradition, so called because he pulls or attracts devotees' *hearts to himself. Some scholars doubt that there was an actual historical person by the name of Krishna whose teachings are recorded in the *Bhagavad-Gītā and other parts of the *Mahābhārata, but this skepticism is proably unwarranted. The

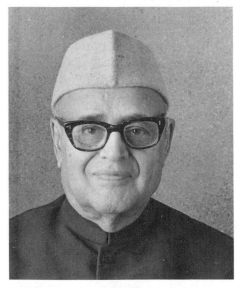
Gopi Krishna

name Krishna first appears in the ancient *Rig-Veda (8.74), where it refers to a sage. In another passage (8.85) it refers to a monster. A reference that is thought more likely to pertain to the *adept Krishna is contained in the *Chāndogya-Upanishad (30.6), where Krishna is called the son of Devakī and the pupil of Ghora Angirasa, a sun priest belonging to the tradition of the *Atharva-Veda. Sarvepalli Radhakrishnan (1948) points out the "great similarity between the teaching of Ghora Angirasa . . . and that of Krishna in the Gītā" (p. 28). It appears that this Krishna was the leader of a branch of the Yādava tribe and a much-revered spiritual teacher. In the course of time, he became deified like so many other masters.

In medieval times, Krishna became associated with the exuberant *bhakti movement, a further development of the bhakti-yoga first taught in the *Bhagavad-Gītā. His fictitious life story is told in the Hari-Vamsha ("*Hari's Genealogy"), an appendix to the *Mahābhārata, and also in the *Bhāgavata-Purāna. There he is celebrated as a full *incarnation (pūrna-avatāra) of *Vishnu. See also avatāra.

KRISHNA, GOPI (1903–1984), a native of Kashmir who in 1937, after seventeen years of practicing *meditation while simultaneously pursuing a career as a government employee, experienced a sudden awakening of the "serpent power" (*kun-dalinī-shakti). For several years this unleashed psychospiritual power played havoc with his *body and *mind until the condition stabilized. His tribulations are recorded in great detail in his autobiography, Kundalini: Evolutionary Energy in Man, which in its first English edition had a psychological commentary by James Hillman. Gopi Krishna's testimony is the most comprehensive descriptive account of the *kundalinī* phenomenon available. In subsequent years he published many other books, in which he expressed the belief that the *kundalinī* is the mechanism responsible for the higher spiritual *evolution of humanity. Gopi Krishna did not found a school or movement, but his work did much to make *kundalinī-yoga* more widely known in the West.

KRITYA ("action"). See *panca-vidha-kritya*.

KRIYĀ ("act" or "rite"), often used synonymously with *karma*. In contemporary *Yoga circles, *kriyā* also stands for involuntary movements of the limbs resulting from the arousal of the "serpent power" (*kundalinī-shakti*). See also *kriyā-yoga*.

KRIYĀ-SHAKTI ("action power"), that aspect of the *Divine that is the source of all dynamism in *nature. See also *shakti*; cf. *icchā-shakti, jnāna-shakti*.

KRIYĀ-YOGA ("Yoga of [ritual] action"). In the *Yoga-Sūtra* (2.1), *kriyā-yoga* stands for the *Yoga of transmutative *action that obliterates the subliminal activators (*samskāra*) through asceticism (*tapas*), study (*svādhyāya*), and devotion to the Lord (*īshvara-pranidhāna*). This Yoga can be contrasted with the *ashta-anga-yoga* whose "limbs" (*anga*) are expounded in aphorisms 2.28–3.8. Even though *Patanjali's Yoga has achieved fame for its eightfold path, it is likely that this particular systematization was merely cited by Patanjali and that his own contribution to Yoga was *kriyā-yoga*.

In the *Tri-Shikhi-Brāhmana-Upanishad* (2.23) the *path of *kriyā-yoga* is contrasted with *jnāna-yoga* and equated with *karma-yoga*. It is also said in verse 24 to consist in the fixation of the *mind upon a particular *object and the adherence of the mind to the moral disciplines enjoined in the scriptures. The last is deemed *karma-yoga* proper.

According to the *Bhāgavata-Purāna* (11.27.49), *kriyā-yoga* can be either *Vedic or *Tantric ritual practice. Both approaches are said to lead to the *Divine.

In modern times, Paramahamsa *Yogananda's Kriya Yoga has won many Western practitioners. Its goal is to awaken the *kundalinī* through mental focusing (*dhāranā*) and breath control (*prānāyāma*) on the basis of *bhakti-yoga*.

KRODHA ("anger"), one of the "gates of hell," together with desire (*kāma*) and greed (*lobha*). In a memorable passage in the *Bhagavad-Gītā* (2.63), anger is said to arise from *desire and to cause bewilderment (*moha*), which in turn leads to confusion of one's *memory and loss of wisdom (*buddhi*), whereupon a person is completely lost.

Yet when one assumes the position of the *witness, that is, the transcendental *Self, in the midst of intense *emotion, one's true nature can manifest in this high-energy state. This teaching is expressed, for instance, in the *Spanda-Kārikā* (1.22), one of the important texts of Kashmiri *Shaivism.

KSHAMĀ ("patience"), often listed among the moral disciplines (*yama*). In the *Yoga-Yājnavalkya* (1.64), it is defined as equanimity (*samatva*) toward all pleasant and unpleasant things. The *Darshana-Upanishad* (1.16–17) explains it as refraining from agitation when provoked by one's enemies. See also *kshānti, titikshā*.

KSHANA ("moment" or "instant"), defined in the *Yoga-Bhāshya* (3.52) as the time taken by an atom (*parama-anu*) to shift from one position to another. See also *kāla*.

KSHĀNTI ("forbearance"), a synonym for *kshamā*. The *Bhagavad-Gītā* (13.7) considers it to be a manifestation of wisdom (*jnāna*).

KSHARA ("mobile"), a common term in *Epic Yoga for *nature, which is constantly in flux, while the ultimate *Reality is perfectly stable. Cf. *akshara*.

KSHEMARĀJA (10th cen. CE), an *adept of Kashmiri *Shaivism and one of the principal disciples of *Abhinava Gupta. He wrote the *Vimarshinī*, an important commentary on the *Shiva-Sūtra* of Vasugupta. He also composed many other celebrated works, including the *Pratyabhijnā-Hridaya*, *Spanda-Samdoha*, and *Spanda-Nirnaya*.

KSHETRA ("field"), a term of *Epic Yoga to denote *nature and/or the body-mind, as opposed to the "field knower" (*kshetra-jna*), or *Self.

KSHETRA-JNA ("field knower"), also called *kshetrin*; the transcendental *Self supporting the individual *consciousness. As the *Mahābhārata* (12.212.40) puts it: "That being (*bhāva*) who abides in the *mind is called 'field knower.' " The *Yoga-Bhāshya* (2.17) emphasizes that the "field knower" is immutable and inactive. According to the *Bhagavad-Gītā* (13.2), the "field knower" of all the "fields" is none other than *Krishna.

KSHUDHĀ ("hunger"), sometimes counted as one of the defects (*dosha*); according to some works of *Postclassical Yoga, it can be combated by *shītalī-prānāyāma.

KSHURIKĀ-UPANISHAD (*Kshurikopanishad*, "Dagger *Upanishad*"), one of the *Yoga-Upanishads, a *Vedānta-based tract of twenty-four stanzas dealing principally with concentration (*dhāranā*). Concentration is called the "knife" or "dagger" (*kshurikā*) by which the *yogin severs the knot of *ignorance. Here *dhāranā is a combination of focusing *mind, breath (*prāna*), and *gaze on specific locations in the *body: the ankles, shanks, knees, thighs, anus, *penis, *navel, central channel (*sushumnā-nādī*), "heart abode" (*hridaya-āyatana*; see *hridaya*), and *throat. According to the commentary by *Upanishad Brahmayogin, two further stations are the middle of the eyebrows (*bhrū-madhya*) and the *sahasrāra-cakra* at the crown of the *head. The text refers to these loci (*desha*) as "joints" (*marman*) that are to be severed. A similar process is described for the 72,000 currents (*nādī*) of the *life force circulating in the body. They have to be "cut off" with the exception of the axial channel (*sushumnā-nādī*). The goal of this *Yoga is absorption (*laya*) into the *Absolute.

KUHŪ-NĀDĪ ("new-moon channel"), one of the fourteen principal channels (*nādī*) through which the *life force flows in the *body. According to the *Shāndilya-Upanishad* (1.4.9), it is situated to the back and side of the central channel (*sushumnā-nādī*) and extends to the *genitals. The *Darshana-Upanishad* (4.8) also places it to the side of the central channel, and the *Yoga-Shikhā-Upanishad* (5.26) associates it with the anus and defecation.

KUKKUTA-ĀSANA (*kukkutāsana*, "cock posture"), described in the *Gheranda-Samhitā* (2.31) thus: Sitting in the lotus posture (*padma-āsana*), one should insert the hands between one's thighs and knees and raise oneself, supporting the *body with the elbows.

KULA, in ordinary contexts, stands for "family," "flock," or "home," thus conveying the idea of the familiar, as in *guru-kula*, "teacher's family," meaning a spiritual lineage. Something of this connotation is preserved in the usage of the term *kula* in the esoteric schools of *Tantrism, where it refers to the divine power (*shakti*), the feminine aspect of the *Absolute. The masculine aspect of the *Divine is known as *akula*. To confuse matters, *kula* is also used to describe the experience of the union between *Shiva and *Shakti, *god and *goddess, power and *Consciousness. See also *kaula*.

KULA-ĀCĀRA (*kulācāra*, "kula conduct"), the liberating approach of the *Kaula school. See also *ācāra*.

KULA-ĀGAMA (*kulāgama*, "kula tradition"), the *Tantric tradition that has the notion of *kula* as its doctrinal mainstay. Also called *kula-ācāra* and *kula-mārga*.

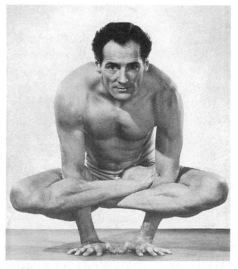

Kukkuta-āsana, demonstrated by Theos Bernard

KULA-AMRITA (*kulāmrita*), the immortal nectar (*amrita*) of the feminine power (*shakti*) of the *Divine.

KULA-ARNAVA-TANTRA (*Kulārnavatantra*, "Flood of Kula Treatise"), a short text of the *Kaula school consisting of sixty stanzas dealing with *concentration on various psychoenergetic centers (*cakra*) of the *body and the paranormal powers (*siddhi*) resulting from this practice.

KULA-KUNDALINĪ, a synonym for *kula* and *kundalinī*.

KULA-MĀRGA ("*kula* path"), a synonym for *kaula-mārga*.

KULASEKHARA (prob. 8th cen. CE), one of the twelve *Ālvārs of Southern *Vaishnavism. A ruler of Kerala, he is remembered more for his devotional poetry than his royal deeds.

KUMBHAKA ("potlike"). *Breath retention is one of the most direct means of effecting changes in *consciousness—a fact that has been exploited in many spiritual traditions around the *world. The term *kumbhaka* can denote both "breath control" (*prānāyāma*) in general and the key practice of "breath retention" in particular. In the latter sense, the term *kumbhaka* refers to the fact that during the suspension of the *breath the trunk of the *body is filled with life energy (*prāna*), which is retained as a pot (*kumbha*) retains liquid. But since this technique also stabilizes the *mind, the *Yoga-Tattva-Upanishad (142) likens *kumbhaka* to a lamp inside a pot that does not flicker because no breeze can reach it.

According to the *Shāndilya-Upanishad (1.7.13.5), *kumbhaka* is of two kinds: "associated" (*sahita*) with inhalation and exhalation, and "isolated" (*kevala*), that is, without either inhalation or exhalation. The latter type of retention is an advanced form of *breath control, which should occur without strain. Whereas the various *sahita* forms of *kumbhaka* attract the "serpent power" (*kundalinī-shakti*) into the central channel (*sushumnā-nādī*), the "isolated" retention is the principal means of forcing that power up along the spinal axis to the center at the crown of the *head. The *Hatha-Yoga-Pradīpikā* (2.72ff.) makes this observation:

So long as [the *yogin* still aspires to] the attainment (*siddhi*) of the *kevala* [type of breath suspension], he should practice the *sahita* [variety]. When the breath (*vāyu*) is easily retained, without exhalation and inhalation . . .

. . . this [type of] breath control is said to be *kevala-kumbhaka*. When this *kevala-kumbhaka* without exhalation and inhalation is attained . . .

. . . nothing in the three worlds is difficult for him to obtain. He who is empowered by means of *kevala-kumbhaka*, through the retention (*dhāranā*) of the breath at will . . .

. . . attains even to the condition of *rāja-yoga*. There is no doubt about this.

According to the *Shiva-Samhitā* (3.53), one must be able to retain the *breath for three *ghatikās* (i.e., seventy-two minutes) before one can hope to obtain paranormal powers (*siddhis*). Elsewhere (3.59) this work states that when one is able to perform *kumbhaka* for a whole *yāma* (i.e., three hours) the *body becomes so light that one is able to balance on one's thumb (see also *lāghava*).

KUNDALA ("ring"). Members of the *Kānphata order wear large earrings requiring the piercing and splitting of the cartilage of both ears. This is said to have a beneficial influence on the flow of the *life force in the *body. These earrings are also called "seals" (*mudrā*).

KUNDALINĪ-SHAKTI ("serpent power"; also called *kundalī*, *kutilangī*, *bhujanginī*, *phanī*, *nāgī*, *cakrī*, *sarasvatī*, *lalanā*, *rasanā*, *samkinī*, *rājī*, *sarpinī*, *mani*, *ashtā-vakrā*, *ātma-shakti*, *avadhūtī*, *kuntī*, and a host of other names), a mysterious psychospiritual force; a conceptual and practical mainstay of *Tantrism and *hatha-yoga. In the *Hatha-Yoga-Pradīpikā* (3.1) it is hailed as the support of all *Yoga treatises (*tantra*). The enigmatic *kundalinī* may have been hinted at already in the *Rig-Veda* (10.189) under the name of Vāc Virāj ("Voice Resplendent"), who is described as a "serpent queen" (*sarpa-rājnī*). Because the *kundalinī* experience is claimed to depend on universal structures of the *body, we can assume that it has been encountered by mystics throughout the ages. It was only with the body-positive esotericism of the *Tantras, however, that this experience was elaborated into a full-fledged conceptual model that then served practitioners as a road map in their efforts to systematically awaken the *kundalinī* power.

On the occult principle that the *body is a microcosm that faithfully reflects the large configurations found in the *macrocosm, the *kundalinī* is envisioned as being the individualized form of the cosmic feminine principle, or *shakti. That divine force is thought to manifest in the form of the *kundalinī*, on the one hand, and the life force (*prāna*), on the other. The *kundalinī*, however, is understood as a more fundamental potency in the spiritual process. Perhaps the relationship between *prāna* and the *kundalinī* can be compared to that of an A-bomb and an H-bomb. It takes the concentrated impact of the *prāna* force, regulated through *breath control, to trigger the *kundalinī* force and make it ascend along the central conduit (*sushumnā-nādī) of the *body.

The kundalinī is pictured as residing in a state of potency, brilliant as a million suns, at the lowest esoteric center (*cakra) of the *body. The kundalinī's state of potency is expressed in the notion of its lying coiled—three and a half, five, and eight coils are often mentioned—at the basal center. This hidden serpent closes off the gate to *liberation, which is the lower entrance to the central channel (*sushumnā-nādī). The *Goraksha-Samhitā (1.47ff.) observes:

The serpent power, forming an eightfold coil above the "bulb" (*kanda), remains there, all the while covering with its face the opening of the door to the *Absolute.

Through that door the safe door to the *Absolute can be reached. Covering with the face that door, the great *Goddess is asleep [in the ordinary person].

Awakened through *buddhi-yoga together with [the combined action of] *mind and *breath, she rises upward through the *sushumnā like a thread [being pushed through] a needle.

Sleeping in the form of a serpent, resembling a resplendent cord, she, when awakened by the Yoga of *fire [i.e., mental *concentration and *breath control], rises upward through the *sushumnā.

Just as one may open a door with a key by force, so the *yogin should break open the door to *liberation with the kundalinī.

The *Tantric yogin's task consists in obliging the kundalinī to "uncoil" and rise to the "thousand-petaled lotus" at the top of the *head, which is the locus of the static pole of the psychospiritual energy. It is the seat of *Shiva. The resulting reunion of Shiva and Shakti, *god and *goddess, is celebrated as the supreme goal of *Yoga. It manifests in a radical switch in *con-sciousness, obliterating the sense of individuation and flooding the *body with divine nectar, the *kula-amrita (or *soma), which is experienced as unsurpassably blissful (*ānanda).

The ascent of the kundalinī from the base *cakra to the *head is associated with a variety of psychic phenomena, notably heat and light (*jyotis) but also different kinds of inner sounds (*nāda). According to the *Yoga-Shikhā-Upanishad (1.114f.), the constant stimulation of the kundalinī produces a sensation in the central channel similar to that of ants crawling up the spine. Some of these physiological side effects can be greatly disturbing, especially when the kundalinī awakening has occurred spontaneously and without adequate preparation or *purification. These have been vividly described by Gopi *Krishna (1971), a modern kundalinī "victim," who gradually learned to master this power. In his autobiography, Kundalini: Evolutionary Energy in Man, he vividly described his experience as follows:

Suddenly, with a roar like that of a waterfall, I felt a stream of liquid light entering my brain through the spinal cord. Entirely unprepared for such a development, I was completely taken by surprise; but regaining self-control instantaneously, I remained sitting in the same posture, keeping my mind on the point of concentration. The illumination grew brighter and brighter, the roaring louder, I experienced a rocking sensation and then felt myself slipping out of my body, entirely enveloped in a halo of light. (pp. 12–13)

The final realization of the *Tantric yogin is thought to be more complete than that of the *rāja-yogin, because it includes the *body. In other words, it is not merely a mind-transcending state but illumines the body itself: The body is experienced as the body of the *Divine. In this way the *Tantric *yogin*, or *sādhaka*, combines the ideal of liberation (*mukti*) with the ideal of world enjoyment (*bhukti*). See also *granthi*.

KUNDALINĪ-YOGA, the *Tantric discipline involving the deliberate arousal of the *kundalinī-shakti*. See also *bhūta-shuddhi*.

KŪRMA ("tortoise"), one of the five secondary forms of the life force (*prāna*). According to the *Tri-Shikhi-Brāhmana-Upanishad* (2.82), it circulates in the skin and bones and is responsible for the closing and opening of the *eyes, which is its widely accepted function.

KŪRMA-ĀSANA (*kūrmāsana*, "tortoise posture"), described in the *Gheranda-Samhitā* (2.32) thus: One should place the crossed heels under the scrotum and keep the *body, *head, and neck aligned. The *Hatha-Yoga-Pradīpikā* (1.22) stipulates that one should press the crossed ankles against the anus. Contemporary manuals explain this posture (*āsana*) differently: Sitting with one's legs stretched out in front, one should bend forward. Then one should insert one's arms beneath one's legs and reach up toward the back, locking one's fingers behind the back. See also *uttāna-kūrma-āsana*.

KŪRMA-NĀDĪ ("tortoise channel"), mentioned in the *Yoga-Sūtra* (3.31) and explained in the *Yoga-Bhāshya* as a structure in the chest. By performing ecstatic "constraint" (*samyama*) on this *nādī, the *yogin achieves a motionless (mental) state like that of a serpent or iguana.

KŪRMA-PURĀNA, originally probably a *Vaishnava work of the fifth century CE that was recast several hundred years later in the light of the *Pāshupata tradition. It contains the *Īshvara-Gītā*.

KUTA-STHA ("summit-abiding"), a term used in the *Bhagavad-Gītā* (6.8), e.g., to designate the perfected *adept and elsewhere (15.16) to refer to the imperishable (*akshara*) dimension of existence.

KUTĪRA ("hut"), a *yogin*'s hermitage. The *Gheranda-Samhitā* (5.5ff.) supplies the following details for its construction: One should construct a solitary hut within an enclosed compound in a good location (*desha*) in a just, donation-friendly (*subhiksha*), and conflict-free state. The hut, smeared with cowdung, should be located neither too high nor too low, and it should be free from insects. The compound should include a well or pond. The *Hatha-Yoga-Pradīpikā* (1.13) recommends that the hermitage (*matha*) should have no windows and only a small door. The *yogin*'s dwelling is also called *mandira*. See also *āshrama*.

KU-YOGIN ("bad *yogin*"), an unsuccessful practitioner who, according to the *Bhāgavata-Purāna* (2.4.14), is unable to attain the *Divine. The *Uddhāva-Gītā* (23.29) says of him that he is led astray by the obstacles (*antarāya*), other human beings, or even *deities.

· L ·

LĀGHAVA, LĀGHUTĀ, or LĀGHUTVA ("lightness"). The sensation of bodily lightness is one of the by-products of regular and advanced *breath control, especially after rubbing one's sweat (*sveda) produced by intensive *prānāyāma into the skin. In the *Gheranda-Samhitā (1.11) this is regarded as the fifth "limb" (*anga) of the sevenfold *path. See also laghiman, Levitation, utthāna.

LAGHIMAN ("levitation"), one of the eight classic paranormal powers (*siddhi). The *Tattva-Vaishāradī (3.45) observes that by means of this ability one becomes airborne like the tuft of a reed. The *Mārkandeya-Purāna (40.31) curiously explains it as swiftness (shīgratva).

LAGHU-ĀHĀRA (laghvāhāra; "scant diet," from laghu, "scant" and āhāra, "eating"), sometimes regarded as one of the component disciplines of self-restraint (*niyama). The *Yoga-Tattva-Upanishad (28) even considers it to be the most important practice of moral discipline (*yama). According to the *Mandala-Brāhmana-Upanishad (1.2.2), a light diet keeps the defects (*dosha) in check. See also āhāra, mita-āhāra; cf. atyāhāra.

LĀGHUTĀ. See lāghava.

LAGHU-YOGA-VĀSISHTHA, a work composed by the Kashmiri scholar *Gauda Abhinanda at the beginning of the tenth century CE, perhaps on the basis of an earlier and no longer extant work; generally considered to be an abridgment of the *Yoga-Vāsishtha, though there are good reasons to assume that the Laghu ("Short")-Yoga-

Vāsishtha is actually an original work that was subsequently cast into the five-times-larger Yoga-Vāsishtha by the same author or another poet-editor. The Laghu-Yoga-Vāsishtha comprises six chapters with a total of some 6,000 verses. It is presented as the composition of the ancient Sage Valmīki, the legendary author of the *Rāmāyana. Vālmīki relates to the seer Bharadvāja a didactic conversation that occurred between *Rāma and *Vashishtha.

As the title indicates, the work purports to expound yogic teachings, though its scope is rather more comprehensive, covering not only spiritual and philosophical matters but also cosmology. The general slant is toward the *Yoga of wisdom (*jnāna-yoga). Its metaphysical basis is *Vedantic nondualism with a prominent presence of *Shaktism. Thus the supreme *Reality is presented (3.7.1) as possessing all potencies (*shakti). Its aspects are said to be the power of awareness (*cit-shakti), the power of motility (spanda-shakti), the power of fluidity (drava-shakti), and the power of the void (shūnya-shakti).

The ultimate *Reality is pure, omniscient, omnipresent Consciousness (*cit, *citta). It is described (6.53.24) as being "like the chest of a stone [sculpture], which is void inside and void outside . . . tranquil, lucid as the vault of the sky, neither visible nor beyond vision."

The phenomenal *world is like a *dream appearing in the vast expanse of pure Awareness, or *Consciousness. Only the unenlightened being deems it to be external to itself. The human *mind alone creates the *illusion of *bondage and the illusion of the process of *liberation. What is to be realized is that ultimately nothing ever happens and that there is simply eternal, objectless *bliss. This extreme idealistic metaphysics has inspired many *Vedānta teachers, including some of the composers of the *Yoga-Upanishads.

LAJJĀ ("shame"), occasionally listed among the defects (*dosha) that foil *progress in *Yoga.

LAKSHANA ("characteristic, sign"), in the *Yoga-Sūtra (3.13), an *object's specific mode of existence. See also parināma.

LAKSHMĪ, also called Shrī Lakshmī; the *goddess of fortune, prosperity, and beauty; the spouse of *Vishnu. Like Venus, she was born from the ocean. The name is mentioned already in the *Vedas, but this graceful *deity became a major figure of the *Hindu pantheon only with the *Mahābhārata and *Rāmāyana. The Agastya-Samhitā (489) notes that Lakshmī attracts the *mind of *yogins by her beauty and youthfulness, as pollen attracts the bee.

LAKSHYA ("perceivable object" or "vision"), in *tāraka-yoga, a meditative visionary state marked by an intense experience of *light. Three variations of this state are distinguished: inner vision (*antar-lakshya), external vision (*bahir-lakshya), and intermediate vision (*madhya-lakshya).

LAKULĪSHA ("Lord of the Club"), also called Lakuli and Nakulīsha; the reputed founder of the *Pāshupata sect, whose distinguishing mark is the club (lakula) carried by all members. He is remembered to have had four main disciples and to have been seated on an "altar of *ashes" when instructing his followers. He lived probably in the first century CE and was soon deified.

LALANĀ-CAKRA ("caressing wheel"), a psychoenergetic center situated in the *head near the uvula. It is also known as the *tālu-cakra. Its curious name is probably explained by the yogic practice of tonguing the *palate or, more specifically, the uvula in order to stimulate the flow of the lunar *nectar. Lalanā is also one of the esoteric designations of *idā-nādī. See also cakra.

LALĀTA ("forehead"), often mentioned in the *Yoga texts as the location of the *ājnā-cakra, though this psychoenergetic center is really in the core of the brain. *Yogins belonging to the various sects of *Hinduism, such as the *Shaivas and *Vaishnavas, paint their respective sect marks on their foreheads. The round dot (*bindu) worn by some on the forehead marks the place of the ājnā-cakra. In the case of women, this ornamental mark is called tilaka (from tila, "sesame").

LALLĀ (14th cen. CE), an *adept of Kashmiri *Shaivism and a practitioner of *laya-yoga. In one of her beautiful poetic sayings she mentions that she was called Lallā (Sanskrit: lalāsa) because she was ever "desirous" of knowing *Reality.

LAMBIKĀ-YOGA ("Yoga of the hanger"). The lambikā ("hanger") is the uvula, which is also called "royal tooth" (*rāja-danta). This anatomical part carries special significance in *hatha-yoga. As the *Goraksha-Paddhati (2.48) explains:

When the *tongue constantly "kisses" the tip of the uvula, [thereby causing] the liquid (*rasa) to flow—[which may taste] salty, pungent, sour, or like milk, honey, or ghee—this leads to the cure of *diseases, prevents ageing, [and grants] immunity to weapons that are hurled [at one's person]. That [*yogin who has mastered this practice] will [enjoy] *immortality and the acquisition of the eight "excellences" (*guna) and obtain ultimate *perfection.

This technique is part of the *khecarī-mudrā. See also lalanā-cakra.

LAMP. See dīpa.

LANGUAGE. Even though the ultimate spiritual realization transcends both the *mind and speech, the practitioners of all the *world's spiritual traditions have consistently endeavored to communicate something about it so that others might be able to duplicate that realization. Language has the curious capacity to both disclose and veil the *truth, and since ancient times the masters of India's spirituality have been especially sensitive to the possibilities and the limitations of linguistic communication. Thus, more than five thousand years ago, the seers (*rishi), whose wisdom is recorded in the *Rig-Veda and the other *Vedic hymnodies, developed a sophisticated symbolic language of extraordinary power and beauty.

Much later, the masters of *Tantrism invented a secret language called *sam-dhya-bhāshā ("twilight language") that served the purpose of concealing spiritual truths from outsiders and to reveal the mysteries to the *initiates. See also Alphabet, vāc; cf. mauna.

LANGUOR. See ālasya, styāna, tandrā.

LAULIKĪ ("rolling"), a synonym for *naulī.

LAULYA ("fickleness"), or **LOLUPTVA** ("rolling-about-ness"); one of the factors detrimental to success in *Yoga, according to the *Hatha-Yoga-Pradīpikā (1.15). Cf. aloluptva, dhairya, dhriti.

LAW. See dharma, sanātana-dharma.

LAWLESSNES. See adharma.

LAYA ("dissolution" or "absorption"). The *Agni-Purāna (368.1ff.) distinguishes between four types of dissolution: (1) nitya-laya, the "daily death" of millions of beings; (2) naimittika-laya, the "incidental dissolution" of all beings into the *Absolute; (3) prākrita-laya, the "material dissolution" of everything at the end of a world period, that is, after a cycle of 4,000 eons (*yuga); and (4) ātyantika-laya, the "ultimate dissolution" of the individual psyche (*jīva) into the *Absolute.

In *hatha-yoga the term laya signifies the immersion or absorption of *attention into *Reality by means of the practice of ecstasy (*samādhi). Occasionally, the term laya is employed as a synonym for *sama-dhi. The *Hatha-Yoga-Pradīpikā (4.34) has this relevant stanza: "They say: 'Dissolution, dissolution.' But what is the nature of dissolution? Dissolution is the nonremembering of things due to the nonarising of previous subliminal traits (*vāsanā) [in the condition of *ecstasy]." The same scripture (4.66) speaks of *Adinātha, the primal god *Shiva, as having taught a crore and a quarter of ways to achieve laya. However, it recommends particularly the "cultivation of the [inner] sound" (*nāda-anusamdhāna).

By contrast, the *Tejo-Bindu-Upanishad (1.41) cites laya as one of the nine obstacles (*vighna) of *Yoga. Here the word is apparently used in the sense of "inertia."

LAYA-YOGA ("Yoga of [meditative] absorption"), any of various *Tantric meditation approaches that seek to dissolve the conditional *mind, often through such means as *breath control and the various "seals" (*mudrā) of *hatha-yoga. In the *Amaraugha-Prabodha (27f.), e.g., laya-yoga is said to be for the middling practitioner and to consist of the *contemplation of the *nectar of immortality in one's *body. This involves visualizing *Shiva in his brilliant phallic (*linga) form in the *kāma-rūpa at the base of the spine. After six months, the text assures the reader, one comes to enjoy paranormal powers (*siddhi) and longevity for up to three hundred years.

The *Yoga-Bīja (142) defines laya-yoga as the "identity (aikya) of 'field' (*kshetra) and 'field knower' (*kshetra-jna)." The text continues (143): "Upon realizing that identity, O Goddess, the *mind dissolves. When the [condition of] laya-yoga ensues, the life force (pavana) becomes stable. Owing to [that condition of] absorption, one reaches *happiness, the bliss (*ānanda) within oneself, the transcendental state."

LAZINESS. See ālasya, styāna, tandrā.

LEFT-HAND PATH, TANTRIC. See vāma-mārga; cf. dakshina-mārga.

LETTERS. See akshara, Alphabet.

LEVITATION. See ākāsha-gamana, bhū-cara-siddhi, khecaratva, lāghava, mano-gati, utkrānti, utthāna.

LIBERATED POSTURE. See mukta-āsana.

LIBERATION. According to *Hinduism, liberation is the highest human potential and value (see purusha-artha). Without it, none of the other values or goals that human beings can pursue make any sense. The pursuit of liberation, which can be equated with spiritual life per se, is not only the noblest but also the most meaningful undertaking of which people are capable. The reason for this is that through liberation we actualize our essential nature, as the *Self. While liberation is interpreted differently in the various schools of thought, it always is held to free the person from all unconscious conditioning, putting him or her in touch with *Reality. See also apavarga, jīvan-mukti, kaivalya, krama-mukti, moksha, mukti, videha-mukti.

LIFE. See jīva, prāna.

LIFE FORCE. See prāna.

LIGHT. "Radiance (*prakāsha) alone is eternal," declares the anonymous author of the *Pāshupata-Brāhmana-Upanishad (2.21), thus reiterating an ancient and worldwide mystical intuition. The *Chāndogya-Upanishad (3.13.7f.) has this memorable passage:

Now, the light (*jyotis) that shines beyond the *heavens, upon the backs of all, upon the backs of everything, higher than the highest—verily, that is the same as the light that is here within the person. It is visible . . .

. . . when one perceives [its] warmth in this *body. It is audible when one closes one's *ears and hears a kind of sound as of a bee, a bull, or a blazing fire. One should reverence that visible and audible light. He who knows this, he who knows this becomes one beautiful to see, one heard of in renown.

The transcendental *Self is luminous, and its experience is vividly described in countless scriptures as being of a blinding light. Luminosity is in fact a characteristic of many spiritual or inner states. It is an attribute of the life force (*prāna), the various psychoenergetic centers (*cakra), and not least the "serpent power" (*kundalinī-shakti), the great agent of transformation according to *Tantrism. See also taraka-yoga.

LIGHTNESS. See lāghava, Levitation.

LĪLĀ ("play"). Some nondualist schools of *Hinduism view the *world as a purely spontaneous, arbitrary creation or divine play. Specifically, *līlā* refers to the love play of *Krishna culminating in the nocturnal dance, the **rasa-līlā*, in which *Krishna multiplied himself so that each shepherdess (**gopī*) thought she alone had his full attention. By contrast, the *dance of *Shiva, as "king of dance" (**nata-rāja*), is one of destruction.

LIMB. See *anga*.

LINGA ("mark" or "sign"), often spelled *lingam* in English. In the *Sāmkhya tradition, this term refers to "that which has characteristics," i.e., the human personality, consisting of the higher mind (**buddhi*), the "I-maker" (**ahamkāra*), the lower mind (**manas*), the five cognitive senses (**jnāna-indriya*), and the five conative senses (**karma-indriya*).

The **Maitrāyanīya-Upanishad* (6.10) applies the term *linga* to the entire *creation extending from the first principle (**mahat*) to the "particulars" (**vishesha*).

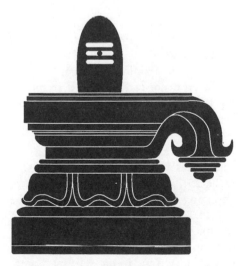

A *shiva-linga*, symbol of universal creativity

It contrasts this with the *linga* that is "without foundation," i.e., the unthinkable *Reality itself.

In the **Mahābhārata* (12.195.15) the *linga* is the vehicle, or *body, of the transmigrating psyche.

The term *linga* can also denote the phallus or, by extension, the cosmic principle of creativity. The worship of the *Divine through the symbol of a phallus dates back to the *Indus-Sarasvati civilization. Early on *Shiva became associated with the symbol of the *linga* and its *worship. It is the god's most common emblem. The *Lingāyatas, a branch of *Shaivism, wear a miniature *linga* as an amulet. Metaphysically, the *linga* stands for the unimaginable potency or power of creativity prior to the *creation of the world. In his *Tantra-Āloka* (5.54), the great scholar and adept *Abhinava Gupta explains the word as follows: "This whole [universe] is dissolved (*līnam*) in that, and this whole [universe] is perceived (*gamyate*) as residing within that." Similarly, the **Amaraugha-Prabodha* (55) offers this etymological definition: "Where the movable and immovable dissolves by force of *laya*, that is [known as] *linga*."

By the occult law of correspondence "as above, so below," the cosmic *linga* also has its representation within the *microcosm of the human *body. Thus the scriptures of *Tantrism and *hatha-yoga describe experiences involving a radiant *linga* that can be seen in different psychoenergetic centers (**cakra*) of the body. For instance, the *Brahma-Upanishad* (80) speaks of three types of *linga* that should be made the object of one's *meditation: (1) the *adho* ("lower")-*linga* at the base of the spine; (2) the *shikhin* ("crest")-*linga* at the upper terminal of the central channel (**sushumnā-nādī*); and (3) the *jyotir* ("light")-*linga* situated in the psychoenergetic center of the *forehead. The *Siddha-Sid-dhānta-Paddhati (2.4) mentions a linga-shaped flame in the *heart. See also yoni.

LINGA-CAKRA ("phallus wheel"), also known as linga-sthāna ("place of the phallus"); a rare synonym for *svādhishthāna-cakra.

LINGA-MĀTRA ("pure sign"), in *Classical Yoga, the level of cosmic manifestation prior to the emergence of specific *objects. The *Tattva-Vaishāradī (1.45) also styles this the "great principle" (mahat-tattva), and *Vyāsa, in his *Yoga-Bhāshya (2.19), speaks of it as "mere being" (*sattā-mātra).

LINGA-PURĀNA, one of the eighteen principal *Purānas. It belongs to the tradition of *Shaivism and discusses *Yoga in many chapters (especially chapters 7–9 and 88) from the perspective of the *Pāshupata school. The text describes the eightfold *path (*ashta-anga-yoga) and furnishes long lists of obstacles (*vighna) and omens (*arishta).

LINGA-SHARĪRA ("body of characteristics"), according to the *Sāmkhya tradition, consists of the constituent parts of the subtle vehicle called *linga, with the addition of the sensory potentials (*tan-mātra). This complex is also known as the "subtle body" (*sūkshma-sharīra) and is contrasted with the "gross body" (*sthūla-sharīra), the physical organism composed of the material elements (*bhūta). The gross *body in itself is thought to be insentient. It becomes animated when it is linked with the linga-sharīra, which is the entity that transmigrates by sheer force of the individual's *karma. See also citta-sharīra, deha.

LINGĀYATA SECT, a moderate religious school within *Shaivism that originated in the twelfth century CE. Its followers are also known as Vīra Shaivas. The founder, or reorganizer, was *Basava or Basavanna (1106–1167 CE). The name Lingāyata (often written Lingayat in English) derives from the custom of worshiping *Shiva in the form of the phallus (*linga), a symbol of creativity. One of the doctrinal innovations of this tradition is the idea of the "six regions" (*shat-sthāla).

LION POSTURE. See simha-āsana.

LISTENING. See shravana.

LOBHA ("greed"), one of the principal defects (*dosha), which must be checked through the constant *practice of "non-grasping" (*aparigraha).

LOCK. See bandha.

LOCUST POSTURE. See shalabha-āsana.

LOIN CLOTH. See kaupīna.

LOKA ("realm"; from the root ruc/loc, "to shine, be bright, visible"), a dimension of cosmic existence or region of the *world. According to *Hindu cosmography, there are seven major realms, each corresponding to a specific state of *consciousness. See also Cosmos.

LOKA-SAMGRAHA ("world gathering"), a compound found in the *Bhagavad-Gītā (3.20, 25), where it stands for the ideal of "bringing together," or harmonizing, the *world. This goal is proposed as an incentive for righteous or lawful (*dharma) *action, and it counterbalances the simultaneous demand in *karma-yoga for "same-mindedness" (*sama-buddhi), or the yogic virtue of regarding everything with inspired indifference. See also *sarva-bhūta-hita, para-artha-ihā*.

LORD. See *īshvara, nātha, pati*.

LORDSHIP. See *aishvarya*.

LOTUS POSTURE. See *kamala-āsana, padma-āsana*.

LOVE. See *bhakti, pranidhāna, prapatti*.

LUMINOSITY. See *dīpti, jyotis*, Light.

LUST. See *kāma*.

· M ·

MACROCOSM. See *brahma-anda*; cf. Microcosm, *pinda-anda*.

MADA ("pride"; also, "exhilaration" or "intoxication"), sometimes listed as one of the defects (**dosha*).

MĀDHU-BHŪMIKA ("he who is on the honey level"). The **Yoga-Bhāshya* (3.51) explains that a **yogin* who has attained to the experience of the truth-bearing wisdom (**ritam-bhara-prajnā*) at the highest level of conscious ecstasy (**samprajnāta-samādhi*) is known as a *mādhu-bhūmika*. This type of practitioner is tempted by higher beings and therefore needs to fix his **mind firmly on the goal of "aloneness" (**kaivalya*), or **liberation. This temptation is referred to in the **Yoga-Sūtra* (3.51), which speaks of high-placed beings (*sthānin*). See also *bhūmi, mādhu-vidyā*; cf. *atikrānta-bhāvanīya, prajnā-jyotis, prathama-kalpika*.

MĀDHU-VIDYĀ ("honey doctrine"), an ancient teaching expounded in the **Bri-had-Āranyaka-Upanishad* (2.5.1ff.). Here *mādhu* ("honey") stands for the nourishing essence of a thing. The underlying idea is that all things participate in the transcendental **Self (**ātman*), which holds together the entire **cosmos. Thus the **ele-ments, the **sun, lightning, **space, and so on have the quality of nutrient honey because of that fundamental **Being. According to the **Tattva-Vaishāradī* (3.54), *mādhu* is the truth-bearing wisdom (**ritam-bhara-prajnā*).

MĀDHURYA ("graciousness"), sometimes counted among the practices of moral discipline (**yama*). See also *mārdava*.

MADHYA-LAKSHYA ("middle vision" or "intermediate sign"), one of three types of visionary experience (**lakshya*) in **tāraka-yoga*. The **Advaya-Tāraka-Upanishad* (7) describes it as the experience of different-colored **light leading to the experience of the five types of luminous "ether-space" (**ākāsha*). Cf. *antar-lakshya, bahir-lak-shya*.

MADHYA-MĀRGA ("middle path"), a synonym for **sushumnā-nādī*.

MADYA or MADĪRA ("wine"), a synonym for **surā*. Wine is one of the five ingredients used in the **Tantric **panca-tattva* ritual, where it is considered a sexual stimulant. The **Kaula-Jnāna-Nirnaya* (18.7–9) gives a symbolic explanation for this practice. It states that a mixture of wine, semen, and female secretion (**rakta*) is the

*Absolute itself. It also states that when the wine is prepared with proper devotion (*bhakti), it is the bliss (*ānanda) of *Consciousness. Resorting to esoteric etymology, the *Kula-Arnava-Tantra (17.63–64) explains that *madya* is so called because it destroys all the nets of illusion (*māyā), reveals the *path to *liberation, and bestows great gifts (*dāna).

MAGARADHVĀJA YOGI 700 (12th cen. CE), a prominent *adept of *Shaivism. The curious name of this *yogin* is found on various inscriptions, the figure 700 apparently referring to the number of his disciples.

MAGIC (Sanskrit: *abhicāra, indra-jāla* ["Indra's net"], or *māyā), the archaic art of influencing one's environment through practices and rites that are based on laws other than the causal laws accepted by the rational *mind. The tradition of *Yoga harbors many magical elements, and throughout the centuries *yogins* have not only been celebrated as masters of their own selves but have also been feared as possessors of extraordinary powers. In fact, the word for spiritual perfection and paranormal power is the same in Sanskrit—*siddhi. The tradition of asceticism (*tapas), which is one of the historical tributaries to Yoga, is essentially a form of magic, since it is based on the direct or indirect coercion of invisible beings, often the deities (*deva) themselves. Magical features are especially prominent in the schools of *Tantrism. Although aspirants are frequently warned against the use of magical powers for selfish ends, numerous stories tell of *yogins* who have fallen from *grace precisely because they failed to heed such warnings.

MAHĀ ("great"), an adjective prefixed to many important Sanskrit words.

MAHĀ-ĀTMAN (*mahātman*, "great self"), refers to a holy person, a "great soul" such as Gandhi. In philosophical contexts, the term stands for the ultimate *Reality.

MAHĀ-BANDHA ("great lock"), described in the *Hatha-Yoga-Pradīpikā (3.19ff.) thus: Place the left foot at the perineum (*yoni) and the right *foot on the left thigh. After inhaling, press the chin firmly against the chest, contract the anal sphincter, and fix the *mind on the central conduit (*sushumnā-nāḍī) of the *life force. Retain the *breath for as long as possible and then exhale gently. Repeat with the right foot placed against the perineum. Some authorities specify that one should not perform the *throat lock (called *kantha-bandha* or *jālandhara-bandha) but simply block the air flow by performing the "tongue lock" (*jihvā-bandha). This is done by pressing the *tongue against the front teeth. The *Shiva-Samhitā (4.21f.) further explains that one should force the *apāna upward and the *prāna downward. This technique is thought to invigorate and rejuvenate the *body, strengthen the bones, gladden the *heart, and most importantly, force the life energy into the central channel (*sushumnā-nāḍī), ultimately awakening the "serpent power" (*kundalinī-shakti).

MAHĀBHĀRATA ("Great [Story of] the Bharatas"), one of India's two great national epics composed in Sanskrit, the other being the *Rāmāyana. Legend attributes both epics to *Vyāsa. Even though the *Rāmāyana* has many stories of ascetics (*tapasvin), it contains virtually no yogic elements in the strict sense. The *Mahābhārata*, however, is replete with references to *Yoga and *Sāmkhya. It is an important document for the schools of *Preclassical Yoga. Three didactic passages are of spe-

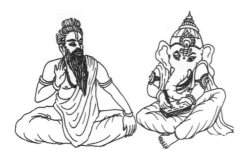

Vyāsa dictating the *Mahābhārata* to Ganesha, who alone could memorize the sage's words

cial significance: the *Bhagavad-Gītā*, the *Moksha-Dharma*, and the *Anu-Gītā*.

Scholars are in disagreement over the age of the *Mahābhārata*. The war between the Kauravas and Pāndavas, which forms the nucleus of this epic, appears to have been fought about 1500 BCE, several centuries after the dispersion of the *Indus-Sarasvati civilization from the Indus River to the fertile area of the Ganges. The Pāndavas had been cheated out of their kingdom and were seeking to win it back. They succeeded in doing so with the assistance of *Krishna, who was Prince *Arjuna's teacher. While this story is undoubtedly very old, the extant version of the epic appears to have been completed about 200 CE.

MAHĀ-BHŪTA ("great element"), the five coarse material elements (*bhūta). Cf. tanmātra.

MAHĀDEVA ("Great God"), a common epithet of *Shiva.

MAHĀ-MUDRĀ ("great seal"), explained in the *Gheranda-Samhitā (3.6f.) as follows: Press the left heel against the buttocks while stretching the right leg and catching hold of one's toes. Then contract the *throat and *gaze at the spot between the *eyebrows. Repeat with the left leg extended. This technique is said to cure all *diseases, particularly consumption, hemorrhoids, and indigestion. The *Shiva-Samhitā (4.16) states that one should press the left heel against the perineum (*yoni). In modern texts, this is also known as the "half back-to-front posture" (*ardha-pashcima-uttāna-āsana).

The *Goraksha-Paddhati (1.76) defines *mahā-mudrā* as the purification (*shodhana) of the entire network of channels (*nādī), and the drying-up (shoshana) of the liquids (*rasa) of the *body. This work also states (1.60) that this technique can transmute the deadliest poison into *nectar. The *Hathu-Yoga-Pradīpikā (3.18) claims that this *mudrā awakens the "serpent power" (*kundalinī-shakti). See also *nabho-mudrā*.

MAHĀN or MAHAT ("great one"), a synonym for *buddhi.

MAHĀNIRVĀNA-TANTRA ("Treatise on the Great Extinction"), a widely esteemed *Tantra dating from the eleventh century CE. A comprehensive work that has been called "the most important Hindu Tantra" (Agehananda Bharati, 1965), it contains fourteen chapters that carefully describe various ritual practices such as the *purification of the location, invocation and *worship of one's chosen *deity, *mantra recitation, the left-handed rite of the "five M's" (*panca-ma-kara), and so on. It also contains valuable *kaula lore (14.179), which is considered superior to any other teaching. In 14.123 this *Tantra* defines *Yoga as the "union of the psyche (*jīva) with the transcendental *Self" and states that he who has realized the *Absolute transcends both Yoga and worship (*pūjā).

MAHĀ-RAJAS ("great *rajas"), the female form of seminal liquid (*bindu), identified as both menstrual blood and vaginal secretion. It is said to be of red color, which is captured in the word *rajas*, from the root raj/ranj ("to be red").

MAHĀRSHI ("great seer"; from *mahā*, "great," and *rishi*, "seer"), a title of respect for an *adept.

MAHĀ-SATTĀ ("great beingness"), in Kashmiri *Shaivism, the highest *Reality. See also *sattā*.

MAHĀ-SIDDHA ("great adept"). Northern *Tantrism knows of eighty-four *mahā-siddhas*, who have realized perfection (*siddhi*), or *enlightenment, and who also possess all the various paranormal powers (*siddhi*). See also Adept, *siddha*.

MAHĀ-SIDDHI ("great power"), *liberation itself, according to the *Yoga-Tattva-Upanishad (76). It is deemed far superior to any of the paranormal powers (*siddhi*) because it is their source.

MAHĀ-SUKHA ("great joy"), the supreme *bliss, or perfect delight, that is realized upon *enlightenment. This term is at home particularly in the *Sahajiyā movement, which teaches the ultimate identity of the transcendental *Reality with the immanent reality. See also *ānanda*, Pleasure, *sukha*.

MAHAT. See *mahān*.

MAHĀ-UPANISHAD (*Mahopanishad*), one of the *Samnyāsa-Upanishads, which deal with the ideal of *renunciation. It defines (5.42) *Yoga as the "pacification of the *mind" and mentions (V.22) seven levels (*bhūmi*) of yogic development.

MAHĀ-VĀKYA ("great saying"). In the *Upanishads, the great sayings are declarations of the ultimate truth (*satya*). The three best known spiritual sayings or axioms are "I am the *Absolute" (*aham brahma asmi*), "You are That" (*tat tvam asi*), and "This self is the *Absolute" (*ayam ātmā brahma*).

MAHĀ-VĀKYA-UPANISHAD (*Mahāvākyopanishad*, "Upanishad of the Great Saying"), one of the *Yoga-Upanishads. It consists of only twelve stanzas and recommends the practice of recitation (*japa*) of the *hamsa. It states that in order to acquire supreme wisdom (*vijñāna*), one must abandon both the "eye of knowledge" (*vidyā-cakshus*), which leads to *liberation, and the "eye of nescience" (*avidyā-cakshus*), which leads to *bondage. The highest *realization has nothing to do with ecstasy (*samādhi*) or the powers (*siddhi*) of *Yoga, or even with the mind's dissolution (*mano-laya*). It is simply one's flawless identity (*aikya*) with the *Absolute.

MAHĀ-VEDHA ("great piercer"), described in the *Hatha-Yoga-Pradīpikā (3.26ff.) as follows: Practicing the "great lock" (*mahā-bandha*), inhale and then apply the "throat seal" (*kantha-mudrā*), that is, *jālandhara-bandha. Repeatedly raise oneself slightly off the ground and allow the buttocks to drop back down. This is thought to force the life energy (*prāna*) into the central channel (*sushumnā-nādī*). As is clear from the *Shiva-Samhitā (4.24), this practice is known as the "piercer" because it forces the concentrated *prāna to pierce the three "knots" (*granthi*). The *Gheranda-Samhitā (3.21ff.) states: "As a *woman's beauty, youth, and charms are in vain without a man [to admire them], so too are the root lock (*mūla-bandha*) and the great lock (*mahā-bandha*) without the great piercer."

MAHĀ-VIDYĀ ("great wisdom"), the liberating wisdom (*jnāna) that reveals the transcendental *Self. Southern *Shaivism knows of ten *goddesses symbolizing various aspects of the great or transcendental wisdom: (1) *Kālī, who is the power behind time (*kāla), the ultimate destructive force, which is also the power of spiritual transmutation; (2) Tārā, who, as the name suggests, is the guiding star (*tāra*) that delivers (*tārayati*) the worshiper from all evil and from the world of change (*samsāra*) itself; (3) Shodashī, who is portrayed as a sixteen-year-old maiden and is the power of *perfection; (4) Bhuvaneshvarī, who governs the created *universe and infuses it with the possibility of *wisdom; (5) Chinnamastā, who, with her severed head, symbolizes the power of self-sacrifice, which is fundamental to the spiritual process; (6) Bhairavī, who inspires *fear because she is the power of *death; (7) Dhūmavatī, who is depicted as a crone, symbol of absolute *renunciation and negation; (8) Bagalā, who is the power behind all *suffering, which, ultimately, leads to spiritual transformation; (9) Mātanginī, who, as the name indicates, is the "elephantine" power of domination by which this *goddess establishes *peace, and (10) Kamalā, who is generally identified with *Lakshmī, because she bestows good fortune on the worshiper.

All ten *goddesses are aspects of the feminine principle, or *shakti, of the *Divine. Together they facilitate the spiritual process of self-understanding, *self-transcendence, and final *Self-realization.

MAHĀ-VRATA ("great vow"), the five constituent practices of moral discipline (*yama), which are to be observed at all times and under all circumstances, according to the *Yoga-Sūtra (2.31). Other Indian traditions and schools list different practices under this heading, which reflects a universal *morality.

MAHĀ-YOGA ("great Yoga") comprises *mantra-yoga, *laya-yoga, *hatha-yoga, and *rāja-yoga, according to the *Yoga-Shikhā-Upanishad (1.129f.). The text emphasizes the central importance of *breath control when it states (1.138) that what all these approaches have in common is the "joining" (*samyoga) of the inbreath (*prāna) and the outbreath (*apāna). The phrase mahā-yoga is also often used synonymously with *samādhi, the great state of *Yoga.

MAHIMAN ("magnification"), the power of infinite expansion; one of the eight classic paranormal powers (*siddhi) recognized in *Yoga and other traditions of India. *Vācaspati Mishra, in his *Tattva-Vaishāradī (3.45), explains it as the ability to become as large as an elephant, a mountain, or a whole town, and so on. The *Mani-Prabhā (3.44), however, defines mahiman as "pervasiveness" (vibhūtva), which suggests that it is not the physical *body that expands but the "subtle body" (*sūkshma-sharīra), or the *mind.

MAITHUNĀ ("intercourse"), also called *ādi-yāga; ritual sex between consecrated male and female initiates; a central practice of left-hand *Tantrism. The woman, who is known as the "seal" (*mudrā), is for the duration of the rite looked upon as the *Goddess or divine *Shakti, whereas the male practitioner is *Shiva. This sacramental intercourse is the climax of the *panca-tattva ceremony. It generally takes place in a circle (*cakra) of initiates with the *teacher present. He is usually seated together with his consort in the center of the circle.

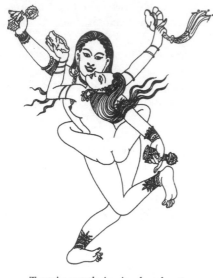

Tantric couple in ritual embrace

This is never intended as an occasion for lustful behavior. Rather, the ceremony comes at the end of a prolonged ritual and is essentially a *meditation exercise. Orgasm is generally bypassed through the diffusion of sexual energy throughout the *body. The psychosomatic energy generated through sexual contact is used to enhance the initiate's complex *visualizations and is transformed into bliss (*ānanda). See also bindu, Sexuality.

MAITRĀYANĪYA-UPANISHAD (*Maitrāyanīyopanishad*), a prose scripture dating from the second or third century BCE. This work, which exists in two recensions and contains numerous interpolations, is the earliest record of a sixfold Yoga (*shadanga-yoga*).

MAITRĪ ("friendliness" or "friendship"), recognized as a virtue in *Classical Yoga. Together with compassion (*karunā), gladness (*mudita), and equanimity (*upekshā), the projection or conscious radiation of friendliness is mentioned in the *Yoga-Sūtra (1.33) as a means of pacifying the *mind. In *Buddhism these four virtues are known as the "brahmic stations" (*brahma-vihāra*).

MA-KARA ("letter *m*"). See *panca-makara*.

MAKARA-ĀSANA (*makarāsana*, "makara posture"), widely known in Western *Yoga circles as the dolphin posture, although the word *makara* generally refers to a dangerous marine creature such as a crocodile or shark. The *Gheranda-Samhitā (2.4) offers this description: Lying face down with both legs extended and spread-eagled, hold the *head with one's hands. According to depictions in modern manuals, the arms form a cradle—hands touching opposite shoulders—in which the *forehead is placed. This practice is said to increase the "bodily *fire," or metabolism.

MALA ("impurity" or "defilement"). All spiritual traditions are agreed that the ordinary person exists in a state of impurity that prevents the dawning of real wisdom (*jnāna). The yogic *path can be viewed as a massive attempt at self-purification. Perfect *purity is equated with *liberation. The *Tattva-Vaishāradī (4.31) identifies the defilements as the "causes of suffering" (*klesha) and *karma.

Kashmiri *Shaivism recognizes three fundamental defilements: (1) āṇava-mala, relating to individuation itself; (2) māyīya-mala, causing the illusion (*māyā) of an external *world populated by a multitude of *objects; and (3) kārma-mala, resulting in motivated *action in that illusory world. All three defilements are coverings surrounding the inherent *light and *bliss of the transcendental *Self. See also antarāya, dosha, nava-mala; cf. shodhana, shuddhi.

MĀLĀ ("garland" or "rosary"). Some *yogins use a rosary for their *mantra recitation. Rosaries can be made of a variety of substances, the favorite substance being rudra-aksha ("*Rudra's eye"), the dried berries of the tree Elaeocarpus Ganitrus. Usually 108 beads are strung together.

MĀLINĪ, one of the many names of the *goddess *Shakti. In Kashmiri *Shaivism, this name stands for a mystical arrangement of the fifty letters of the Sanskrit *alphabet, which are said to form the *body of the deity. This highly esoteric teaching is expounded, for instance, in the Mālinī-Vijaya-Uttara-Tantra.

MĀMSA ("meat" or "flesh"), one of the five ingredients of the *panca-tattva ritual of left-hand *Tantrism. *Meat, which is strictly forbidden to orthodox *Hindus, is here taken as a stimulant together with *wine and other taboo substances, culminating in sexual congress (*maithunā) between the male and female participants.

MANAS ("mind"), the lower mind that deals with organizing the information received from the senses (*indriya), as opposed to the higher intuitive mind (*buddhi), the source of *wisdom. Because of its proximity to sensory functions, it is viewed as a sense. In the *Brihad-Āranyaka-Upanishad (1.5.3) its operational modes are said to be desire (*kāma), volition (*samkalpa), doubt (vicikitsā), faith (*shraddhā), lack of faith (ashraddhā), resolution (*dhriti), irresolution (adhriti), shame (hrī), knowledge (*dhī), and fear (bhī).

The *Yoga scriptures emphasize the volitional and doubting disposition of the *mind. The universal recommendation is that the mind, as the *Shvetāshvatara-Upanishad (2.9) puts it, should be restrained "like a chariot pulled by unruly horses." The *Laghu-Yoga-Vāsishtha (6.9.367) compares the mind to a tree that should be cut not merely at the branches but at the root. "The *bliss that arises upon the dissolution of the mind," states the *Maitrāyanīya-Upanishad (6.24), "is the Absolute (*brahman)." The same scripture (4.6) declares that the mind can be either pure or impure, depending on whether or not it is riddled with *desires. According to another stanza (4.11), when the mind is turned toward sensory *objects it leads to *bondage; when it is turned away from them it is the cause of *liberation. The *Hatha-Yoga-Pradīpikā (4.26) likens the manas to mercury, which is quite unsteady. In verse 4.29 it is called the "lord" (*nātha) of the *senses, whereas the life force (*prāna) is said to be the "lord" of the mind. The connection between the *breath and the mind is one of the great discoveries of *Yoga, and much is made of it in *hatha-yoga. See also citta.

MANAS-CAKRA ("mind wheel"), one of the psychoenergetic centers of the *body, depicted as a white six-petaled lotus in the *head. It is situated above the *ājnā-cakra and is also called sūrya-mandala ("solar orb") and jnāna-netra ("eye of wisdom"). See also cakra, jnāna-cakshus.

MANA-UNMANĪ (manonmanī, "mental exaltation"), sometimes used in *Tantrism and *hatha-yoga as a synonym for *samādhi (ecstasy). The *Hatha-Yoga-Pradīpikā (4.3) contains this stanza: "When the life force (*prāna) flows in the *sushumnā, the [condition of] mana-unmanī is accomplished. Otherwise the other practices are only an exertion for *yogins." See also amanaskatā, unmanī.

MANDALA ("circle" or "orb"), in general terms, a region, often inside the *body;

more specifically, a circular arrangement similar to the *yantra that serves as a tool of *concentration. It contains three principal geometric elements. In the center is the "seed" (*bindu), representing the point of potentiality of both the *cosmos and the *mind. The surrounding circles represent various levels of existence. They are in turn encompassed by a square with open "gates." Beyond this can be a variety of other elements. In Tibetan *Buddhism, such mandalas can be complex pictorial representations. However complicated or simple a mandala may be, it always represents consecrated space and is thought to be the body of one's chosen deity (*ishta-devatā). The mandala is used to *worship that deity and, through complex *visualization practices, to become one with it.

MANDALA-BRĀHMANA-UPANISHAD (Mandalabrāhmanopanishad), one of the *Yoga-Upanishads, consisting of eighty-nine paragraphs divided into five sections. Sections 3–5 appear to be an independent text. The teachings of this *Upanishad are linked with the name of *Yājnavalkya. He expounds an eightfold *Yoga (*ashta-anga-yoga) whose component practices differ from *Patanjali's path. Yājnavalkya also speaks of the five defects (*dosha): lust (*kāma), anger (*krodha), faulty breathing (*nishvāsa), fear (*bhaya), and sleep or drowsiness (*nidrā). These are conquered by abstention from volition (*samkalpa), patience (*kshamā), a scanty diet (*laghu-āhāra), attentiveness, and the cultivation of *truth. This work also refers to the three visionary experiences (*lakshya) and the five types of "ether-space" (*ākāsha) known in *tāraka-yoga. It further mentions three types of gaze (*drishti) during *meditation. The goal of this *Yoga is "transmindedness" (*amanaskatā), the condition of "living liberation" (*jīvan-

mukti), also known as "Yoga sleep" (*yoga-nidrā).

MANDAVYA, mentioned in the *Tattva-Vaishāradī (4.1) as an example of a *yogin who uses potions (*aushadhi). He is mentioned in many *Purānas, and the *Mahābhārata (1.107f.) relates an incident in which he was impaled by robbers and kept himself alive through his yogic powers. He was feared for the potency of his curses.

MANDIRA ("dwelling" or "temple"). See deva-mandira, kutīra.

MANDUKA-ĀSANA (mandukāsana, "frog posture"), a posture (*āsana) mentioned already in the *Mahābhārata (12.292.8) and sketchily described in the *Gheranda-Samhitā (2.34) as follows: Place the (wide-apart) knees forward and the feet backward so that the toes touch each other. In other words, the practitioner almost sits on the heels. Cf. uttāna-manduka-āsana.

MĀNDUKĪ-MUDRĀ ("frog seal"). According to the *Gheranda-Samhitā (3.62f.), this practice is done by closing one's mouth and twirling the *tongue (like a leaping frog) against the *palate. This stimulates the production of the ambrosial liquid (*amrita) and prevents *illness and aging. See also khecarī-mudrā, lambikā-yoga.

MĀNDŪKYA-KĀRIKĀ of *Gaudapāda, a verse commentary on the Māndūkya-Upanishad of the second or third century BCE. The Kārikā, which has a valuable subcommentary by *Shankara, includes an exposition of the "intangible Yoga" (*asparsha-yoga).

MANIFEST. See vyakta; cf. avyakta.

MANIFESTATION. See Appearance, Cosmos, Creation.

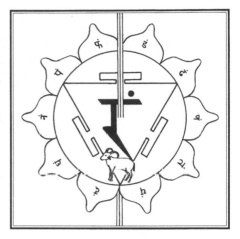

Manipura-cakra, the psychoenergetic center located at the navel

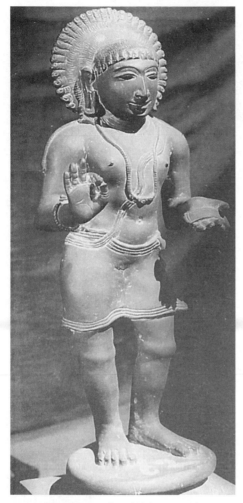

Manikkavācakar (13th century)

MĀNIKKAVĀCAKAR (Sanskrit: Manikavā-caka, "He whose words are jewels"), one of the great *Shaiva saints and masters of *bhakti-yoga. He lived (mid-9th cen. CE) in South India. It appears that at the time of his *renunciation he was a junior minister of King Varaguna II. His devotional poetry forms the eighth book (*Tiruvāca-kam*, "Sacred Words") of the *Tirumurai*, the canon of southern *Shaivism. See also Nayanmārs.

MANIPURA-CAKRA ("wheel of the jeweled city"), also known as *manipuraka*; the psychoenergetic center (*cakra*) located at the *navel, generally depicted as a ten-petaled lotus the color of rain clouds. According to the *Shat-Cakra-Nirūpana* (19), there is a triangular region (*mandala*) of *fire within this *cakra. The center's presiding *adept is *Rudra; the presiding *goddess is the four armed, dark hued Lākinī. The "seed syllable" (*bīja-mantra*) is *ram*, which pertains to the fire element. The *Goraksha-Paddhati* (1.23) fancifully derives the name *mani-pura* from the fact that this is also the location of the "bulb" (*kanda*), which is pierced by the central channel (*sushumnā-nādī*) "like a gem (*mani*) by a string."

According to the *Shiva-Samhitā* (5.81), the *yogin* who contemplates this esoteric structure not only conquers *disease and *death but also acquires the ability to enter another *body, as well as to make gold, discover medical remedies, and locate hidden treasures. See also *nābhi-cakra*.

MANI-PRABHĀ ("Jewel Luster"), a six-teenth-century subcommentary by Rāmā-nanda Sarasvatī on the *Yoga-Bhāshya.

MANLINESS. See paurusha.

MANO-GATI ("mind walk"), the paranor-mal power (*siddhi) to go in one's *mind wherever one wishes. See also ākāsha-ga-mana, khecaratva.

MANO-JAVITVA ("fleetness [as of] the mind"), a paranormal power (*siddhi) that enables the *adept to move about at the speed of the *mind, i.e., instantane-ously. It is referred to, e.g., in the *Yoga-Sūtra (3.48), which states that this ability is acquired in conjunction with complete mastery of the matrix of *nature.

MANO-LAYA ("dissolution of the mind"). See laya.

MANO-MAYA-KOSHA ("sheath composed of mind"), one of the five "envelopes" (*kosha) occluding the *Self; otherwise known as the lower mind (*manas). See also deha.

MANTHANA, mentioned in the *Hatha-Yoga-Pradīpikā (1.6) as an *adept of *hatha-yoga. He may be identical with Manthana Bhairava, who authored a work on *alchemy entitled Ānanda-Kānda.

MANTRA (from the root man, "to think," and the suffix tra, suggesting instrumen-tality), thought or intention expressed as

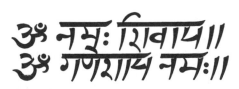

The mantras "Om namah shivāya" and "Om ganeshāya namah"

*sound. Thus the word mantra denotes "prayer," "hymn," "spell," "counsel," and "plan." In yogic contexts, mantra stands for numinous phonemes that may or may not have communicable meaning. The *Kula-Arnava-Tantra (17.54) defines it as follows: "A mantra is so called because it saves one from all *fear through ponder-ing (*manana) the luminous *deity who is of the form of *Reality." However, this is only one of the purposes to which mantras are put. They are also frequently employed as simple magical devices to achieve worldly ends.

A mantra is a mantra by virtue of its having been communicated in an initia-tory setting. Thus even the most famous of all mantras, the sacred syllable *om, be-comes a mantra only when it has been em-powered by one's teacher (*guru). Every mantra is associated with a particular in-visible power, or *deity. Some mantras, such as om, designate the *Absolute as such.

A mantra can consist of a single sound or a string of phonemes that have no ap-parent meaning. It can also consist of a whole meaningful sentence, as in the case of the ancient *gāyatrī-mantra. Of special significance are the *bīja- or "seed" man-tras, which express the quintessence of a mantra and of the corresponding *deity. Thus the bīja-mantra of *Kālī is krīm, of *Shiva hrīm, of Mahālakshmī (see Lak-shmī) shrīm, and so on. See also nāda, mantra-shāstra, mantra-yoga, shabda.

MANTRA-MAHODADHI ("Ocean of Man-tras"), an encyclopedic work on *mantra-yoga, consisting of twenty-five chapters with over 3,300 stanzas. The text was com-pleted in May–June 1889 CE by Mahi-dhara, a renowned commentator on the *Yajur-Veda who also wrote an autocom-mentary called Naukā ("Boat").

MANTRA-SHĀSTRA ("teaching on *mantras*"; also known as *mantra-vidyā*, "science of *mantras*"), the body of speculations about the numinous potential of human sounds. See also *nāda*, *shabda*.

MANTRA-YOGA, one of the principal branches of the *Yoga tradition. The *Yoga-Tattva-Upanishad* (21f.) defines it as the recitation (*japa*) of various *mantras* made up of the "matrices" (*mātrikā*), that is, the primary sounds of the Sanskrit *alphabet. This discipline, which is said to be suitable for the inferior practitioner who has little insight into spiritual life, should be pursued for twelve years. It gradually leads to wisdom (*jnana*) as well as the classic paranormal powers (*siddhi*). That the *Yoga of the recitation of numinous sounds has its roots in the spells of archaic *magic is evident from the *Rig-Veda*, whose *mantras* are presented as having magical properties. Mantric recitation, an important ingredient of the sacrificial cult, became an exact and exacting science at the hands of the *brahmins*, for the invisible powers have to be worshiped and invoked with precision lest they should turn against the sacrificer.

The practice of mantric recitation is one of the earliest components of *Yoga. Even though *mantras* retained their original character as magical tools for achieving one's *desires in the Yoga tradition, they acquired a new function, namely, to aid the *yogin*'s spiritual maturation. In other words, *mantras* became instruments of *Self-realization. *Mantra-yoga* as an independent branch of Yoga is, however, a relatively late development in the long *history of Yoga. Its appearance is closely connected with the emergence of *Tantrism. It is treated in numerous scriptures belonging to that cultural movement. There are also a number of works that spe-cifically expound *mantra-yoga*, notably the encyclopedic *Mantra-Mahodadhi*, the *Mantra-Yoga-Samhitā*, the *Mantra-Mahārnava* ("Great Flood of *Mantras*"), the *Mantra-Mukta-Āvalī* ("Independent Tract on *Mantras*"), the *Mantra-Kaumudī* ("Moonlight on *Mantras*"), and the *Tattva-Ānanda-Tanginī* ("River of the Bliss of Reality").

According to the *Mantra-Yoga-Samhitā*, *mantra-yoga* has sixteen "limbs" (*anga*): (1) *bhakti*, or "devotion," which is threefold—"prescribed devotion" (*vaidhi-bhakti*) consisting of ceremonial worship, "devotion involving attachment" (*rāga-ātmika-bhakti*), and "supreme devotion" (*para-bhakti*); (2) *shuddhi*, or "purification," which consists in ritual cleansing of the *body and *mind, the use of a specially consecrated environment (*desha*) for *practice, and facing in the right direction during *recitation; (3) *āsana*, or "posture"; (4) *panca-anga-sevana*, or "serving the five limbs," which consists in the daily practice of reading the *Bhagavad-Gītā* ("Lord's Song") and the *Sahasra-Nāma* ("Thousand Names [of the *Divine]"), reciting songs of praise, protection, and heart opening; (5) *ācara* ("conduct"), which is of three kinds, "divine" (*divya*), "left-hand" (*vāma*) involving worldly activity, and "right-hand" (*dakshina*) involving *renunciation; (6) *dhāranā*, or "concentration"; (7) *divya-deva-sevana*, or "serving the divine space," which consists of sixteen practices that convert a given place into consecrated space (*desha*) suitable for mantric *recitation; (8) *prāna-kriyā*, or "breath ritual," which is the *sacrifice of one's *breath into the *Divine and is accompanied by a number of rites, including the "placing" (*nyāsa*) of the life force (*prāna*) into different parts of the *body; (9) *mudrā*, or "seal," which consists of a variety of hand gestures that focus the *mind; (10) *tarpana*, or "satisfaction," which is the practice of offering libations of *water to the invisible powers in order to make them favorably disposed; (11) *havana*, or "invocation," which is the calling upon one's chosen deity (*ishta-devatā*) by means of *mantras; (12) *bali*, or "offering," consisting in the giving of gifts of fruit or flowers to one's chosen deity; (13) *yāga*, or "sacrifice," which can be external or internal, the latter being thought superior to the former; (14) *japa*, or "recitation"; (15) *dhyāna*, or "meditation"; and (16) *samādhi*, or "ecstasy," which is also called the "great condition" (*mahā-bhāva*) in which the *mind dissolves in the *Divine.

It is clear from these practices that *mantra-yoga* is pronouncedly ritualistic, reflecting not only its origins in the sacrificial cult of ancient India but also its *Tantric provenance.

MANTRA-YOGA-SAMHITĀ ("Compendium on Mantra-Yoga"), a systematic exposition of *mantra-yoga* comprising 566 stanzas. Its date is unknown, though it can tentatively be assigned to the seventeenth or eighteenth century CE. The "Yoga of sound" is defined (1.4) thus: "The *Yoga that is practiced by means of the support of [the right] disposition (*bhāva*) and sound (*shabda*) and [by means of the support] of the self [composed of] 'name and form' (*nāma-rūpa*) is called *mantra-yoga*."

This work discusses the qualifications of the teacher (*guru*) and the aspirant (*shishya*), ritual *purification practices, *breath control, projection (*nyāsa*) techniques, various kinds of worship (*pūjā*), and how to determine the right kind of *mantra for the student by means of a diagnostic diagram (called *cakra*).

MANU-SMRITI, also known as the *Mānava-Dharma-Shāstra*, a work composed of 2,685 verses dealing with the obligations of the various social classes (*varna*) of *Hinduism. It is ascribed to Manu, the ancestor of the human race in the present world cycle (*manvantara*), which comprises 311,040,000 human years. However, scholars regard this scripture as the product of several authors and assume that it was probably not completed until the beginning of the common era. While the *Manu-Smriti* focuses on the practicalities of *dharma for priests, rulers, and ordinary citizens, it also affords a valuable glimpse into the archaic tradition of *asceticism. The word *yoga* is primarily used in the sense of "harnessing" the senses. In one place (6.65) the *brahmin is exhorted to contemplate the subtleness of the supreme *Self by means of *Yoga. The compound *karma-yoga*, which occurs several times, refers to ritual performance rather than the Yoga of self-transcending *action, as taught in the *Bhagavad-Gītā*. The yogic process consists in kindling inner heat (*tapas*), which makes the Yoga of the *Manu-Smriti* consistent with the archaic Yoga of the *Vedas. See also *dharma-shāstra*.

MANVANTARA (from *manu* and *antara* or "period"), a world cycle ruled by a special Manu, or progenitor of the human race. According to the *Manu-Smriti* (1.79), these cycles are countless and consist of 852,000 "divine" years (71 × 12,000). The present cycle is the seventh in the dynasty of Manu Svayambhū and is governed by Manu Vaivasvat. See also *kalpa*, World ages.

MARANA-SIDDHI ("death power"), the paranormal power (*siddhi*) to kill through mere thought; mentioned in the *Kaula-Jnāna-Nirnaya* (4.14).

MĀRDAVA ("gentleness"), sometimes counted among the practices of moral discipline (*yama). See also mādhurya, maitrī.

MĀRGA ("way"). See bhakti-mārga, kaula-mārga, nivritti-mārga, Path, pravritti-mārga.

MĀRGA-ANURAKTI (mārgānurakti, "adherence to the path"), mentioned in the *Mandala-Brāhmana-Upanishad (1.1.4) as one of the constituent practices of self-restraint (*niyama). See also mumukshutva.

MĀRKANDEYA, a renowned *adept mentioned in the *Mahābhārata and in many *Purānas, notably the *Mārkandeya-Purāna. It is probable that there was more than one sage by this name.

MĀRKANDEYA-PURĀNA, one of the earliest extant *Purānas, perhaps dating from the third century BCE. It deals with *Yoga specifically in chapters 36–44, which in the main consist of a long dialogue between *Dattātreya and Alarka. This work prescribes a rather ritualistic lifestyle for the *yogin, which in some scriptures of *Postclassical Yoga is called *kriyā-yoga.

MARKATA-ĀSANA (markatāsana, "monkey posture"), described in the *Hatha-Ratna-Āvalī (3.55) thus: Pressing the feet with the hands and firmly grasping the toes, place the *head between the feet, like a bow.

MARMAN ("joint"), any of the several particularly vital spots in the *body, reminiscent of acupuncture points. Indian medicine (*Āyur-Veda) knows of 107 such places in the body, the principal marman being the *heart. The *Yoga scriptures generally speak of eighteen marmans. Thus the *Shāndilya-Upanishad (1.8.1f.) names the feet, big toes, ankles, shanks, knees, thighs, anus, *penis, *navel, heart, *throat, the "well" (kūpa, meaning the "throat well" or jugular notch), the palate (*tālu), *nose, *eyes, the middle between the eyebrows (*bhrū-madhya), *forehead, and *head. According to the *Kshurikā-Upanishad (14), one should cut through these vital spots by means of the "mind's sharp blade." The underlying practice is to focus *attention and *breath on each marman and to free it from tensions so that the life force (*prāna) can flow freely through the subtle channels (*nādī).

The word marman can also signify "measure of fingers," as in *Abhinava Gupta's Parā-Trishikā-Vivarana (p. 82), where it is applied to the extent of the inner space of a particular *visualization practice. See also desha, sthāna.

MASTERY OVER FOOD. See āhāra-jaya.

MASTERY OVER SENSES. See indriya-jaya.

MASTERY OVER THE FOUNDATION (OF NATURE). See pradhāna-jaya.

MĀTANGINĪ-MUDRĀ ("elephant seal"), described in the *Gheranda-Samhitā (3.88ff.) thus: Standing up to the neck in *water, draw in the water through both nostrils and expel it again through the mouth, then suck it up through the mouth and expel it through the *nose. It is said that by regularly repeating this cycle several times one becomes as strong as an elephant.

MATHA ("hut" or "monastery"). See āshrama, kutīra.

MATI ("conviction"), sometimes regarded as one of the practices of self-restraint (*niyama); explained in the *Darshana-

Upanishad (2.11) as "faith" (*shraddhā) in the *Vedic teachings and avoidance of any doctrines that run counter to the *Vedas.

MĀTRĀ ("measure"), a unit of measurement that has traditionally been used to calculate the duration of various exercises, particularly breath control (*prānāyāma). A mātrā is defined in the *Yoga-Cūdāmani-Upanishad (100) as the time taken by a single breath (*shvāsa) to occupy the "space" above and below, that is, to fill the lungs. According to the *Yoga-Tattva-Upanishad (40), however, it is the time it takes to snap one's fingers after circling the knee with one's hand. The *Tattva-Vaishāradī (2.50) specifies that the knee must be circled three times to arrive at the correct duration. The *Mārkandeya-Purāna (39.15) states that a mātrā is the time taken to open and close one's *eyes.

In earlier works, such as the *Bhagavad-Gītā (2.14), the term mātrā can stand for "matter" or "material *object."

MĀTRIKĀ-NYĀSA ("placing the mothers"). The mātrikās (lit. "little mothers") are the letters of the Sanskrit *alphabet, which are the foundation of all *mantras. In depictions of the different "lotuses" (*padma) representing the psychospiritual centers (*cakra) of the *body, the fifty letters of the alphabet are often seen inscribed in the petals. In the ritual of mātrikā-nyāsa, the Sanskrit alphabet is placed in the body of the initiate, thereby investing him or her with the power of the deity (*devatā). See also nyāsa.

MĀTSARYA ("envy" or "jealousy"), often mentioned as an undesirable character trait that must be overcome. Especially the practitioner of the left-hand *path (*vāma-mārga) of *Tantrism—the "hero" (*vīrya)—must have conquered sexual jealousy, because during the sacred rite of intercourse (*maithunā) his female partner is rarely the same person twice. No *attachment must be formed between the participants of this *Tantric ceremony. A synonym for mātsarya is īrshyā.

MATSYA ("fish"), one of the five ingredients of the *Tantric *panca-tattva ritual, where fish is taken as a stimulant.

MATSYA-ĀSANA (matsyāsana, "fish posture"), described in the *Gheranda-Samhitā (2.21) thus: Assume the lotus posture (*padma-āsana) and then lie back while cradling the *head with one's arms.

MATSYENDRA ("Lord of Fish," from matsya, "fish," and indra, "lord"), or MATSYENDRANĀTHA, remembered as one of the eighty-four great adepts (*mahā-siddha). Although some scholars place him in the fifth century CE, the consensus of opinion favors the tenth century CE. An earlier date seems, however, increasingly likely. He appears to have been the founder of the Yoginī branch of the *Kaula school of *Tantrism in Assam. In Tibet he

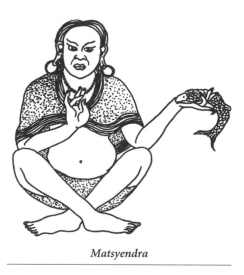

Matsyendra

is known as Mīnanātha or Luipā (probably a shortened version of Lohipāda ("He who hails from the river Lohit in Assam"), and in Nepal he is venerated as the deity Avalokiteshvara. He is traditionally regarded as the first human *teacher of *hatha-yoga and may have been the originator of the *Nātha sect. Matsyendra is said to have had twelve (or twenty-two) disciples, the most famous being *Goraksha. In Northern India there are many legends about him and Goraksha. Matsyendra is credited with the authorship of a number of works, including the old *Kaula-Jnāna-Nirnaya, which, however, was probably written a century after his time. According to some scholars, matsyendra and goraksha are titles suggesting specific initiatory levels.

MATSYENDRA-ĀSANA (matsyendrāsana, "Matsyendra's posture"), described in the *Gheranda-Samhitā (2.22f.) as follows: While sitting, twist the trunk sideways. Place the left leg next to the right thigh and the right elbow on the same thigh, holding the chin with the right hand. Repeat in the other direction. According to the *Hatha-Yoga-Pradīpikā (1.27), this ex-

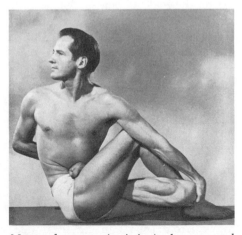

Matsyendra-āsana (variation), demonstrated by Theos Bernard

ercise fans the gastric *fire, cures all *diseases, and awakens the "serpent power" (*kundalinī-shakti).

MAUNA ("silence"), the characteristic condition of the *muni, the silent sage. According to the *Bhagavad-Gītā (17.16), mauna is an aspect of mental austerity (*tapas). It is occasionally counted among the constituent practices of moral discipline (*yama) as well as self-restraint (*niyama). The *Yoga-Bhāshya (2.32) distinguishes between kāshtha-mauna, "stock-stillness," and ākāra-mauna, "formal silence." *Vācaspati Mishra, in his *Tattva-Vaishāradī (2.32), explains the former as the practice of abstaining from signaling one's intentions even by means of gestures, while the latter is simply abstention from speech. In the *Laghu-Yoga-Vāsishtha (4.5.29), mauna is equated with *liberation. The *Shiva-Samhitā (5.4), however, considers it to be one of the possible obstacles (*vighna) on the spiritual *path. Cf. katthana.

MAUNI, an *adept in the lineage of *Goraksha; said to have been the *teacher of Vāmanayya, a minister of King Cola, who ascended the throne in 1012 CE.

MĀYĀ ("she who measures"), a key concept of the *Vedānta tradition. The term is generally translated as "illusion." In such early *Yoga and *Sāmkhya scriptures as the *Bhagavad-Gītā (7.14) and the *Shvetāshvatara-Upanishad (4.10), however, the word is used in the sense of "creative power," referring to the three primary constituents (*guna) of *nature. By the māyā of the Lord (*īshvara), states the Gītā (18.61), all beings are whirled about as if they were mounted on a machine.

Only in some radical idealist schools of later *Vedānta did the word acquire the meaning of "illusion" or "phantom existence." For instance, in the *Shiva-Samhitā* (1.64) *māyā* is called the "mother of the universe" (*vishva-janani*), the universe being a "play of illusion" (*māyā-vilāsitā*). More moderate nondualist schools understand *māyā* as "relative existence" rather than "hallucination." It is used in contrast to the absolute *Reality, which is nondual. See also *līlā, parināma, sat-kārya-vāda.*

MĀYĪYA-MALA. See *mala.*

MAYŪRA-ĀSANA (*mayūrāsana,* "peacock posture"), described in the *Gheranda-Samhitā* (2.29f.) thus: Placing one's palms on the ground, balance the *body with one's stomach resting on the elbows. Then raise the legs in the air. This is said to stimulate digestion and cure abdominal *diseases.

MEANNESS. See *kārpanya.*

MEANS, SPIRITUAL. See *upāya*; see also *anga, sādhana.*

MEASURE. See *mātra, pramāna.*

MEDHRA ("penis," from the root *mih,* "to make water," and the suffix *tra*), a synonym for *linga or *upastha.*

MEDICINE. The links between Indian medicine and *Yoga are manifold. Yoga makes use not only of medical concepts but also has adopted a number of procedures described in the *Āyur-Veda scriptures. Examples are the notion of the different forms of life energy (*prāna), bodily humors (*dhātu), vital areas (*marman), the signs (*arishta) of approaching *death, and *dietary considerations, as well as the use of enemas (*vasti) and sniffing water (*neti). The Yoga tradition has, in turn, in-

fluenced the medical authorities both conceptually and technologically. Many *yogins past and present have had a background in the healing arts. Thus the members of the *Kānphata order have a considerable reputation in the practice of medicine.

Works that illustrate well the close relationship between Yoga and *Āyur-Veda are the *Mishraka and the *Sat-Karma-Samgraha *Cidghanānanda. See also Anatomy.

MEDITATION, the practice of systematically vacating and unifying *consciousness. Even though the meditative state is structured differently from the ordinary *waking state, it is nonetheless accompanied by *awareness. In fact, it is characterized by an unusual degree of lucidity. See also *dhyāna, jhāna, nididhyāsana, samādhi.*

MEDITATOR. See *dhyātri.*

MEMORY. See *smriti.*

MERIT. See *punya.*

MERU, the golden mountain that, according to *Hindu mythology, exists in the center of the *earth. It is supposed to be 350,000 miles high and as many miles deep. This mountain serves as the pleasure ground of the *deities of the Hindu pantheon. In *Yoga and *Tantrism, *meru* is a secret term for the central axis of the human *body, the spinal column, and is often also called *meru-danda* ("*meru* staff"). *Meru* is also the designation for the central bead of a rosary (*mālā). See also Cosmos.

MEYKANDAR (mid-13th cen. CE), a famous *adept of the *Shaiva-Siddhānta tradition; author of the *Shiva-Jnāna-Bodha*

("Illumination of the Wisdom of *Shiva"), consisting of only twelve verses based on the *Raurava-Āgama*. This is the first Tamil attempt at a systematic exposition of the theological doctrines of Southern *Shaivism. Meykandar had forty-nine *disciples.

Microcosm (Sanskrit: *pinda-anda*), the human *body, which is born of an egg (*anda*) yet contains the entire *universe within itself. *Yoga subscribes to the archaic notion that body and *cosmos are structurally homologous. Therefore the *world can be transcended by transcending the body in all its aspects. Cf. Macrocosm.

Mīna ("Fish"; also known as Mīnanātha), mentioned in the *Hatha-Yoga-Pradīpikā* (1.5) as an early master of *hatha-yoga*. Some traditions identify him with *Matsyendra.

Mind. See *buddhi, citta,* Consciousness, *manas.*

Mishraka ("Mixture"), a work by *Cidghanānanda dealing with *diseases due to faults in one's *Yoga practice. See also *Sat-Karma-Samgraha.*

Mistress, Tantric. See *nāyikā.*

mita-āhāra (*mitāhāra,* "moderate diet"), sometimes considered to be one of the practices of moral discipline (*yama*). The *Hatha-Yoga-Pradīpikā* (1.58) defines it as agreeable and nutritious *food that is consumed in order to delight *Shiva. This work echoes widespread dietary wisdom when it stipulates that one should fill half the stomach with food, one quarter with liquid, and leave one fourth empty. The *Gheranda-Samhitā* (5.16ff.) states: "He who practices *Yoga without moderation in *diet incurs various *diseases and obtains no success." See also *āhāra, laghvāhāra*; cf. *atyāhāra.*

Modesty. See *hrī.*

moha ("delusion"), frequently counted among the defects (*dosha*). The *Yoga-Vārttika* (2.34) explains it as a mistaken notion, such as the idea that merit accrues from sacrificing animals. The most serious form of *moha* is the self-delusion that one is a limited ego personality rather than the transcendental *Self.

moksha ("liberation"), explained in the *Laghu-Yoga-Vāsishtha* (5.9.48) as follows: "*Liberation is neither beyond the sky nor in the netherworld nor on *earth. Liberation is said to be the dissolution of the *mind upon the obliteration of all aspirations (*āshā*)." In other words, *liberation is an intrapsychic event, not a locality. It is a shift in *consciousness whereby one transcends all *duality. The event of liberation, paradoxically, coincides with the realization that both liberation and *bondage are merely conceptual constructs and hence of no ultimate significance. The *Laghu-Yoga-Vasishtha* (6.13.25) puts it this way: "There is neither bondage nor liberation. There is only the *Absolute beyond ill." The same scripture (VI.13.93) emphatically states: "What is called 'liberation' does not have *space or time or any other state." See also *apavarga, jīvan-mukti, kaivalya, krama-mukti, mukti, videha-mukti.*

Moksha-Dharma ("Liberation Doctrine"), a remarkable didactic section in the *Mahābhārata* (12.168–353) that records teachings of many schools of *Preclassical Yoga and *Sāmkhya.

Monkey posture. See *markata-āsana.*

Moon. See *candra*; cf. *sūrya*.

Morality, a vital aspect of spiritual life, though it must not be equated with spirituality in general. A moral, or "good," way of life—embodying such values as love (*bhakti*), forgiveness, generosity (*dāna*), etc.—is the foundation on which all higher spiritual practice can thrive. Whereas morality prevents the accumulation of further *karmic demerit, or *sin, spiritual practice aims at the *transcendence of both good and evil. See also Ethics, *yama*.

Mrigendra-Tantra (from *mriga*, "deer," and *indra*, "lord"), an authoritative scripture of the *Pāshupata tradition, composed between 500 and 800 CE. It deals with *Yoga in a special chapter in two apparently independent passages. One passage mentions a yogic *path consisting of the following "limbs" (*anga*): *breath control, *sense withdrawal, *concentration, *meditation, "inspection" (*vīkshana*), and *ecstasy. Yoga itself, as the *angin* or "possessor of the limbs," is said to be the eighth component.

mrita-āsana (*mritāsana*, "corpse posture"), also known as *shava-āsana*, "dead pose", described in the *Gheranda-Samhitā (2.19) as lying flat on the ground like a corpse. This is said to remedy fatigue and also to quieten an agitated *mind.

mrityu ("death"), sometimes regarded as one of the defects (*dosha*) of human existence. See also Death, *kāla*.

muditā ("gladness"), or a positive state of *mind, is to be consciously projected. See also *karunā*, *maitrī*, *upekshā*.

mudrā ("seal"). This word has a number of different connotations in *Yoga and *Tantrism. Thus in *hatha-yoga it stands for practices similar to the postures (*āsana*). The *Gheranda-Samhitā (3) knows of twenty-five such "seals," which include the "locks" (*bandha*) and, curiously, also five concentration practices (*panca-dhāranā*): *ashvinī-mudrā, *bhujanginī-mudrā, *jālandhara-bandha, *kākī-mudrā, *khecarī-mudrā, *mahā-bandha, *mahā-mudrā, *mahā-vedha, *māndukī-mudrā, *mātangī-mudrā, *mūla-bandha, *nabho-mudrā, *pāshinī-mudrā, *sahajolī-mudrā, *shakti-cālanī-mudrā, *shāmbhavī-mudrā, *tādāgī-mudrā, *uddīyāna-bandha, *vajrolī-mudrā, *viparīta-karanī-mudrā, and *yoni-mudrā, as well as *pārthavī-mudrā, *āmbhasī-mudrā, *vāyavī-mudrā, *āgneyī-mudrā, and *ākāshī-mudrā. All these "seals," the text states, are to be kept secret with great care. They should especially not be taught to a rogue *disciple or one lacking in *devotion. These *mudrās give both enjoyment (*bhoga*) and liberation (*mukti*). They have great curative and rejuvenating power and also increase the gastric fire (*jāthara-agni*). The *Hatha-Yoga-Pradīpikā (3.8) calls them "divine" (*divya*) because they lead to liberation and also produce the classic paranormal abilities (*siddhi*) of a liberated being. Another important "seal," not named in the *Gheranda-Samhitā, is the *shan-mukhī-mudrā.

The term *mudrā*, moreover, denotes certain hand gestures used during yogic rituals and in the course of the performance of particular postures (*āsana*) and *meditation. The *Soma-Shāmbhu-Paddhati* describes no fewer than thirty-seven hand *mudrās*. The best known in yogic circles are *abhaya-mudrā, anjali-mudrā (performed by joining the palms in front of the chest), *cin-mudrā, *dhyāna-mudrā, and *jnāna-mudrā.

In *Tantrism two further meanings of

mudrā are current. Here the term can refer to the female participant in the sexual ritual (**maithunā*) as well as to parched grain, one of the five ingredients of the **panca-tattva* rite, which is thought to have aphrodisiac properties. Finally, the **hatha-yogins* also apply the term *mudrā* to the large *earrings worn by members of the *Kānphata order. See also *bhairava-mudrā*.

MUHŪRTA, a period of forty-eight minutes, consisting of two *ghatikās*. See also *brahma-muhūrta, kāla*.

MUKTANANDA, SWAMI (1908–1983), a great contemporary *adept of *kundalinī-yoga*, which he called *siddha-yoga*. A *disciple of Bhagawan *Nityananda, he in turn had a large following in India and Western countries, initiating thousands of men and women through direct spiritual transmission (**shakti-pāta*). Among his more

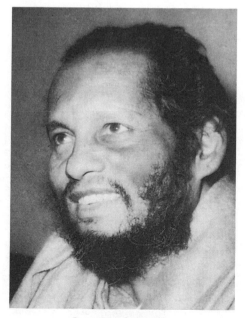

Swami **Muktananda**

prominent American students was the late "Rudi" (Swami Rudrananda), who taught Swami Chetanananda and Franklin Jones (alias Da Free John, alias Da Avabhasa), who was also initiated by Swami Muktananda himself. Philosophically, Swami Muktananda was at home in Kashmiri *Shaivism.

MUKTA-ĀSANA (*muktāsana*, "liberated posture"), described in the *Gheranda-Samhitā* (2.11) thus: Place the left heel at the root of the *genitals and the right heel above the genitals. The *Yoga-Yājnavalkya* (3.14) gives this alternative: Place the left ankle above the genitals and the right ankle above that.

MUKTI ("release"), a synonym for *moksha*. The *Mārkandeya-Purāna* (39.1) understands it as the separation (*viyoga*) from spiritual *ignorance upon the dawn of true wisdom (**jnāna*) and as one's identity (**aikya*) with the *Absolute and nonidentification with the primary constituents (**guna*) of *nature. The *Shiva-Purāna* (4.41.3) lists four types or degrees of such release: (1) *sālokya-mukti*, release through dwelling in the same realm (**loka*) as *God; (2) *sāmnidhya-mukti*, release through proximity to God; (3) *sārū-pya-mukti*, release through assuming the same form as God; and (4) *sāyujya-mukti*, release through being perfectly yoked to God. See also *jīvan-mukti, krama-mukti, videha-mukti*.

MUKTIKĀ-UPANISHAD (*Muktikopanishad*), a *Vedānta scripture dating from the late fourteenth century CE and consisting of two parts. In the second part various yogic processes are mentioned.

MŪLA-BANDHA ("root lock"), one of the three "locks" (**bandha*) employed in *hatha-yoga. It is described in the *Ghe-

randa-Samhitā (3.14ff.) as follows: With the aid of the left heel placed against the perineum (**yoni*), contract the perineum and carefully press the **navel against the spinal cord. The right heel should be placed against the genitals. This technique is said to lead to the mastery of the **breath and bring about the rejuvenation of the **body. According to the **Yoga-Kundalī-Upanishad* (1.42ff.), the naturally downward-moving **apāna* breath is forced upward by contracting of the anal sphincter muscle. The **Hatha-Yoga-Pradīpikā* (3.61ff.) notes that the *mūla-bandha* helps the **prāna* and **apāna* to unite with the **nāda* and **bindu*. This "lock" is also thought to stimulate the **body's inner **fire and to arouse the dormant "serpent power" (**kundalinī-shakti*). One of the side effects of this practice is the diminution of urine and feces. The **Tejo-Bindu-Upanishad* (1.27) furnishes a symbolic definition, stating that the *mūla-bandha* is that which is the root of all the **worlds.

MŪLĀDHĀRA-CAKRA ("root-prop wheel"), the lowest of the seven psychoenergetic

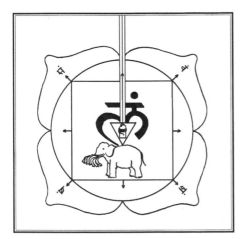

Mūlādhāra-cakra, the psychoenergetic center located at the base of the spine

centers (**cakra*) of the **body. Most schools depict this center as a four-petaled lotus situated at the anus or the perineum (**yoni*). The petals are generally described as being of crimson hue. Its "seed syllable" (**bīja-mantra*) is *lam*, which pertains to the **earth element. The center's presiding **adept is Dviranda, and its presiding **goddess is Dākinī. This center contains the radiant triangle called **kāma-rūpa* ("desire-formed"), within which is found the golden phallus (**linga*) of **Shiva. This *cakra* is the source of the central channel (**sushumnā-nādī*) of the **life force, and the resting place of the "serpent power" (**kundalinī-shakti*). Regular **contemplation of this psychoenergetic center yields, among many other things, the paranormal ability to jump like a frog and, in advanced stages, to actually perform **levitation.

MŪLA-SHODHANA ("root cleansing"), one of the four kinds of "washing" (**dhauti*) used in **hatha-yoga*. It is described in the **Gheranda-Samhitā* (1.42ff.) thus: So long as the rectum is not properly cleansed, the **apāna* breath does not circulate freely. Hence one should carefully cleanse the rectum with **water by means of a stalk of turmeric or one's middle finger. See also *cakrī-karma*.

MUMUKSHUTVA ("desire for liberation"), a **Vedānta term adopted by some **Yoga authorities. The desire to transcend the ego personality is an essential prerequisite for spiritual growth. Without it a person's commitment to the trials of discipline is apt to be weak. On the other hand, the desire for **liberation must be free of any neurotic urge to escape the **world or oneself. The person aspiring to **liberation is called *mumukshu*, as opposed to the "pleasure seeker" (*bubhukshu*). See also *mārga-anurakti*.

MUNI ("sage"), a word etymologically related to *mauna ("silence"). Apparently this designation was originally used in ancient *Vedic times to refer to religious ecstatics outside the circles of orthodox *Brahmanism. The word is probably related to the Greek term *mania* ("exaltation"). By the time of *Shankara (ca. 800 CE), however, the *muni* was regarded as representing the highest type of spiritual *perfection.

In the *Laghu-Yoga-Vāsishtha* (6.7.3) two types of *muni* are distinguished. The ordinary type is known as *kāshtha-tapasvin* or the "ascetic who stands stock-still." The second, superior type is the *jīvan-mukta*, who, as the name indicates, is liberated while still embodied. See also *keshin*.

MŪRCHĀ ("fainting") can occur during some yogic practices, notably *breath control. According to the *Yoga-Mārtanda* (55), it can be overcome by practicing the *khecarī-mudrā*.

Mūrchā is also the name of one of the eight types of breath retention (*kumbhaka*) described in the *Hatha-Yoga-Pradīpikā* (2.69): At the end of inhalation one should firmly practice the throat lock (*jālandhara-bandha*) while exhaling slowly. This is so called because it causes the *mind to swoon into *happiness.

MŪRTI ("form"), the visible manifestations of the deities (*devatā*) that are to be worshiped, invoked, or *meditated upon. Often this is an image of the *Divine or one's teacher (*guru*), who is venerated as an embodiment of the transcendental *Reality.

MUSIC has played an important role in the religious and spiritual life of the *Hindus ever since the time of the *Vedas. The *Sāma-Veda*, one of the four *Vedic hymnodies, is to this day employed by the *udgātri* priests during the sacrificial *rituals. Its hymns are chanted or sung according to the heptatonic melodies fixed in special songbooks called *Gānas*. *Breath control was clearly important in this practice. Little is known about the early development of Indian music, but by the beginning of the common era India had a full-fledged system of music theory, as is evident from the *Bhārata-Nātya-Shāstra*. Especially the various schools of the Yoga of devotion (*bhakti-yoga*) favored music as an expression of the spiritual impulse. Thus chants and songs were and still are employed by the South Indian *Vaishnavas and the *Bāuls of Bengal. See also *kīrtana*.

MYSTERY. See *guhya*, Secret.

MYSTICISM. *Yoga has often been characterized as a form of mysticism. This is correct, providing we understand mysticism as a systematic approach to *self-transcendence in order to achieve a deeper connection with, or awakening of oneself as, the ultimate *Reality. Yoga is not mystical in the sense of being nebulous; rather its orientation is thoroughly pragmatic or experiential. Perception (*pratyaksha*) is deemed an important means of knowledge (*pramāna*), though the Yoga authorities operate with an extended concept of perception, allowing for what they call *yoga-pratyaksha*. This includes the kind of suprasensory knowledge (*atīndriya-jnāna*) that modern *parapsychology is only beginning to explore.

MYTHOLOGY. Myths and legends form an integral part of the heritage of *Yoga and are used for edification and instruction about yogic principles. Their symbolism is incredibly rich and offers a valuable entrance into the Yoga tradition. The folklore of the *Purānas makes for an especially rewarding study, as does the much more elaborate and obscure mythology of the *Vedas upon which many Purānic stories are based.

· N ·

NĀBHI ("navel"), one of the sensitive areas (*marman) of the *body.

NĀBHI-CAKRA ("navel wheel"), a synonym for *manipura-cakra. It is the only *cakra referred to by name in the *Yoga-Sūtra (3.29), which states that by practicing ecstatic "constraint" (*samyama) upon this psychoenergetic center, one acquires *knowledge about the *body's *anatomy. According to the *Shāndilya-Upanishad (1.4.6), it is here that the psyche (*jīva) resides "like a spider in its web."

NĀBHI-KANDA ("navel bulb"). See kanda.

NABHO-MUDRĀ ("ether-space seal"). The term nabhas (changed to nabho in front of a soft consonant) is a synonym for *ākāsha. This "seal" (*mudrā) is described in the *Gheranda-Samhitā (3.7) as follows: Regardless of the activities one is engaged in, one should always turn the *tongue backward against the *palate and restrain one's *breath. This can be called *khecarī-mudrā in daily life. According to the *Yoga-Cūdā-manī-Upanishad (45), however, nabho-mudrā is a synonym for *mahā-mudrā.

NĀDA ("sound"), the inner sound (*shabda or *dhvani) that becomes audible when the network of psychoenergetic currents (*nādī) has been duly purified. According to the *Yoga-Shikhā-Upanishad (3.3), it is the second level of manifestation of the "Absolute as sound" (*shabda-brahman). This sound manifests in a variety of ways. The *Darshana-Upanishad (6.36) distinguishes three degrees of it, resembling the sound of a conch, a thundercloud, and a mountain cataract respectively. The *Nāda-Bindu-Upanishad (34f.) compares the first degree of sound manifestations to the sound produced by the ocean, a thundercloud, a kettledrum, or a waterfall. The second degree is said to resemble the sound made by a drum, a big drum, or a bell. The third degree is likened to the sound of a small bell, a bamboo flute, a lute, or a bee.

The *Hamsa-Upanishad (16) speaks of ten modes of the inner sound, the last being called the "sound of the thundercloud" (megha-nāda), which is the only fit focus for *concentration. Certain other phenomena are said to be associated with the different levels of the inner sounds, and they become significant from the fourth level on. In ascending sequence, the phenomena described are as follows: tremor of the *head, the profuse production of the "nectar of immortality" (*amrita), enjoyment of the ambrosial liquid, the acquisition of secret *knowledge, "higher speech" (parā-vācā), the ability to make oneself invisible and to see infinitely, and finally identification with the *Absolute. The *Hamsa-Upanishad (43), furthermore, compares the nāda to a snake charmer, since it captivates the fickle mind (*manas).

The *Hatha-Yoga-Pradīpikā (3.64) speaks of a union of the *prāna and *apāna with the nāda and *bindu. That is to say, through controlled breathing and mental *concentration a conjunction between the outbreath and the inbreath is effected. This occurs in the central channel (*sushumnā-nādī) and produces the inner sound. That inner sound, riding on the focused *breath, then proceeds to the *bindu, which is the inaudible aspect of sound, envisioned to exist above the *heart. This work (4.90ff.) states:

As a bee drinking the nectar cares not for the scent, so the *mind absorbed in the nāda does not crave for sense *objects.
The sharp hook of the nāda effectively curbs the mind, [which is like] a mad elephant, roaming in the garden of the sense objects.
When the mind is bound by the noose of the nāda and has discarded [its habitual] restlessness, it reaches full *steadiness, like a bird with clipped wings.
The nāda is the snare by which the deer is bound within, and it is the hunter who slays the deer within.

The nāda is thought to originate in the center of the spine, which the *Dhyāna-Bindu-Upanishad (95) calls the "fiddle-stick" (vīnā-danda). In order to elicit the inner sound more readily, some *yogins practice what is known as the "six-openings seal" (*shan-mukhī-mudrā), blocking off the *nostrils, *eyes, and *ears.
The nāda is represented in writing as a crescent or semicircle (*ardha-candra), as in the sacred syllable *om (see illustration at om).

NĀDA-ANUSANDHĀNA (nādānusandhāna, "cultivation of the [inner] sound"), also called nāda-upāsana (nādopāsana, "worship through sound"), the primary means of accomplishing mental absorption (*laya), according to the *Hatha-Yoga-Pradīpikā (4.66), This discipline is said to have four stages (*avasthā).

NĀDA-BINDU-UPANISHAD (Nādabindū-panishad), one of the *Yoga-Upanishads. Consisting of only fifty-three stanzas, it expounds a *Vedānta-based *nāda-yoga. The inner sound (*nāda) is stated (31ff.) to be the vehicle that will transport the *yogin beyond the ocean of phenomenal existence; it drowns all external noises and focuses the *mind. The practice of *vaishnavī-mudrā is recommended. The ultimate goal of this *Yoga is *liberation, which is accomplished after shedding the physical *body.

NĀDA-SPHUTATVA ("explosion of the [inner] sound"), mentioned in the *Hatha-Yoga-Pradīpikā (2.78) as one of the signs of *perfection. See also nāda.

NĀDA-YOGA, a prominent teaching in the *Yoga-Upanishads. It is indirectly referred to already in the *Maitrāyanīya-Upanishad (6.22), which speaks of those who listen to the sound (*shabda) inside the *heart by placing the thumbs against the *ears. The subtle sound (*nāda) that becomes thus audible must not be confused with the thumping of the heart muscle or ringing in the ears. *Kabir referred to this practice as surati-shabda-yoga, an expression that has been retained by the Rādhāsvāmi school. See also Yoga.

NĀDĪ ("conduit," "channel," "vein," or "artery"), any of the blood-carrying veins or arteries; also, any of the subtle (*sūkshma) channels in or along which the life force (*prāna) circulates. A more sophisticated interpretation understands the nādīs as the flow patterns of the psychosomatic

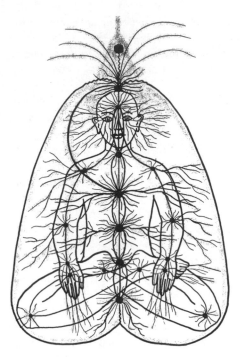

The network of subtle energy channels (*nādī*) that sustain the physical body

teaches that only one of these 101 channels passes to the crown of the *head and leads to *immortality. This teaching is reiterated in some of the *Yoga-Upanishads*. Thus the *Yoga-Shikhā-Upanishad* (6.5) identifies the *nādī* extending to the head as the *para-nādī*, otherwise known as the *sushumnā-nādī*.

Among this multitude of pathways of the *life force, three have special esoteric significance: the central channel called *sushumnā-nādī* and the two channels that wind around it in helical fashion, which are known as the *idā-nādī* and the *pingalā-nādī*.

The *Vāraha-Upanishad* (5.28) describes the twelve main channels as a "multicolored cloth" in whose middle is the *nābhi-cakra*. In the *Shāndilya-Upanishad* (1.4.11) and the *Yoga-Yājnavalkya* (4.46), both of which acknowledge fourteen principal *nādīs*, this network of channels is likened to the *ashvattha*, the sacred fig tree. All the *nādīs* are said to originate in the "bulb" (*kanda*). They are the locus of the psyche (*jīva*).

The *Laghu-Yoga-Vāsishtha* (6.9.111) states that the *nādīs* bind the *body like creepers. This, however, is only true so long as they are laden with impurities (*mala*). In that case, the life force (*prāna*) cannot circulate freely in them, and especially it cannot enter the central channel. Hence the *yogin* is advised to practice exercises for their *purification. The *Shāndilya-Upanishad* (1.7.1) promises results after only three months. See also *amrita-nādī*, *nādī-shodhana*, *nādī-shuddhi*, *rākā-nādī*.

energy. Other technical terms for *nādī* are *hita* ("beneficial") and *sira* ("stream").

Their number is generally affirmed to be 72,000, although, as the *Tri-Shikhi-Brāhmana-Upanishad* (2.76) assures us, they are really countless. The *Shiva-Samhitā* (2.13) claims the existence of 350,000 *nādīs* in all. Some works state that 72 *nādīs* are particularly important, but most mention only 10, 12, or 14 by name. Thus according to the *Darshana-Upanishad* (4.6ff.), the 14 major conduits of the life force are: *sushumnā, *idā, *pingalā, *sarasvatī, *pūshā, *varunā, *hasti-jihvā, *yashasvinī, *ālambusā, *kuhū, *vishva-udārā, *payasvinī, *shankhinī, *gāndhārā.

An earlier tradition, recorded in the *Brihad-Āranyaka-Upanishad* (4.2.3) and the *Chāndogya-Upanishad* (8.6.6), speaks of 101 *nādīs*. The *Katha-Upanishad* (6.16)

NĀDĪ-CAKRA ("wheel of channels"), the entire network of conduits (*nādī*) of the *life force; also, the "heart lotus" (*hridaya-pundarīka*, see *hrit-padma*).

NĀDĪ-SHODHANA ("purification of the channels"), an essential prerequisite of advanced breath control (*prāṇāyāma*). The higher breathing practices and techniques for awakening the "serpent power" (*kundalinī-shakti*) are dangerous so long as the *nāḍīs* have not been thoroughly purified. According to the *Gheranda-Samhitā* (5.36), the purificatory practices are of two basic types: *samanu* and *nirmanu*. The former is done by means of a "seed-" or *bīja-mantra* and is really a more advanced *meditation and breathing practice. The latter consists in the six "washing" (*dhauti*) practices, which should precede the *samanu* exercise. For the *samanu* process, one should assume the lotus posture (*padma-āsana*), place the teacher (*guru*) in one's *heart, and contemplate the "seed" syllable of the *wind element, which is *yam*. This exercise has the following stages: (1) inhale through the left *nostril while repeating the sound *yam* sixteen times; (2) restrain the *breath for sixty-four repetitions; (3) slowly exhale through the right nostril over a period of thirty-two repetitions; (4) raise the "fire" (*agni*) from the region of the *navel toward the *heart; (5) inhale through the right nostril while repeating sixteen times the "seed" syllable of the *fire element, which is *ram*; (6) retain the breath for sixty-four repetitions; (7) exhale through the left nostril over a period of thirty-two repetitions; (8) while contemplating the luminous reflection of the "moon" (*candra*) at the tip of the nose, inhale through the left nostril while repeating sixteen times the "seed" syllable *tham*; (9) retain the breath for sixty-four repetitions while contemplating the "nectar" (*amrita*) flowing from the "moon"; and (10) exhale through the right nostril while repeating thirty-two times the syllable *lam*.

According to the *Hatha-Yoga-Pradīpikā* (1.39), the *nāḍīs* are purified by means of the regular practice of the adept's posture (*siddha-āsana*), though this scripture (2.7ff.) also recommends a form of alternate breathing. The *Darshana-Upanishad* (5.10) stipulates that one should practice alternate breathing while in seclusion three to four times daily for a period of three to four days. See also *nāḍī-shuddhi*.

NĀDĪ-SHUDDHI ("purity of the channels"), sometimes used synonymously with *nāḍī-shodhana*, though strictly speaking, it refers to the end state of *purity. Among the signs of a purified system of *nāḍīs* are bodily lightness (*lāghava*), increased glow of the "*fire" in the abdomen, and the manifestation of the inner sound (*nāda*). See also *cihna*.

NĀGA ("serpent"), one of the secondary types of life force, or *upaprāna*. Most texts ascribe to it the function of belching and vomiting. According to the *Siddha-Siddhānta-Paddhati* (1.68), it is present in all the limbs and is responsible for motion and discharge.

NĀGOJĪ BHATTA (late 16th cen. CE), also known as Nāgesha, one of the great *Hindu scholars; author of many original works on *Vedānta and also a larger and a shorter commentary on the *Yoga-Sūtra*.

NAISHKARMYA-KARMAN ("actionless action"), a key concept of *karma-yoga. First taught in the *Bhagavad-Gītā (3.4), this doctrine states that a person is not karmically affected by his or her *actions if those actions are done in the spirit of *sacrifice. *Naishkarmya-karman* is ego-transcending activity and must be carefully distinguished from mere action (*karman*) and inaction (*akarman*).

NAKULĪSHA. See Lakulīsha.

NALAYIRA-DIVYA-PRABANDHAM. See
Divya-Prabandham.

NĀMADEVA (1270–1350 CE), a contemporary of *Jnānadeva, whose work he continued. Traditional accounts state that in his
early life Nāmadeva was a highway robber
and that he was brought to his senses by
the tears of a *woman whose husband he
had killed. After his conversion, he became
one of the great spokesmen for the medieval *bhakti* movement. He left behind a
large number of instructional verses (*abhanga*). See also Ekanātha, Gahinīnātha.

NĀMA-RŪPA ("name [and] form"), a
*Vedānta phrase that denotes the phe-
nomenal universe, which is a mental construct (*samkalpa*) and hence distinct from
*Reality. It is the conventional reality to
which Goethe poetically referred as "Schall
und Rauch" (sound and smoke). The Ultimate is nameless and formless. See also
Appearance; cf. Name.

NAME. Although most schools of *Hinduism deem the *Divine in itself to be nameless and formless, it has traditionally been
worshiped under many names (*nāman*),
which are all sacred. In fact, there are
compilations known as *Sahasra-Nāma*
("Thousand Names") that are entirely
dedicated to listing the many names by
which the Divine may be invoked. This is a
form of *mantra* practice. Cf. *nāma-rūpa.*

NAMM ("Our," in Tamil; prob. late 9th
cen. CE), one of the *Ālvārs; the last and
also the most revered of the *Vaishnava
poet-saints of South India. He composed
numerous hymns (*āruvāymoli*) that are
part of the *Vaishnava canonical literature
and a love poem entitled *Tiru-Virutta*, as
well as two other minor works. He has at
times been considered as an incarnation

(*avatāra*) of *Vishnu, whom he worshiped. His poetry epitomizes the devotional (*bhakti*) approach to *enlightenment.

NĀNAK (1469–1539 CE), the first of the
ten *gurus* of *Sikhism. He taught his followers through songs that are at once simple and beautiful. His teaching is a synthesis of *Hindu devotionalism (*bhakti*) and
Muslim Sufism. For him there were no
Hindus and Muslims but only the divine
truth. According to Sikh tradition, Nānak
disappeared for three days at the age of
thirty. During this period, he was in the
presence of *God, who charged him with
the mission to teach humanity how to pray
and to be an example to all by praising the
divine *name and by practicing *charity,
ablutions, and service.

NANDIKESHVARA-KĀSHIKĀ, the only
surviving work of Nandikeshvaranātha
(ca. 250 BCE). Consisting of twenty-six
verses, it is an exposition of *Shaiva philosophy. Its author is traditionally said to
have been the teacher (*guru*) of *Patanjali
and Vyāghrapāda.

NĀRADA. There were probably several individuals by this name, unless we doubt
Nārada's historicity altogether, for which
there are no stringent reasons. A seer
called Nārada is mentioned already in the
Atharva-Veda (5.19.9) and again in the
old *Chāndogya-Upanishad* (7.1ff.). It is
unlikely that this Nārada is identical with
the sage who, for instance, figures so
prominently in the *Mahābhārata* and in
many of the *Purānas*, or with the Nārada
who composed one of the two extant
Bhakti-Sūtras.

NĀRADA-PARIVRĀJAKA-UPANISHAD, the
most extensive text of the group of *Sam-

nyāsa-Upanishads; prob. composed ca. 1200 CE. It describes (5.11ff.) six classes of ascetics: *kutīcaka, bahūdaka, *hamsa, *par-ama-hamsa, *turīya-atīta,* and **avadhūta.* Only the last two are said to enjoy the "aloneness" (**kaivalya*) of the *Self. This work (5.26) decries the value of the disci-plines prescribed in *Yoga and *Sāmkhya scriptures, though in chapter 6 it speaks of the "knower of *Vedānta" (*vedānta-vid*) as a *yogin. Its Yoga is clearly of the *nondu-alist variety.

NĀRADEVA, mentioned in the *Hatha-Yoga-Pradīpikā* (1.8) as one of the masters of *hatha-yoga.

NĀRAKA ("pertaining to the human," from *nara* and the suffix *ka*), hell. Refer-ences to hell are found already in the an-cient *Rig-Veda* (7.104, etc.), but the first clear picture of what this entails is given in the *Upanishads*. The *Yoga-Bhāshya* (3.26) reflects popular notions when it speaks of the seven hell realms. These are, in ascending order: *avīci* ("that which is waveless [i.e., static]"), *mahā-kāla* ("great death/blackness"), *ambarīsha* ("frying pan"), *raurava* ("that which pertains to *ruru* [a demon]"), *mahā-raurava* ("that which pertains to the great *ruru*"), *kāla-sūtra* ("thread of death/blackness"), and *andhatā-mishra* ("thick darkness"). These names are in part explained by the pre-dominant *element that characterizes each of those hellish regions or states of being. In these realms, creatures suffer the conse-quences of their own misdeeds in other lives. See also Cosmos, *pātāla*; cf. *svarga*.

NĀRAKA-DVĀRA ("gate of hell"). The *Bhagavad-Gītā* (16.21) speaks of three gates of *hell: desire (*kāma*), anger (*krodha*), and greed (*lobha*).

NĀRĀYANA ("Man's Abode"), one of *Vishnu's many names.

NĀRĀYANA TĪRTHA (prob. 18th cen. CE), a great *Vedānta scholar; author of two commentaries on the *Yoga-Sūtra*: the *Sūtra-Artha-Bodhinī* and the *Yoga-Sid-dhānta-Candrikā*, in which he interprets *Classical Yoga from a *Vedantic point of view, drawing especially on the discipline of devotion, or *bhakti-yoga.

NĀSA ("nose"), one of the loci (*desha*) for *concentration.

NĀSA-AGRA-DRISHTI (*nāsāgradrishti*, "gaze at the tip of the nose"), prescribed for a variety of postures (*āsana*) and *meditation practices. See also *drishti*.

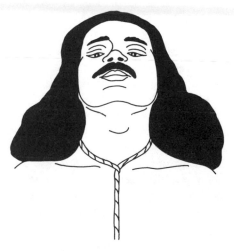

Nāsa-agra-drishti, the yogic concentrative gaze at the tip of the nose

NĀTHA ("lord"), the distinguishing title of *adepts of the *Nātha sect and members of the *Kānphata order, notably *Matsyendra and *Goraksha.

NĀTHA SECT, or **NĀTHISM**; a teaching lineage within *Shaiva *Tantrism. Although the origins of Nāthism are obscure, it has correctly been described as a particular phase of the *Siddha cult, whose members aspired to the *transubstantiation of the human *body. It was within the Nātha sect that *hatha-yoga came to be developed. Its two most outstanding *adepts are *Matsyendra and his disciple *Goraksha. Northern India knows of a tradition of nine nāthas. Different lists name different individuals. The best-known list has the names of Matsyendra-, Goraksha-, *Carpata-, Mangala-, Ghugo-, *Gopī-, Prāna-, Sūrata-, and Cambananātha.

The success of this sect was partly due to its *teachers' refusal to recognize caste barriers, and their teachings were adopted by outcastes and kings alike. In the course of time, the followers of Nāthism became a "casteless" caste of spinners, weavers, and metal workers. See also Kaula.

NĀTHAMUNI (prob. 10th cen. CE), was the first learned sage of the *Vaishnava tradition of South India. He is said to have been a practitioner of the eightfold *path (*ashta-anga-yoga) and to have often walked about naked, living on food thrown to him. Among the scriptures authored by him is the *Yoga-Rahasya. This widely traveled teacher had eleven principal disciples. He was the grandfather of *Yamunācārya, *Rāmānuja's teacher.

NĀTHISM. See Nātha sect.

NATURE. See Cosmos, prakriti, World.

NAULĪ, also known as laulikī ("rolling"); described in the *Hatha-Yoga-Pradīpikā (2.33f.) thus: With the shoulders bent forward, vigorously rotate the abdominal muscles. This practice, which is one of the "six acts" (*shat-karma), is said to be the "crown" of *hatha-yoga, stimulating the gastric *fire and curing all disorders of the bodily *humors. The *Hatha-Ratna-Āvalī (1.31ff.) distinguishes between an inner (antara) and an outer (bāhya) naulī. The latter is the familiar rotation of the abdominal muscles. The former is explained as the vigorous rotation of the *idā-nādī and the *pingalā-nādī, the two currents flowing in helical fashion around the central channel (*sushumnā-nādī) of the *life force. It is not clear what is meant by this, though probably the intended practice is a form of alternately activating these two currents by means of *visualization and/or *breathing alternately through the left and the right *nostril. Some *Yoga authorities interpret antara-naulī as consisting in the vertical movement of the abdominal muscles.

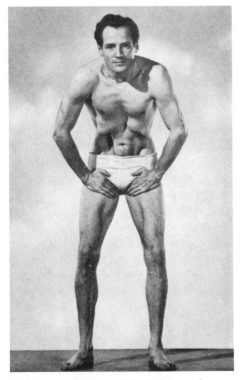

Naulī, a technique of hatha-yoga, demonstrated by Theos Bernard

NAVA-CAKRA ("nine wheels"). Some traditions speak of a system of nine psychoenergetic centers (*cakra), which generally includes the well-known set of seven plus the "palate center" (*tālu-cakra) and the "ether center" (*ākāsha- or vyoma-cakra), which is part of the *sahasrāra-cakra.

NAVA-DVĀRA ("nine gates"), the nine bodily apertures. The *Mahābhārata (12.203.35) speaks of the *body as the "virtuous city with nine gates." This notion was already current in ancient *Vedic times. In *Yoga, these nine openings are to be shut "like a tortoise withdrawing its limbs," as the *Yoga-Tattva-Upanishad (141) puts it. See also dvāra.

NAVA-KĀRANA ("nine causes"). According to an abstruse philosophical doctrine expounded in the *Yoga-Bhāshya (2.28), there are nine types of cause: (1) utpatti-kārana, "generative cause" (e.g., the *mind as the cause of mental processes); (2) sthiti-kārana, "permanent cause" (e.g., the mind whose permanence alone can fulfill the *Self's innate purposiveness); (3) abhivyakti-kārana, "cause of manifestation" (e.g., the Self's continuous apperception of all mental processes creates, for instance, the experience of color); (4) vikāra-kārana, "modifying cause" (e.g., fire is the cause that modifies the food to be cooked); (5) pratyaya-kārana, "cause of presentation" (e.g., the notion of smoke is the cause of the notion of fire); (6) prāpti-kārana, "cause of attainment" (e.g., the performance of *Yoga is the cause of *liberation); (7) viyoga-kārana, "cause of disunion" (e.g., the performance of Yoga is the cause of the Self's disjunction from the impure psyche); (8) anyatva-kārana, "cause of otherness" (e.g., a goldsmith is the cause of the gold's transformation into

jewelry); and (9) dhriti-kārana, "cause of sustenance" (e.g., the *body is the cause that sustains the senses). See also Causation.

NAVA-MALA ("nine blemishes"), a synonym used in the *Yoga-Bhāshya (1.3) for the obstacles (*antarāya) on the yogic *path. See also mala.

NAVA SHAKTI-SHATKA ("Eight [stanzas] on the Nine Powers"), a short work of two folios ascribed to *Goraksha.

NAVEL. See nābhi.

NAYANMĀRS, a group of sixty-three male and female South Indian *Shaiva saints who lived between the fourth and the ninth century CE. Some came from *brahmin families, others belonged to the merchant class, while yet others were low-caste individuals. However, all social distinctions were melted by their all-consuming love (*bhakti) for *Shiva, which they expressed in poetry and songs. Best known are *Tirumūlar, *Sambandhar, *Appar, *Mānikavācakar, and *Sundarar. Cf. Ālvārs.

NĀYIKĀ ("mistress"), the *Tantric consort, also called *mudrā.

NECESSITY. See niyati.

NESCIENCE. See ajnāna, avidyā.

NETI, one of the "six acts" (*shat-karma) of *hatha-yoga. According to the *Gheranda-Samhitā (1.49), this practice is performed by inserting a fine thread nine inches in length into one *nostril and pulling it out through the mouth. According to the *Hatha-Ratna-Āvalī (1.37), the length of the thread should be six vitastas,

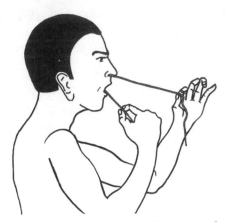

Neti, cleansing of the sinuses by means of a thread (*sūtra*)

i.e., fifty-four inches. This practice is thought to cure disorders of phlegm (*kapha*), improve one's eyesight, and facilitate the practice of *khecarī-mudrā*. Modern *yogins* use a thin rubber thread. A preparatory practice, or an alternative, is *jala-neti*, which consists in sniffing up water (*jala*) through the *nose.

NETI-NETI (composed of *na iti*, "not thus"), a well-known *Upanishadic response to the inquiring student who desires a positive description of the transcendental *Self. Whatever can be said of *Reality is not ultimately true. Descriptions are merely pointers to that which is beyond all mental constructs. See also Language.

NIDIDHYĀSANA (from the desiderative of the root *dhyai*, "to meditate, contemplate"), a *Vedānta term for *dhyāna.

NIDRĀ ("sleep"), widely considered one of the great enemies of *Yoga practice and hence often listed among the defects (*dosha*). Already the *Mahābhārata (12.209.1) states that one should abandon

it. Elsewhere (12.263.46) this work lists sleep among such defects as desire (*kāma*), anger (*krodha*), greed (*lobha*), and fear (*bhaya*).

In *Classical Yoga *sleep is considered to be one of the five "fluctuations" (*vritti*) of *consciousness. *Patanjali, in his *Yoga-Sūtra (1.10), defines it as that mental state which is based on the experience (*pratyaya*) of the nonoccurrence of other mental phenomena. This means it is a kind of rudimentary awareness. That sleep is not simply the absence of conscious activity is, according to the *Yoga-Bhāshya (1.10), demonstrated by the fact that when one wakes up, one remembers "I have slept well." The *Yoga-Sūtra* (1.38) also states that insights derived from sleep can be made a topic of *meditation. A variety of yogic techniques can be used to combat sleep, including *breath control, particularly the *sīt-karī-prānāyāma, and the *khecarī-mudrā. See also Dream, *sushupti, svapna, yoga-nidrā*.

NIDRĀ-JAYA ("conquest of sleep"), listed in the *Siddha-Siddhānta-Paddhati (2.32) as one of the practices of moral discipline (*yama*).

NIGRAHA ("restraint"). See *indriya-nigraha*.

NIHSANGATĀ ("noncontact" or "nonattachment"), mentioned in the *Siddha-Siddhānta-Paddhati (2.33) as one of the practices of self-restraint (*niyama*). Socializing is typically felt to be detrimental to the *yogin*'s inner work. *Attachment tends to be reinforced through contact with others. See also *sanga, sat-sanga*.

NIMESHA ("closing [of the *eyes]"), in Kashmiri *Shaivism, the process of involution by which the *world of multiple *objects participates in, or is reabsorbed into, the *Divine. The term also refers to the ecstatic *awareness of the inherence of all things in the *Divine. Cf. unmesha.

NIMĪLANA-SAMĀDHI ("ecstasy with closed [eyes]"), in Kashmiri *Shaivism, the type of ecstasy (*samādhi) in which *attention is turned inward and which is accompanied by the closing of the *eyes. This practice is referred to in the *Vijnāna-Bhairava (34): "Fixing the mind (*manas) upon the interior of the cranium (*kapāla) while seated with closed eyes (mīlita-locana), one should, through the steadiness of the mind, gradually perceive the supreme vision (*lakshya)." See also pratimīlana-samādhi; cf. unmīlana-samādhi.

NIRĀLAMBANA-ĀSANA (nirālambanāsana, "unsupported posture"), described in the *Hatha-Ratna-Āvalī (3.60) thus: Making the hands like a lotus, rest on the elbows and raise oneself up easily. This seems to be a preparatory practice for the cobra posture (*bhujanga-āsana).

NIRĀNANDA-SAMĀPATTI ("coinciding beyond bliss"), a level of ecstatic realization (*samādhi) mentioned by *Vācaspati Mishra in his *Tattva-Vaishāradī (1.41) as following upon *sa-ānanda-samāpatti. This stage of the ecstatic experience is, however, explicitly denied by *Vijnāna Bhikshu in his *Yoga-Vārttika (1.41). It is possible that Vācaspati Mishra, who does not appear to have been a *yogin, invented this type of ecstasy as a logical complement to *nirvitarka- and *nirvicāra-samāpatti. See also Bliss, samāpatti.

NIRANJANA, mentioned in the *Hatha-Yoga-Pradīpikā (1.7) as an *adept of *hatha-yoga.

NIRASMITĀ-SAMĀPATTI ("coinciding beyond 'I-am-ness' "), a form of conscious

ecstasy (*samprajnāta-samādhi) proposed by *Vācaspati Mishra in his *Tattva-Vaishāradī (1.41) as the stage following upon *sa-asmitā-samāpatti. The weighty authority of *Vijnāna Bhikshu, as expressed in his *Yoga-Vārttika (1.41), however, goes against accepting this type as a legitimate level of ecstasy (*samādhi). See also asmitā, samāpatti.

NIRBĪJA-SAMĀDHI ("seedless ecstasy"), *Patanjali's term for that supreme state of *consciousness resulting from the total restriction (*nirodha) of all conscious processes. This *ecstatic condition is called "seedless" in the *Yoga-Sūtra (1.51) because it transcends the "causes of affliction" (*klesha) in their latent form as "subliminal activators" (*samskāra). According to the *Yoga-Bhāshya (1.18), however, it is to be explained as lacking any objective prop (*ālambana) on which *attention could be fastened. This state is also called "supraconscious ecstasy" (*asamprajnāta-samādhi) but, more accurately, represents the final phase of that elevated ecstatic state, the *dharma-megha-samādhi. See also bīja, samādhi.

NIRGARBHA-PRĀNĀYĀMA ("breath control without seed"; occasionally also referred to as agarbha-prānāyāma), *prānāyāma that is not combined with the recitation of *bīja-mantras. Here garbha is a synonym for *bīja. Cf. *sagarbha-prānāyāma, sahita-prānāyāma.

NIRGUNA ("unqualified") applies to the transcendental *Reality, which eternally abides beyond the qualities (*guna), or primary constituents, of *nature. The manifest *world, by contrast, is said to be "qualified," or saguna.

NIRGUNA-BRAHMAN ("unqualified *Absolute"), the ultimate *Reality, to which no qualities can be attributed (see *neti neti*). Cf. *saguna-brahman*, *shabda-brahman*.

NIRLIPTA ("undefiled," sometimes "non-defilement") the seventh aspect of the sevenfold discipline (*sapta-sādhana*), according to the *Gheranda-Samhitā* (1.9). See also *shauca*.

NIRMĀNA-CITTA ("created consciousness"), a term appearing in the *Yoga-Sūtra* (4.4) and traditionally interpreted in the sense of "artificially created mind." It seems to have a more philosophical meaning, however, standing for the "individualized consciousness" that evolves out of the ontological principle (*tattva*) of "pure I-am-ness" (*asmitā-mātra*). See also *citta*.

NIRMĀNA-KĀYA ("created body"), in Mahāyāna *Buddhism, the earthly *body of the *Buddha. In *Yoga, however, the term refers to a magical ability (*siddhi*), as is clear from the following stanza of the *Mahābhārata* (12.289.26): "O Bull of Bharata, having obtained power (*bala*), the Yoga [follower] should fashion for himself many thousands [of bodies], and he should roam the *earth with all of them." The *Tattva-Vaishāradī* (3.18) mentions the *adept Avatya as an example of a master who, by means of his yogic powers, created an "artificial" body for himself.

NIRMANU. See *nādī-shodhana*.

NIRODHA ("restriction"). In *Classical Yoga, four levels of restriction of *consciousness are recognized: (1) *vritti-nirodha*, "restriction of the fluctuations (*vritti*)," which is achieved by means of meditation (*dhyāna*); (2) *pratyaya-nirodha*, "restriction of the presented ideas

(*pratyaya*)," which is accomplished on the level of conscious ecstasy (*samprajnāta-samādhi*); (3) *samskāra-nirodha*, "restriction of the [subliminal] activators (*samskāra*)," which occurs on the level of supraconscious ecstasy (*asamprajnāta-samādhi*); and (4) *sarva-nirodha*, "complete restriction," which coincides with the realization of the "cloud of *dharma* ecstasy" (*dharma-megha-samādhi*).

The term *nirodha* is also sometimes used as a synonym for *kumbhaka*.

NIRVĀNA ("extinction" or "blowout"), a term generally associated with *Buddhism, where it refers to the cessation of all *desire, a condition synonymous with *enlightenment. However, the term is also employed in some schools of *Yoga. Thus, e.g., already the *Bhagavad-Gītā* (2.72) speaks of the *yogin*'s "extinction in the Absolute" (*brahma-nirvāna*). The *Gītā* (6.19) also has this pertinent stanza: " 'As a lamp standing in a windless [place] flickers not'—that simile is recalled [when] a *yogin* with yoked attention (*citta*) practices the union (*yoga*) of the self [with the transcendental *Self]."

NIRVĀNA-CAKRA ("wheel of extinction"), a synonym for *sahasrāra-cakra*. The specific location of this psychoenergetic center (*cakra*) is at the upper termination point of the central channel (*sushumnā-nādī*), also known as the "brahmic fissure" (*brahma-randhra*).

NIRVĀNA-KALĀ, one of the three aspects of the "serpent power" (*kundalinī-shakti*). According to the *Shat-Cakra-Nirūpana* (47), it is situated within the *amā-kalā* and is like "a thousandth part of the tip of a hair" and as "lustrous as the light of all the suns shining simultaneously." Cf. *nirvāna-shakti*.

NIRVĀNA-SHAKTI, the highest of the three aspects of the "serpent power" (*kundalinī-shakti). It is the divine power stationed in the transcendental seed point (*para-bindu*). In the *Shat-Cakra-Nirūpana* (48) it is said to be "lustrous like ten million suns" and to be the "mother of the three worlds" who "graciously carries the knowledge of truth (*tattva-bodha*) to the mind of the sages." Within it is the "ever-flowing stream of love (*prema*)." Cf. *amā-kalā*, *nirvāna-kalā*.

NIRVICĀRA-SAMĀPATTI ("suprareflexive coincidence"), one of the forms of conscious ecstasy (*samprajnāta-samādhi*) in *Classical Yoga. This *ecstatic state is de void of the cognitive elements, called "reflection" (*vicāra*), that characterize the condition of "reflexive coincidence" (*savicāra-samāpatti*). It thus corresponds to *nirvitarka-samāpatti* on a higher level. See also *samādhi*, *samāpatti*.

NIRVICĀRA-VAISHĀRADYA ("suprareflexive lucidity"), the culmination of *nirvicāra-samāpatti*. According to the *Yoga-Sūtra* (1.47), it is coterminous with the state of perfect clarity of the inner being known as *adhyātma-prasāda*.

NIRVIKALPA-SAMĀDHI ("formless ecstasy"), the *Vedānta equivalent of the supraconscious ecstasy (*asamprajnāta-samādhi*) in *Classical Yoga. As the *Laghu-Yoga-Vāsishtha* (5.10.81) puts it, this state obliterates all the subconscious traits (*vāsanā*), leading to *liberation. According to the *Mandala-Brāhmana-Upanishad* (5.2), the experience of this *ecstatic condition reduces urine, feces, and *sleep. See also *samādhi*; cf. *savikalpa-samādhi*.

NIRVITARKA-SAMĀPATTI ("supracogitative coincidence"), one of the forms of

conscious ecstasy (*samprajnāta-samādhi*) in which all cogitation (*vitarka*) has ceased. It follows upon the *ecstatic state of "cogitative coincidence" (*savitarka-samāpatti*) and is analogous to *nirvicāra-samāpatti*. See also *samādhi*, *samāpatti*.

NISHADANA ("seat"), a rare synonym for *āsana*.

NISHCAYA ("determination"), one of the factors conducive to success in *Yoga, according to the *Hatha-Yoga-Pradīpikā* (1.16).

NISHKALA ("impartite"), a synonym for *akala*.

NISHKARMA-KARMAN. See *naishkarmya-karman*.

NISHPATTI-AVASTHĀ (*nishpattyavasthā*, "state of maturity"), the fourth and final stage (*avasthā*) of the yogic *path. The *Vāraha-Upanishad* (5.75) states that on this level of spiritual accomplishment the *yogin reaps, by means of the "Yoga of spontaneity" (*sahaja-yoga*), the fruit of "liberation while alive" (*jīvan-mukti*). The *Shiva-Samhitā* (3.66) notes that spiritual maturity is reached through gradual practice. The *Hatha-Yoga-Pradīpikā* (4.76f.) has these stanzas:

Having pierced Rudra's knot (*rudra-granthi*) [situated in the *ājnā-cakra*], the *life force reaches the seat of the All [i.e., the *Lord]. Then a flutelike *sound or the sound of a lute is heard.

When the *mind has become unified (*ekī-bhūta*), which is called *rāja-yoga*, the *yogin becomes equal to the Lord (*īshvara*) in that he is able to create and destroy [whole worlds].

NISHVĀSA ("[faulty] breathing"), one of the defects (*dosha*) mentioned in the

Mandala-Brāhmana-Upanishad (2.1). This presumably refers to the shallow, irregular breathing of the ordinary person, which must be corrected through breath control (*prānāyāma*).

NITYANANDA, BHAGAWAN (d. 1961), Kashmiri *Shaiva adept; the teacher of Swami *Muktananda. His date of birth is unknown, though he took up the life of a renouncer (*samnyāsin*) at the early age of twelve. Born in the south of India, he spent his early years wandering in the Himalayas, acquiring the reputation of a great spiritual master, healer, and miracle worker. For several years he lived in trees or, when not wandering about, in caves. For the last twenty-five years of his life Bhavavan Nityananda could be found in his hermitage in the small town of Ganeshpuri, near Bombay. He was an *avadhūta*, often going about naked and using highly unconventional behavior to instruct others in the illusoriness of ordinary life.

NITYANĀTHA (ca. 1300 or 1400 CE), mentioned in the *Hatha-Yoga-Pradīpikā* (1.7) as a master of *hatha-yoga*. He may be identical with the author of a work on *alchemy and *medicine entitled *Rasa-Ratna-Ākāra* and a work on *magic entitled *Kaksha-Pūta-Samhitā*.

NIVRITTI-MĀRGA ("path of cessation"), the spiritual orientation of the *yogin*, who has renounced the *world. Cf. *pravritti-mārga*.

NIVRITTINĀTHA, the elder brother and *guru of *Jnānadeva.

NIYAMA ("restraint"), the second "limb" (*anga*) of the eightfold path (*ashta-anga-yoga*) taught by *Patanjali. According to his *Yoga-Sūtra* (2.32), it has five constituent practices: purity (*shauca*), contentment (*samtosha*), asceticism (*tapas*), study (*svādhyāya*), and devotion to the Lord (*īshvara-pranidhāna*). In the *Tri-Shikhi-Brāhmana-Upanishad* (2.29) *niyama* is defined as one's "continuous attachment to the supreme *Reality." This scripture also mentions that *niyama* encompasses the following ten practices: asceticism (*tapas*), contentment (*samtushti*), affirmation (*āstikya*) of the *Vedic heritage or of the existence of the *Divine, liberality (*dāna*), adoration (*ārādhana*), "listening to [the scriptures of] *Vedānta" (*vedānta-*shravana*), modesty (*hrī*), conviction (*mati*), recitation (*japa*), and vow (*vrāta*).

The *Uddhāva-Gītā* (14.34) furnishes a list of twelve practices: bodily and mental purity (*shauca*), which are counted separately; recitation (*japa*); asceticism (*tapas*); sacrifice (*homa*); faith (*shraddhā*); hospitality (*atithya*); worship (*arcanā*); pilgrimage (*tīrtha-atana*); exertion for the good of others (*para-artha-iha*); contentment (*tushti*); and service to one's teacher (*ācārya-sevana*). The *Linga-Purāna* (1.8.29f.) additionally mentions "control over the penis" (*upastha-nigraha*) and fasting (*upavāsa*), bathing (*snāna*), and silence (*mauna*). The *Siddha-Sid-dhānta-Paddhati* (2.33) adds to the above: living in solitude (*ekānta-vāsa*), noncontact (*nihsangatā*), indifference (*audāsi-nya*), dispassion (*vairāgya*), and "following the teacher's footsteps" (*guru-carana-avarūdhatva*). Cf. yama.

NIYATI ("necessity"), in Kashmiri *Shaivism, one of the five coverings (*kancuka*) around the transcendental *Self, produced by the power of illusion (*māyā*). It limits the freedom and all-pervasiveness of the Self.

NONATTACHMENT. See *asanga, vairāgya*.

NONBEING. See *abhāva-yoga, asat*.

NONDUAL. See *advaya*.

NONDUALITY. See *advaita*.

NON-SELF. See *anātman*; cf. *ātman*.

NONVIOLENCE. See *ahimsā*; cf. *himsā*.

NONWAVERING. See *aloluptva*.

NOSE, NOSTRILS. See *nāsa*.

NRITI ("dance"). Restraint of the *life force in the lowest psychoenergetic center of the *body, the *mūlādhāra-cakra*, sometimes leads to spontaneous dancing. See also Dance.

NYĀSA ("casting" or "placing"), the focusing of *attention to the point where *subject and *object merge; used synonymously with *samyama* in the *Yoga-Sūtra (3.25). In other contexts, especially in *Tantrism, *nyāsa* refers to a variety of rites designed to gradually assimilate the *body into the body of one's chosen deity (*ishta-devatā*) or one's *teacher by touching specific parts of the body and reciting empowering *mantras. These rites are usually preceded by the purification of the elements (*bhūta-shuddhi*).

The first step in the *nyāsa* ritual is *jīva-nyāsa*, the infusion of the life (*jīva*) of the *deity into one's *body. This is followed by *mātrikā-nyāsa*, placing the fifty letters of the Sanskrit *alphabet into one's body. Then the practitioner salutes various deities associated with different parts of the body, which is known as *rishi-nyāsa*. Next comes the "placing of the six limbs" (*shad-anga-nyāsa*), which consists of placing the limbs (*anga-nyāsa*) and placing the hands (*kara-nyāsa*). The former rite is done by touching various places on the *head while reciting specific *mantras. The latter rite consists in assigning *mantras to the various parts of one's hands. Thus *nyāsa* is an esoteric means of distributing psychospiritual power (*shakti*) in the body and thereby creating a new inner and outer reality for oneself.

NYĀYA, one of the six classical systems (*darshana*) of *Hinduism. The Nyāya tradition seeks to ascertain truth by means of correct logical procedures or rules (*nyāya*). The origins of this school of thought are obscure, though there appears to have been a historical connection to the *Yoga tradition. The founder of Nyāya was Gautama, who probably lived during the early common era and is credited with the authorship of the *Nyāya-Sūtra*.

· O ·

OBEDIENCE. See *guru-shushrūshā*.

OBJECT. Whether the *world of objects is viewed to be real, as in *Classical Yoga, or illusory, as in most schools of *Vedānta, all traditions of *Hinduism concur that the universe of forms is inferior to the formless *Reality, because forms inevitably undergo change (*parināma*), whereas the Formless is eternally stable. For the human being, change implies varying degrees of suffering (*duhkha*); hence only the realization of the unchanging *Being promises abiding *happiness. See also Appearance, *artha, drishya, vishaya*; cf. Subject.

OBSERVANCES, MORAL. See Morality, *vidhi, yama*.

OBSTACLES. See *upasarga, vighna*; see also *dosha*.

OCCULTISM. Even the most intellectually sophisticated schools of *Yoga contain elements of *magic or occultism. One may be tempted to view these features as simply being dysfunctional remnants of an earlier, uninformed age. Any attempt to demythologize Yoga is doomed to failure, however, because it would involve the obliteration of vital aspects of this ancient tradition.

The new discipline of *parapsychology has so far been too busy defending itself against the consensus opinion of the scientific establishment to proceed much beyond statistical experiments of no ultimate conclusiveness. No overarching model has yet been formulated that could accommodate and satisfactorily interpret all known facts, whether tested or alleged. Until such a model is available a more appropriate orientation would be to adopt a stance of epistemological humility toward matters that are not immediately intelligible from within the framework of "objective" science. We can, after all, place a certain *faith in the fact that *Yoga looks back on a much longer *history of experimentation than modern science, and in an area that hitherto science has almost completely ignored—namely, the area of our species' higher psychospiritual capacities. See also *siddhi*.

OFFERING, SACRIFICIAL. See *bali, dāna, havis, homa, pushpa*.

OJAS ("force," "strength," or "vitality"; from the root *vaj*, "to be strong"), in *Āyur-Veda, the quintessence of the constituents (*dhātu*) of the *body. Some modern interpreters deem it to be albumen or glycogen, but *yogins* assure us that it is rather a subtle force that is distributed over the entire body and nourishes it incessantly. *Ojas* is the vital principle that is contained or stored in the seven *dhātus*.

The greatest concentration of *ojas* is found in semen (*bindu, *shukra*), which explains why all traditions recommend, if not total abstention, at least stringent sexual economy. The underlying idea is that the conservation of semen increases the *ojas* store and thus enhances not only one's *health but also the quality of one's *consciousness. See also *brahmacarya*.

OM, sacred monosyllable symbolizing the *Absolute; the oldest and most venerated of all *Hindu *mantras*, also employed in *Buddhism. It is only hinted at in the *Vedas and makes its first appearance in the *Brāhmanas*. It is also called the "root-" or *mūla-mantra* and often pre-

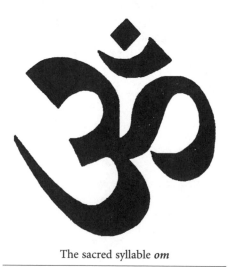

The sacred syllable *om*

cedes other *mantras*. The *Maitrāyanīya-Upanishad* (6.22) refers to it as the *sound of the soundless *Absolute. It is by means of this numinous sound that the *yogin focuses his *attention to the point where he can transcend the finite *consciousness in its entirety. The aforementioned *Upanishad (6.24) likens the *body to a bow, the syllable *om* to an arrow, the focused *mind to the arrow's tip, and the ultimate *Mystery as the target. This scripture also observes, "Just as a spider climbing up by means of its threads finds open space, so indeed the meditator climbs up by means of *om* and finds autonomy (*sva-tantrya*)."

The *Mandukya-Upanishad, which is entirely dedicated to an analysis of the theology and esotericism of the monosyllable *om*, opens with the following passage: "*Om!* This syllable (*akshara*) is this whole *world. Its further explanation is: The past, the present, and the future—everything is but the sound *om*. And whatever else that transcends triple time—that, too, is but the sound *om*." This same scripture explains that *om* is composed of four parts, or "measures" (*mātra*): *a, u, m*, and the aftersound (*anusvāra*), represented by a dot placed above the letter *m* in Sanskrit, which signifies a nasal humming. These four parts are compared to the four states of *consciousness: *waking, *dreaming, *sleeping, and the "fourth" (*turīya*), which is the transcendental *Self beyond the *mind. See also *bindu, catur-tha, hamsa-mantra, nāda, pranava*.

OMENS. See *arishta, cihna*.

OMNISCIENCE. See *sarva-jnātva*.

ONE, THE. See *eka*.

ONE-POINTEDNESS. See *ekāgratā*.

ONTOLOGY, the philosophical discipline concerned with *Being and its categories. *Hindu philosophy, including *Yoga, is largely grounded on the ontological conceptions developed in the influential *Sāmkhya tradition. The ontology of *Classical Yoga, however, is quite original and conceptually and terminologically distinct from that of Classical Sāmkhya, as encoded in the *Sāmkhya-Kārikā. See also *tattva*.

ORDER, MORAL. See *dharma*.

OSHADHI. See *aushadhi*.

OSTENTATION. See *dambha*.

OUT-OF-BODY EXPERIENCE, also called "astral projection" or "astral travel" in Western occult circles; the temporary relocation of *consciousness from the physical *body to the subtle body (*sūkshma-sharīra*). Accomplished *yogins are able to leave the physical body at will and to roam in the subtle dimensions of existence. Some *adepts are even said to be able to disconnect from the physical body completely and to transfer their *consciousness to another body—a feat known as *para-deha-pravesha. See also *ākāsha-gamana, khecaratva*.

OVEREXERTION. See *prayāsa*.

· P ·

PADA has numerous meanings, including "foot," "footstep," "home," "mark," and "word."

PĀDA ("foot" or "quarter"). See Feet.

PADA-ARTHA (*padārtha*, "thing [corresponding to] the word [*pada*]"), the ultimate *Reality; the term can be translated as "essence."

PADA-ARTHA-BHĀVANĀ-BHŪMI ("level of the realization of the essence"), one of the seven levels of wisdom (*sapta-jnāna-bhūmi*); explained in the *Vāraha-Upanishad* (4.2.9) as the apperception (*avabodhana*) of the ultimate *Reality, following the prolonged focusing of the *mind on that Reality.

PADA-CANDRIKĀ ("Moonlight on the Words [of *Patanjali]"). See *Yoga-Sūtra-Artha-Candrikā*.

PĀDA-PĪTHA-ĀSANA (*padapīthāsana* "foot bench posture"), described in the *Hatha-Ratna-Āvalī* (3.71) thus: Stand on one leg, encircle the body with the hands, and vigorously pull the other leg toward the back. This appears to be the same as the *nata-rāja-āsana* ("king of dance posture") mentioned in some contemporary manuals of *hatha-yoga*.

PĀDA-PŪJĀ ("worship of the feet"), a synonym for *pāda-sevana*.

PĀDA-SEVANA ("service at the feet [of *God]"), one of the "limbs" (*anga*) of the *Yoga of devotion (*bhakti-yoga*); part of the ritual *worship of the *Divine installed in the shrine as an image (*mūrti*) or as a symbol, such as the phallus (*linga*).

PADDHATI (from *pad-hati*, "foot tread"), a class of manual. See, e.g., *Goraksha-Paddhati*.

PADMA ("lotus"), a synonym for *cakra*.

PADMA-ĀSANA (*padmāsana*, "lotus posture"; also called *kamala-āsana*), described in the *Gheranda-Samhitā* (2.8) as follows: Placing the right *foot on the left thigh and the left foot on the right thigh, cross the hands behind the back and catch hold of one's big toes. Place the chin on the chest and fix the *gaze on the tip of the nose (*nāsa-agra*). This posture (*āsana*) is said to cure all *diseases. The *Hatha-Yoga-Pradīpikā* (1.45f.) gives an alternative version: Place the feet, soles up, on the op-

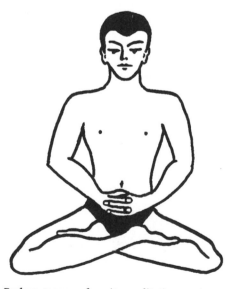

Padma-āsana, a favorite meditation posture

posite thighs and place the hands, palms up, between the thighs. Both versions are commonly recommended for the practice of breath control (*prānāyāma*).

PĀDUKĀ ("sandals"). The *guru*'s sandals are considered to be a sacred object or symbolic substitute for the teacher, and in many schools are treated reverentially in the course of the ceremonial worship of the teacher (*guru-pūjā*).

PĀDUKĀ-PANCAKA ("Five [Verses on] the Footstool"), a work of only seven stanzas describing the *meditation on the five esoteric loci of *kundalinī-yoga*: (1) the twelve-petaled lotus at the *heart; (2) the triangle (*trikona*) in its pericarp; (3) the region of the *nāda* and *bindu*; (4) the "jewel seat" (*mani-pītha*) within it; and (5) the *hamsa* below that seat, together with the triangle above it.

PAIN. See *duhkha*; cf. Pleasure.

PAKVA ("ripe" or "mature"). In *hatha-yoga*, the ordinary *body is thought to be "immature" or "unbaked" (*apakva*). The purpose of the various practices of this *Yoga is to strengthen the body and help it ripen into a "divine body" (*divya-deha*). See also *hatha-pāka*, Transubstantiation.

PALATE, an important esoteric location (*desha*) of the *body. See also *tālu*.

PANCA-ĀKĀSHA (*pancākāsha*, "five ether-spaces"). See *ākāsha*.

PANCA-AKSHARA-MANTRA (*pancākshara-mantra*, "five-syllable *mantra*"), the most sacred *Shaiva *mantra: *om namah shivāya*, "*Om*, obeisance to *Shiva*." See also *akshara*.

PANCA-ANGA-SEVANA (*pancāngasevana*, "serving the five limbs"), a constituent practice of *mantra-yoga*. The five "limbs" (*anga*) of one's chosen deity (*ishta-devatā*) are said to be the daily ritual reading of the *Bhagavad-Gītā* and the *Sahasra-Nāma* ("Thousand Names [of *God]"), singing songs of praise, reciting formulas of protection, and opening one's *heart.

PANCA-AVASTHĀ (*pancāvasthā*, "five states"). See *avasthā*.

PANCA-BHŪTA ("five elements"). See *bhūta*.

PANCA-DASHA-ANGA-YOGA (*pancadashāngayoga*, "fifteenfold Yoga"). The *Tejo-Bindu-Upanishad* (1.15ff.) teaches a yogic *path consisting of the following fifteen "limbs" (*anga*): (1) moral discipline (*yama*); (2) self-restraint (*niyama*); (3) abandonment (*tyāga*); (4) silence (*mauna*); (5) place (*desha*); (6) time (*kāla*); (7) posture (*āsana*); (8) "root lock" (*mūla-bandha*); (9) bodily equilibrium (*deha-samya*); (10) steadiness of vision (*drik-sthiti*); (11) breath restraint (*prāna-samyamana*), which is the same as *prānāyāma*; (12) sense withdrawal (*pratyāhāra*); (13) concentration (*dhāranā*); (14) meditation on the *Self (*ātma-dhyāna*); and (15) ecstasy (*samādhi*). The anonymous author of this *Upanishad* interpets most of these practices symbolically rather than literally. Cf. *ashta-anga-yoga, sapta-sādhana, shad-anga-yoga*.

PANCA-DHĀRANĀ ("five concentrations"), the *Tantric and *hatha-yoga* practice of concentration (*dhāranā*) on the five material elements (*bhūta*). This can be done by focusing either on the symbols of these elements or on their associated deities (*devatā*). Thus, according to the

Tri-Shikhi-Brāhmana-Upanishad (2.133ff.), the *earth element is to be visualized as a yellow square, the *water element as a silvery crescent, the *fire element as a red flame, the *air element as a smoke-colored sacrificial altar, and the *ether element as lustrous deep black *space. Their presiding *deities are Aniruddha, *Nārāyana, Pradyumna, Samkarshana, and Vasudeva respectively. In each case, *concentration must be accompanied by breath retention (*kumbhaka). Concentration on the earth element is supposed to be two hours in duration, with each subsequent concentration lasting two hours more than the preceding one.

The *Yoga-Tattva-Upanishad* (69ff.) explains that one should retain the *breath in the bodily region (*sthāna) governed by each of the five elements. The five elemental regions of the *body are as follows: (1) *prithivī-sthāna* ("earth area"), extending from the soles of the *feet to the knees; (2) *apam-sthāna* ("water area"), from the knees to the hips; (3) *vahni-sthāna* ("fire area"), from the hips to the *navel; (4) *vāyu-sthāna* ("wind area"), from the navel to the *nose; and (5) *ākāsha-sthāna* ("ether area"), from the nose to the top of the *head.

These five types of *concentration, which may have been practiced already at the time of the *Shvetāshvatara-Upanishad* (2.13), are listed in the *Gheranda-Samhitā* (3.68ff.) as "seals" (*mudrā) and are respectively called *pārthivī-, *āmbhasī-, *āgneyī-, *vāyavī-, and *ākāshī-dhāranā-mudrā*. They lead to bodily firmness and, in addition, each concentration is said to yield certain paranormal powers (*siddhi).

PANCA-MA-KARA ("five *m* letters," or "five *m*'s"), also known as *panca-tattva*, stands for the five core practices of the left-hand *Tantric ritual, which all have names starting with the letter *m*. These are *madya* ("wine"), *māmsa* ("flesh"), *matsya* ("fish"), *mudrā* ("parched grain"), and *maithunā* ("intercourse"). The consumption of wine, meat, fish, and parched grain is thought to stimulate the sexual drive, and *maithunā*, as the crowning practice of this *ritual, is the means of employing the accumulated sexual energy for the arousal of the "serpent power" (*kundalinī-shakti).

PĀNCARĀTRA ("Relating to five nights"), a monotheistic *Hindu tradition that worships Vasudeva, or *Vishnu, and is at least as old as *Buddhism. Originally a marginally *Vedic religious culture, the Pāncarātra tradition, whose followers called themselves *Bhāgavatas, gave rise to *Vaishnavism. Apart from its emphasis on monotheistic *worship, it also introduced into *Hinduism the idea of temples and images and challenged the existing caste system by its ideal of equality among people. The name *pāncarātra* is obscure but suggests the kind of syncretism that characterizes this tradition.

There are said to be 108 "compilations" (*samhitā*) of the Pāncarātra tradition, though in effect over 200 titles are known. These works ideally treat of four topics: (1) wisdom (*jnāna); (2) *Yoga; (3) cultic activity (*kriyā*), such as the construction of temples or the creation of images of the *Divine; and (4) ritual conduct (*caryā*).

PANCASHIKHA ("Five-Tufted"; fl. prob. 1st cen. CE), a renowned authority of the *Sāmkhya tradition. References to him are found in a number of works on *Yoga, including the *Yoga-Bhāshya*.

PANCA-TATTVA ("five principles"), a synonym for *panca-ma-kara*.

PANCA-VIDHA-KRITYA ("fivefold activity"), the five principal functions credited to *Shiva in *Shaiva Siddhānta: (1) *srishti* ("creation," lit. "ejection"), the emanation of the *world; (2) *sthiti* ("stability"), the maintenance of the created or emanated universe; (3) *samhāra* ("withdrawal"), the reabsorption of the emanated world; (4) *vilaya* ("resorption"), the latency of the world in Shiva's infinite being; and (5) *anugraha* ("grace," lit. "dispensation"), Shiva's blessing power by which all beings are liberated. In the *Shaiva-Paribhāshā* (2.9), an important manual of Shaiva Siddhānta, *Shivāgrayogin explains: "His agency (*kartatva*) with regard to the fivefold activity is by mere proximity, like the sun's proximate activity of causing a lotus or lily to bloom or close [its petals], liquifying butter, or drying a bog." In other words, the Lord himself is perfectly immutable in the midst of these creative functions. See also Shaivism, *shakti*.

PANCA-VYOMAN ("five ether-spaces"). See *ākāsha*.

PANDITA ("pundit" or "scholar"). The *Bhagavad-Gītā* (4.19) describes the true pundit as one whose *actions are devoid of desire (*kāma*) and egoic motive (*samkalpa*), i.e., who is a genuine practitioner of *karma-yoga. See also *grantha, shāstra*.

PĀNI-PĀTRA-ĀSANA (*pānipātrāsana*, "hand vessel posture"), described in the *Hatha-Ratna-Āvalī* (3.49) thus: Place the ankles at the *navel and then form the hands into a vessel (cradling the *feet). This exercise should be done gradually but with *effort. This appears to be the same as the *kandaāsana* mentioned in some contemporary manuals of *hatha-yoga.

PĀPA or PĀPMAN ("sin" or "evil"). The related concepts of sin and evil played an important role already in the moral life of the ancient *Vedic people. The *Rig-Veda* contains many *prayers for the forgiveness of sin. The Vedic seers (*rishi*) accepted sin as part of the human condition. Sin is the inevitable by-product of the experience of separation between I and you. Only the *breath, which is frequently equated in the *Rig-Veda* with the *Self (*ātman*), is not overcome by evil. Hence attunement to the Self is the only means of combating sin and evil.

This *Vedic understanding of sin also informs later *Hindu thought. Thus the *Bhagavad-Gītā* (3.36f.) has the following exchange between *Krishna and his disciple *Arjuna:

Now, by what is this man impelled to commit evil, even unwittingly, O Varshneya [i.e., *Krishna]? As though constrained by force?

It is desire (*kāma*), it is *anger born of the dynamic quality (*rajo-*guna*), alldevouring and greatly evil—know this as the enemy here [on earth].

*Desire, then, is at the root of all evil. But desire is itself rooted in the ego sense (*ahamkāra*), the *illusion that one is divorced from the rest of existence. Only *wisdom, or gnosis (*jnāna*), can move a person beyond sin, for through wisdom is one made whole. As *Krishna explains in the *Bhagavad-Gītā* (4.36ff.):

Even if you were the most evil of all evildoers, you will cross all crooked [streams of life] with the raft of wisdom.

As a kindled fire reduces its fuel to *ashes, O Arjuna, so does the fire of wisdom reduce all actions to ashes.

For nothing here [on earth] purifies like wisdom; and this [person] perfected in *Yoga will find of himself in time within himself.

Already in the ancient ethical literature (*dharma-shāstra*) sin is said to be atoned by means of strenuous *breath control, as a high form of austerity (*tapas). This idea is repeated in many later *Yoga texts. Controlled breathing is a form of self-sacrifice, the application of *wisdom. See also a-dharma, dosha, kilbisha, pātaka, prāyash-citta; cf. dharma, punya.

PARA-ARTHATVA (parārthatva, "other-purposiveness"). In the *Yoga-Sūtra (3.35) this term is used to express the notion that *nature exists solely for the purposes of the *Self, which, by contrast, has no purpose beyond itself. The two primary purposes of nature are to serve either the worldly enjoyment (*bhoga) or the liberation (*moksha) of the Self.

PARA-ARTHA-IHA (parārtheha, "exertion for the weal of others"), listed in the *Ud-dhāva-Gītā (14.34) among the practices of self-restraint (*niyama). See also loka-sam-graha.

PARA-BRAHMAN ("supreme Absolute"), the unqualified ultimate *Reality, about which nothing can be said. See also Absolute, brahman; cf. shabda-brahman.

PARA-CITTA-JNĀNA ("knowledge of another mind"), one of the paranormal powers (*siddhi). According to the *Yoga-Sūtra (3.19), it is acquired by direct perception (*sākshātkārana) of the contents of another person's *consciousness. See also Mind.

PARA-DEHA-PRAVESHA ("entering another body"; also called para-kāya-pravesha or -āvesha), an important yogic power (*siddhi) claimed for many *adepts. It results from intense *contemplation on the *ājñā-, the *anāhata-, or the *mūlā-dhāra-cakra. The *Laghu-Yoga-Vāsishtha (6.9.117) mentions that this can be accom-

plished by means of exhalation (*recaka), when the steadied life force (*prāna) is kept at a distance of twelve digits from the face. This, however, presupposes an awakened "serpent power" (*kundalinī-shakti). A well-known story, told in the Shankara-Dig-Vijaya, relates how *Shankara entered the corpse of a king in order to experience the *pleasures of his harem so that he, Shankara, a renouncer with no knowledge of *sexuality, might win an intellectual tournament.

According to the *Kaula-Jnāna-Nirnaya (20.8), this ability extends to animal bodies. Thus in the *Mahābhārata (12.260.5–262.45) there is the story of Syūmarashmi, who entered the *body of a cow in order to converse with the sage *Kapila. This paranormal ability has sometimes been equated with the phenomenon of *astral projection, though a more complex process is involved.

PARĀNTA-JNĀNA ("knowledge of the end [of one's life]," from para, "ultimate," and anta, "end") is, according to the *Yoga-Sūtra (3.22), acquired from omens (*arishta) or by practicing ecstatic "constraint" (*samyama) in regard to one's *karma. See also anta-kāla, Death.

PARAMA-ANU (paramānu, "superatom"). In the *Yoga-Sūtra (1.40) this phrase simply means the "most minute." *Vyāsa, in his *Yoga-Bhāshya (1.43), however, borrows the *Vaisheshika idea that everything consists of atoms (*anu). He thus regards *objects as "conglomerations of atoms" (anu-pracaya). In his comments on this passage, *Vācaspati Mishra introduces the concept of parama-anu or "superatoms," which he seems to use interchangeably with anu. See also bhūta.

PARAMA-ĀTMAN (paramātman, "supreme Self"), the transcendental *Self, as opposed to the psyche (*jīva) or "living self" (*jīva-ātman).

PARAMA-GURU ("supreme teacher"), one's teacher's teacher or, in theological contexts, the *Divine itself, which is the source of all spiritual *knowledge and teachings. See also *īshvara.*

PARAMA-HAMSA ("supreme swan"), honorific applied to an *adept who enjoys *liberation, or *enlightenment. See also *avadhūta, buddha, hamsa.*

PARAMA-ĪSHVARĪ (*parameshvarī,* "supreme goddess"), a synonym for *kundalinī.*

PARAMPARĀ ("[from] one [to] another"), the chain of oral transmission and *empowerment from teacher (*guru) to disciple (*shishya). It is traditionally considered auspicious and important to be a member of such a teaching lineage, though there have always been *adepts who became *enlightened without the benefit of a human teacher.

PARANORMAL POWERS. See Parapsychology, *siddhi, vibhūti.*

PARANORMAL PERCEPTION. See *divya-cakshus, divya-darshana, divya-shrotra, pratibhā.*

PARAPSYCHOLOGY. Claims of paranormal abilities and occurrences are a "universal constant" of the world's psychospiritual traditions. The literature of *Yoga is replete with references to numerous major and minor powers (*siddhi) that the *yogin is thought to acquire in the course of his spiritual discipline. Almost an entire chapter of the *Yoga-Sūtra is dedicated to para-

normal abilities and the techniques by which they can be acquired. The method recommended by *Patanjali is known as "constraint" (*samyama), which is the combined practice of *concentration, *meditation, and *ecstasy with regard to the same *object of contemplation. This method is said to yield a special kind of *knowledge, and it is recognized as a form of valid cognition (*pramāna) by most other schools of *Hindu philosophy. It is also known as *yogi-pratyaksha, "yogin's perception."

There is probably no psychic phenomenon known today that is not mentioned somewhere in the vast spiritual literature of India, but the most spectacular claims revolve around the doctrine of the eight major paranormal powers or *mahā-siddhis,* also known as "lordly powers" (*aishvarya): *animan, *mahiman, *lāghiman, *prāpti, *prākāmya, *vashitva, *īshītritva,* and *kāma-avasāyitva. These are said to be by-products of an *adept's highest spiritual realization. Most *Hindu authorities understand these major paranormal powers literally, but some interpret them symbolically, and a few regard them as pertaining only to the "subtle body" (*sūkshma-sharīra). While we must remain alert to the ever-present readiness of the human *mind to delude itself and engage in fantasies, modern parapsychology has amassed enough evidence for the existence of paranormal phenomena. Therefore, today some of the claims of *Yoga and other similar spiritual traditions seem no longer implausible. See also Psychology.

PARA-SHARĪRA-ĀVESHA (*parasharīrāvesha,* "entering another body"), a synonym for *para-deha-pravesha.*

PARA-SHIVA ("Transcendental Shiva"), or **PARAMA-SHIVA** ("Highest Shiva"), one of the many designations of *Shiva as the ultimate *Reality.

PARA-VAIRĀGYA ("superior renunciation"), in *Classical Yoga, the higher form of dispassion (*vairāgya), defined in the *Yoga-Sūtra (1.16) as the *yogin's "non-thirsting for the primary constituents" (*guna-vaitrishnya) of *nature. It is a final no to the *world in its entirety. Unlike ordinary dispassion, this superior form is realizable only after experiencing the ecstatic condition (*samādhi). It results from the "vision of the Self" (*purusha-khyāti). In the *Mani-Prabhā (1.51) it is paraphrased as "eagerness for the so-called *dharma-mega[-samādhi]."

PARICĀYA-AVASTHĀ (paricāyāvasthā, "accumulation state"), the third of four stages of yogic development. The *Hatha-Yoga-Pradīpikā (4.74f.) describes it as follows: One hears a *sound like that of a drum in the "ether-space" of the *ājnā-cakra. Then the life force (*prāna) reaches the "great void" (mahā-shūnya), which is the seat of all powers (*siddhi). When one has transcended "mind(-generated) bliss" (citta-ānanda), there arises "spontaneous bliss" (sahaja-ānanda), whereupon one becomes free from *pain, aging, *disease, *hunger, and somnolence (*nidrā). According to the *Shiva-Samhitā (3.60), this stage is characterized by the life force entering into the central channel (*sushumnā-nādī) and is accompanied by the awakening of the "serpent power" (*kundalinī-shakti).

PARIDHĀNA ("putting around"), a secret process referred to in the *Hatha-Yoga-Pradīpikā (3.112) by which the "serpent power" (*kundalinī-shakti) can be awakened. This practice may be the same as *nauli.

PARINĀMA ("transformation"), a key term in the philosophy of *Patanjali, de-

notes serial change. According to the *Yoga-Sūtra (3.13), transformation is of three basic types: (1) dharma-parināma, change in the form of a substance; (2) laksh-ana-parināma, change implicit in the fact that time (*kāla) consists of past, present, and future; and (3) avasthā-parināma, qualitative change due to the effects of *time (i.e., aging), as when an earthen vessel breaks and turns to dust. Patanjali seeks to apply these insights to *consciousness and its transmutation through the techniques of *Yoga. Patanjali's philosophy of change disallows permanency to the phenomena of *nature. Only the transcendental Self (*purusha) is considered to enjoy immutability (aparināmitva). See also Evolution.

PART, DIVINE. See amsha.

PART, SIXTEENTH. See kalā.

PĀRTHAVĪ-DHĀRANĀ-MUDRĀ ("earthy concentration seal"; also called adho-dhā-ranā), one of the five *concentration techniques described in the *Gheranda-Samhitā (3). It consists in focusing *mind and *life force on the *earth element held at the *heart for a period of 150 minutes. This is said to cause steadiness (stambha) and give the *yogin control over the earth itself. See also dhāranā, mudrā, panca-dhā-ranā.

PARTICULARIZED. See vishesha; cf. avi-shesha.

PARVAN ("joint"). In his *ontology, *Patanjali distinguishes four levels (parvan) of manifestation or layers of *nature: *vi-shesha ("particularized"), *avishesha ("un-particularized"), *linga-mātra ("differenti-ated"), and *alinga ("undifferentiated"). These levels are distinct but interrelated functional spheres of the three primary qualities (*guna) composing all phenomena. The *Self is the *witness consciousness beyond these levels.

PARYANKA ("couch"), a posture (*āsana) mentioned, e.g., in the *Yoga-Bhāshya (2.46). According to *Vācaspati Mishra's commentary on this passage, it is executed by holding the knees with one's arms while reclining. Modern manuals describe this posture differently: Starting in the hero posture (*vīra-āsana), arch backward until the *head rests on the ground. The arms are to cradle the head.

PĀSHA ("noose" or "fetter"), an important concept of *Shaivism, which distinguishes the divine Lord (*pati) from the creatures (*pashu)—hence *Pashupati. The word refers to the fact that all creatures are bound by *karma, which has its root in spiritual ignorance (*avidyā). Also, *Shiva is iconographically depicted as holding a noose by which he fetters those who transgress the moral order (*dharma).

PASHCIMA-TĀNA-ĀSANA (pashcimatānāsana, "back extension posture"), described in the *Tri-Shikhi-Brāhmana-Upanishad (2.51) as follows: Seated with the legs stretched out in front, bend forward until one can grasp the big toes with one's hands and the *head comes to rest on one's knees. As the anonymous author of the *Yoga-Cūdāmanī-Upanishad (49) observes, this is really a "lock" (*bandha) because of the constriction in the abdominal area achieved by this posture. The *Shiva-Samhitā (3.92) states that this is also called *ugra-āsana. See also āsana.

PASHCIMA-UTTĀNA-ĀSANA (pashcimottānāsana, "back stretching posture"), a common synonym for *pashcima-tāna-āsana.

PĀSHINĪ-MUDRĀ ("bird-catcher seal"; also known as *phanīndra), described in the *Gheranda-Samhitā (3.65) thus: Place one's legs around the back of the neck, holding them firmly like a noose (*pāsha). This not only gives strength (*bala) and vigor (pushti) but also awakens the "serpent power" (*kundalinī-shakti).

PASHU ("beast" or "creature"), a *Shaiva synonym for *jīva, the individuated self, or psyche. The *Shiva-Purāna (7.1.5.61) describes all beings—from the Creator God *Brahma down to the least creature—as animals bound by a noose (*pāsha), whose fodder is *pain and *pleasure. In reality, however, the pashus are identical with *Shiva, or *Pashupati, representing the transcendental *Self. Only profound ignorance (*avidyā) blinds them to their inherent *freedom and *bliss.

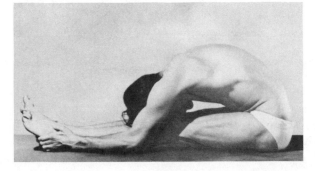

Pashcima-uttāna-āsana, demonstrated by Theos Bernard

PĀSHUPATA SECT, the earliest and most influential sect or school of *Shaivism, whose members worship *Shiva as *Pashupati. Its founder is *Lakulīsha and its teachings are codified in the *Pāshupata-Sūtra. Another important work of this tradition, which was most prominent in Gujarat, is Haradatta's ninth-century Gana-Kārikā, consisting of merely eight verses. This text is often wrongly attributed to Bhāsarvajna, who wrote the commentary Ratna-Tīkā on it. See also Kālāmukha, Kāpālika sect.

PĀSHUPATA-BRĀHMANA-UPANISHAD (Pāshupatabrāhmanopanishad), one of the *Yoga-Upanishads, consisting of seventy-eight verses distributed over two sections. It presents a symbolic sacrificial philosophy exalting the inner *sacrifice. It recommends a form of *nāda-yoga in which the *mind is to be applied to the *hamsa. The specific approach put forward in this scripture (2.6) is called hamsa-arka-pranava-dhyāna or "meditation on the humming sound [i.e., *om] of the radiant swan." It enjoins (2.21) silence (*mauna) on the grounds that *light (*prakāsha) alone exists. This text further states (2.31) that the person who knows the *Self is neither *liberated nor unliberated, since such ideas pertain only to those who are still bound. For the same reason prohibitions about food (*anna) are said not to apply to the Self-realized *adept, who is both food and the eater of food (in the spirit of the ancient *Taittirīya-Upanishad).

PĀSHUPATA-SŪTRA ("Aphorisms on the Pāshupata [Teachings]"), the main scripture of the *Pāshupata school of thought; attributed to Lakulīsha and discovered only in 1930. It deals with *Yoga in its fifth chapter and has an extensive treatment of the moral disciplines (*yama) and the practices of self-restraint (*niyama). It recommends detachment from all past, present, and future things and attachment to the *Divine. Its yogic *path, which is highly ritualistic, must be distinguished from the *pāshupata-yoga described in the *Purānas, which is more akin to the *Classical Yoga of *Patanjali. The Pāshupata-Sūtra has a valuable commentary by Kaundinya entitled Panca-Artha-Bhāshya ("Discussion on the Five Topics [of Pāshupata Philosophy]").

PĀSHUPATA-YOGA, the collective name given to a variety of post-Patanjali *Shaiva teachings. The yogic doctrines are expounded in such scriptures as the *Shiva-, *Linga-, and *Kūrma-Purāna. Their avowed goal is union with *Shiva.

PASHUPATI ("Lord of Beasts"), one of the names of *Shiva, who, in *Shaivism, is deemed the master of all creatures (*pashu). During the excavations at Mohenjo Daro, one of the big cities of the *Indus-Sarasvati civilization, a terra-cotta

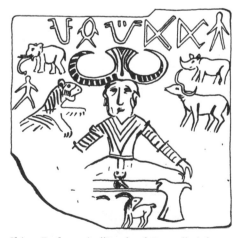

Shiva Pashupati, "Lord of Beasts" (after a terra-cotta seal from the Indus-Sarasvati civilization)

seal was discovered that depicts a figure seated cross-legged upon a platform, endowed with what appears to be an erect phallus (*linga*), wearing a two-horned headdress adorned with jewelry, and surrounded by various animals. This figure has frequently been thought to be the earliest representation of Pashupati, though this interpretation has not remained unchallenged. See also Divine, God, *pancakritya*.

PASSION. See *kāma, rāga, rajas, rati.*

PĀTĀLA ("nether region"), one of the seven nether regions above the seven hells (*nāraka*), according to the *Yoga Bhāshya* (3.26). The others are *mahā-tāla, rasa-tāla, atāla, sutāla, vitāla,* and *tāla-atāla,* the word *tāla* meaning "plane." See also Cosmos.

PĀTAKA ("sin"), the kind of sin (*pāpa*) that is so serious that it deprives one of one's caste membership, which means one's livelihood. According to the *Yoga-Cūdāmanī-Upanishad* (108), the practice of *breath control can expiate even a cardinal sin.

PĀTANJALA-DARSHANA ("Patanjali's view"), the native *Hindu term for what modern scholars call *Classical Yoga.

PĀTANJALA-RAHASYA ("Patanjali's Secret"), a short subcommentary on the *Tattva-Vaishāradī* that offers many concise definitions and quotations from other works. Its author is Rāghavānanda Sarasvatī (19th cen. CE).

PĀTANJALA-SŪTRA. See *Yoga-Sūtra.*

PĀTANJALA-YOGA-SŪTRA differs from the well-known work of *Patanjali. This

text, which comprises 501 aphorisms, was dictated by the blind pundit Dhanraj of Benares to Bhagavan Das in 1910.

PATANJALI. Several men named Patanjali have been prominent in the history of *Hindu thought. The famous grammarian by that name, who wrote a learned commentary on Pānini's *Ashta-Adhyāyī* ("Eight Lessons [in Grammar]"), lived some time in the second century BCE. He is different from the Patanjali who wrote the *Nidāna-Sūtra* ("Aphorisms on Origin"), an important work for the study of the *Vedic ritual literature. A third Patanjali was a well-known teacher of *Sāmkhya. All of these are very probably different from their namesake who composed

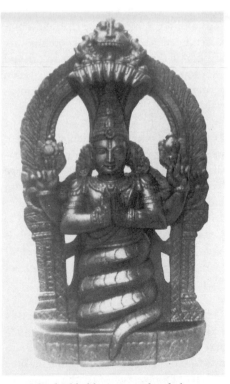

Patanjali, shielded by a many-headed serpent, guardian of esoteric lore

217

the *Yoga-Sūtra, although native Indian tradition maintains that the grammarian and the *Yoga writer are identical. From internal evidence of the *Yoga-Sūtra and general historical considerations, Patanjali the Yoga authority may have lived in the second century CE.

Virtually nothing is known about him. According to *Hindu tradition, he was an incarnation of *Ananta, or Shesha, the thousand-headed ruler of the serpent race. Ananta, desiring to teach *Yoga on earth, is said to have fallen (*pat*) from *heaven onto the palm (*anjali*) of a virtuous woman named Gonikā. He was clearly an *adept of Yoga with a penchant for philosophy. Often wrongly regarded as the "father of Yoga," Patanjali's great contribution was to have compiled and systematized existing knowledge and given Yoga a philosophical shape that allowed it to compete with other contemporary schools of thought. According to an oral tradition of South India, Patanjali was a master of *Shaivism. See also Hiranyagarbha.

PATANJALI-CARITA ("Patanjali's Life"), an eighteenth-century narrative by Rāmabhadra Dīkshita that speaks of the sage *Patanjali as the author of the *Yoga-Sūtra and a medical treatise of uncertain title.

PATANJALI-SŪTRA of *Umāpati Shivācārya, a work describing procedures of *worship and festivities at the temple of Cidambaram in South India.

PATH. Spiritual life is almost universally represented as a path that leads from a state of spiritual ignorance (*avidyā*) to *wisdom or *enlightenment. Only in some radical schools, such as the *Sahajiyā movement, is this metaphor rejected. See also *mārga*, *sādhana*.

PATI ("lord") refers to *Shiva, who is considered the master of all creatures (*pashu*) bound by the noose (*pāsha*) of ignorance (*avidyā*). See also Pashupati.

PATIENCE. See kshamā, kshānti, titikshā.

PAURUSHA ("manliness" or "valor"), an important notion in the *Yoga-Vāsishtha (2.4.10ff.), where manly *effort is placed above *fate. Without effort, suffering (*duhkha*) cannot be overcome. As this work (2.7.31) affirms, one must not depend on *destiny. Cf. Grace.

PAVANA ("wind"), a synonym for *prāna and *vāyu.

PAVANA-VIJAYA ("Conquest of the Wind"), a modern work on *breath control, consisting of 349 stanzas distributed over nine chapters.

PĀYASVINĪ-NĀDĪ ("watery current"), a channel of the life force (*prāna*) situated between the *pūshā- and the *sarasvatī-nādī and extending to the right *ear.

PEACOCK POSTURE. See mayūra-āsana.

PENANCE. See prayashcitta.

PERCEPTION. See drishti, grahana, pratyaksha, sākshātkāra.

PERFECTION. See siddhi.

PERFECTION OF THE BODY. See kāya-sampat, kāya-siddhi.

PERINEUM. See yoni.

PERIYA ĀLVĀR (also known in Sanskrit as Vishnucitta), one of the great South Indian *adepts who worshiped *Vishnu. He was born into a brahmin family around 800 CE in the village of Puduvaiyaru and achieved local fame for his devotional poetry. He composed the ten opening verses—known as *Pallāntu*—of the Tamil canon and also authored the fifty poems of the *Tirumoli* celebrating *Krishna's infancy and childhood. According to Tamil tradition, he remained single all his life but in his later years found and adopted an abandoned baby girl who was to become the famous *Āndāl.

PERIYA-PURĀNAM, the twelfth book of the *Tirumurai, composed in the Tamil language. It tells the stories of the sixty-three *Nāyanmārs, and was authored by Sekkilar in the twelfth century CE.

PERPLEXITY. See *bhrama*.

PERSPIRATION. See *prasveda, sveda*.

PHALA ("fruit"), the moral reward, or *karmic payoff, of one's *actions. According to the *Bhagavad-Gītā* (18.12), this fruition is threefold: (1) *anishta* ("undesirable"), or, as *Shankara explains in his *Gītā* commentary, leading to a future existence in *hell; (2) *ishta* ("desirable"), or leading to a future existence in some heavenly realm; and (3) *mishra* ("mixed"), or presumably leading to a future human existence. The practice of *karma-yoga*, as taught in the *Bhagavad-Gītā*, consists principally in the inward *renunciation of the fruit of one's deeds. As this scripture (2.47) puts it: "In *action alone is your rightful interest (*adhikāra*), never in its fruit. Let not your motive be the fruit of action, nor let your *attachment be to inaction (*akarman*)." A related concept is *vipāka* ("fruition").

PHALLUS. See *linga*.

PHANĪNDRA (from *phani*, "serpent," and *indra*, "lord"), a synonym for *pāshinī-mudrā*, according to the description found in the *Hatha-Ratna-Āvalī* (3.64).

PHLEGM. See *kapha*.

PILGRIMAGE. See *tīrtha-gamana, yātrā*.

PINDA ("lump"), a term used in many *hatha-yoga* texts to denote the human *body. The *Siddha-Siddhānta-Paddhati* (1) speaks of six *pindas*, of which the physical body, called "embryonic body" (*garbha-pinda*) is the coarsest manifestation. See also *deha, kosha, sharīra*.

PINDA-ANDA (*pindānda*, "lump egg"), the human *body as an exact replica of the *macrocosm. Thus, according to the *Siddha-Siddhānta-Paddhati* (3.2ff.), the entire *cosmos is faithfully reflected in the body. For instance, the mythological tortoise that upholds the universe resides at the sole of the feet, the different nether regions (*pātāla*) are at the toes, the knees, and the thighs. The realms of the earth world (*bhū-loka*) are to be found in various parts of the trunk, while the heavenly realms are located in the *head. See also Microcosm.

PINGALĀ-NĀDĪ ("tawny current"), one of three primary channels of the life force (*prāna*), situated to the right of the central conduit (*sushumnā-nādī*) and terminating in the right *nostril, according to most scriptures, though the *Shiva-Samhitā* (2.26) has it end in the left nostril. It is associated with the sun (*sūrya*) and is responsible for heating the *body. It corresponds on the physical level to the sympathetic nervous system. According to the *Hatha-Ratna-Āvalī* (2.143), it is also called *dumbhinī, sūryā, yaminā, aksharā, kāla-agni, rudrī*, and *candī*. Cf. *idā-nādī*.

PĪTHA ("seat"), sometimes used synonymously for *āsana. The term can also refer to a sacred site (*tīrtha), such as a temple, or a special locus of spiritual energy (*shakti) within the *body, corresponding to a *cakra. The *Laghu-Yoga-Vāsishtha (6.2.100f.), e.g., speaks of the thirty-six tīrthas in the body in which *God should be worshiped.

Moreover, in one of its several classification systems, *Shaiva *Tantrism employs the term pītha to denote a certain type of scripture (*Āgama), analogous to the categories of *āmnāya and *srota. There are four such pīthas: vidyā-, mantra-, mudrā-, and mandala-pītha. While the scriptures of a particular class deal chiefly with the subject matter indicated by the name of their category (such as *mantras or *mandalas), each scripture covers all the important *Tantric principles.

PITRI-YĀNA ("way of the ancestors"). The pitris are one's distant ancestors, whereas the word *preta refers to a recently departed ancestor. Because, according to *Hindu eschatology, *death does not imply the final annihilation of a being, the ancestors are thought to inhabit the nether regions (*pātāla) or, if they were evildoers, the realms of hell (*nāraka). The pious *Hindu remembers his ancestors in daily rites and feeds them through sacrificial offerings. Ever since the time of the earliest *Upanishads, however, the "way of the ancestors" has been described as a way of "return" (āvritti), that is, *rebirth. In the *Bhagavad-Gītā (8.25) it is known as the "dark course" (krishna-gati). The ancestral *destiny is contrasted with the "way of the gods" (*deva-yāna). See also ātivāhika-deha, Liberation.

PITTA ("gall"), one of the three humors (*dhātu) recognized in *Āyur-Veda and

*Yoga. It is associated with the following qualities: fat, hot, pungent, and liquid. Some works recommend *bhastrikā-prānāyāma for the removal of excess gall. See also kapha, vāta.

PĪYŪSHA ("milk" or "cream"), a synonym for *amrita.

PLACE. See desha, pītha, sthāna, tīrtha.

PLANET. See graha.

PLĀVINĪ ("floater"), one of the eight types of breath retention (*kumbhaka) taught in *hatha-yoga. The *Hatha-Yoga-Pradīpikā (2.70) describes it as follows: By generously inhaling and filling the abdomen (i.e., the lower half of the lungs) with *air, one can float on water as easily as a lotus. See also prānāyāma.

PLAY. From the vantage point of *enlightenment, or *liberation, conditional existence appears inconsequential (alpa), and the individual's struggle for continuity seems even absurd. Everything in *nature's orbit is bound to change and ultimately disintegrate. The *ego's desperate bid for survival is doomed to be frustrated, and no lasting *happiness can be found even in the highest dimensions of the multilevel *cosmos. Yet this fait accompli does not disturb the enlightened *adept, who has realized the permanent *Reality, the *Self, beyond the phenomenal world of constant *change. On the contrary, because of his realization of the innate bliss (*ānanda), he is able to reengage life with all its absurdities; knowing that the *body and the *mind are destined to die, together with all their *dreams and *hopes, he places no great store in them, but meets all experiences as a play (*līlā) of the *Divine. Play is an appropriate metaphor for the world process, since it is utterly spontaneous, inconsequential, and beyond anyone's control. This notion is particularly at home in the schools of nondualism, or *Advaita Vedānta: The world and its countless events are the sport of the singular Reality. See also Dance.

PLEASURE. Ordinary life revolves around the maximization of pleasure (*sukha) and the minimization of pain (*duhkha). While it is clearly desirable to avoid *pain, the *Yoga authorities also enjoin that one should overcome pleasure. Like pain, pleasure has a binding effect on the *mind. It calls for its repetition and in due course leads to addiction. The Yoga masters propose an ideal that is quite different from the "pleasure principle." They claim that we find ultimate fulfillment only in the personal realization of the transcendental *Reality, which is inherently blissful (*ānanda).

PLOW POSTURE. See hala-āsana.

POSTCLASSICAL YOGA encompasses many different schools and yogic traditions that flourished after the time of *Patanjali, including the teachings of *Tantrism, *hatha-yoga, the *Yoga-Upanishads, and the *Yoga-Vāsishtha. In contrast to the dualistic metaphysics espoused by Patanjali, these later teachings are based on the kind of nondualist (*advaita) philosophy that also characterizes *Preclassical Yoga.

POSTURE. See āsana, bandha, mudrā, nishadana, pītha.

POWERS. See bala, Parapsychology, siddhi, vibhūti.

PRABHUDEVA. See Allāma Prabhudeva.

PRACTICE. See abhyāsa, sādhana.

PRACTITIONER. See abhyāsin, sādhaka, yogin, yoginī.

PRADAKSHINA, the clockwise circumambulation of an icon (*mūrti), shrine, or venerated person such as a *guru.

PRADHĀNA ("foundation"), the transcendental matrix of *nature as apart from the multiple monads of *Consciousness, or Selves (*purusha). In the *Tattva-Vaishāradī (2.23), the term, common to *Yoga and *Sāmkhya, is explained as "that by which the host of evolutes (*vikāra) is brought forth (pradhīyate)." See also prakriti.

PRADHĀNA-JAYA ("mastery over the foundation [of *nature]"), mentioned in the *Yoga-Sūtra (3.48) as one of the fruits of practicing ecstatic "constraint" (*samyama) upon the perceptual process (*grahana). This paranormal power (*siddhi) makes the *yogin a master of the entire *cosmos. It is also called *aishvarya. *Vācaspati Mishra, in his *Tattva-Vaishāradī (3.18), observes that an *adept with this power is able to create thousands of bodies for himself and to freely roam through *heaven and *earth.

PRADĪPIKĀ. See Hatha-Yoga-Pradīpikā, Yoga-Anushāsana-Sūtra-Vritti, Yoga-Pradīpikā.

PRAHLĀDA, an *adept of the early *Vaishnava tradition, mentioned already in the *Bhagavad-Gītā (10.30). Legend has it that his father, Hiranyakashipu, ordered Prahlāda to be killed because he was enraged by his son's devotion (*bhakti) to *Krishna. In later times Prahlāda came to be associated with the myth of *Vishnu's incarnation as Nara-Simha ("Man-Lion"). He is a prominent figure in the *Bhāga-

vata-Purāna and a universal model of *de-votion.

PRAJALPA ("talkativeness"), according to the *Hatha-Yoga-Pradīpikā* (1.15), one of the factors by which *Yoga is foiled. Cf. *mauna*.

PRAJĀPATI ("Lord of Creatures"), the creator of the *worlds. In later *Hinduism, this name is also used as a title for various high beings endowed with the powers commonly attributed to the divine creator. See also Brahma.

PRAJNĀ ("wisdom" or "knowledge"), a synonym for *jnāna*; insight leading to *liberation or even the essence of *libera-tion itself. The *Mahābhārata extolls *wis-dom as the highest *virtue: "Wisdom is the foundation of beings. Wisdom is deemed the highest acquisition. Wisdom is the greatest good in the *world. Wisdom is deemed *heaven by the virtuous (12.173.2)." According to the *Yoga-Sūtra (1.49), *prajnā* is gnosis obtained in the ec-static condition (*samādhi*) and is quite distinct from *knowledge gained by *in-ference or from *tradition. It is based on direct perception (*sākshātkāra*). On the highest level, this superknowledge is desig-nated as being "truth-bearing" (*ritam-bhara*).

PRAJNĀ-ĀLOKA (*prajnāloka*, "luster of wisdom") results, according to the *Yoga-Sūtra* (3.5), from one's mastery of the practice of ecstatic "constraint" (*sam-yama*).

PRAJNĀ-JYOTIS ("he who has wisdom's light"), a type of *yogin who, according to the *Yoga-Bhāshya* (3.51), has subjugated the *elements and *senses and who can preserve his spiritual accomplishments and build on them to achieve *liberation.

Cf. *atikrānta-bhāvanīya, mādhu-bhūmika, prathama-kalpika.*

PRĀKĀMYA ("wish fulfillment"), one of the great paranormal powers (*siddhi*). The *Yoga-Bhāshya* (3.45) explains it as the "nonobstruction of one's will." As *Vyāsa elucidates in this text, this power enables the *yogin, e.g., to dive into solid *earth as if it were liquid.

PRAKĀSHA ("brightness" or "luminos-ity"), an essential characteristic of the *Di-vine; also, one of the qualities of *sattva, the cosmological principle of lucidity. See also Light, *vimarsha*.

PRAKRITI ("creatrix"), the *Yoga and *Sāmkhya term for *nature, or creation. Although the word does not appear prior to the *Bhagavad-Gītā* (3.39) and the *Sh-vetāshvatara-Upanishad* (4.10), the under-lying concept was known much earlier and was often termed *avyakta* ("unman-ifest"). The designation *prakriti* was origi-nally also used for the eight principal evo-lutes of *nature: the unmanifest (*avyakta*) dimension, which *Patanjali calls *alinga*; the higher mind (*buddhi*); the "I maker" (*ahamkāra*); and the five elements (*bhūta*). In the *Bhagavad-Gītā* (7.4) *Krishna speaks of these eight divisions or principles (*tattva*) as his "lower nature," whereas his "higher nature" is the "life principle" (*jīva-bhūta*), meaning the Self (*purusha*).

*Hinduism views *nature as a multilevel hierarchic organization extending from the visible realm composed of the five *el-ements to the transcendental foundation (*pradhāna*), or "root nature" (*mūla-pra-kriti*). The visible dimension is designated as "coarse" (*sthūla*), and all the other, hidden dimensions are called "subtle" (*sūkshma*). The *Sāmkhya tradition has developed the most sophisticated model explaining the gradual evolution (*pari-nāma) from the transcendental core of nature to the manifest realm accessible to the five senses (*indriya). This model has been adopted and adapted by most of the *Yoga and *Vedānta schools. In its various forms it serves as a kind of map for the *yogin, who seeks to proceed in *consciousness from the external to the internal, then to the transcendental dimension of nature, and at last, beyond Nature's orbit, to the supraconscious *Self.

According to the metaphysics of *Classical Yoga and *Sāmkhya, *nature in all its aspects is utterly insentient. Only the transcendental Self, the *purushu, enjoys *Consciousness. Whereas the Self is perfectly and eternally immobile, a pure witness (*sākshin), nature is inherently in motion. Its dynamics is due to the interplay of its three types of primary constituent (*guna): *sattva, *rajas, and *tamas. In combination, they weave the entire pattern of cosmic existence, from high to low. The gunas underlie all material and psychic realities. The *mind and the *ego are counted among the material phenomena, which are illumined by the unchanging transcendental Consciousness, or *cit.

The relationship between the supposedly insentient nature and the exclusively sentient *Self has proved a philosophical stumbling block. In the *Mahābhārata (12.303.14ff.) this relationship is compared to the relationship between fly and fig, fish and water, fire and fire basin. Later thinkers wrestled with the epistemological question of how a radically transcendent Self-monad could possibly experience anything.

In *Classical Yoga *nature is also called the "visible" (*drishya), while the *Self is known as the "seer" (*drashtri) or the "power of seeing" (*drik-shakti). The relationship between these two ultimate principles is said to be one of "preestablished harmony" (*yogyatā). In the literature of commentary on the *Yoga-Sūtra, this fit between prakriti and *purusha is explained by the doctrine of reflection (*pratibimba): The "*light" of the transcendental Self is mirrored in the highest, or most subtle, aspect of nature, namely, the *sattva. When the sattva of *consciousness is as pure as the transcendental Self, the condition of "aloneness" (*kaivalya), or *liberation, obtains.

PRAKRITI-LAYA ("absorption into *nature"), mentioned in the *Yoga-Sūtra (1.19) as the *destiny of those who fail to transcend the "notion of becoming" (bhava-pratyaya) and achieve a kind of pseudoliberation in a disembodied (videha) state at the core of nature. This describes the condition of the *deities who, compared to human beings, live immeasurably long lives but who are nevertheless doomed to die. As *Vyāsa explains in his commentary on the above aphorism, the pressure of the rudimentary *consciousness of the prakriti-layas sooner or later forces them to experience renewed *embodiment in one or the other realm of nature. Genuine *liberation, which transcends nature completely, is forever. See also laya.

PRALAYA ("dissolution"), the disappearance of the material universe at the end of its cycle of manifestation. *Hindu cosmomythologists have calculated this duration to be 2.16 billion years. This is thought to be the length of a single waking day, or *kalpa, in the life of *Brahma. During his sleep, which has the same duration, only the subtle dimensions of the *cosmos, inhabited by the *deities and sages, exists. When Brahma awakens from his sleep, the *world is created anew. Upon completing his hundredth year, Brahma himself dies, and the entire universe, with all its coarse and subtle dimensions, dissolves into the *Divine. This moment is known as the "great dissolution" (*mahā-pralaya*). See also *kāla*, *manvantara*, World Ages, *yuga*.

PRAMĀDA ("heedlessness"), inattention; one of the obstacles (*antarāya*) mentioned in the *Yoga-Sūtra* (1.30). *Vyāsa, in his *Yoga-Bhāshya* (1.30), defines it as the lack of cultivation of the means to ecstasy (*samādhi*). In the *Yoga-Kundalī-Upanishad* (1.59) the synonym *pramattatā* is employed, which is said to be one of the ten obstructions (*vighna*) on the yogic *path.

PRAMĀNA ("measure" or "standard"), in *Classical Yoga, valid cognition. Like all the other schools of *Hinduism, *Yoga does not bypass the important philosophical issue of the possibility and scope of *knowledge. Thus *Patanjali recognizes three sources of valid cognition: perception (*pratyaksha*), inference (*anumāna*), and testimony (*āgama*).

PRĀNA ("life"; lit. "breathing forth," from the prefix *pra* and the root *an*, "to breathe"), in the *Rig-Veda* (10.90.13, e.g.), stands for the breath of the cosmic *purusha* and for the *breath of life in general. Early on it came to be equated with the Absolute (*brahman*) as the transcendental source of all life. In secular contexts, *prāna* denotes "air." In the sacred scriptures of *Hinduism, however, *prāna* almost invariably signifies the universal life force, which is a vibrant psychophysical energy similar to the *pneuma* of the ancient Greeks. The *Yoga-Vāsishtha* (3.13.31) tellingly defines *prāna* as the "vibratory power" (*spanda-shakti*) that underlies all manifestation.

Later writers distinguish between the universal or "primary life force" (*mukhya-prāna*) and the life force as it enlivens the individual being. The individuated *prāna*, which is also identified with the psyche (*jīva*, *hamsa*), is said to reside at the *heart; its color is red. In the *Tri-Shikhi-Brāhmana-Upanishad* (2.79ff.), however, the *prāna* force is said to circulate in the mouth, the *nose, the *heart, the *navel, and the big toes and to be responsible for the assimilation of *food. According to the *Yoga-Yājnavalkya* (4.58f.), it is situated in the middle of the abdomen and has the function of separating *water, solid food, and their "essence" (*rasa*).

The individuated type of *prāna* has from the earliest times been thought to have five aspects: (1) *prāna*, the ascending *breath issuing from the *navel or the *heart and including both inhalation and exhalation; (2) *apāna*, the breath associated with the lower half of the trunk; (3) *vyāna*, the diffuse breath circulating in all the limbs; (4) *udāna*, the "up-breath" held responsible for eructation, *speech, and the ascent of *attention in higher states of *consciousness; and (5) *samāna*, the breath localized in the abdominal region, where it is connected with the digestive processes. *Prāna* and *apāna* also frequently stand for inhalation and exhalation respectively. Common synonyms for *prāna* are *marut*, *vāta*, *vāyu*, and *pavana*.

In the period following *Shankara (early 9th cen. CE), the authorities of *Yoga and *Vedānta often added a set of five secondary breaths (*upaprāna*) comprising the following: *nāga* ("serpent"); *kūrma* ("tortoise"); *kri-kara* ("*kri* maker"); *deva-datta* ("God-given"); and *dhanamjaya* ("conquest of wealth").

These ten types of life force are generally thought to circulate in, or along, 72,000 channels (*nādī*) that feed all the organs of

the *body. Already in the ancient *Taittirīya-Upanishad (2) this intricately pat-
terned life energy is conceived as forming
a distinct field, *prāna-maya-kosha.

In the *Chāndogya-Upanishad (2.13.6)
the five principal *breaths are referred to
as the "gatekeepers to the heavenly
world," suggesting an esoteric understanding of the close relationship between
breath and *consciousness, which led to
the invention of the various techniques of
breath control (*prānāyāma). See also
svara.

PRĀNA-DHĀRANĀ ("holding the life
force"), the technique of projecting the life
force (*prāna) into specific parts of the
*body in order to restore a particular
organ to *health. This practice, which is
mentioned in the *Tri-Shikhi-Brāhmana-
Upanishad (2.109), is said to conquer all
illnesses (*roga) and fatigue (klama).

PRĀNA-LINGA, a term of the *Vīra-Shaiva
sect for "living sign," meaning one's personal experience of *Shiva in the *linga.

PRĀNA-MAYA-KOSHA ("sheath composed
of the life force"), one of the five "sheaths"
(*kosha) covering the innate luminosity of
the transcendental *Self. Some modern oc-
cultists equate this field with the *aura.

PRĀNA-RODHA or PRĀNA-SAMRODHA
("restraint of the life force"), a synonym
for *prānāyāma. Complete restraint of the
life force (*prāna), also known as prāna-
jaya ("conquest of the life force"), is usually gauged by the *yogin's capacity to hold
his *breath for prolonged periods of *time.
In order to demonstrate this extraordinary
ability, some yogins have let themselves be
buried for several hours and even days at
a time in allegedly airtight containers underground.

PRĀNA-SAMYAMA ("constraint of the life
force"), a synonym for *prānāyāma. According to the *Brihad-Yogi-Yājnavalkya-
Samhitā (9.35), it is the fourth "limb"
(*anga) of *Yoga, whereas the *Tejo-
Bindu-Upanishad (1.31) lists it as the
eleventh "limb" of its fifteenfold Yoga
(*panca-dasha-anga-yoga). The *Tri-
Shikhi-Brāhmana-Upanishad (2.30) gives
it a symbolic meaning, defining it as the
conviction that the *world is false (mithyā).

PRĀNA-SPANDA ("quiver of the life
force"). According to the *Laghu-Yoga-
Vāsishtha (5.9.78), when the ever-dynamic
life force (*prāna) is stopped, the movements of the *mind are likewise arrested.
See also spanda.

PRANAVA ("humming"), the esoteric designation of the sacred syllable *om, which
is recited with a nasalized hum. According
to the *Yoga-Sūtra (1.28), the pranava
should be recited and its inner meaning
should be contemplated for the cultivation
of "inward-mindedness" (*pratyak-cet-
ana). Since it is the primary *mantra, it is
also known as "primal seed" (ādi-bīja).
The *Shiva-Purāna (1.17.4) offers the following imaginative etymology: pra from
*prakriti ("nature") and nava ("boat"),
because the pranava is the boat by which
the *yogin can safely cross the ocean of existence and reach the shore of the *Absolute. See also bīja, bindu, japa, nāda.

PRĀNĀYĀMA ("breath control"), the
fourth "limb" (*anga) of the eightfold
*path taught by *Patanjali. The word is
composed of prāna ("breath" or "life
force") and āyāma ("extension"), which
hints at the principal objective of breath
control, the phase of retention (*kumbhaka). Prolonging the duration of the with-
held *breath is thought to prolong life

itself. *Prānāyāma* is recognized as one of the chief means of rejuvenating and indeed immortalizing the *body. The ultimate purpose of *prānāyāma*, however, is to control the movement of the *mind. As the *Yoga-Shikhā-Upanishad* (1.61) states, the life force cannot be controlled by mere speculation, talk, the snare of books, contrivances, spells, or medications. It must be checked through the practice of *prānāyāma*. The *yogin who attempts to practice *Yoga without controlling the breath is compared (1.62f.) to a person who wants to cross the ocean in an unbaked earthen vessel, which soaks up water and is bound to sink.

Prānāyāma is the main technique of *hatha-yoga by which the "serpent power" (*kundalinī-shakti) is forced to enter the central channel (*sushumnā-nādī) and begin its ascension to the *head. The scriptures of *hatha-yoga know of eight kinds of *breath control, which are also called "retentions" (*kumbhaka, lit. "pots"): *sūrya-bedha or -bedhana ("sun-piercing"); *ujjayī ("victorious"); *sīt-karī ("sīt maker"); *shītalī ("cooling"); *bhastrikā ("bellows"); *bhrāmarī ("humming"); *mūrchā ("swooning"); and *plāvinī ("floater"). In place of the *sīt-karī* and *plāvinī* forms of breath control, the *Gheranda-Samhitā* (5.46) mentions *sahita ("combined") and *kevalī ("absolute") *prānāyāma* instead.

Breath control has three phases: inhalation (*pūraka), retention (*kumbhaka), and exhalation (*recaka). In addition, the *Hatha-Yoga-Pradīpikā* (2.72) distinguishes between *sahita- and *kevala-kumbhaka. Whereas the former practice involves deliberate inhalation and exhalation, the *kevala-kumbhaka* is breath retention on the spot.

Before *prānāyāma* can be started, the aspirant must engage in various purificatory practices (called *dhauti). Some of the types of *prānāyāma* also serve this purpose. Upon mastery of *breath control, the *yogin is fit to proceed to the higher stages of *Yoga. The *Gheranda-Samhitā* (5.1) mentions four essential prerequisites for the practice of *prānāyāma*: *sthāna, or right place; *kāla, or right time; *mita-āhāra, or moderate diet; and *nādī-shuddhi, or purity of the channels (*nādī) through which the *life force flows. The *Shiva-Samhitā* (3.37) recommends that *prānāyāma* should not be practiced shortly after a meal or when one is hungry. Also it states that one should take some milk and butter before starting. These restrictions do not apply, however, to a practitioner who is accomplished.

The *Hatha-Yoga-Pradīpikā* (2.15) advises caution in performing breath control: "Just as a lion, an elephant, or a tiger is tamed gradually, so should the *life force be controlled; else it will kill the *practitioner." Properly executed, however, *prānāyāma* has great curative value, and the texts mention hiccup, cough, asthma, and pain in the *head, *ears, and *eyes among the *diseases that can effectively be healed through breath control. *Prānāyāma* is also said to reduce feces, urine, and phlegm (*kapha). Furthermore, it strengthens and invigorates the body-mind and is even claimed to have a rejuvenating effect.

The practice of *prānāyāma* is associated with a variety of psychosomatic phenomena. The *Shiva-Samhitā* (3.40ff.) mentions four stages in this process. In the first stage, perspiration (*sveda) is caused, and the sweat should be massaged into the limbs. In the second stage, the *yogin experiences trembling (*kampa). In the third stage, he begins to jump "like a frog." In the fourth stage, he experiences great lightness (*lāghutā) and is able to walk on air. See also *shīt-krama*.

PRANIDHĀNA ("devotion" or "dedication"), one's whole-hearted application to the spiritual process. See also *īshvara-pranidhāna*.

PRAPATTI ("resignation" or "surrender"), a key concept of the *Pāncarātra or *Vaishnava tradition; unconditional surrender to the *Divine in which the devotee (*bhakta) drops all concern even about *liberation, instead trusting entirely the mercy of *God. This attitude of radical devotion (*bhakti) is epitomized in the final admonition of *Krishna in the *Bhagavad-Gītā (18.66): "Relinquishing all teachings (*dharma), come to me alone for shelter. I will deliver you from all *sin. Do not grieve!" The *practitioner cultivating *prapatti* starts from the recognition of his or her own insignificance and helplessness. Gradually the devotee grows more deeply attached to the *Divine until his or her self-effacement leads to perfect ecstatic oblivion in *God.

Some scriptures, such as the *Yati-Indra-Mata-Dīpikā* (7.28), regard *prapatti* as an alternative to the arduous discipline of the sevenfold practice (*sapta-sādhana) and the eightfold *path (*ashta-anga-yoga). The devotee has to surrender himself or herself to the *Divine only once to be assured of *God's saving grace (*prasāda). There is no evidence that *Rāmānuja, the great medieval proponent of devotion (*bhakti), taught this total surrender to the will of God. Yet some 150 years after Rāmānuja's death, his followers split into two groups, known respectively as the Southern and the Northern school (Tamil: *tengalai* and *vadagalai*). The adherents of the former school explain *prapatti* as sheer receptivity to the grace of God, whereas the authorities of the latter school believe that the devotee must take certain positive steps to deserve that *grace, including the

recitation of sacred *mantras. Throughout his writings, Rāmānuja emphasized the importance of meditation (*dhyāna, *upāsana) on the Divine. Cf. Effort, *paurusha*.

PRĀPTI ("attainment"), the ability to expand infinitely, one of the classic paranormal powers (*siddhi). The *Yoga-Bhāshya* (3.45) seriously suggests that the *yogin who enjoys this power can touch the moon with his fingertips.

PRĀRABDHA-KARMAN ("started action"), *karma, or *destiny, in progress, which cannot be prevented.

PRASĀDA ("clarity," "tranquillity," or "grace"). In the sense of "clarity" or "serenity," *prasāda* is sometimes listed among the practices of moral discipline (*yama). According to the *Bhagavad-Gītā (17.16), *prasāda* is an aspect of austerity (*tapas). In another stanza from this work (2.64), serenity is said to be the gift of the *yogin who has brought his self (or *ego) under control. Through serenity, he becomes free from all sorrow (*duhkha). This is also the contention of the *Mahābhārata (12.238.10), which states that through mental tranquillity (*citta-prasāda*) one leaves behind both the auspicious (*shubha*) and the inauspicious (*ashubha*). In the *Yoga-Sūtra (1.47) "clarity of the inner being" (*adhyātma-prasāda) is said to result from the "suprareflexive lucidity" (*nirvicāra-vaishāradya), a high-level *ecstatic experience. Thus *prasāda* is sometimes regarded as one of the signs (*cihna) of *progress on the *path. In aphorism 1.33 *Patanjali recommends the practice of projecting the sentiments of friendship (*maitrī), compassion (*karunā), gladness (*muditā), and equanimity (*upekshā) for the pacification (*prasādana*) of *consciousness.

It is easy to see why the word *prasāda* should also have acquired the meaning of "grace," since mental tranquillity is a precondition for one's entrance into higher states of *consciousness. This event is often experienced as being given "from above," that is, as an act of *grace. Thus the *Linga-Purāna (1.7.4) reassures us: "Through grace, wisdom (*jnāna) is born; through wisdom, *Yoga comes about. By means of Yoga, *liberation is procured. Thence through grace, everything [is accomplished]." This position is maintained already in the ancient *Katha-Upanishad (2.23), which has this verse: "This *Self is not to be attained through instruction, nor by the intellect, nor by much learning. It is to be attained only by the one whom it chooses. To such a one that Self reveals itself (tanu)." The same view is expressed by *Shankara in his learned commentary on the Brahma-Sūtra (1.1.4): "The knowledge of the Absolute (*brahman) is not dependent on human activity. What then? Just like *knowledge of an *object that is an object of *perception and of other means of knowledge, this [knowledge of the Absolute] also depends solely on that [transcendental] Object."

See also anugraha, kripā; cf. Effort.

PRASAMKHYANA ("elevation"), a high-level *ecstatic state, consisting in the vision of discernment (*viveka-khyāti). The *yogin must be "nonusurious" (akusīda) toward this experience so that he may realize the "cloud of dharma ecstasy" (*dharma-megha-samādhi). According to the *Yoga-Bhāshya (1.2), however, it is another name for the dharma-megha-samādhi. In another passage (2.2) the same work states that it is the fire of prasamkhyāna that burns the "causes of affliction" (*klesha), rendering them sterile. *Shankara, in his *Vivarana (2.4), interprets the term as "perfect vision" (samyag-darshana).

PRASHVĀSA ("breathing forth"), listed by *Patanjali in his *Yoga-Sūtra (1.31) as one of the symptoms accompanying the obstacles (*antarāya); here it probably has the meaning of "faulty breathing." Elsewhere (2.49), however, the term occurs in the sense of "exhalation." See also shvāsa; cf. nishvāsa.

PRASVEDA ("sweat" or "sweating") sometimes designates profuse perspiration. See sveda.

PRATHAMA-KALPIKA ("he who is of the first form"), the neophyte in the first stage of yogic *practice for whom, as the *Yoga-Bhāshya (3.51) puts it, the *light is just dawning. Cf. atikrānta-bhāvanīya, mādhu-bhūmika, prajnā-jyotis.

PRATIBHĀ ("shining forth"), explained in the *Yoga-Bhāshya (3.33) as "a preliminary form of the *knowledge born of discernment (*viveka), just as the light at dawn [heralds] the *sun." *Vyāsa also calls this the "deliverer" (*tāraka). The *Yoga-Sūtra (3.36) mentions "flashes of illumination" (pratibhā) in regard to hearing, sensing, sight, taste, and smell. According to the *Yoga-Bhāshya (3.36), these are the "supersenses" (ati-indriya) possessed by the *adept. *Patanjali states (3.37) that these phenomena are powers (*siddhi) in the *waking state but *obstacles on the *path to attaining ecstasy (*samādhi). Already the *Mahābhārata (12.232.22) advises that these "flashes of illumination" arising from one's spiritual practice should be ignored. In another passage of the same work (12.266.7) we read: "The knower of truth (tattva-vid) [should conquer] sleep (*nidrā) and pratibhā through the practice of wisdom (*jnāna)." See also divya-cakshus, divya-samvid, divya-shrotra.

PRATIBIMBA ("reflection"), an important epistemological concept of *Classical Yoga that attempts to explain how the transcendental *Self, which is thought to be eternally distinct from *nature and thus from the human body-mind, can possibly apperceive mental states. While the second-century *Yoga-Sūtra makes no reference to pratibimba at all, the *Yoga-Bhāshya (4.23) mentions the term once and understands it as the "reflection" of the *object in *consciousness. The *Tattva-Vaishāradī (2.17), written several hundred years later, makes a distinction between *bimba, or the mirroring of the object in consciousness, and pratibimba ("countermirroring"), or the reflection of that content of consciousness to the transcendental *Self. In this text, however, both terms are frequently used interchangeably. According to *Vācaspati Mishra, consciousness is like a mirror (darpana) in which the Self's awareness (*caitanya) is reflected. This idea is found fully developed in the *Yoga-Vārttika (1.4) by *Vijñāna Bhikshu, who speaks of a "mutual reflection" (parasparam pratibimbam).

PRATIMĪLANA-SAMĀDHI, the experience of both introvertive and extravertive ecstasy in succession. See also nimīlana-samādhi, unmīlana-samādhi.

PRATIPAKSHA-BHĀVANĀ ("cultivation of the opposite"), a method suggested by *Patanjali in his *Yoga-Sūtra (2.33) to combat negative mental states characterized by him as "unwholesome deliberations" (*vitarka). At the simplest level, this could consist in the mere recollection of the opposite of whatever negative or undesirable intentions or thoughts are assailing one's *mind. But it is easy to see how this could be developed into a full-fledged *contemplation. Thus the *Yoga-Bhāshya (2.33) advises the *practitioner who is troubled by harmful thoughts to ponder as

follows: "Boiled by the terrifying coals of existence (*samsāra), I take my refuge in the precepts of *Yoga by bestowing fearlessness on all creatures. Having cast off [all] unwholesome deliberations, I betake myself to them again like a dog: As a dog [devours] its vomit, so do I betake myself to [that which I have] cast off." See also bhavana.

PRATIPRASAVA ("counterflow"), in *Classical Yoga, the involution of the primary constituents (*guna) of *nature. Prasava signifies the "streaming forth" of the ultimate building blocks of nature into the multiple forms of the universe in all its dimensions. Pratiprasava, on the other hand, denotes the process of dissolution of those forms relative to the *microcosm of the *adept who is about to win liberation (*kaivalya). In Classical Yoga, which subscribes to the ideal of disembodied liberation (*videha-mukti), this coincides with the psychophysical *death of the individual. Cf. Evolution.

PRATĪTI ("conviction" or "faith"). The *Yoga-Shikhā-Upanishad (1.132) declares that when *faith is merged with the *recitation of one's *mantra, this becomes *hatha-yoga. See also shraddhā.

PRATYABHIJÑĀ SCHOOL, the most prominent school of the North Indian branch of *Shaivism. Founded by *Vasugupta (770–830 CE), the "discoverer" of the *Shiva-Sūtra, this school gets its name from its central tenet, that the individual being is able to "re-cognize" himself or herself as *Shiva, the *Absolute. This notion was first philosophically elaborated by Somānanda, a disciple of Vasugupta, in his Shiva-Drishti ("View on Shiva"). The most popular textbook expounding this philosophy, which is still in use among

Kashmiri pundits today, is the *Pratyabhi-jnā-Hridaya* ("Heart of Recognition") by *Kshemarāja, a pupil of the renowned *adept *Abhinava Gupta.

*Yoga played a significant role among the Pratyābhijna adherents. In fact, the *Shiva-Sūtra* can be considered a manual of Yoga similar to the *Yoga-Sūtra. *Vasugupta and his commentators emphasize the importance of *grace, as manifested in the "descent of the power" (*shakti-pāta), proper initiation (*dīkshā), and "illumined knowledge" (*bodha-jnāna*). The yogic technology employed in this school is close to that of early *hatha-yoga.

PRATYĀHĀRA ("withdrawal"), sensory inhibition; the fifth "limb" (*anga) of the eightfold *path (*ashta-anga-yoga) of *Patanjali. In the *Yoga-Sūtra* (2.54) *pratyāhāra* is defined as the imitation of the nature of *consciousness by the *senses insofar as they disunite themselves from their respective *objects. This is said to result in the supreme "obedience" (*vashyatā*) of the senses, which is the ability to "switch off" and produce a state of extreme inward-mindedness at will. *Vyāsa, in his *Yoga-Bhāshya* (2.54), gives the following simile: "As when the queen bee flies up and the bees swarm after her, and when she settles down and they also settle down: similarly, the senses are controlled when consciousness (*citta) is controlled."

The *Maitrāyanīya-Upanishad* (6.25) compares *pratyāhāra* to the retraction of our sensory awareness in *sleep. This comparison is somewhat unfortunate, however, because *pratyāhāra* is a completely voluntary process and does not lead to a state of diminished *awareness but one of intensified *consciousness. The *Yoga-Cū-dāmanī-Upanishad* (121) likens this process to the *sun withdrawing its luster in the third quarter of the day. The *Shāndil-ya-Upanishad* (1.8.1) offers a symbolic interpretation of *pratyāhāra*: everything that is seen should be looked upon as the *Self. This scripture also defines it as the mental performance of the prescribed daily rites, and as the holding of the breath (*vāyu) in the eighteen sensitive places (*marma-sthāna*) in sequence.

A favorite image for describing the process of sensory inhibition is expressed, e.g., in the *Goraksha-Paddhati* (2.24): "As the tortoise retracts its limbs into the middle of the *body, so the *yogin should withdraw the *senses into himself." This scripture (2.25ff.) continues as follows:

Knowing that whatever he hears, [be it] pleasant or unpleasant, is the *Self: the Yoga-knower withdraws [his senses].

Knowing that whatever scent he smells with the *nose is the Self: the Yoga-knower withdraws.

Knowing that whatever he sees with the *eyes, [be it] pure or impure, is the Self: the Yoga-knower withdraws.

Knowing that whatever he senses with the skin, tangible or intangible, is the Self: the Yoga-knower withdraws.

Knowing that whatever he tastes with the *tongue, [be it] salty or not salty, is the Self: the Yoga-knower withdraws.

According to the *Tejo-Bindu-Upanishad* (1.34), *pratyāhāra* is the twelfth "limb" of the fifteen-limbed Yoga (*panca-dasha-anga-yoga*). It is defined here as the "pleasant consciousness" (*citta-ranjaka*) that beholds the *Self in all things. This is in contrast to most other definitions, which suggest a state of acute inwardness. Thus the *Tri-Shikhi-Brāh-mana-Upanishad* (2.30) defines *pratyāhāra* as the condition of the "inward-facing" (*antar-mukhin*) consciousness. Elsewhere (130) the same text speaks of it as the withdrawal of the *life force from different places in the *body. See also *indriya-jaya*, *marman*.

PRATYAKSHA ("perception"; lit. "having before one's *eyes [aksha]"), in *Classical Yoga, one of the three means of valid cognition (*pramāna*), the other two being inference (*anumāna*) and tradition (*āgama*). The *Mahābhārata* (12.211.26), which is representative of *Preclassical Yoga, states that perception is the foundation of the other two epistemological means. Elsewhere (12.289.7) in this scripture, *pratyaksha* is used to contrast *Yoga with the more theory-dependent approach of the *Sāmkhya tradition, which is characterized as resting upon the ascertainment of the *knowledge taught in the books (*shāstra-vinishcaya*).

Pratyaksha also figures as the sixth "limb" (*anga*) of the sevenfold discipline (*sapta-sādhana*) and in this connection is defined in the *Gheranda-Samhitā* (1.11) as the perception of the *Self, resulting from meditation (*dhyāna*). More commonly, this higher spiritual perception is called *sākshātkāra* to emphasize the fact that *Self-realization is not *knowledge based on any sensory input but direct perception. Cf. *viparyaya*.

PRATYAYA In the *Yoga-Sūtra*, this term very probably has the meaning of "notion," or "idea," throughout, although classical commentators interpret some of its occurrences in the sense of "cause." The word denotes any content of *consciousness and is thus more comprehensive than either the five types of mental fluctuation (*vritti*) or the higher intuitions (*prajnā*) of ecstasy (*samādhi*). Both these mental phenomena are in fact "presented-ideas" (*pratyaya*), which are continuously apperceived by the transcendental *Self.

PRAVRITTI ("activity"), that mental disposition which is due to the influence of *rajas* and, according to the *Tattva-Vaishāradī* (1.2), consists in such states as distress and grief (*shoka*). In the *Yoga-Sūtra* (1.35) the term also refers to a special mental phenomenon that in the *Yoga-Bhāshya* (3.25) is explained as a kind of "divine perception" (*divya-samvid*), or what we might call heightened sensory awareness. As Vyāsa points out, such paranormal phenomena are useful insofar as they dispel the aspirant's doubts (*samshaya*).

PRAVRITTI-MĀRGA ("path of activity"), the orientation of the person who does not renounce the *world, which consequently leads to rebirth after rebirth (*punar-janman*) punctuated by repeated *deaths (*punar-mrityu*). Cf. *nivritti-mārga*.

PRAYĀNA-KĀLA ("time of departure"), the moment of *death. See also *anta-kāla*.

PRAYĀSA ("overexertion"), one of the factors that impede *progress in Yoga, according to the *Hatha-Yoga-Pradīpikā* (1.15). See also Effort, *vighna*.

PRĀYASHCITTA (lit. "departure mind," from *prāyash*, "going forth," and *citta*, "mind") penance, or atonement; *discipline undertaken to atone for a transgression of a moral rule or failure to fulfill an obligation on the spiritual *path; penance by which shortcoming is to be corrected. Since *Vedic times, such corrective disciplines have played an important role in the spiritual life of the Indians. The famous physician Caraka (see *Caraka-Samhitā*) considered it to be equivalent to a medical remedy (*bheshaja*), since it removes the *diseases or disorders caused by wrongful *action, or *sin. The purpose of *prāyashcitta* is to restore moral and ritual *purity.

PRAYATNA ("effort"), an essential prerequisite for success in *Yoga, according to the *Yoga-Tattva-Upanishad (81). As the *Bhagavad-Gītā (6.45) affirms, this *effort may have to be kept up over many lifetimes until *perfection is reached. In the *Yoga-Sūtra (2.47), however, *prayatna* stands for "tension," which must be released for the accurate performance of the postures (*āsana). See also *paurusha, yatna*; cf. Grace.

PRAYER. Many of the hymns (*sūkta*) of the ancient *Rig-Veda are prayers that combine praise with petition. In some contexts, the *Vedic Sanskrit word *brahman* means as much as "prayerful meditation." Later it came to stand for the ultimate *Reality to which the seers (*rishi) aspired. Prayer is intimately connected with the *worship of the *Divine as a personal force. Thus it is a prominent element in the theistic schools of *Vaishnavism and *Shaivism, notably *bhakti-yoga. The purer the prayer, or the less amount of self-will it expresses, the more it approximates meditation (*dhyāna), which is the absorption of the individual *consciousness into the transcendental Consciousness (*cit).

PRECEPTOR. See *ācārya*.

PRECLASSICAL YOGA, a broad historical category that refers to the numerous *Yoga teachings found in scriptures such as the *Katha-, Maitrāyanīya-, and *Shvetāshvatara-Upanishad, as well as the *Mahābhārata, especially the *Bhagavad-Gītā, the *Moksha-Dharma, and the *Anu-Gītā sections of that epic. The metaphysics of Preclassical Yoga is essentially *Vedantic. Cf. Classical Yoga, Epic Yoga, Postclassical Yoga.

PRETA ("departed [spirit]"), the postmortem entity of a recently deceased person. The *Yoga-Vāsishtha (3.55.27ff.) states that the *pretas* experience themselves in a new *body created out of the *offerings of their living relatives. Later they meet the messengers of *Yama, the god of death. The virtuous souls get snatched away in heavenly carriages, whereas the sinners have to walk through snow and dangerous forests. Upon arrival in the world of Yama, they are judged and then transported either to *heaven or to *hell. After a period of time in either realm, they reincarnate. See also *deva-yāna, pitri-yāna*.

PRIDE. See *abhimāna, darpa, dambha, mada, smaya*.

PRITHIVĪ ("earth," from *prithu*, "wide"), one of the five material elements (*bhūta) that compose the densest level of the *cosmos. See also *tattva*.

PRITHU, an ancient *Vedic emperor of Ayodhya (Audh) and a great sage who is remembered in many *Purānas, especially the *Vāyu-Purāna*. He appears to have been closely connected with the *Vrātya brotherhoods, from which he learned the secret *knowledge about the syllable *om. According to the *Bhāgavata-Purāna (4.23), he was initiated into *Yoga by *Sanatkumāra.

PRĪTI ("satisfaction"), sometimes counted among the principles of moral discipline (*yama). See also *samtosha, tushti*.

PROGRESS. Most esoteric traditions depict spiritual life as a winding *path that, step by step, brings the practitioner (*yogin, *sādhaka) closer to the summit, which is *liberation. A few schools understand liberation as a sudden, spontaneous event, but even then some form of preparation or discipline is thought to be necessary.

Those who view spiritual life as a graduated process (*krama) of increasing self-understanding or self-surrender often distinguish between distinct states (*avasthā) or stages (*bhūmi) of maturation. The texts differ in their assessment of how quickly certain stages can be reached. The *Amrita-Nāda-Upanishad (28f.), e.g., proposes the following sequence: after three months, wisdom (*jnāna) dawns; after four months, the deities (*deva) can be seen; after five months, the resplendent principle called *virāj becomes visible; after six months "aloneness" (*kaivalya), or *liberation, is attained. This optimistic view is not shared, for example, by the anonymous author of the *Yoga-Tattva-Upanishad (21), who states that *wisdom is gained after twelve years of practicing *mantra-yoga, though he concedes that the purification of the channels (*nādī-shuddhi) can be accomplished within three months.

Since most *Yoga authorities believe that *liberation is, in the final analysis, a matter of *grace that descends on the well-prepared practitioner, these computations must not be taken too literally. Presumably, their purpose is to encourage the aspirant. Spiritual progress depends very much on the individual's dedication to the process of *self-transcendence and *karmic (genetic, psychomental) strengths and liabilities.

PROXIMITY OF SELF. See samnidhi.

PSYCHOLOGY. While the aspects and phenomena of the ordinary *consciousness are analyzed in unparalleled detail in *Buddhism, *Hindu *Yoga has developed a comprehensive phenomenology of extraordinary states of *consciousness, called *samādhi, for which there is no equivalent even in modern psychology. Especially the

notion of the transcendental *Self as "witness" (*sākshin) deserves our close attention.

*Yoga psychology is therapy, or healing, in the broadest sense of the word. However, whereas modern psychotherapy has grown out of the clinical treatment of cases that *medicine was unable to help, Yoga from the beginning has been a system of spiritual catharsis and transformation intended to restore the individual to primordial wholeness rather than mere physical or mental *health. The *yogins have always endeavored to transcend the ordinary *consciousness, with its sense of self-dividedness and *suffering, and to realize the undiminishable *bliss of the Self (*purusha, *ātman). In the course of their spiritual disciplines, comprising both bodily and mental techniques, they inevitably encountered the habit patterns of the psyche (*jīva), which tend toward conventional modes of motivation and perception. Long before Sigmund Freud, they discovered the reality of the subconscious. Thus the authorities of *Classical Yoga speak of the "subliminal activators" (*samskāra) that combine into "traits" (*vāsanā) through which the conventional (i.e., unenlightened) personality system is maintained.

The purpose of *Yoga is nothing less than the complete transmutation of the subconscious *mind through the transcendence of the ego mechanism, called "I maker" (*ahamkāra) or "I-am-ness" (*asmitā). This goal, which coincides with *enlightenment, or *liberation, is alien to the worldview of modern psychology and psychotherapy. Nevertheless, humanistic psychology, which was ushered in by Abraham Maslow, and especially transpersonal psychology are more sympathetic toward the yogic ideal of *Self-realization and also appreciate that the ecstatic states (*samādhi) are, as the *yogins claim, suprawakeful rather than unconscious states. See also Parapsychology.

PŪJĀ ("worship") is to *Tantrism what the sacrifice (*yajna) is to mainstream *Vedic religion, or *Brāhmanism. It signifies primarily, though not exclusively, the daily worship of one's chosen deity (*ishta-devatā). It involves the following *ritual components: (1) *āsana, the "seat" of the image of the *deity; (2) svāgata, bidding welcome to the deity; (3) pādya, water for the washing of the deity's *feet; (4) arghya, the offering of unboiled rice, flowers, etc.; (5) ācamana, water for sipping, which is offered to the deity twice; (6) mādhuparka, honey, milk, or ghee; (7) *snāna, bathing; (8) vasana, cloth; (9) ābharana, jewels for beautifying the image (*mūrti) of the deity; (10) gandha, scents and sandalwood paste; (11) *pushpa, flowers; (12) *dhūpa, incense; (13) *dīpa, light; (14) naivedya, food; and (15) *vandana or namaskāra, worshipful praise. The ceremony also includes the use of *mantra recitation, *breath control, and *meditation.

PŪJANA ("worship" or "reverence"). The *Bhāgavata-Purāna (17.14) speaks of the reverence of *deities, *teachers, sages, and "twice-born" (dvija) members of *Hindu society (i.e., brahmins, warriors, and merchants) as physical austerity (*tapas). See also guru-pūjā, īshvara-pūjana.

PŪJARIN, the person who performs a ritual of worship (*pūjā).

PŪJYAPĀDA, mentioned in the *Hatha-Yoga-Pradīpikā (1.7) as an *adept of *hatha-yoga. He is probably different from the Karnataka mystic and philosopher by the same name who authored a work on *medicine called the Kalyana-Karaka and whom some scholars place around 600 CE.

PUNAR-JANMAN ("rebirth"). The idea that a person has more than one lifetime is common to most schools of Indian thought. This notion seems to have been an integral part of the *Vedic belief system but was first talked about more openly in the oldest *Upanishads, which nevertheless treated it as a secret teaching. The *Chāndogya-Upanishad (5.10.7), e.g., has this passage: "Thus those whose conduct here [on earth] is pleasing quickly enter a pleasing womb—the womb of a *brahmin [woman], the womb of a [woman of the] warrior [estate], or the womb of a merchant [woman]. But those whose conduct here [on earth] stinks quickly enter a stinking womb—the womb of a dog, the womb of a swine, or the womb of an outcast."

The notion of punar-janman is associated with the idea, first expressed in the *Brihad-Āranyaka-Upanishad (4.4.5), that the quality of one's being is determined by the quality of one's *actions, so that the doer of good deeds becomes good, whereas the doer of *evil becomes evil. The doctrine of reembodiment extends this idea beyond the orbit of the present lifetime. The connecting link between the various *embodiments is *karma.

The ultimate purpose of *Yoga is to escape this neverending cycle of births and *deaths, to put a stop to the generation and fruition of karma, and to awaken, or reawaken, to one's identity as the transcendental Self (*ātman, *purusha).

PUNYA ("merit"), the fruit of *actions or volitions (*samkalpa) that are morally good, that is, in keeping with the cosmic order (*rita, *dharma). Cf. pāpa, phala.

PUPIL. See shishya.

PŪRAKA ("inhalation"), one of the three phases of breath control (*prānāyāma).

The *Brihad-Yogi-Yājnavalkya-Samhitā (8.19) defines it as that restriction of the *breath that fills all the subtle channels (*nādī). This implies that inhalation is more than the intake of *air. It is the attraction into the *body of the universal life force (*prāna). Cf. kumbhaka, recaka.

PURĀNA ("Ancient [Story]"), a type of popular encyclopedia that, at least theoretically, deals with five topics: the original *creation of the *world, the world's re-creation after its destruction, the great *world ages, the genealogy of *deities and sages, and dynastic history. Eighteen major works of this genre, called mahā-purāna, are known, which include the *Mārkandeya-, *Vishnu-, *Bhāgavata-, *Kūrma-, *Linga-, and *Agni-Purāna. Although most of these Purānas were composed in the common era, in some instances they draw on traditions that flourished as far back as the *Vedic age. Thus statements about Purānas can be found already in the *Brāhmana texts.

The yogic teachings in the Purānas belong to *Postclassical Yoga and are thus broadly nondualist (*advaita). They generally make use of the formulations of *Patanjali but tend more toward ritualism. Especially the later Purānas show *Tantric influence. There are also secondary scriptures of this literary genre, known as Upa-Purānas. Traditionally, eighteen Upa-Purānas are listed, though their number is much greater. Of these, the Kālikā-Purāna, which is counted as one of the sacred texts of *Shāktism, is dedicated to the worship of the goddess *Kālī, or *Durgā.

PURASHCARANA ("preparatory ritual"), in *Tantrism, the practice of reciting a *mantra a large number of times in order to activate it. This *ritual is combined with other practices, such as dietary restrictions and the use of consecrated space (*desha). See also japa.

PURIFICATION. See dhauti, shauca, shodhana.

PURIFICATION OF CHANNELS. See nādī-shodhana.

PURITY, or shuddhi, a notion that is central to all spiritual traditions. The transcendental *Reality is commonly conceived as being perfectly pure, in stark contrast with the human *mind, or *consciousness, which is tainted by the mechanism of the *ego. The spiritual *path consists in the progressive *purification of the body-mind until it is cleansed of all defects (*dosha) and becomes capable of flawlessly reflecting the *light of the *Divine, or *Self. In *Yoga and *Sāmkhya, this process is understood as the gradual emergence of the *sattva aspect of *nature.

The *Vijnāna-Bhairava (123) states that conventional purity is still impurity from a spiritual point of view, because it does not destroy the karmic seeds (see karma). True purity is achieved when the *mind has been cleansed of all limiting ideas (*vikalpa).

PŪRNA ("full" or "whole"), an ancient *Vedic designation for the *Absolute. The *Yoga-Shikhā-Upanishad (1.19) speaks of the fullness (pūrnatva) of the Absolute, which allows it to be both divided (sakala) and impartite (nishkala). The much older Kaushītaki-Upanishad (4.8) observes that by worshiping that plenum, one becomes filled with splendor (yashas) and the "*brahmic luster" (brahma-varcasa).

PŪRNA-YOGA, the Sanskrit term for Sri *Aurobindo's Integral Yoga, which is based on the metaphysics of *Vedānta merged with the Western notion of *evolution. According to Aurobindo's philosophy, the singular *Being manifests in the material realm and is liberated from the unconsciousness of matter through the evolutionary process, which caused life, then created the *mind, and finally challenges us to conscious participation so that the "Supermind" can emerge. Thus the world of *appearance is not merely illusory but an essential part of the process of divine unfolding.

Integral Yoga differs from traditional forms of Yoga in that it does not encourage any *abandonment of the *world or worldly obligations but seeks to realize the supramental consciousness through a world-affirmative attitude. In other words, the *pūrna-yogin* not merely raises his consciousness to the level of the transcendental Self, or Spirit, but also endeavors to bring the Spirit into the material realm as a potent transformative power. To the degree that traditional yogic methods are useful to this transmutation, they are integrated into the path of *pūrna-yoga*.

In his *Synthesis of Yoga* (1965) Aurobindo sees perfection in *Yoga (*yoga-siddhi*) as the ultimate fruit of the synergy of *shāstra (by which he means knowledge of the principles of the yogic process, as revealed in one's own *heart), *utsāha (patient and persistent effort), *guru (teacher, understood as the inner guide), and *kāla (time, in the sense of ripening through the flow of the *Divine itself).

PURUSHA ("male"), the *Yoga and *Sāmkhya term for the transcendental *Self, or pure Spirit, generally called *ātman in the *Vedānta tradition. The *Brihad-Āranyaka-Upanishad (1.4.1) furnishes the following fanciful etymology: "Because he, being prior (*pūrva*) to everything, consumed (*aushat*) all *evils, he is [called] *purusha*." The *Go-Patha* ("Cow Path")-*Brāh-

mana (1.1.39), a work more than 3,000 years old, defines the word *purusha* as "he who rests in the castle" (*puri-shaya*), the "castle" being the *body. This is also the explanation of the *Linga-Purāna* (1.28.5), a medieval scripture. More likely than either etymology is the derivation of *purusha* from *pu* ("male") and *vrisha* ("bull").

The *purusha*, as the transcendental *Consciousness, is the "witness" (*sākshin*) of all psychomental experiences. In the *Yoga-Sūtra* (1.3) the *Self is called the "seer" (*drashtri*). *Shankara, in his *Vivarana* (1.3), names it the "cognizer" (*boddhri*) of cognitions (*buddhi*). In *Epic Yoga it is widely referred to as the "knower" (*jna*) or the "field knower" (*kshetra-jna*), the "field" being *nature in the form of the individual *body and *mind.

In *Classical Yoga the *purusha*, which is styled the "power of Awareness" (*citishakti*), is conceived as being absolutely distinct from nature (*prakriti*), which lacks all *awareness. Yet what we call *consciousness is due to a curious correlation (*samyoga*) between the *purusha* and *prakriti*. That correlation is to be undermined through the processes of *Yoga, until the *Self shines forth in its original splendor.

The *Katha-Upanishad* (5.3) also refers to the *purusha* as the "dwarf" (*vāmana*) who dwells in the middle of the *body, i.e., at the *heart. This work (4.12) also states that the *purusha*, in its association with the body-mind, is "thumb-sized." In its transcendental status, however, the *purusha* is infinite. This dual nature of the *Self—in its bound and liberated form—has led to the question of whether there are many transcendental Selves or, as the *Vedānta tradition postulates, only a single Self (*ātman*). The *Mahābhārata* (12.338.2) states that both *Yoga and *Sāmkhya proclaim the existence of multiple *purushas* in the world but that these many *purushas* all have their origin in the single Self, which is eternal, immutable, and incommensurable. That Self is described in the same section as being both the "seer" (*drashtri*) and the "seen" (*drashtavya*). This view is characteristic of the schools of *Epic or *Preclassical Yoga. It is not, however, the stance of *Classical Yoga.

Thus the *Yoga-Bhāshya* (1.24) clearly announces that there are numerous *purushas*, or Spirits, who enjoy the condition of *liberation. They are called *kevalins*, as in *Jainism. Nevertheless, the *Tattva-Vaishāradī* (1.41) emphasizes that there is no distinction between these many Selves. Logic dictates that if there is more than one omnipresent and omnitemporal being, they must all coincide in eternity. This argument has escaped both *Patanjali, the author of the textbook on *Classical Yoga, and *Īshvara Krishna, the founder of *Classical Sāmkhya.

PURUSHA-ARTHA (*purushārtha*, "human purpose"). According to *Hinduism, there are four goals to which people can dedicate themselves: (1) *artha*, or material welfare, prosperity; (2) *kāma*, or pleasure, i.e., the quest for physical comfort, emotional well-being, and intellectual delight; (3) *dharma*, or virtue, justice—a moral way of life; and (4) *moksha*, or *liberation. *Yoga is concerned with assisting in the realization of liberation, as the summum bonum of human life. The Marathi *adept *Jnānadeva postulated a fifth goal of human endeavor—love or devotion (*bhakti*) to the *Divine.

PURUSHA-KHYĀTI ("vision of the Self"), the essence of the supraconscious ecstasy

(*asamprajnāta-samādhi*). See also *ātmadarshana, khyāti*.

PURUSHA-UTTAMA (*purushottama*, "supreme male"), a *Vaishnava theological term for the *Divine. According to the *Bhagavad-Gītā* (15.18), the *purusha-uttama* is beyond the *kshara-purusha* ("mobile self"), which is the individual psyche, and the *akshara-purusha* ("immobile *Self"), which is the transcendental Spirit, or the Self upon *liberation, also known as the principle that is "summit-abiding" (*kutastha*).

PURYASHTAKA ("eightfold city," from *puri*, "city," and *ashtaka*, "eightfold") consists, according to the *Laghu-Yoga-Vāsishtha* (6.5.5f.), of the "I maker" (*ahamkāra*), the lower mind (*manas*), the higher mind (*buddhi*), and the five senses (*indriya*). This is also called the "subtle *body" (*sūkshma-sharīra*). See also *linga-sharīra*.

PŪSHĀ-NĀDĪ ("nourishing current"), one of the subtle channels (*nādī*) of the life force (*prāna*), generally thought to be situated to the rear of the *pingalā-nādī* and to terminate in the right *eye or *ear, though sometimes the left eye is specified.

PUSHPA ("flower [offering]"), part of the *Tantric ritual. According to the *Kaula-Jnāna-Nirnaya* (3.24), this should be a mental act consisting of such spiritual practices as nonharming (*ahimsā*), sense restraint (*indriya-nigraha*), patience (*kshamā*), and meditation (*dhyāna*).

The term *pushpa* is also used to designate the female semen (*bindu*), which is also called *kusuma* ("flower").

· Q ·

QUALIFICATIONS, SPIRITUAL. See *adhikāra*.

QUALIFIED PRACTITIONER. See *adhikārin*.

QUALITIES OF NATURE. *Yoga and *Sāmkhya cosmology pictures the *cosmos as made up of many levels of existence—from the "coarse" (*sthūla*) material realm to the "subtle" (*sūkshma*) psychic realms, to the unmanifest (*avyakta*) dimension of nature (*prakriti*). The "stuff" of which all these levels and their respective phenomena are composed are the three types of fundamental qualities (*guna*). Everything is formed by their interplay. Only the transcendental *Reality, or *Self, is eternally beyond these primary constituents of *prakriti* and hence is said to be *nirguna*.

QUALITY. See *dharma*.

QUIESCENCE. See *shama*.

QUIETUDE. See *shānti*.

· R ·

RĀDHĀ, the spouse of the *Krishna and to this day the symbol of spiritual womanhood for *Hindus. For the pious followers of *Vaishnavism, Rādhā has served for centuries as the great ideal of the passionate woman whose love (*bhakti*) is so full and deep that it transcends the mere carnal and touches the spiritual core of her own and her lover's being. The spiritual love story between the shepherdess (*gopī*) and Krishna is touchingly told in the *Bhāgavata-Purāna* and, in more openly erotic fashion, in the *Gītā-Govinda*.

RĀGA ("passion" or "attachment"), in *Classical Yoga, one of the five "causes of affliction" (*klesha*); defined in the *Yoga-Sūtra* (2.7) as one's dwelling upon the pleasurable. It is often paired up with *dvesha*, meaning "repulsion" or "hatred." The *Bhagavad-Gītā* (3.34) calls these the two "waylayers" (*paripanthin*). See also *kāma, rajas, rati*.

RAHASYA ("secret"). Even today, the essential teachings of the spiritual traditions of India are transmitted by word of mouth in *secrecy. In former times, oral *transmission was the exclusive mode in which a teacher (*guru*) would impart higher *knowledge to a *disciple. Thus the *Upanishads have traditionally been characterized as secret teachings par excellence. See also Secret.

RAISED POSTURE. See *utkata-āsana*.

RĀJA-DANTA ("royal tooth"), the esoteric designation for the uvula, which plays an important role in the practice of the *khecarī-mudrā*. By stimulating the uvula, the "nectar" (*amrita*) is said to flow more profusely. See also *lambikā-yoga*.

RĀJA-MĀRTANDA ("Royal Sun"), also called *Bhoja-Vritti*; a commentary by King *Bhoja on the *Yoga-Bhāshya*. While largely concurring with the interpretations of the *Tattva-Vaishāradī*, Bhoja occasionally offers original exegetical observations.

RAJAS (from the root *raj/ranj*, "to be colored, affected, excited, charmed"), a term with several important meanings. First, it designates one of the three primary constituents (*guna*) of *nature. *Rajas* is the dynamic principle, whose aspects are listed in the *Maitrāyanīya-Upanishad* (3.5) as follows: thirst (*trishnā*), affection (*sneha*), passion (*rāga*), greed (*lobha*), violence (*himsā*), lust (*rati*), false vision (*drishti*), contradictoriness (*vyāvritatva*), jealousy (*īrshyā*), desire (*kāma*), instability (*asthiratva*), fickleness (*cāncalatva*), possessiveness (*jihīrshā*), material acquisitiveness (*artha-uparjana*, written *arthoparjana*), nepotism (*mitra-anugrahana*), dependence on one's environment (*parigraha-avalamba*), repulsion from undesirable sense objects (*anishteshu indriya-artheshu dvishti*), and fondness for what is desirable (*ishteshu abhishu anga*).

Second, *rajas* denotes the mental or emotional disposition of *passion and as such counts as one of the defects (*dosha*). The *Bhagavad-Gītā* (14.7) describes it as being of the nature of attraction (*rāga*), springing from thirst (*trishnā*) and attachment (*sanga*). It is also said to produce *bondage through one's clinging to *action.

A third connotation of *rajas* is "blood," and in this sense is used to refer to the female "semen," or vaginal secretion. In *Tantrism and some schools of *hatha-yoga*, this *rajas* fluid is sucked up through the *penis by means of the *vajrolī-mudrā*. By extension, *rajas* also stands for the female principle, or *shakti*, in general.

Thus the *Yoga-Shikhā-Upanishad* (1.136) states: "In the middle of the perineum (*yoni*), the great place, dwells the well-concealed *rajas*, the principle of the *Goddess, resembling the *japa* and *bandhuka* [flowers]." See also *mahā-rajas*, *retas*; cf. *bindu*.

RĀJA-YOGA ("royal Yoga"), the *yoga-darshana*, or *Classical Yoga, as pithily expounded in *Patanjali's *Yoga-Sūtra*. It is often contrasted with *hatha-yoga*, in which case *rāja-yoga* stands for the higher spiritual practices, whereas *hatha-yoga* is seen as a preparatory discipline. This distinction came into vogue in about the eleventh century CE as part of an attempt to integrate the more *meditative, renunciative approach of the eightfold *path (*ashta-anga-yoga*) with the new body-positive teachings of *Tantric *hatha-yoga*.

The *Hatha-Yoga-Pradīpikā* (3.126), which seeks to build a bridge between these two approaches of *Yoga, affirms: "Without *rāja-yoga*, the earth (*prithivī*) is inauspicious. Without *rāja-yoga*, the night (*nishā*) [is inauspicious]. Without *rāja-yoga*, even the different seals (*mudrā*) [are inauspicious]." This couplet contains a subtle pun on the word *rāja*, which suggests the sovereign's rule, the *moon (*rāja*), and the king's (*rāja*) seal. The *Jyotsnā* commentary on this medieval text understands the words "earth" and "night" symbolically. It takes the former to stand for the quality of stability (*sthairya*) of the yogic postures (*āsana*) and the latter for the absence of the flow of the *life force in the practice of breath retention (*kumbhaka*).

The *Yoga-Shikhā-Upanishad* (1.137) explains *rāja-yoga* as the union (*yoga*) between *rajas and *retas, or the male and female creative principle. By practicing this union, we are told, the *yogin "shines" (*rājate*).

RĀJA-YOGIN (masc.), or RĀJA-YOGINĪ (fem.), a practitioner of *rāja-yoga.

RĀKĀ-NĀDĪ ("full-moon channel"), a current of the *life force, mentioned in the *Yoga-Shikhā-Upanishad (5.24). It is said to fill the *nose with rheum and to cause sneezing after sipping water. See also nādī.

RĀMA or RĀMACANDRA, the ruler of the ancient kingdom of Kosala. According to some scholars, he may have lived in the eighth century BCE; others put him much earlier. He is the celebrated hero of the *Rāmāyana and in the *Vaishnava tradition is worshiped as one of the incarnations or "descents" (*avatāra) of *Vishnu. Rāma, as the name suggests, is generally described as having been of dark color and is frequently depicted carrying a bow and arrow. His wife *Sītā is the personification of marital *devotion and fidelity.

RAMAKRISHNA (1836–1886), widely recognized as one of the greatest spiritual ge-

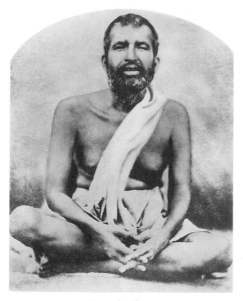

Ramakrishna

niuses of modern *Hinduism. The son of a poor Bengali brahmin, he had his first spiritual experience at the age of six or seven. Throughout his life he worshiped the goddess *Kālī and at one point was initiated into *Tantric practice. Subsequently his teacher Tota Puri instructed him in *Advaita Vedānta and the practice of formless ecstasy (*nirvikalpa-samādhi), which Ramakrishna succeeded in accomplishing in a single day. He lived the life of a renouncer (*samnyāsin) and temple priest at the Kālī temple of Dakshineshvar near Calcutta. Ramakrishna was married, though the marriage was never consummated. His wife, Sarada Devi, was to him the *Goddess incarnate, and she looked upon her husband as her spiritual teacher (*guru). Ramakrishna, a "fool of God" who was oriented more toward mystical experiences than learning, submitted himself to various religious disciplines—including Christianity and Islam—and became convinced that all *paths lead to the same end, namely, *God-realization. Ramakrishna had numerous disciples, among them the world-renowned Swami *Vivekananda.

RAMALINGA SWAMI (1823–1874). Born in the village of Marudur, ten miles north of Chidambaram in South India, Ramalinga was brought up in Madras after his father's premature death. Even as a young boy he composed devotional hymns, and he began to teach formally at the age of twelve. He soon achieved fame for his wisdom and compassionate activity. He founded the Sanmarasa Veda Sanmarga Sangam (later renamed Sanmarasa Suddha Sanmarga Satya Sangam). His Tiru-Varulpa ("Sacred Song of Grace") is counted as one of the great works of Tamil literature. Toward the end of his earthly life, Ramalinga is said to have achieved the complete *transubstantiation of his *body. On January 30, 1874, after announcing that he would enter all bodies, he had himself locked up in his room. While devotees were chanting outside his door, a sudden flash of violet light emanated from his room. When the door was eventually opened, the saint had disappeared without a trace. Ramalinga chronicled in some detail the transmutation of his body first into a "pure" (*shuddha*) or "golden" (*suvarna*) body, then into a graceful (*pranava*) body that was visible but intangible, and finally into an omnipresent gnostic body (*jnāna-deha*).

RAMANA MAHARSHI (1879–1950), born in Venkataraman; one of the twentieth century's greatest adepts of *jnāna-yoga*. Inspired by the *Periya-Purānam*, a Tamil work recounting the lives of South India's

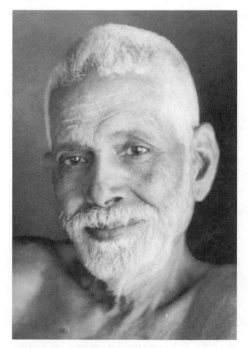

Ramana Maharshi

illustrious saints and sages, he was moved to spiritual life early on. One day he suddenly experienced an intense fear of death, which prompted him to picture his own cremation and dissolution. This imaginative exercise led to his discovery of the Self beyond the physical body. In this way he became Self-realized at the age of sixteen. After his enlightenment he settled for the remainder of his life on the sacred hill of Arunachala in Tiruvannamalai. At first he lived in various caves but later, at the request of a growing number of devotees, reluctantly agreed to move into a hermitage (*ashrama*). His peaceful presence attracted thousands of seekers from around the world. His fame in the West was primarily due to the advocacy of Paul Brunton (1898–1981), who wrote about his encounter with Ramana Maharshi in *A Search in Secret India* (1934).

He most often recommended to seekers the method by which he himself had become enlightened, namely, to ponder the question "Who am I?" This meditative inquiry (ātma-vicāra) is a version of the Vedantic method of *neti neti* ("not thus, not thus") and is intended to gradually penetrate the many false identities obscuring the real Self (*ātman*) beyond the ego personality.

RĀMĀNUJA (born in South India 1017 CE; said to have died 1137 CE, the founder of the Vishishta-Advaita ("Qualified Nondualism") school of *Vedānta and the leading theologian and philosopher of the medieval *bhakti* movement. A zealous proponent of *Vaishnavism, Rāmānuja converted numerous people to his religion and reportedly counted among his followers 700 ascetics as well as 12,000 monks and 300 nuns. His keen intellect and missionary enthusiasm made him the chief opponent of *Shankara's philosophy. Rāmānuja wrote brilliant commentaries on the *Brahma-Sūtra*, the **Bhagavad-Gītā*, and the major **Upanishads*, all of which occasioned a vast literature of subcommentary.

Rāmānuja taught that the *Absolute is not merely impersonal and unqualified but includes in its being the phenomenal *world as a part (**amsha*) of itself. He regarded the changeable world as the body of the *Divine and rejected the idealist notion that the universe is unreal (*mithyā*) or illusory (**māyā*). *God, whom Rāmānuja calls the "Lord" (**īshvara*), is the foundation of everything. God's existence cannot be inferred but must be accepted on the basis of revelation. Even though everything is dependent on God, there is also free will. A creature can turn toward or away from God. Those who turn to the *Divine with devotion (**bhakti*) receive God's favor (**prasāda*), which draws them ever closer to *liberation. For Rāmānuja, *bhakti* is not a state of emotional effusiveness but one of wisdom (**jnāna*). See also *prapatti*.

RĀMĀYANA ("Life of Rama") of Vālmīki, one of India's two national Sanskrit epics, the other being the **Mahābhārata*. The *Rāmāyana*, a tragic love story whose hero is *Rāma, was probably composed a little before the beginning of the common era, though its nucleus is very much older. It has served countless generations as a repository of folk wisdom. In its present form, the epic consists of seven chapters with a total of ca. 24,000 stanzas. The spiritual ideal of the *Rāmāyana* is that of asceticism (**tapas*) rather than *Yoga.

RAMDAS, SWAMI (1884–1963), a revered modern saint who taught a form of simple *japa-yoga*, the *Yoga of the constant *recitation of the name Rām (Sanskrit: Rāma). He renounced the world in 1922 and six years later founded the Ananda Ashram. He is the author of several books.

RASA ("essence") has several connotations. First, in the sense of "taste," it is associated with the *tongue and the *water element and thus is one of the functions of the cognitive senses (**indriya-jnāna*). By extension, *rasa* is one's "taste" for the objective *world, which, as the **Bhagavad-Gītā* (2.59) observes, lingers even after one abstains from "feeding" on the world. However, this subconscious relish—which is equivalent to the notion of **vāsanā*—disappears when the transcendental *Reality is realized.

Second, *rasa* is the "essence" of pure *bliss in the highest state of devotional surrender to the *Divine. It is the culmination of *bhakti-yoga. Third, in *alchemy, *rasa* refers to mercury. Fourth, in yogic alchemy, it stands for the "nectar of immortality" (**amrita*), the great life-giving elixir, hidden in the *body. According to the **Goraksha-Paddhati* (2.48), *rasa* can be made to flow copiously by "kissing," that is, stimulating the uvula (**rāja-danta*) with the *tongue. At first it tastes salty, pungent, and sour, but as the body becomes purified, it tastes like milk, honey, and ghee.

Finally, *rasa* stands for bodily liquid in general and the humors (**dosha*) in particular. Their "drying up" (*shoshana*) is effected by means of the "great seal" (**mahā-mudrā*).

RASA-ĀYANA (*rasāyana*). See Alchemy.

RATI (from the root *ram*, "to be delighted"), passionate love, as experienced by *Rādhā in relation to *Krishna. *Rati* is aesthetic *pleasure and its refined distillate of spiritual delight, the basic emotion of

the erotic spirituality of the *Bhāgavata religion. Thus the *Krishna followers made
a virtue out of what in other, more body-
negative schools is viewed as a vice. See
also *bhakti*.

RAVI ("sun"), a synonym for *sūrya*. Cf.
candra.

REALITY. See Absolute, Being, Divine,
God, *tattva*.

REASON. Even though most schools of
*Hinduism place great store in revelation
(*shruti*) and faith (*shraddhā*), it is readily
apparent from the available literature that
the Indians did not indulge in amorphous
irrationalism. The theological and philosophical masterpieces of *Shankara, *Rāmānuja, and *Vijnāna Bhikshu, e.g., compare in their acuity, learning, and lucidity
with the great works of Aristotle, St. Au-
gustine, and St. Thomas of Aquinas.
   The *Hindu authorities have shunned
neither reason nor intellect but merely determined and delimited their function and
usefulness. They clearly understood that
*Reality lies beyond reason, beyond the
mind (*manas*), even beyond illumined
reason or wisdom ("*buddhi*). Therefore
they have used rational arguments to show
the limits inherent in reason and to point
out a practical, experiential way by which
one's innate desire for *truth can be fulfilled—the demanding spiritual *paths of
*self-transcendence and self-transforma-
tion to the point of *Self-realization, or
*enlightenment. See also *tarka*.

REBIRTH. See *punar-janman*.

RECAKA ("exhalation"), also called *reca*
and *recya*; the expulsion, or outward flow,
of the life force (*prāna*); one of three aspects of breath control (*prānāyāma*). Cf.
kumbhaka, pūraka.

RECTITUDE. See *ārjava*.

REFLECTION. See *bimba, pratibimba*.

REFLECTION (consideration). See *tarka,
vicāra, vitarka*.

REFUTATION. See *apavāda*.

RELAXATION is fundamental to *meditation and other yogic disciplines. It implies
a loosening of the fixation of *attention on
the ego identity (*ahamkāra*), which represents a *contraction that conceals the
true nature of the *body and *mind (as
omnipresent). See also *shaithilya*.

RENUNCIATION. See Abandonment, *samnyāsa, tyāga*.

RESPIRATION. See Breath, *prāna, shvāsa*.

RESTRAINT. See *dama, niyama*.

RESTRAINT OF LIFE FORCE. See *prāna-
rodha*.

RESTRICTION. See *nirodha*.

RETAS ("semen"), a synonym for *bindu*.
According to the *Goraksha-Paddhati
(2.49), when the *body is filled with the
"nectar of immortality" (*amrita*), the
retas rises. This rising of the semen is a
psychosomatic process that is only inadequately characterized as sublimation. It
involves higher states of *consciousness.
See also *ūrdhva-retas*; cf. *rajas*.

REVELATION. See *shruti*; cf. Reason.

RIBHU, a *Vaishnava sage, referred to and
quoted in some of the later *Upanishads.
His nondualist teaching is also spoken of
in the *Vishnu-Purāna (1.15–16).

RIG-VEDA ("Knowledge of Praise"), the oldest of the four *Vedic collections (*samhitā*). Its date is in dispute, but it may be as far back as 3000 BCE or earlier still. It comprises ten chapters (called *mandala*) with a total of 1,028 hymns (*sūkta*, *mantra*). This work is the fountainhead of *Brāhmanism. The word *yoga* and its root *yuj* occur frequently in the *Rig-Veda* and generally have the meaning of "yoke" or "discipline," though there is as yet no systematic *path of *Yoga. Several important ideas and practices of later Yoga are foreshadowed in this hymnody, however, and these spiritual teachings can with some justification be referred to as "Archaic Yoga." See also History of Yoga, Indus-Sarasvati civilization, Preclassical Yoga, Veda.

RIJU-KĀYA ("erect body"), one of the characteristics of correct posture (*āsana*), according to the *Bhāgavata-Purāna (3.28.8). The *Yoga-Tattva-Upanishad (36) treats it as a requirement for the practice of *breath control.

RISHABHA, the name of several sages and kings. A Rishabha is remembered in the *Bhāgavata-Purāna (5.5.28ff.) as an *adept who besmeared himself with his own excreta but still emitted a sweet fragrance. In the *Shiva-Purāna (3.4.35) he is introduced as an incarnation of *Shiva. Rishabha is also the name of the first *tīrthankara of *Jainism.

RISHI ("seer"), the title of the *Vedic bard, who "sees" the hymn (*sūkta*, *mantra*) before composing it. *Rishi* and *mahārshi* (from *mahā* + *rishi*, "great seer") are honorific titles that are bestowed on saintly folk even today. A female seer is known as a *rishikā*. Three classes of *rishi* are generally recognized: *brahmarshi*

(from *brahma* + *rishi*), *rājarshi* (from *rāja* + *rishi*), and *devarshi* (from *deva* + *rishi*). *Vashishtha belonged to the first class, *Vishvāmitra to the second, and *Kāshyapa to the third. In each world cycle (*manvantara*) there are said to be seven great seers (known as the *saptarshis, from *sapta* and *rishi*). See also *keshin, muni*.

RITA ("truth" or "order"), a synonym for *satya. It is one of the key concepts of *Vedic times and expresses the universal harmony, both cosmic and moral. See also *dharma*.

RITAMBHARA-PRAJNĀ ("truth-bearing wisdom") is, as mentioned in the *Yoga-Sūtra (1.48), discovered by the *yogin at the culmination of the "ultrareflexive ecstasy" (*nirvicāra-samādhi). This special *knowledge is said to be "truth-bearing" because it discloses the contemplated *object as it is, without any mental distortions.

RITUAL, RITUALISM. *Yoga has always been connected with some form of religious or magical ritualism. However, certain schools are more ritualistic than others and include rites (*kriyā) as a significant aspect of their spiritual discipline. Particularly the yogic teachings mentioned in the *Purānas and *Tantras are pronouncedly ritualistic in their orientation. By contrast, the literature of *Classical Yoga, which inclines more toward the philosophical end of the spectrum, is relatively free of the ritual component.

RITUAL, PREPARATORY. See *purashcarana*.

ROGA ("illness"). For the *Yoga authorities, illness or disease (*vyādhi) confirms the fundamental insight of *Patanjali and Gautama *Buddha that "everything is suffering" (*sarvam duhkham*). As the *Mahābhārata* epic (12.318.3) puts it: "Bodily and mental illnesses pierce the *body like sharp-pointed arrows shot by a skilled archer." Although *Yoga is first and foremost a spiritual discipline leading to *self-transcendence and *Self-realization, health (*ārogya*) is valued, and some of the yogic practices clearly have prophylactic and therapeutic value. Especially many techniques of *hatha-yoga* are directly concerned with creating a "divine body" (*divya-deha*) that is absolutely immune to *disease.

According to the *Hatha-Yoga-Pradīpikā* (2.16f.), *breath control can cure all illnesses but when improperly practiced will cause all sorts of maladies, including asthma, cough, hiccup, and pain in the *head. Similar claims are made for certain cleansing practices (*dhauti*), "locks" (*bandha*), "seals" (*mudrā*), and even postures (*āsana*). Faulty yogic discipline can produce illnesses of its own. These are discussed together with their remedies in such works as the *Sat-Karma-Samgraha* and the *Mishraka*. See also *Āyur-Veda*, Medicine.

ROSARY. See *mālā*.

RUDRA ("Howler"), an independent *deity in *Vedic times, later became assimilated into *Shiva. In the *Shiva-Purāna* (7.1.32.36) the name is explained as "he who quells misery (*rud*)." Rudra appears to have been one of the deities invoked by the *Vrātya brotherhoods. See also *deva*.

RUDRA, a rare synonym for *prāna* or *vāyu*.

RUDRA-AKSHA (*rudrāksha*, "Rudra's eye"), the "third eye" in the middle of the *forehead, signifying the *ājnā-cakra*. See also *mālā*.

RUDRA-GRANTHI ("Rudra's knot"), one of the three "knots" (*granthi*) that block the flow of the *life force through the central channel (*sushumnā-nādī*) of the *body. It is located at the *ājnā-cakra* in the *head.

RULE. See *vidhi*.

RŪPA ("form"), a multipurpose word. It can denote the *body, physical beauty, a visible thing, or a psychic phenomenon, or "sign" (*cihna*). The last-mentioned meaning is found, for instance, in the *Mahābhārata* (12.228.18f.), which mentions the following visionary signs that can occur during *meditation: smoke, *water, *fire, an appearance "like a yellow garment," a phenomenon the color of wool. The *Shvetāshvatara-Upanishad* (2.11) lists phenomena resembling fog, smoke, *sun, fire, *wind, fireflies, lightning, crystal, and the *moon, which are said to be preliminary to the ultimate realization of *enlightenment. See also *mūrti*.

· S ·

SA-ĀNANDA-SAMĀPATTI (*sānanda-samāpatti*, "coinciding with bliss"), one of the subforms of conscious ecstasy (*sampra-jnāta-samādhi*) mentioned by *Vācaspati Mishra in his *Tattva-Vaishāradī* (1.44). It consists in the experience of bliss (*ān-

anda) as a result of practicing ecstatic "constraint" (*samyama*) with regard to the sense organs (*indriya*). See also *samādhi, samāpatti*; cf. *nirānanda-samāpatti*.

SA-ASMITĀ-SAMĀPATTI (*sāsmitā-samāpatti,* "coinciding with I-am-ness"), a subform of conscious ecstasy (*samprajñāta-samādhi*), according to the *Tattva-Vaishāradī* (1.44). It is the ecstatic experience of being present without any other mental content. See also *samādhi, samāpatti*; cf. *nirasmitā-samāpatti*.

SABĪJA-SAMĀDHI ("ecstasy with seed"), in *Classical Yoga, the technical name for various types of conscious ecstasy (*samprajñāta-samādhi*). According to the *Yoga-Bhāshya* (1.46), the "seed" (*bīja*) is the *object of *concentration. As *Vijnāna Bhikshu notes in his *Yoga-Vārttika* (1.46), however, the objects themselves are the seeds of *suffering. Thus they must ultimately be transcended in the state of supraconscious ecstasy (*asamprajñāta-samādhi*). See also *samādhi*; cf. *nirbīja-samādhi*.

SAC-CID-ĀNANDA ("existence, consciousness, bliss," from *sat, *cit, and *ānanda), the three essential aspects of the *Absolute, as taught in *Vedānta. These are not qualities, however, for the Absolute is unqualified (*nirguna*) and impartite (*akala*). Thus *bliss is not a state of *mind but the condition that remains when all psychomental phenomena, including the experience of *joy, have been transcended. See also Being.

SACRIFICE. The notion of sacrifice (*yajna, *hotra, *huta, *ijyā) is central to *Hinduism. The early *Vedic religion has rightly been characterized as one of sacrificial ritualism. During the period of the *Brāhmanas* this was developed into a full-fledged sacrificial *mysticism, which served as a bridge to the "inner sacrifice" of the *Upanishads* and later *Yoga. If the external sacrifice, involving a variety of *rituals, was the way to *heaven for the Vedic people, the sacrifice of the *self, or *ego, is the way to *liberation for the *yogin. Of course, the Vedic concept of heaven entailed more than the Christian elysium and in some passages of the *Vedas* appears to be understood in a sense similar to the later notion of *liberation.

SADĀ-SHIVA ("Eternal Shiva"), one of the many names of *Shiva as the ultimate *Reality.

SAD-GURU ("true teacher" or "teacher of the true"), an authentic spiritual *teacher who is *enlightened, or has realized the *Self. The *Kula-Arnava-Tantra* (13.104ff.) has these pertinent stanzas:

There are many teachers (*guru*), like lamps in house after house; but hard to find, O *Devī, is the teacher who lights up all like the sun.

There are many teachers who are proficient in the *Vedas* and the textbooks (*shāstra*); but hard to find, O Devī, is the teacher who has attained to the supreme *Truth.

There are many teachers on earth who give what is other than the *Self; but hard to find in all the worlds, O Devī, is the teacher who reveals the *Self.

Many are the teachers who rob the disciple of his wealth; but rare is the teacher who removes the *disciple's afflictions.

He is a [true] teacher by whose very contact there flows the supreme bliss (*ānanda*). The intelligent man should choose such a one as his teacher and none other.

SĀDHAKA, (masc.), or SĀDHIKĀ, (fem.; "accomplisher"), the *Tantric designation for the spiritual practitioner (*yogin or yoginī). According to the *Shiva-Samhitā (5.10), there are four types of practitioner, depending on their enthusiasm and commitment to the spiritual process: (1) The mridu-sādhaka ("soft practitioner") lacks zeal, is dull witted, sickly, greedy, attached to his wife, fickle, timid, ill, cruel, dependent on others, and given to evil deliberations; he finds fault with his *teacher and is a miracle monger (bahu-āshin, written bahvāshin). Such an individual is said to be fit for *mantra-yoga and may succeed after twelve years of diligent application. (2) The madhya-sādhaka ("middling practitioner") is even minded, patient, desirous of *virtue, soft spoken, and moderate in all undertakings. He is suited for *laya-yoga. (3) The adhimātra-sādhaka ("ardent practitioner") is fit for *hatha-yoga and may obtain success after six years of *practice. He is steady minded, disciplined, self-reliant, energetic, compassionate, patient, honest, courageous, mature, and filled with *faith; he also has high expectations, worships his teacher's *feet, and is constantly engaged in *Yoga practices. (4) The adhimātratama-sādhaka ("most ardent practitioner"), who qualifies for any type of Yoga and meets with success after only three years of practice, is highly energetic, zealous, agreeable, valiant, informed about the teachings (*shāstra), eager to practice, not deluded, not confused, in the prime of his youth, moderate in his *diet, with his *senses under control, fearless, clean, skillful, charitable, a support to all people, competent, firm, wise, content with his lot, forbearing, good natured, virtuous, well-spoken, and free from major *illnesses; he can also keep his endeavors secret, has faith in the teachings, worships his *teacher and the *deities, avoids public gatherings, and practices all forms of *Yoga.

SĀDHANA or SĀDHANĀ ("means of realization"), the spiritual *path, especially of *Tantrism, that leads to perfection (*siddhi). Although all authorities of *Yoga subscribe to the view that we are inherently free, they also concur that in order to realize that native *freedom, one must cultivate self-knowledge and an attitude of *dispassion. In other words, one must live from a disposition that is analogous to inherent freedom, or *enlightenment. This process of imitating the *Divine (imitatio Dei) is the very essence of the spiritual *path. See also ashta-anga-yoga, sapta-sādhana, shad-anga-yoga, yoga-kritya.

SĀDHIKĀ. SEE sādhaka.

SĀDHU (masc.), or SĀDHVĪ (fem.; "virtuous"), a saintly person who may or may not be a practitioner of *Yoga. Association (*sanga or sangama) with saintly folk has traditionally been considered to be one of the most rewarding practices. Sādhu-sanga, as the *Yoga-Vāsishtha (2.16.9) notes, "removes the darkness in one's *heart and is the lamp for the right *path in the world." See also sat-sanga.

SAGARBHA-PRĀNĀYĀMA ("breath control with seed"), the practice of breath control in conjunction with the mental or vocal recitation of a *bīja-mantra. Here the "seed" or bīja is called *garbha. Cf. a-garbha-prānāyāma, nirgarbha-prānāyāma.

SAGE. See muni; cf. keshin, rishi.

SAGUNA-BRAHMAN ("qualified Absolute"), the phenomenal dimension of *Reality composed of the three primary constituents (*guna) of *Nature. See also brahma-loka, brahman; cf. nirguna-brahman.

SAHAJA ("innate" or "spontaneous," from saha and ja, "to be born," lit. "together born" or "coemergent"), the idea that *freedom is not external to us but our very condition, that the phenomenal reality (*samsāra) arises simultaneously with, and within, the transcendental *Reality (*nirvāna), and that the conditional *mind and *enlightenment are not mutually exclusive principles. According to this teaching, true spontaneity or naturalness is an expression of *Reality, and enlightenment is always close at hand. The great Buddhist adept Sarahapāda calls this the "straight path" (uju-patha) or "royal path" (rāja-patha). This is a key notion of Mahāyāna *Buddhism and the *Sahajiyā movement.

SAHAJA-KARMAN ("spontaneous action"), a phrase found in the *Bhagavad-Gītā (18.48). It refers to *action that is in keeping with one's essential nature (*svabhāva). The Gītā is adamant that it is preferable to perform, even if only imperfectly, actions that are true to oneself rather than to perform perfectly actions that are true to another person's inner law (*svadharma). See also karma-yoga.

SAHAJA-SAMĀDHI ("spontaneous ecstasy"), explained in the Tri-Pura-Rahasya (17.107), an exceptional *Vedānta work, as the realization of unbroken transconceptual ecstasy (*nirvikalpa-samādhi) while being engaged in external activities. Supraconscious ecstasy (*asamprajnāta-samādhi), which is the yogic term for this elevated state of *consciousness, implies an extreme focusing of *attention with a concomitant withdrawal of one's awareness from the physical *body. As a result, this condition has often been con-fused with trance. However, the external "stonelike" existence fails to convey the *yogin's inner realization of the transcendental *Consciousness. By contrast, the sahaja-samādhi brings that realization down into the *body. The *yogin lives, as it were, in both worlds—the dimension of unqualified (*nirguna) existence and the dimension of relativity. Sahaja-samādhi is equivalent to full and permanent *enlightenment, or "liberation while being alive" (*jīvan-mukti). Within that condition, the liberated yogin may experience a variety of states of consciousness, including *savikalpa- or *samprajnāta-samādhi and *nirvikalpa- or *asamprajnāta-samādhi. See also sahaja, samādhi.

SAHAJIYĀ MOVEMENT, a development within the medieval *Vaishnava tradition that originated in Bengal and was associated with Sahajayāna *Buddhism on the one hand and Hindu *Tantrism on the other. As the name suggests, this movement was dedicated to the cultivation of the *sahaja state, primarily through the transmutation of sexual pleasure (*rati) into transcendental bliss (*ānanda or *mahā-sukha). *Yoga, in the form of *bhakti-yoga as spiritual eroticism, played a significant role in this movement. The ideal of sexual pleasure with a *woman other than one's wife—parakīya-rati—best expresses the spirit of the Sahajiyā teachings. The greatest figure of this movement is the fourteenth-century adept-poet *Candīdāsa. The *Bauls also belong to this remarkable manifestation of *Hindu spirituality, though they conceive of the sexual-spiritual union as occurring within one's own *heart rather than externally through intercourse (*maithunā). See also rasa, sama-rasa.

SAHAJOLĪ-MUDRĀ ("*sahajolī* seal"), a variation of the *vajrolī-mudrā* described in the *Hatha-Yoga-Pradīpikā* (3.92ff.). It consists in besmearing the *body, after intercourse (*maithunā*), with a mixture of water and *ashes obtained from the burning of cow dung. This process is said to succeed only in the case of a virtuous practitioner who is brave and free from *jealousy. See also *mudrā*; cf. *amarolī-mudrā*.

SĀHASA ("boldness"), one of the six factors that promote *Yoga, according to the *Hatha-Yoga-Pradīpikā* (1.16). Timidity clearly has no place in Yoga, which is experiential and even experimental, one's own body-mind being the laboratory. Boldness is not, however, recklessness.

SAHASRĀRA-CAKRA ("thousand-spoked wheel," from *sahasra* and *ara*), the topmost center (*cakra*) of the body's psychospiritual energy (*prāna*). It is situated at

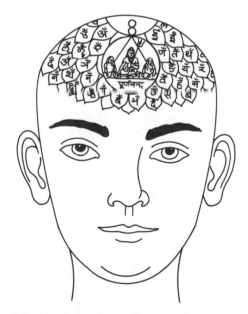

Sahasrāra-cakra, the psychoenergetic center at the crown of the head

the crown of the *head and is also called the "thousand-petaled lotus" (*sahasra-dala-padma*), the "great seat" (*mahā-pītha*), and the "ether wheel" (*ākāsha-cakra*). The *Kaula-Jnāna-Nirnaya* (5.8) describes it as a white lotus floating in the middle of the universal "milk ocean" in whose center resides the *Self. The *Shiva-Samhitā* (5.102, 122f.) gives three different locations for it: the root of the palate (*tālu*), the "brahmic fissure" (*brahma-randhra*), and outside the *body (above the head). Only the last two locations are generally accepted.

The *Shaiva adherents visualize the *sahasrāra-cakra* as Mount Kailāsa, the abode of *Shiva and his spouse, *Pārvatī (or simply *Devī). For the *Vaishnavas it is the locus of the "supreme person" (*parama-purusha*), i.e., *Vishnu. This is the upper terminal point of the central channel (*sushumnā-nādī*) and the final destination of the awakened "serpent power" (*kundalinī-shakti*). When the *kundalinī*, the force of Devī, reaches this center, this signals the merging of *Shiva and *Shakti.

The thousand spokes or petals of this bell-shaped psychospiritual center are arranged in twenty layers, with fifty petals each. Each petal is visualized as having one letter (*mātrikā*) of the Sanskrit alphabet inscribed in it, forming a ring, which is known as the "five-crested garland" (*panca-shikhā-mālā*). In the pericarp of the lotus is the "lunar region" (*candra-mandala*), which emits nectarine *light. It contains a luminous triangle within which is the void (*shūnya*), also called the "supreme seed point" (*parama-bindu*), the abode of transcendental *Consciousness-Bliss. See also *dvādasha-anta*.

SAHITA-KUMBHAKA ("combined retention"), one of the eight types of *breath control mentioned in the *Gheranda-Samhitā (5.47f.). It is of two kinds: *sagarbha* ("with seed") and *nigarbha* ("without seed"). The "seed" or "womb" (*garbha) is the sacred syllable *om. The former type is practiced together with the *recitation of the syllable *om (as *aum*), whereby one inhales (reciting *a*) for 16 measures, retains the breath (reciting *u*) for 64 measures, and exhales (reciting *m*) for 32 measures. One should alternate nostrils. *Nigarbha-kumbhaka* consists simply in controlling the *breath without repetition of the *bīja-mantra*, and inhalation, retention, and exhalation can be regulated from 1 to 100 measures (*mātra), which are to be counted by circling the left knee with the palm of the left hand. See also *kumbhaka, prānāyāma.*

SĀKSHĀT-KĀRANA or SĀKSHĀT-KĀRA ("sensing with the eyes," from *sa*, "with," and *aksha*, "eye"), also known as "*yogin*'s perception" (*yogi-pratyaksha); the unmediated *perception of things in the state of ecstasy (*samādhi). Although no sensory input is involved, the *yogin, through the ecstatic process, becomes identical with the *object, thereby experiencing it from within itself. This term is often applied to *Self-realization. Cf. *grahana.*

SĀKSHIN ("witness"), a common designation for the transcendental *Self. The *witness consciousness has been hailed as the great discovery of Indian spirituality. See also *drashtri.*

SAMA ("same" or "equal"), a favorite expression of the *Bhagavad-Gītā, where it is used on its own and in conjunction with nouns, especially as *sama-darshana. The underlying idea is conveyed in stanza 9.29 thus: "I [*Krishna] am the same in all beings. To Me none is hateful or dear."

The *Absolute, or *Divine, is omnipres-

ent. All things are arising in and as it. Hence nothing in the *world is alien to it, and such notions as hateful rejection or passionate favoritism do not apply. The *yogin is asked to emulate this spirit of perfect equality (*samatva). Thus the *Bhagavad-Gītā (12.18f.) states:

He who is the same toward friend and foe and also toward fame and ill-fame, the same in cold and heat, *pleasure and *suffering, without *attachment;

who is the same in blame and praise, is silent and content with everything, "homeless" and of steady *mind, and who loves [me]—that man is dear to me.

On the surface, this statement seems to contradict *Krishna's claim to flawless impartiality. However, what is spoken of here is an esoteric fact rather than a theological doctrine: Through love-devotion (*bhakti), the *yogin can directly participate in the blissful being of the *Divine. He opens himself to the ever-present divine grace (*prasāda), experiencing the love of *Krishna.

SAMA-BUDDHI ("same-mindedness"), the attitude of inner aloofness by which the *yogin comes to regard a clod of earth or a piece of gold with equal *tranquillity. This yogic ideal of sublime indifference is balanced by the positive orientation toward the common weal (*sarva-bhūta-hita), which is likewise recommended in the *Bhagavad-Gītā (12.4).

SAMA-CITTATVA ("same-mindedness"), a synonym for *sama-buddhi. The *Bhagavad-Gītā (13.8–9) regards this mature attitude as a manifestation of wisdom (*jnāna).

SAMA-DARSHANA ("even vision" or "vision of the same"), the state of the person who beholds the *Self in everything. The *Bhagavad-Gītā (6.32) celebrates such a person as the foremost of *yogins.

SAMĀDHĀNA ("collectedness"), a synonym for *samādhi.

SAMĀDHI ("ecstasy"), the final "limb" (*anga) of the yogic *path. The *Gheranda-Samhitā (7.1) speaks of samādhi as a "great *Yoga," which is acquired through good fortune and through the *grace and kindness of one's *teacher and by virtue of one's *devotion to him. The *Tri-Shikhi-Brāhmana-Upanishad (2.31) describes ecstasy as the "perfect forgetting" of the state of *meditation, which precedes it. The *Yoga-Sūtra (3.3) speaks of it as that condition in which consciousness (*citta) shines forth as the intended object. That is to say, in samādhi there is a merging of subject and object. The *Kūrma-Purāna (2.11.41) explains this state as being one of "uniformity" (eka-ākāra). The Paingalā-Upanishad (3.4) offers this explanation: "Ecstasy is [that condition where] *consciousness ranges only with the object of meditation (dhyeya) and, like a lamp placed in a windless [spot], is oblivious of meditator (dhyātri) and meditation (*dhyāna)."

Ordinarily, ecstasy is accompanied by complete sensory inhibition, as effected through the techniques of sense withdrawal (*pratyāhāra) and meditation. Some works, such as the *Mani-Prabhā (3.12) and various *Purānas, explain that samādhi has the duration and intensity of twelve *meditations, which implies abstraction from the external environment. Ecstasy is thought to have magical properties as well. This is made clear in the *Hatha-Yoga-Pradīpikā (4.108ff.):

The *yogin yoked by ecstasy is not devoured by time (*kāla), is not bound by [his] actions (*karman), and cannot be overpowered by others.

The yogin yoked by ecstasy knows neither himself nor others and does not [experience] smell, taste, sight (*rūpa), touch, or *sound.

The yogin yoked by ecstasy does not experience cold or heat, *sorrow or *joy, honor or contempt.

The yogin yoked by ecstasy is immune to [magical influences from] *mantras and *yantras and is invulnerable to any weapon and unassailable by any person.

All traditions distinguish at least between two major types of ecstasy: *savikalpa- or samprajnāta-samādhi, the samādhi involving identification with an *object and accompanied by higher thought forms (called *prajnā), and *nirvikalpa- or *asamprajnāta-samādhi, the samādhi that consists in one's identification with the transcendental *Self and is devoid of any content of *consciousness. Only the second variety can lead to *Self-realization, or *liberation, by way of the complete transmutation of consciousness. Some schools also know of a third type of ecstatic condition: "spontaneous ecstasy" (*sahaja-samādhi), which is equivalent to liberation while still in the embodied state, or *jīvanmukti.

According to the *Yoga-Cūdāmanī-Upanishad (110), samādhi leads first to "wondrous consciousness" (caitanya-adbhuta) and subsequently to liberation (*moksha). The wonders of *consciousness are indeed accessed through the various states of *samprajnāta-samādhi. In fact, these states are the *yogin's way of doing research, as is evident from the third chapter of the *Yoga-Sūtra, which introduces examples of the method of ecstatic "constraint" (*samyama). But ultimately, all forms of yogic gnosis (*prajnā) must be transcended as well, so that only the vision of the *Self remains. As the *Garuda-Purāna* (49.36) puts it, *samādhi* is that condition in which the *yogin* realizes "I am the *Absolute." Hence *samādhi* is often defined in the *Vedānta and Vedānta-dependent schools as the "union of the psyche (*jīva*) with the Self (*ātman*)." For "union" (*samyoga*), some authorities substitute "sameness" (*samatva*) or "identity" (*aikya*). The *Hatha-Yoga-Pradīpikā* (4.5ff.) has the following famous simile:

As salt mingles with and dissolves in water, similarly the merging of the *mind and the *Self is ecstasy.

When the life force (*prāna*) is compressed [in the central channel, or *sushumnā-nādī*] and the mind is dissolved, then there is coessentiality (*sama-rasatva*), which is designated as ecstasy.

That equilibrium (*sama*) or identity of the individual self and the supreme Self [in which] all volition is absent is designated as ecstasy.

This event of *Self-realization alone destroys, in the words of the *Yoga-Yājnavalkya* (10.1), the "noose of existence" (*bhava-pāsha*). Therefore *samādhi* is occasionally equated with *liberation, or *enlightenment.

The most complete model of ecstatic states is that of *Classical Yoga. The following forms of *samādhi* are given in descending order: (1) supraconscious ecstasy (*asamprajnāta-samādhi*); and (2) conscious ecstasy (*samprajnāta-samādhi*), with its subforms (a) suprareflexive clarity (*nirvicāra-vaishāradya*), (b) suprareflexive ecstasy (*nirvicāra-samādhi*), (c) reflexive ecstasy (*savicāra-samādhi*), (d) supracogitative ecstasy (*nirvitarka-samādhi*), and (e) cogitative ecstasy (*savitarka-samādhi*).

The different forms of conscious ecstasy also bear the technical designation of "coincidence" (*samāpatti*), referring to the coinciding between subject and object, which is the hallmark of true ecstatic states. Some authorities, such as *Vācaspati Mishra, insert the following additional states before the above-mentioned subcategories of conscious ecstasy: (a) ecstasy beyond I-am-ness (*nirasmitā-samāpatti*), (b) ecstasy with I-am-ness (*sa-asmitā-samāpatti*), (c) ecstasy beyond bliss (*nirānanda-samāpatti*), and (d) ecstasy with bliss (*sa-ānanda-samāpatti*). The legitimacy of this scheme is doubtful and was rejected already by *Vijnāna Bhikshu.

The term *samādhi* is also used to denote the circular grave of the *yogin. In India ascetics are buried in the cross-legged position, whereas the ordinary person is cremated. Cremation is seen as a rite of passage for those who have not been purified by the fire of *Yoga. See also *nimīlana-samādhi*, *pratimīlana-samādhi*, *unmīlana-samādhi*.

SAMA-DRISHTI ("even vision"), a synonym for *sama-darshana*.

SAMA-KĀYA ("even body"), one of the results of correct *Yoga practice and one of the positive signs (*cihna*).

SAMĀNA (from the prefix *sam*, "together," and the root *an*, "to breathe"), one of the principal currents of the life force (*prāna*), which pervades all limbs and is responsible for nourishing the *body by distributing food as *rasa. According to the *Linga-Purāna* (1.8.65), it normalizes the bodily functions. Many *hatha-yoga texts place it in the region of the *navel, but the *Mahābhārata* (12.177.24) assigns it to the *heart. According to the *Yoga-Sūtra* (3.40), mastery of the *samāna* current leads to "effulgence" (*jvalana*).

SAMANU. See *nādī-shodhana*.

SAMĀPATTI ("coincidence"), in *Classical Yoga, the ecstatic identification with the object of *contemplation. In this sense, it is synonymous with or the underlying process of *samādhi. See also *ananta-samāpatti, nirānanda-samāpatti, nirasmitā-samāpatti, nirvicāra-samāpatti, nirvitarka-samāpatti, sa-ānanda-samāpatti, sa-asmitā-samāpatti, savicāra-samāpatti, nirvicāra-samāpatti.

SAMA-RASA ("even essence" or "equilibration"), the process and state of resonating bodily in harmony with the *Divine; an important concept of the *Siddha movement, especially *hatha-yoga. According to the *Siddha-Siddhānta-Paddhati (5.4), this condition presupposes yogic *knowledge of the *body's structure and the *grace of one's *teacher.

SAMA-RASATVA ("equilibrium"), a synonym for *sama-rasa.

SAMA-SAMSTHĀNA ("even position"), a posture (*āsana) mentioned in the *Yoga-Bhāshya (2.46). It is described by *Vācaspati Mishra in his commentary thereon as follows. Pull in the *feet and press them against each other at the heels and the toes.

SAMATVA or SAMATĀ ("evenness" or "equanimity"), an important concept in the *Bhagavad-Gītā, which (2.47) defines *Yoga as equability (samatva). Because the same transcendental *Absolute underlies all phenomenal forms, to realize that fundamental sameness through the attitude of equanimity and even-mindedness is deemed the greatest spiritual *virtue. The *Shiva-Samhitā (3.18) regards this orientation as a precondition for success in Yoga. According to the *Laghu-Yoga-Vāsishtha (4.5.12), samatā is what remains when

all volitional activity (*samkalpa) has ceased. The *Yoga-Tattva-Upanishad (107) understands the term as the "sameness," or union, of the individual psyche (*jīva) with the transcendental *Self.

SĀMA-VEDA ("Knowledge of Songs," from sāman, "song" or "chant"), one of the four *Vedic hymnodies. This collection contains 1,875 verses, of which 1,800 were adopted from the *Rig-Veda. The hymns of the Sāma-Veda were chanted during the sacrificial *rituals, and this practice became early on associated with breath control (*prānāyāma), one of the most important aspects of *Yoga. See also Veda.

SAMĀVESHA or ĀVESHA ("entering"), in Kashmiri *Shaivism, the *adept's ecstatic absorption into the divine *consciousness; thus, a synonym for the highest form of *samādhi.

SAMBANDHAR, one of the greatest and still one of the most revered *Shaiva worshipers of South India. He was a contemporary of the seventh-century adept *Appar, with whom he traveled for several months. One of Sambandhar's verses opens the entire Shaiva canon, and his devotional songs show his extraordinary mystical intimacy with *Shiva and his divine spouse, *Pārvatī. He composed more than 4,000 verses, all of which were set to music, and he was largely responsible for the revival of Tamil musical poetry. He also was a great miracle worker, and among his finest miracles was the conversion to *Shaivism of the hunchbacked Jaina ruler Kun Pandya, whom he relieved of his ugly disfigurement. See also Nayanmar.

SAME-MINDEDNESS. See sama-buddhi, sama-cittatva.

SAMHĀRA ("retraction"), the destruction of the *cosmos at the end of an eon (*kalpa); also, the dissolution of the *elements in the course of *meditation, in which case it is a synonym for *laya.

SAMHITĀ ("collection"), the title given to a genre of sacred works in the tradition of *Vaishnavism. The four *Vedic hymnodies also carry this designation, as do a number of *Yoga manuals, such as the *Gheranda-Samhitā and the *Shiva-Samhitā.

SAMKALPA ("volition," "intention," or "fancy"), sometimes listed as one of the functions of the "inner instrument" (*antahkarana), or *mind. According to the *Shvetāshvatara-Upanishad (5.8), volition and "I maker" (*ahamkāra) together characterize the finite personality. The *Yoga-Vāsishtha (6b.1.27) defines it as "mental bondage" (mano-bandha), while the absence of volition is said to be *liberation (vimuktatā). The *Bhagavad-Gītā (6.2) notes that one becomes a *yogin by renouncing all volitional activity, which breeds desire (*kāma). The *Varāha-Upanishad (2.45), again, speaks of samkalpa as the real origin of the *world and states that it should be abandoned in favor of *nirvikalpa (-samādhi).

SAMKATA-ĀSANA (samkatāsana, "critical posture") described in the *Gheranda-Samhitā (2.28) thus: Place the left foot on the ground and encircle the left leg with the right leg, placing the hand on one's knees.

SAMKETA ("convention"), a technical term employed in the *Yoga-Shāstra (41ff.) of *Dattātreya to denote specific foci of *concentration, such as the *contemplation of the void (*shūnya) or the space in front of one's *nose. See also desha.

SĀMKHYA ("number"), an archaic form of ontology; also, an adherent of Sāmkhya. The name derives from the Sāmkhya authorities' enumeration of the categories (*tattva) of existence. Sāmkhya distinguishes between twenty-four or twenty-five major ontic categories, the two principal categories being that of the transcendental *Self (*purusha) and that of *nature (*prakriti). The remaining categories pertain to the different levels of manifestation in nature. The spiritual *path of Sāmkhya consists in the careful differentiation between purusha and prakriti and the complete *renunciation of everything that is other than the Self, which is the only principle endowed with *consciousness. This practice of discernment (*viveka) hints at the other meaning of the term samkhyā: "insight" or "investigative understanding."

Like *Yoga, the Sāmkhya tradition has a protracted history whose beginnings can-

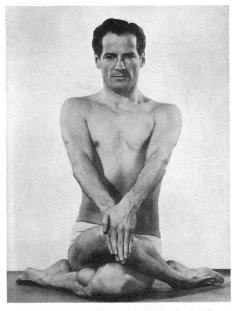

Samkata-āsana, demonstrated by Theos Bernard

not be precisely determined. Proto-Sāmkhya elements can be found already in the hymns of the *Rig-Veda and *Atharva-Veda. The *Mahābhārata (notably the *Bhagavad-Gītā and *Moksha-Dharma sections) and such esoteric texts as the *Katha-, *Shvetāshvatara-, and *Maitrāyanīya-Upanishad represent preclassical schools of Sāmkhya, which developed in the period between 500 and 200 BCE. These schools show a close connection with the tradition of Yoga, to the degree that both are often mentioned together, as *sāmkhya-yoga. However, there are also passages in the *Moksha-Dharma that make a clear distinction between Sāmkhya and Yoga, though emphasizing that both lead to the same goal. Thus one passage of the *Mahābhārata (12.289.7) delineates the two traditions by stating that whereas Yoga relies on perception (*pratyaksha), Sāmkhya is based on tradition (or the testimony of *adepts). In the *Bhagavad-Gītā (5.4) Yoga is equated with *karma-yoga and Sāmkhya with the path of renunciation (*samnyāsa), though in the next stanza their essential unity is stressed.

The sage *Kapila is celebrated as the founder of Sāmkhya, though nothing definite is known about him. This ramified and once obviously influential tradition reached its zenith in the classical formulations of *Īshvara Krishna, author of the *Sāmkhya-Kārikā. There is also an aphoristic (*sūtra) compilation, the Sāmkhya-Sūtra, ascribed to Kapila, but this is generally thought to be of a much later date (prob. 14th cent. CE), and it differs philosophically in many respects from Īshvara Krishna's teachings. From about 1000 CE on, the Sāmkhya tradition declined until *Vijñāna Bhikshu's valiant attempts at reviving Sāmkhya metaphysics in the light of *Vedānta nondualism. Often *Patanjali's *yoga-darshana is wrongly held to have

been simply grafted onto Sāmkhya metaphysics, whereas in fact his teachings represent an original yogic point of view.

SĀMKHYA-YOGA, a spiritual approach based on insight into the nature of worldly existence and the transcendental *Self, as characteristic of Preclassical *Sāmkhya. In the *Matsya-Purāna (52.2) it is equated with *jnāna-yoga and contrasted with *karma-yoga, or "ritual *Yoga." In the *Laghu-Yoga-Vāsishtha (6.7.13) the sāmkhya-yogin is juxtaposed to the yoga-yogin. The same distinction is made in the Anna-Pūrna-Upanishad (5.49), where the former is said to awaken by means of ecstasy (*samādhi) and the complete restriction of *knowledge, whereas the latter reaches *liberation through the tranquilization of the life force (*prāna).

SAMKOCA ("contraction"). According to Kashmiri *Shaivism, the transcendental creativity of *Shiva, known as visarga, consists of two movements: expansion (vistāra, also called vikāsa) and contraction (samkoca). The *world is the direct result of the self-contraction within the infinite body of Shiva. Only in its form as spiritual ignorance (*ajnāna) is this contraction binding and therefore must be removed through *Yoga.

SAMMOHA ("confusion") arises, according to the *Bhagavad-Gītā (2.63), from contact with the sense objects (*vishaya). The *Maitrāyanīya-Upanishad (3.2), which employs the synonym sammūdhatva, declares that as a result of this fundamental confusion, one cannot behold the *Lord.

SAMNIDHI ("proximity"), a technical term used in the *Yoga-Bhāshya (1.4) to describe the transcendental closeness between the *Self and consciousness (*citta) by virtue of which it is possible for the Self to apperceive the cognitions (*buddhi) of the finite *mind. See also samyoga.

SAMNYĀSA ("renunciation"), a fundamental orientation within *Hinduism, which, like *Yoga, has produced its own values, practices, and literature (e.g., the *Samnyāsa-Upanishads). It is as old as the oldest *Upanishads. The *Bhagavad-Gītā (18.2) explains samnyāsa as the *renunciation, or inner *sacrifice, of *actions dictated by *desire, or (6.2) as the renunciation of volition (*samkalpa). This is contrasted with *tyāga, or the relinquishing of the fruit (*phala) of all one's actions, which is essential to *karma-yoga. Mere renunciation is held (5.2) to be inferior to *karma-yoga. See also Abandonment.

SAMNYĀSA-YOGA ("Yoga of renunciation"), a compound found in several works of *Preclassical Yoga, including the *Bhagavad-Gītā (9.28) and the *Mundaka-Upanishad (3.2.6). It simply refers to the practice of *renunciation.

SAMNYĀSA-UPANISHADS (Samnyāsopanishads), *Upanishads that specifically expound renunciation (*samnyāsa). Generally nineteen such works are mentioned, several of which are approximately 1,000 years old.

SAMNYĀSIN ("renouncer"), typified in the *Bhagavad-Gītā (5.3) as the person who neither hates nor desires anything and who is above the "pairs of opposites" (*dvandva). See also samnyāsa.

SAMPRAJÑĀTA-SAMĀDHI ("conscious ecstasy"), in *Classical Yoga, a range of ecstatic experiences that have an objective prop (*ālambana) with which conscious-

ness (*citta) becomes identified and which is associated with superior knowledge (*prajñā). According to the *Yoga-Sūtra (1.17), the principal forms of conscious ecstasy are *vitarka-, *vicāra-, *ānanda-, and *asmitā-samāpatti (or -samādhi). The *Yoga-Bhāshya (1.17) proposes the following schema to understand the composition of each of these four forms:

vitarka ("cogitation") =
   vitarka + vicāra + ānanda + asmitā
vicāra ("reflection") =
               vicāra + ānanda + asmitā
ānanda ("bliss") =
                        ānanda + asmitā
asmitā ("I-am-ness") =
                                  asmitā

Thus the coarser (*sthūla) aspects contain the subtler aspects, whereas the grosser aspects fall away as the more subtle aspects are reached in the state of ecstasy. *Vācaspati Mishra suggests in his *Tattva-Vaishāradī (1.47) that the focus of the

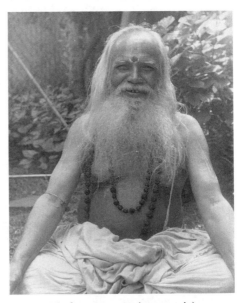

Hindu renouncer (samnyāsin)

first two types are the coarse and the subtle objects of existence, whereas the focus of the third type are the *senses and of the fourth type the ego principle (*asmitā). Vācaspati further argues that each of these four forms has a higher form in which all conscious content is stilled: *nirvitarka-, *nirvicāra-, *nirānanda-, and *nirasmitā-samāpatti. However, this typology of eight forms of conscious *ecstasy is explicitly denied by *Vijñāna Bhikshu, who admits of only six types. He states that the object of "coinciding with bliss" (*ānanda-samā-patti) is *bliss itself, and the object of "co-inciding with 'I-am-ness' " (*asmitā-sam-āpatti) is the intuition (*samvid) of the absolute *Self (kevala-purusha). Thus there are no nirānanda and nirasmitā forms of ecstatic mergence.

These six (or eight) types of sampra-jnāta-samādhi correspond to the *savi-kalpa-samādhi in *Vedānta. Superior to them is the supraconscious ecstasy (*asamprajnāta-samādhi), which reveals the transcendental *Self. See also samādhi, samāpatti.

SAMPUTA-YOGA ("bowl union"), a technical term in *Abhinavagupta's writings signifying the perfect self-containedness of the ultimate *Reality, which is called *Shiva. This term also refers to the practice of samputī-karana, which consists in "enclosing" a principal *mantra with another mantra. Finally, it refers to the sexual union (*maithunā) between male and female partners in the *Tantric ritual.

SAMRAMBHA-YOGA ("Yoga of hatred"). In the *Vaishnava tradition, the strong emotion of hatred, like *love, is sometimes regarded as a means of *Self-realization. A classic example is Hiranyakashipu, the father of *Prahlāda, whose abiding hatred of the *Divine finally led to his spiritual *lib-eration. Hatred can thus be a form of involuntary spiritual practice, based on the esoteric principle that one becomes what one meditates on. See also dvesha.

SAMSĀRA ("flow"), the phenomenal *world, as opposed to the transcendental or noumenal *Reality, whether it be called *nirvāna, *brahman, or *ātman. The word samsāra (from the root sri, "to flow") conveys well the idea that finite existence is a constant flux of events in which no permanence and security can be found. The eternal, transcendental *Self alone serves as a refuge to those wishing to escape the changeability of nature (*prakriti). Samsāra is, above all, the domain of *karma and *rebirth and thus of unmitigated suffering (*duhkha). The *Varāha-Upanishad (2.64) describes it as a long dream (*svapna), a protracted delusion of the *mind, and a sea of *sorrow. As the *Mai-trāyanīya-Upanishad (6.28) puts it, those who are *liberated look down upon the samsāra as upon a dizzily revolving wheel (*cakra). The *Yoga-Bhāshya (4.11) explains that this world wheel, which turns owing to the power of spiritual ignorance (*avidyā), has six spokes: virtue (*dharma) and vice (*adharma), pleasure (*sukha) and pain (*duhkha), and attachment (*rāga) and aversion (*dvesha).

SAMSĀRIN ("worldling"), the being, or psyche (*jīva), who is entrapped in the ever-changing world (*samsāra) of natural and moral *causation. Cf. Self.

SAMSHAYA ("doubt"), a major obstacle (*antarāya) on the yogic *path. It is named in the *Yoga-Kundalī-Upanishad (1.59) as one of the ten obstructions (*vighna) foiling spiritual growth. The *Yoga-Bhāshya (1.30) defines it as a kind of thought (*vijñāna) that touches both alternatives of a dilemma. This work (1.35) also claims that doubt can be effectively dispelled by suprasensory awareness (*divya-sampad*), which creates *faith in the practitioner. According to the *Bhagavad-Gītā (4.40), doubt afflicts the person who lacks faith (*shraddhā*) and ultimately can destroy him or her. As the *Matsya-Purāna (110.10) notes laconically, a person who is inclined toward doubt merely reaps *pain, not *Yoga. Availing itself of a popular image, the *Bhagavad-Gītā (4.42) states that only the sword of wisdom (*jnāna*) can cut through the doubts harbored in one's *heart.

SAMSKĀRA ("activator"), in the general sense of "ritual," denotes any of such rites of passage as the birth ceremony, tonsure, and marriage. In *Yoga, however, the word has a psychological significance. It stands for the indelible imprints in the *subconscious left behind by our daily experiences, whether conscious or unconscious, internal or external, desirable or undesirable. The term *samskāra* suggests that these imprints are not merely passive vestiges of a person's *actions and *volitions but highly dynamic forces in his or her psychic life. They constantly propel *consciousness into action. The *Yoga-Sūtra (3.9) distinguishes two varieties of subliminal activators: those that lead to the externalization (*vyutthāna*) of *consciousness and those that cause the inhibition (*nirodha*) of the processes of consciousness. The *yogin must cultivate the latter type of *samskāra* in order to achieve the condition of ecstasy (*samādhi*), which prevents the renewed generation of subliminal activators. According to the *Yoga-Sūtra (1.50), at the highest level of conscious ecstasy (*samprajnāta-samādhi*) a subliminal activator is generated that obstructs all others and thus leads over into

the condition of supraconscious ecstasy (*asamprajnāta-samādhi*). See also *āshaya*, *karma*, Unconsciousness, *vāsanā*.

SAMTOSHA ("contentment") ranks among the constituent practices of self-discipline (*niyama*) in *Classical Yoga and, according to the *Yoga-Sūtra (2.42), leads to unexcelled joy (*sukha*). The *Darshana-Upanishad (2.4–5) explains it as delight with whatever *fate may bring. This medieval work also speaks of supreme contentment (*para-samtosha*), which is that agreeable condition that results from perfect indifference (*virakti*) and terminates in the realization of the *Absolute. The *Mahābhārata (12.21.2) praises contentment as follows: "Contentment is indeed the highest *heaven. Contentment is supreme joy. There is nothing higher than satisfaction (*tushti*). It is complete in itself." The *Laghu-Yoga-Vāsishtha (2.1.73) explains it as "evenness" (*samatā*) toward hardship and ease, as well as toward things one has obtained and things that are far from one's reach.

SAMVID ("consciousness" or "awareness"), a synonym for *cit. In Kashmiri *Shaivism, it is short for *parā-samvid* or "supreme Consciousness." See also *ahamtā*.

SAMYAG-DARSHANA ("perfect vision"), according to the *Yoga-Bhāshya (2.15), the means to *liberation from pain (*duhkha*), following upon the obliteration of the five causes of suffering (*klesha*). The *Manu-Smriti (6.74) declares that he who is endowed with perfect vision is never bound by his *actions. See also *jnāna*, *vidyā*, *viveka*, Wisdom.

SAMYAMA ("constraint"), explained in the *Yoga-Sūtra (3.4) of *Patanjali as the continuous practice of concentration (*dhāraṇā*), meditation (*dhyāna*), and ecstasy (*samādhi*) upon the same *object. This technique is the *yogin's way of doing research, since it yields all kinds of suprasensuous knowledge (*prajñā). The term *samyama* is also sometimes used in the sense of "control," particularly in connection with the mastery of the *senses.

SAMYOGA ("correlation" or "connection"), in *Classical Yoga, the correlation that exists between the transcendental Self (*purusha*) and nature (*prakriti*), i.e., between transcendental *Awareness and empirical consciousness (*citta*). This correlation, or connection, is at the root of all suffering (*duhkha*). It is caused by spiritual nescience (*avidyā*) and is removed through wisdom (*prajñā*). *Patanjali maintains that the contact between the *Self and the experienced object (*drishya*) is merely an apparent junction, since both the Self and experiential *nature are by definition utterly distinct. He does not analyze this epistemological problem further. This has led to a great deal of speculation in the literature of commentary on the *Yoga Sūtra. Thus *Vācaspati Mishra speaks of that enigmatic relationship in terms of a special fitness (*yogyatā*) between the Self and consciousness. As he elucidates in his *Tattva-Vaishāradī (2.17), the *sattva* aspect of the *mind contains the reflection (*bimba*) of the transcendental Awareness (*caitanya*), which yields the illusion of the empirical consciousness. *Vijnāna Bhikshu even speaks of a "counter-reflection" (*pratibimba*) of the mental states in the Self.

The historical germ for these philosophical speculations can be found in the literature of *Preclassical Yoga. Thus the *Bhagavad-Gītā (13.26) mentions the connection between the "field" (*kshetra*) and

the "field knower" (*kshetra-jna*), which underlies the coming into being of all creatures. This scripture (5.14) also employs the word *samyoga* in regard to the causal nexus between action (*karman*) and its fruit (*phala*). See also *samnidhi*.

SANĀTANA-DHARMA ("eternal teaching"), the traditional name given to *Hinduism by its adherents.

SANATKUMĀRA, apparently the name of several sages. Sanatkumāra is first mentioned in the ancient *Chāndogya-Upanishad (7.1ff.). The *Mahābhārata (12.327.64) lists Sanatkumāra together with the sages Sana, Sanaka, Sānandana, Sanātana, and Sanatsujāta, as a knower of *Yoga and *Sāmkhya. He also figures as a renowned teacher in some of the *Purānas and later *Upanishads.

SANCITA-KARMA ("accumulated karma"). See *karma*.

SANDALS. See *pādukā*.

SANDHĀ-BHĀSHĀ ("intentional language") or SANDHYA-BHĀSHĀ ("twilight language"), the technical name given to the symbolic language of *Tantrism, both in its *Hindu and *Buddhist variety. The texts seem to prefer the former reading, though there has been controversy in scholarly circles regarding which of the two expressions is more accurate (see, e.g., Agehananda Bharati, 1965). Examples of Tantric symbolic language are words like *vajra* ("thunderbolt," standing for the *penis), *bodhicitta* ("enlightenment mind," representing *semen), *kapāla* ("skull," standing for the universe), *lalanā* ("wanton woman," symbolizing *wisdom or the left channel (*nādī*), *rasanā* ("tongue," representing *upāya*, or the means of realization). See also Language.

SANGA ("attachment"), a great stumbling block on the spiritual *path. In this regard, it is synonymous with *rāga. In the *Bhagavad-Gītā (2.47) sanga denotes specifically a person's "clinging" to the fruit (*phala) of one's *actions, which produces adverse *karmic effects and is therefore to be renounced. In some contexts, sanga stands for "socializing," which, according to the *Shiva-Samhitā (5.185), should be avoided. Occasionally it also stands for *sat-sanga, or the beneficial association with sages and *adepts. Cf. nihsangatā.

SANKATA-ĀSANA (sankatāsana, "dangerous posture"), described in the *Gheranda-Samhitā (1.26) thus: Placing the left foot on the ground, twine the right leg around the left leg and place one's hands on the knees. Modern manuals of *hatha-yoga observe that this practice should be repeated while standing on the right foot.

SANTĀNA ("continuity"). *Vācaspati Mishra, in his *Tattva-Vaishāradī (1.4), employs this term to designate the beginningless nexus that exists between spiritual nescience (*avidyā) and the subconscious traits (*vāsanā). See also samyoga.

SAPTA-ANGA-YOGA (saptāngayoga, "sevenlimbed Yoga"). See sapta-sādhana.

SAPTADHA-PRAJNĀ ("sevenfold wisdom"), a term occurring in the *Yoga-Sūtra (2.27) that is left unexplained by *Patanjali. The *Yoga-Bhāshya (2.27), the oldest extant commentary, supplies a probable elucidation, however, stating that at the culmination of conscious ecstasy (*samprajnāta-samādhi) the *yogin has the following immediate insights: (1) That which was to be prevented, i.e., future suffering (*duhkha), has been prevented. (2) The causes of *suffering have been elimi-

nated. (3) Complete cessation (*hāna) has been accomplished. (4) The means for effecting cessation, i.e., the vision of discernment (*viveka-khyāti), has been applied successfully. (5) Sovereignty of the highest mental faculty, the *buddhi, has been achieved. (6) The primary constituents (*guna) of *nature have lost their foothold and, "like rocks rolling down the mountain slope," incline toward dissolution (*pralaya). (7) The *Self abides in its essential nature as primordial light (*jyotis), undefiled and solitary (*kevalin).

Vyāsa further explains that the first four insights, or spontaneous realizations, are called "release of the tasks" (kārya-vimukti), while the last three insights are known as "release of consciousness" (citta-vimukti).

SAPTA-JNĀNA-BHŪMI ("seven stages of wisdom"), a model associated with some schools of *Postclassical Yoga, notably the *Yoga-Vāsishtha in its shorter and longer versions. Thus, according to the *Laghu-Yoga-Vāsishtha (6.13.56ff.), the seven levels are as follows: (1) Shubha-icchā ("desire for the splendid") is the impulse on the part of the *Yoga novice (nava-yogin) to cultivate a positive spiritual attitude and outlook through the *study of the sacred teachings and the application of understanding. (2) Vicārana ("discrimination") is the practice of discernment in daily life, leading to the gradual abandonment of self-will (*abhimāna), *pride, *jealousy, *delusion, etc., and yielding the ability to comprehend the hidden (rahasya) meaning of the sacred teachings. (3) Asanga-bhāvanā ("cultivation of nonattachment"): At this level the practitioner lives in a hermitage (*āshrama) and seriously engages the practice of listening (*shravana) to the sacred lore about self-knowledge and *self-transcendence. This naturally leads to the pacification of the *mind and the inclination to perform only virtuous *actions. (4) *Vilāpinī* ("lamenting"): Here the practitioner looks with *tranquillity upon everything, and his *mind "perishes like a bank of clouds in autumn." (5) *Shuddha-samvin-maya-ānanda-rūpa* is, as the name indicates, the level "formed of *bliss and composed of pure awareness." On this stage of spiritual unfolding, the *yogin* lives in the perpetual certainty of the truth of nonduality (*advaita*). This level coincides with the condition known as "living liberation" (*jīvan-mukti*). (6) *Asamvedana-rūpa* is the level that goes beyond sensation (*samvedana*) and yields the constant experience of bliss (*ānanda*). This stage is said to resemble deep sleep (*sushupti*), though it is associated with wakefulness. (7) *Turya-avasthā-upashānta* (written *turyāvasthopashānta*) is the stage of the "tranquil fourth state," coinciding with "disembodied liberation" (*videha-mukti*) or supreme extinction (*para-nir-vāna*).

Following one of three versions found in the *Yoga-Vāsishtha*, the *Varāha-Upanishad* (4.1.1ff.) gives the seven stages as follows: (1) *Shubha-icchā* (see above); (2) *vicārana* (see above); (3) *tanu-mānasī* ("fine-minded [stage]"); (4) *sattva-āpatti* ("acquisition of *sattva*"); (5) *asamsakti* ("[perfect] detachment"); (6) *padārtha-bhāvanā* ("realization of the essence [of existence]"); and (7) *turīya-ga* ("entering the *fourth"). The last four stages are said to pertain to the *adept who is liberated while yet alive (*jīvan-mukta*).

SAPTA-RISHI (*saptarshi*, "seven seers"), an ancient concept going back to the *Vedic age. In each world cycle (*manvantara*), a different heptad of great seers governs from within the subtle realms of existence. In the present cycle, the seven seers are Marīci, *Angiras, Atri, Pulastya, *Vasishtha, Pulaha, and Kratu. They have anciently been associated with the seven major planets (*graha*) as sources influencing the *destiny of humankind. In *Yoga, the seers are visualized as residing within the human *body itself.

SAPTA-SĀDHANA ("sevenfold discipline") consists, according to the *Gheranda-Samhitā* (1.9), of cleanliness (*shodhana*), firmness (*dridhatā*), stability (*sthairya*), constancy (*dhairya*), lightness (*lāghava*), perception (*pratyaksha*), and nondefilement (*nirlipta*). In *Vedānta, *sapta-sādhana* refers to a different set of disciplines.

SARASVATĪ ("She who flows"). In *Vedic times the Sarasvatī was the mightiest river and its banks formed the heartland of the *Indus-Sarasvatī civilization. This river dried out around 1900 BCE, causing the Vedic peoples to relocate *en masse* to the fertile valley of the Ganges (Gangā) River.

Named after the river, the goddess Sarasvatī presided over speech, learning, and the fine arts, as suggested by her traditional iconographic attributes, which include a lute, a book, and a rosary. In later *Hinduism she also came to be associated with the esoteric center at the base of the spine called *mūlādhāra-cakra*, and with the central channel (*sushumnā-nādi*) in which the *Kundalinī-shakti* ascends.

SARASVATĪ-CĀLANA ("stirring the *sarasvatī*"), the practice in *kundalinī-yoga* of forcing the life energy (*prāna*) into the central channel (*sushumnā-nādī*). The *Yoga-Kundalī-Upanishad* (1.10ff.) describes this esoteric process as follows: Seated in the lotus posture (*padma-āsana*), one should, while the life force is circulating through the *idā-nādī, lengthen the life force (i.e., the *breath) from the normal four digits to twelve digits and "surround" the sarasvatī-nādī with that elongated breath. Then one should hold the life force (through breath retention) in that nādī, and, closing all apertures of the *head with one's fingers, force the *prāna repeatedly from the right nādī into the left nādī for forty-five minutes. Next one should "draw up" the *sushumnā-nādī, which forces the *kundalinī-shakti toward the mouth of the sushumnā conduit. Then one should practice the neck "lock" (*jālandhara-bandha) and the abdominal "lock" (*uddīyāna-bandha), referred to in the text as tāna. This will force the *prāna current upward. Finally, one should expel the life force through the "solar" channel, that is, the *pingalā-nādī to the right of the central channel. See also shakti-cālana.

SARASVATĪ-NĀDĪ ("sarasvatī channel"), a channel (*nādī) of the life force (*prāna), generally said to be situated in front of the central channel (*sushumnā-nādī)—but sometimes equated with it—and to extend to the *tongue. This channel, or flow of life energy, must be activated before the "serpent power" (*kundalinī-shakti) can ascend along the central channel.

SARGA ("creation"). The *Hindu philosophers have always been acutely interested in the origins of the *cosmos, because they have rightly intuited that *knowledge of this kind provides important clues about our personal origins and functions, since *microcosm and *macrocosm are mirrored in each other. See also World ages.

SARVA-ANGA-ĀSANA (sarvāngāsana, "all limbs posture"), what modern manuals of *hatha-yoga call the shoulder stand. It has a number of variations, depending on the position of the legs and arms. Cf. shīrsha-āsana.

SARVA-ARTHATĀ (sarvārthatā, "all-objectness"), a technical expression found in the *Yoga-Sūtra (3.11) that describes the status of the ordinary *consciousness. Cf. eka-agratā.

SARVA-BHĀVA-ADHISHTHĀTRITVA (sarvabhāvādhishthatritva, "supremacy over all states [of existence]") is, according to the *Yoga-Sūtra (3.49), acquired by that *adept who is constantly aware of the distinction between the transcendental *Self and the *sattva aspect of *nature.

SARVA-BHŪTA-HITA ("the good of all beings"), according to the *Mahābhārata

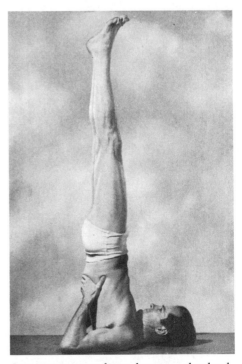

Sarva-anga-āsana, better known as the shoulder stand, demonstrated by Theos Bernard

(12.187.3), one of the outcomes of realizing the *Self. As the *Bhagavad-Gītā (12.4) insists, the sage should actually take delight (*rati) in promoting the weal of everyone. This does not conflict with the call for even-mindedness (*sama-buddhi). See also loka-samgraha.

SARVA-JNATVA or SARVA-JNĀTRITVA ("omniscience"), according to the *Yoga-Sūtra (3.49), the product of the perfected vision of discernment (*viveka-khyāti). The *Shiva-Samhitā (5.65), however, claims that it results from contemplating the *mūlādhāra-cakra, the psychoenergetic center at the base of the spine. The *Yoga-Shikhā-Upanishad (3.25) regards omniscience as the fruit of one's remembrance of the *Absolute. This work makes the same claim for omnipotence (sarva-sampūrna-shakti).

SAT. See Being, sac-cid-ānanda; cf. asat.

SATISFACTION. See prīti, tarpana, tushti.

SAT-KARMA-SAMGRAHA ("Compendium of Right Action"), a work by Cidghanānanda, a disciple of Gaganānanda of the *Nātha sect. It is concerned with the therapeutic aspects of *hatha-yoga and describes a whole range of purificatory techniques, especially for *illnesses resulting from carelessness in the execution of yogic practices or laxity in observing the dietary and other rules. Cidghanānanda advises the *yogin to first try postures (*āsana) and occult remedies to cure himself before resorting to the practices disclosed in his work.

SAT-KĀRYA-VĀDA ("doctrine of the [pre-]existent effect"), a *Sāmkhya and *Yoga teaching according to which all effects are potentially contained in their causes (*kār-ana). The sat-kārya doctrine explicitly rejects the notion of creation ex nihilo. Creation is always only the manifestation (āvirbhāva) of latent possibilities. The ultimate cause is thought to be *prakriti ("creatrix"), or *nature. All unmanifest (invisible) and manifest (visible) forms are simply transformations (vikriti, *vikāra, *parināma) of that primal supersubstance. See also Evolution.

SAT-SANGA ("contact with the Real"), the time-honored practice of associating with *adepts and saintly folk (*sādhu). Contact with them is thought to be purifying and uplifting and to stimulate the spiritual process. See also shakti-pāta.

SATTĀ ("realness" or "beingness," from sat and the suffix tā), a synonym for *sattva. It can denote existence in general or ultimate *Being in particular.

SATTĀ-ĀPATTI (sattāpatti, "attainment of *sattā") one of the seven levels of wisdom (*jnāna). See sapta-jnāna-bhūmi.

SATTĀ-MĀTRA ("mere being"), in the *Yoga-Bhāshya (?.19), a synonym for *linga-mātra, or what the *Tattva-Vaishāradī (2.19) calls the "great mind" (mahad-buddhi). It is the first evolute of nature (*prakriti). The Yoga-Vāsishtha (5.10.86), a *Vedānta work, however, employs this term to designate the transcendental *Reality itself. Sattā-mātra is said to have two aspects: homogeneity (eka-rūpa) and heterogeneity (vibhāga). The latter is created by temporality (kāla-sattā), fragmentation (kala-sattā), and objective existence (vastu-sattā).

SATTVA ("beingness"), "being" in general or "a being" in particular. In the *Yoga and *Sāmkhya traditions, the term also stands for one of the three primary constituents (*guna) of nature (*prakriti). The *Bhagavad-Gītā (14.6) characterizes it as "immaculate, illuminating, without ill." However, sattva, by virtue of being one of the *gunas, also has a binding effect and, as the Gītā notes, can cause attachment to *joy and *knowledge. Nevertheless, it is only by overcoming *rajas (the dynamic principle) and *tamas (the principle of inertia) through the magnification of sattva that *liberation, or *enlightenment, is possible.

Sattva is the psychocosmic principle of lucidity or mere existence devoid of conceptual filters and emotional overlays. *Classical Yoga seeks to purify the sattva aspect of the psyche to the point where its lucidity matches the inherent clarity of the transcendental Self (*purusha), which is pure *Consciousness. See also sapta-jnāna-bhūmi, sattā.

SĀTTVIKA, the adjectival form of *sattva; generally rendered as "sattvic."

SATYA ("truth" or "truthfulness"), in the sense of "truthfulness," one of the constituent practices of moral observance (*yama). The *Mandala-Brāhmana-Upanishad (1.4) lists it among the practices of self-restraint (*niyama). This shows the high regard in which truthfulness is held in the spiritual traditions. The *Mahānirvāna-Tantra (4.75ff.) extols truthfulness thus:

No virtue (*dharma) is more excellent than truthfulness, no *sin greater than [promoting] the untruth. Therefore the [virtuous] man should seek refuge in truthfulness with all his *heart.
Without truthfulness, worship (*pūjā) is futile. Without truthfulness the recitation (*japa) [of sacred *mantras] is useless. Without truthfulness, [the practice of] asceticism (*tapas) is as unfruitful as seed on barren soil.
Truthfulness is the form of the supreme Absolute (*brahman). Truly, truthfulness is the best *asceticism. All *actions [should be] rooted in truthfulness. Nothing is more excellent than truthfulness.

According to the *Yoga-Sūtra (2.36), the *yogin who is grounded in this virtue acquires the paranormal power (*siddhi) by which the fruit of his *actions depends entirely on his will. The *Yoga-Bhāshya (2.36) takes this to mean that whatever the *adept says comes true. Elsewhere in this work (2.3), *Vyāsa states that if one speaks at all, it should be for the communication of one's *knowledge and as a *service to others, and hence the communication should not be deceitful, erroneous, or barren. This definition combines personal integrity with fidelity to facts. Expressing a common sentiment, the Garuda-Purāna (49.30) similarly understands truthfulness as "speech that is beneficial to beings (*bhūta-hita)." The *Darshana-Upanishad (1.9f.) notes that truth is what is based on the evidence of the *senses but that the highest truth is the conviction that everything is the Absolute (*brahman).

SAUMANASYA ("gladness"), one of the fruits of purity (*shauca), according to the *Yoga-Sūtra (2.41). Cf. daurmanasya.

SAURA-ĀSANA (saurāsana, "solar posture"), performed, according to the *Hatha-Ratna-Avalī (3.62), by extending the sole of one foot and placing it on the other foot. This practice is not listed by this name in the list of eighty-four postures (*āsana) furnished by the same text.

SAVICĀRA-SAMĀPATTI ("reflexive coinciding"), a subtype of conscious ecstasy (*samprajnāta-samādhi) in which *attention is focused on a subtle (*sūkshma) object. See also samādhi, samāpatti; cf. nirvicāra-samāpatti.

SAVIKALPA-SAMĀDHI ("ecstasy with form"), the *Vedānta equivalent of the yogic *samprajnāta-samādhi. The word vikalpa can mean both "form" and "ideation." This type of *ecstasy involves a higher mental process that can be called thinking, though the thoughts that spontaneously arise have a clarity and an immediacy that distinguishes them markedly from the thoughts of the ordinary, discursive *mind. See also samādhi, samāpatti; cf. nirvikalpa-samādhi.

SAVITARKA-SAMĀPATTI ("cogitative coinciding"), the lowest form of conscious ecstasy (*samprajnāta-samādhi). Here *attention is concentrated on the coarse (*sthūla) aspect of a thing, such as the visible shape of a *deity as represented iconographically. See also samādhi, samāpatti; cf. nirvitarka-samāpatti.

SCRIPTURE. See shāstra, shruti, smriti, sūtra.

SEAL. See mudrā.

SEAT. See nishadana, pītha.

SECRECY is enjoined by many texts. Those who do not heed this injunction are often threatened with dire consequences, not least ultimate spiritual misfortune. The *Brahma-Vidyā-Upanishad (47), e.g., demands that its teachings should only be imparted to a devoted *disciple, lest the *teacher should be cast into hell (*nāraka). Similarly, the *Mahā-Vākya-Upanishad (2) asks that its most esoteric knowledge should be divulged only to a sattvic (*sātt-

vika) student who is properly introspective (antar-mukha). Secrecy is frequently enjoined regarding specific practices, notably the *khecarī-mudrā. The *Yoga-Shikhā-Upanishad (1.156) demands secrecy with respect to the paranormal powers (*siddhi), which should not be displayed. The *Hatha-Yoga-Pradīpikā (1.11), again, declares that the *yogin who wishes for perfection (*siddhi) should keep the science of *hatha-yoga carefully concealed, for it is potent only so long as it is kept secret but becomes quite inefficacious when disclosed to unworthy people. This demand for secrecy is characteristic of initiatory traditions in general. See also sandhā-bhashā.

SECRET. The ultimate secret, or mystery, is the *Divine itself. It is secret because it is hidden from the view of the ordinary person. Only in the case of the enlightened *adept, who has become one with the Divine or transcendental Self, is the veil of mystery lifted. See also guhya.

SEED. See bīja, bindu.

SEER. See drashtri, rishi.

SELF, TRANSCENDENTAL, the essential core of one's being; what in the Christian tradition is known as the eternal soul. The Self (*ātman, *purusha) is one's authentic identity apart from all one's roles and is deemed immortal and immutable. Moreover, in most spiritual traditions of *Hinduism, it is considered to be suprasensuous (atīndriya) and pure *Awareness (*cit, *citi, cetana, or *caitanya—words that all have the same root).

The transcendental Self is distinct from but lies hidden within or behind the empirical self, or ego (*ahamkāra, *asmitā). It is also different from C. G. Jung's notion of the Self, which is a psychic archetype responsible for the psychospiritual maturation of the personality to the degree that the *ego is sensitive and willing to respond to the messages of the Self. Jung's notion corresponds more to the idea of the "inner controller" (*antaryāmin), one of the aspects of the transcendental Self according to *Vedānta.

All *Hindu traditions are agreed that the realization of the transcendental Self is the noblest and worthiest object of human aspiration. See also adhyātman, purusha-artha.

SELF-OFFERING. See ātma-nivedana.

SELF-REALIZATION (*ātma-jnāna, "Self-knowledge," or *ātma-darshana, "Self-vision"), the recovery of one's authentic identity as the transcendental *Reality, rather than the ego personality. This is not a cognitive process, or mere experience, but a radical shift at the root of *consciousness, which involves the transcendence of the human *mind as well as the *body. It is synonymous with *enlightenment, or *liberation.

SELF-RECOGNITION. See ātma-pratyā-bhijna.

SELF-RELIANCE. See svatantrya.

SELF-SURRENDER, in the language of devotion (*bhakti), the attitude of *self-transcendence, which has as its focus the *Divine or transcendental *Self. See also ātma-nivedana.

SELF-TRANSCENDENCE, the practice of going beyond the limitations of the *ego habit in all matters. It is the ideal and foundation process of spiritual life. A self-transcending attitude is to be applied not only to ordinary situations but also to visions, paranormal abilities (*siddhi), and the different forms of ecstasy (*samādhi). This orientation of *self-surrender, or self-sacrifice, fulfills itself in the great event of *Self-realization, or *liberation.

SELF-VISION. See ātma-darshana.

SEMEN. See bindu, retas, shukra; cf. rajas.

SENSE CONTROL. See indriya-jaya, in-driya-nigraha.

SENSES. See indriya.

SENSE WITHDRAWAL. See pratyāhāra.

SERPENT POSTURE. See bhujānga-āsana.

SERPENT POWER. See kundalinī-shakti.

SERPENT SEAL. See bhujānginī-mudrā.

SERVICE. See sevā.

SEVĀ or **SEVANA** ("service"), an important aspect of discipleship. Since ancient times, the pupil (*shishya) hoping for higher initiation (*dīkshā) has had to prove himself or herself through steadfast service to the teacher (*guru). See also ācārya-sevana, guru-sevā, pāda-sevana, panca-anga-sevana.

SEXUALITY. The spiritual traditions of India fall into two categories: those that espouse a body- and sex-positive orientation, like most schools of *Tantrism, and those that look upon sexuality as an inevitable stumbling block on the spiritual *path. The latter, which are in the majority, demand that the aspirant (nava-yogin) should abstain from all sexual activity and cultivate chastity (*brahmacarya) in the strict sense. Concessions are usually made for the householder (*grihastha) who endeavors to engage spiritual life. Even the householder, however, should strive toward perfect sexual abstinence in thought, word, and deed. The reason for this counsel is that the discharge of one's sexual energies in orgasm involves a loss of life energy (*prāna), or vitality, which is needed for the arduous and lifelong task of transforming the personality through the yogic disciplines. Sublimation is understood as a psychosomatic process that leads to the actual refinement of the seminal substance into what is known as *ojas.

The sex-positive schools are not merely hedonistic, licentious adventures. They also generally do not favor orgasm and the concomitant loss of vitality. Yet they permit and even recommend sexual activity as a valid means of spiritual transmutation. Sexual desire (*kāma) is seen as a normal, if particularly potent, function of the finite personality, which should not be repressed but properly harnessed. In fact, the left-hand branch of *Tantrism offers a battery of methods that specifically seek to stimulate the sexual urge. The core ritual of this Tantric orientation is known as the "five m's" (*panca-ma-kara), of which sexual intercourse (*maithunā) is the fifth and final ceremonial practice. Its purpose is to achieve the ecstatic state (*samādhi) through physical union. This approach is based on the notion that sexual pleasure (*sukha, *rati) is a manifestation of transcendental bliss (*ānanda) and hence can be experienced as such. This orientation is epitomized in the religious motif of the love play between *Krishna and the shepherdesses (*gopī).

India's predominant mood has always been puritanical, and the sex-positive schools for the most part have had to exist underground. Today a decidedly anti-Tantric attitude prevails. On the other side, Tantrism has come to the West, and a number of neo-Tantric schools have sprung up. In most cases, however, these have little more in common with traditional Tantrism than the name. See also *bindu, rasa, Sahajiyā, Semen.

SHĀBARA, mentioned in the *Hatha-Yoga-Pradīpikā (1.5) as a master of *hatha-yoga.

SHABDA ("sound"), one of the principal and oldest means by which *yogins have sought to focus their *attention. Their hard-won experimental findings and theories about the transformative nature of sound are embodied in what is known as *mantra-vidyā or the "science of sacred utterances." Shabda can be lettered (varna-ātmaka) and endowed with meaning, or it can be meaningless sound (dhvani), such as the roar of a waterfall. In addition, there is suprasensuous or inner sound (*nāda). The ultimate ground in and from which all types of sound arise is called the *shabda-brahman. Audible sound is the end product of a whole process of *evolution by which the transcendental vibration (*spanda) of shabda-brahman is gradually made manifest. Generally, four stages are distinguished: (1) Para-shabda ("supreme sound"), the most subtle form of sound, is associated with the psychoenergetic center at the base of the spine, the *mūlādhāra-cakra. (2) Pashyantī-shabda ("visible sound"), which is associated with the *heart, can be heard as the sacred syllable *om (or *pranava). (3) Madhyama-shabda ("middle sound") refers to a variety of basic sounds, such as the fifty sound values (varna) of the Sanskrit *alphabet, known as "matrices" (*mātrikā). This is also the level on which *mantras are revealed to the *adept. Each of these sound units has three aspects:

*bīja, *nāda, and *bindu. (4) Vaikhāra-shabda ("manifest sound"), which is the coarsest aspect of sound, is expressed in speech. See also mantra-yoga; cf. mauna.

SHABDA-BRAHMAN ("Absolute as sound" or "sonic Absolute"), the ground of all sound (*shabda), whether audible or unmanifest. In *Hinduism, it is indicated by the sacred sound *om. See also Absolute, akshara; cf. para-brahman.

SHAD-ANGA-YOGA ("six-limbed Yoga"), first taught by the anonymous author(s) of the *Maitrāyanīya-Upanishad (6.18) as consisting of breath control (*prānāyāma), sense withdrawal (*pratyāhāra), meditation (*dhyāna), concentration (*dhāranā), examination (*tarka), and ecstasy (*samādhi). Noteworthy are the sequence of *meditation and *concentration (reversed in later sources) and the mention of tarka. Similar sixfold arrangements are presented in a variety of scriptures of *Postclassical Yoga. An interesting variant is found in the Garuda-Purāna (227.18), which includes recitation (*japa) as the second component, following *breath control. All these schemas have in common the absence of any mention of moral observance (*yama) and self-discipline (*niyama), which are the foundation of the "eight-limbed Yoga" (*ashta-anga-yoga) of *Patanjali. However, this does not mean that the moral rules of yama are disregarded; they are merely not formalized.

SHADOW. See chāyā, chāyā-purusha.

SHAD-VIMSHA or SHAD-VIMSHAKA ("twenty-sixth [principle]"), a term of *Preclassical Yoga used in several places in the *Mahābhārata. It denotes the transcendental *Reality, the "Lord" (*īshvara). The assumption of a twenty-sixth ontolog-

ical principle (*tattva) distinguishes the *Epic Yoga schools from the rival *Sāmkhya schools of that era. The adherents of Sāmkhya know of only twenty-five principles; twenty-four pertain to insentient nature (*prakriti), and the twenty-fifth is the supraconscious transcendental Self (*purusha). See also budhyamāna.

SHAITHILYA ("relaxation"). Patanjali's *Yoga-Sūtra (2.47) states that posture (*āsana) must be performed while relaxing all effort (*yatna), so that, as the *Yoga-Bhāshya explains, there is no agitation (ejaya) in the *body.

SHAIVA ("pertaining to *Shiva"), an adjective also employed as a noun to denote an adherent of *Shaivism.

SHAIVA SIDDHĀNTA, the southern branch of the ramifying tradition of *Shaivism. Partly based on the twenty-eight Sanskrit *Āgamas composed in the North, it has spawned a huge literature of its own in the Tamil language, beginning with the poetry of such Shaiva saints as *Appar, *Manikkavacakar, *Sambandhar, *Sundarar, and *Tirumūlar. The first systematic Tamil exposition of the doctrines of Shaivism is the thirteenth-century Shiva-Jnāna-Bodham ("Awakening to the Knowledge of Shiva") of *Meykandar, a commentary on the Shaiva-Siddhānta, a work consisting of twelve *sūtras apparently excerpted from the Sanskrit Raurava-Āgama.

The tradition of Shaiva Siddhānta, which espouses a nondualist (*advaita) metaphysics, distinguishes between the *Divine, called *pashupati (i.e., *Shiva); the individual psyche, called *pashu; and insentient *nature, which is referred to as the "fetter" (*pāsha). This religiophilosophical system also recognizes thirty-six principles (*tattva) of existence, which include the twenty-four principles of the *Sāmkhya tradition. The other twelve principles are said to be "pure" or transcendental categories.

Although this school, which is still active today, emphasizes devotional *worship and *ritual, *Yoga also plays a significant role, as can be seen from such works as the *Shiva-Jnāna-Siddhi and the *Shiva-Yoga-Ratna ("Jewel of Shiva-Yoga") of *Jnānaprakasha. See also Pashupata, Pratyābhijna school, Lingāyata sect.

SHAIVISM, the name given to a number of schools—notably *Kāpālika, *Kālāmukha, *Pāshupata, *Krama, *Pratyabhijnā, *Trika, *Spanda, *Shaiva Siddhānta, and *Vīra Shaivism (or Lingāyata)—which cover a wide range of doctrinal outlooks and practical approaches. The common denominator is the *worship of the transcendental *Reality as *Shiva. The origins of Shaivism lie in the obscure past. Shiva is mentioned already in the *Rig-Veda, but the earliest evidence of this deity's full-fledged monotheistic *worship can be found in the *Shvetāshvatara-Upanishad (3d or 4th cen. BCE or earlier). The *Mahābhārata reflects the emergent importance of Shiva, who begins to seriously rival *Vishnu. The common era witnessed the gradual flowering of both Shaivism and its competitor *Vaishnavism, reaching its culmination around the turn of the first millennium CE. The adherents of Shaivism in Northern and Southern India, called Shaivas, produced a vast literature in a variety of languages (notably Sanskrit and Tamil), only a fraction of which is extant today and which is still only poorly researched. They were instrumental in the development of *Yoga, especially along more ascetic lines. Not surprisingly, the Jaina writer Rājasekhara rightly styles Shaivism a "Yoga tradition" (yoga-mata)

in his Shad-Darshana-Samuccaya ("Compendium of the Six Systems"). Cf. Shaktism, Vaishnavism.

SHAKTI ("power"), the dynamic or creative principle of existence, envisioned as being feminine and personified as *Shakti, the divine consort of *Shiva. This concept is intended to explain how the undifferentiated singular *Reality can produce the multidimensional *cosmos with its infinite forms. The transcendental static principle, personified as *Shiva, is in itself incapable of creation. As a popular doctrinal maxim has it: "Shiva without *Shakti is unable to effect anything." Shiva apart from Shakti is likened to a corpse. The *Shiva-Purāna (7.2.4.10) resorts to this poetic metaphor: "Just as the moon does not shine without moonlight, so also Shiva does not shine without Shakti."

*Shiva is called shaktimān, or the "possessor of power," whereas Shakti is like the bride whose life is made complete by the bridegroom. Shiva and Shakti, *god and *goddess, are inseparable principles, and the *Kaula-Jnāna-Nirnaya (17.8) compares their relationship to that between fire and smoke. Some authorities explain that the *Absolute includes an infinite number of shaktis. Frequently, however, three or more principal types of shakti are differentiated. Thus the *Kaula-Jnāna-Nirnaya (2.6) reiterates a popular *Shaiva teaching when it speaks of three fundamental aspects of shakti: the *kriyā-shakti ("power of action"); the *icchā-shakti ("power of intention"), whose essence is sometimes said to be astonishment (*camatkāra); and the *jnāna-shakti ("power of knowledge"). These respectively represent the conative, volitional, and cognitive side of the incomprehensible being of *Shiva. At the time of the dissolution of the universe, the former two aspects resolve into the third aspect. Occasionally two more aspects are listed: the *cit-shakti ("power of awareness") and the *ānanda-shakti ("power of *bliss"). In another passage, the *Kaula-Jnāna-Nirnaya (20.10) mentions nine kinds of shakti, and other works offer still more complicated models.

The *Siddha-Siddhānta-Paddhati (1.5ff.) mentions the following five aspects of the shakti: nijā-shakti ("innate power"); para-shakti ("higher power"); apara-shakti ("lower power"); sūkshma-shakti ("subtle power"); and *kundalinī-shakti ("serpent power"). Elsewhere this scripture (4.2) furnishes a different list: para-shakti ("higher power"); sattā-shakti ("power of being"); ahantā-shakti ("power of 'I-ness' "); sphurattā-shakti ("power of manifestation"); and kalā-shakti ("power of partial existence"). All these refer to the shakti as it relates to specific levels of the process of psychocosmic *evolution.

The *Laghu-Yoga-Vāsishtha (6.2.28) makes the important point that all these shaktis reside within the human *body; i.e., they are both cosmological and psychological realities. However, not only is the shakti responsible for *creation, but it is also the agent of change and destruction. It is the power behind cosmic existence as well as *liberation. Practically speaking, the most significant form of the shakti is the *kundalinī-shakti.

The term shakti is also used in *Tantrism to refer to the female initiate into the sexual practices. See also citi-shakti.

SHAKTI, the personification of the feminine form of the *Divine. See also Devī, shakti; cf. Shiva.

SHAKTI-CALA- or SHAKTI-CĀLANA-MUDRĀ ("power-stirring seal"), described in the *Gheranda-Samhitā (3.49ff.) thus: Smear the *body with *ashes and then wrap a piece of soft cloth four digits (ca. three inches) wide and one span (ca. nine inches) long around one's waist and hold it firmly in place with a piece of string. Sitting in the adept's posture (*siddha-āsana), inhale and energetically mingle the inbreath (*prāna) with the outbreath (*apāna). Then contract the anus slowly by means of the *ashvinī-mudrā until the breath (*vāyu) reaches the central channel (*sushumnā-nādī). The *Hatha-Yoga-Pradīpikā (3.104ff.) offers a different description: Seated in the adamantine posture (*vajra-āsana), hold one's ankles and press them against the "bulb" (*kanda). Next, perform the bellows breathing (*bhastrikā-prānāyāma) and contract the "sun" (i.e., the *navel region). In this manner, fearlessly stir the "serpent power" (*kundalinī-shakti) for an hour and a half

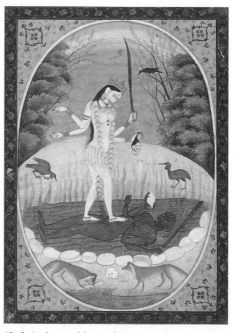

Shakti, the goddess of power, who is associated with the cremation ground, symbolizing the finitude of all creation

270

until it enters the central channel. Celibate practitioners are said to gain perfection (*siddhi*) within forty days. According to the *Yoga-Kundalī-Upanishad* (1.8), this "seal" (*mudrā*) involves the rousing of the *sarasvatī-nādī* followed by *breath retention. This is said to make the *kundalinī* "erect" (*rijvi*).

Essentially, the *shakti-cālana-mudrā* uses the *apāna* form of the life force to awaken the *kundalinī*. The *Goraksha-Paddhati* (1.74) notes that this brings about the union of semen (*shukla*) and blood (*rajas*). See also *sarasvatī-cālana*.

SHAKTI-PĀTA or SHAKTI-NIPĀTA ("descent of power"), the *transmission of psychospiritual energy (*shakti*) from the *adept to the disciple (or any other person). This is generally effected by touch, as in the case of *Ramakrishna, who placed his foot on his favorite disciple Naren (the later Swami *Vivekananda) and plunged him into deep ecstasy (*samādhi). But spiritual transmission can also take place through a mere glance. See also *dīkshā*.

SHAKTISM refers to a large number of schools and traditions within *Hinduism that revolve around the cultic "worship of the *Divine in its feminine form as *Shakti. Going back into the dim prehistoric past, *Goddess worship has always flourished among the lower classes of Indian society but, from about the fifth century CE on, also won the hearts of a large section of the literate population. The Goddess is understood as the active aspect of the transcendental *Reality, which is essentially quiescent and unapproachable. Some of the most popular goddesses (*devī*) of the *Hindu pantheon are *Kālī, *Durgā, *Sarasvatī, Annapūrnā, Cāndī, Lakshmī, Pārvatī, Umā, Satī, *Rādhā, and *Shrī-Vidyā. The sacred scriptures of the *shaktas*, or followers of Shaktism, are generally known as the *Tantras*, but *Tantrism should be distinguished from Shaktism.

SHALABHA-ĀSANA (*shalabhāsana*, "locust posture"), described in the *Gheranda-Samhitā* (2.39) thus: Lying belly down on the ground with one's hands placed near the chest, raise one's legs in the air by one span (ca. nine inches).

SHAMA ("quiescence"), regarded as one of the gatekeepers to *liberation in the *Laghu-Yoga-Vāsishtha* (2.1.64): "He who upon hearing, touching, seeing, tasting, and smelling pleasant or unpleasant [things] neither delights in nor regrets them, is said to be tranquil (*shānta*)."

According to the *Bhagavad-Gītā* (6.3), *shama* is the very essence of the spiritual practice of the accomplished *yogin*, whereas *karma-yoga* is said to be the way for the aspirant. The *Uddhāva-Gītā* (14.36) explains it as the mind's (*buddhi*) "intentness on me" (*man-nishthatā*), the "me" being *Krishna, the transcendental *Reality.

SHAMANISM, the name given to tribal traditions revolving around specialists of ecstasy, called shamans, who use various magical and spiritual practices to enlist the hidden powers of the universe in order to benefit members of their tribe. In particular, shamans are healers, who are called upon to cure physical and mental *diseases. But they also are consulted for divination and guidance in all matters relating to the hereafter. Shamanism shares many elements with *Yoga, notably the shaman's ability to enter at will into ecstatic states of *consciousness and thereby retrieve paranormal *knowledge and *wisdom. It seems probable that Shamanism, in the broadest sense of the term, was one of the roots of the Yoga tradition. The difference between Yoga and shamanism is significant, however, inasmuch as *yogins aspire to *liberation rather than *paranormal abilities or knowledge. It is true, though, that at the highest level of spirituality, the *yogins* also place the welfare of other beings above all else. This is captured in the Buddhist ideal of the *bodhisattva*, who spares no effort to realize *enlightenment so he can best serve others in their own struggle for *awakening and freedom from *suffering. See also Asceticism.

SHĀMBHAVĪ-MUDRĀ ("seal pertaining to Shambhu [i.e., to *Shiva]"), one of the most important "seals" (*mudrā*) of *Tantrism and *hatha-yoga. The texts typically enjoin complete *secrecy about it. The *Gheranda-Samhitā* (3.65), e.g., says that this *mudrā* should be "guarded like a bride of noble lineage" and that by comparison with it, the *Vedas*, textbooks (*shāstra*), and *Purānas* are "like courtesans." The same work (3.64ff.) states that one should fix one's *gaze between the *eyes and behold the *Self's "grove/delight" (*ārāma*). The *Gheranda-Samhitā* (1.54) also notes that this *mudrā* can be induced by means of steady gazing (*trātaka*). The *Hatha-Yoga-Pradīpikā* (4.36) adds that *mind and *breath should be absorbed in the "inner sign" (*antar-lakshya*), with one's open pupils fixed and unseeing. In another verse, this scripture (4.39) refers to a variant practice, which involves gazing at the *light (at the tip of the *nose), otherwise known as the "external sign" (*bahir-laksh-ya*). This technique is claimed to quickly yield the realization of the state of exaltation (*unmanī*). See also *vaishnavī-mudrā*.

SHAME. See *lajjā*.

SHĀNDILYA, the name of several teachers, including a famous authority of the *Pān-

carātra tradition who lived prior to *Rāmā-nuja, who defended the *Vedic legitimacy of his teachings. He is mentioned already by *Shankara in his commentary on the *Brahma-Sūtra* (2.2.45), where a stanza is cited that claims of Shāndilya that he turned to the Pāncarātra tradition because he did not find the highest *bliss through the *Vedas*. Probably a different Shāndilya authored the *Bhakti-Sūtra*, and the teachings of two other well-known *adepts by that name are recorded in the ancient *Chāndogya-Upanishad* (3.14) and the *Mahābhārata* (e.g., 12.47.6).

SHĀNDILYA-UPANISHAD (*Shāndilyopanishad*) is one of the *Yoga-Upanishads*. It consists of three chapters and comprises well over thirty printed pages. This scripture is named after the sage *Shāndilya, who figures in it as the disciple of Atharvan (who is associated with the *Atharva-Veda*). The first chapter defines the "limbs" (*anga*) of the eightfold *path

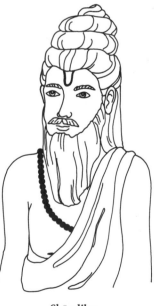

Shāndilya

(*ashta-anga-yoga*), mentioning ten components each for moral observance (*yama*) and self-discipline (*niyama*) and describing five phases of sense withdrawal (*pratyāhāra*) and five types of concentration (*dhāranā*), as well as two forms of meditation (*dhyāna*). It also discusses esoteric *anatomy and the appropriate environment (*desha*) for yogic practice at some length. The short second chapter and the third chapter contain an exposition of *Vedānta metaphysics, which forms the philosophical basis of this scripture's teaching. Many of the stanzas are also to be found in the *Yoga-Yājnavalkya*, and the text generally has the appearance of being a composite with probably numerous interpolations.

SHANKARA, the celebrated preceptor (*ācārya*) of *Advaita Vedānta; born probably in the village of Kaladi in Kerala, South India. He is traditionally said to have lived 788–822 CE, though some modern scholars take the first date to be his year of initiation as a renouncer. Legend describes him as a precocious child who could read at the age of two and had mastered the *Vedas* at the age of eight. Shankara's *Advaita-Vedānta teacher was Govinda, a disciple of *Gaudapāda. Shankara, who traveled widely in India, founded four monastic orders: at Dvarākā in the West, at Pūri in the East, at Badrī in the North and at Shringeri in the South. His exposition of Advaita Vedānta, as preserved in many extant works of great erudition, was chiefly responsible for the renaissance of that ancient tradition and the decline of *Buddhism in India. In addition to his scholarly commentaries on the *Brahma-Sūtra*, the principal *Upanishads*, and the *Bhagavad-Gītā*, he also apparently wrote a number of popular didactic works, notably the *Upadesha-Sahasrī* ("Thousand In-

structions"). A large number of devotional hymns are also attributed to him. Shankara's legendary life story is related in the famous biography by Mādhava, *Shankara-Dig-Vijaya*.

The German Indologist Paul Hacker (1968) put forward good reasons for assuming that prior to his conversion to *Advaita Vedānta, Shankara had been a follower of *Yoga, more specifically of *Patanjali's school. This would support the indigenous claim that Shankara Bhagavatpāda authored an important but little known (and probably suppressed) subcommentary on the *Yoga-Sūtra*, entitled *Vivarana*.

Shankara ("Benevolent") is also one of the many names of *Shiva, of whom Shankara the sage is widely regarded as a partial incarnation (*avatāra*). The name is also occasionally spelled Shamkara, which is explained in the *Spanda-Kārikā*

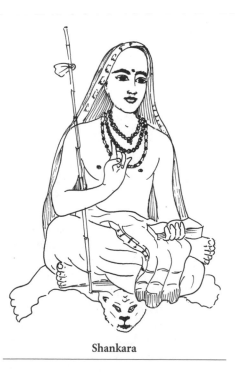

Shankara

(1.1) as "he who makes *sham*," the word *sham* being explained as a synonym for *anugraha, or "grace."

SHANKHINĪ-NĀDĪ ("mother-of-pearl channel"), one of the principal channels of the life force (*prāna), situated between the **gāndhārā-* and the *sarasvatī-nādī and extending to the right (or the left) ear. See also *nādī*.

SHAN-MUKHĪ-MUDRĀ ("six-openings seal"), referred to, e.g., in the **Goraksha-Paddhati* (2.16), where it is said to consist in the blocking of one's *ears, *eyes, and nostrils with one's fingers. This "seal" (*mudrā) is correctly executed by covering the ears with one's thumbs, the eyes with one's index fingers, and the nostrils with the middle fingers. This practice is recommended for the manifestation of the inner sound (*nāda).

SHĀNTI ("peace"), sometimes cited as one of the components of moral observance (*yama); in this context it denotes mental equilibrium. As is clear from the *Bhagavad-Gītā (5.29), however, the word can also stand for the highest condition of extinction in the *Absolute (*brahma-nir-vāna).

SHARĪRA ("body"; from the root *shri*, "to fall apart"), the "wretched *body." The **Maitrāyanīya-Upanishad* (2.3ff.) compares the body to an insensate cart and to a potter's wheel that is whirled about by the *Self. This *Upanishad (3.4) also offers the following classic denunciation of *embodiment: "This body, arising from sexual congress (*maithunā), grows in the [uterine] *hell and emerges from the urinary opening. It is made up of bones, smeared over with flesh, covered with skin, filled with feces, urine, *bile, *phlegm, marrow,

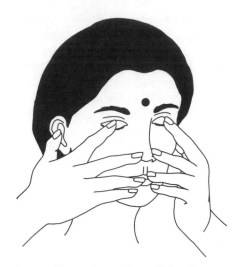

Shan-mukhī-mudrā, sealing off the six openings of the head

fat, and grease, and [endowed] with numerous *diseases, like a treasury with wealth." As the *Shiva-Purāna (5.23.9) puts it succinctly, there is not a single clean spot on the body. See also *deha*, *kosha*, *pinda*.

SHARĪRIN ("embodied one"), a synonym for *dehin.

SHASHI-MANDALA ("lunar circle") or SHASHI-STHĀNA ("lunar place"). See *candra*; cf. *sūrya*.

SHĀSTRA ("teaching" or "textbook"). While most authorities consider the *study of the textbooks essential to successful spiritual *practice, some question or even deny outright the value of written teachings. The **Laghu-Yoga-Vāsishtha* (6.2.130) observes that the *Self cannot be realized without a qualified teacher (*guru) and knowing the content of the textbooks. The *Bhagavad-Gītā (16.24) states that the *shāstras* should guide a person in determining appropriate (*kārya*) and inappropriate behavior, because those who live as they please can never find perfection (*siddhi) or joy (*sukha). The *Mahābhārata (12.245.12) even has the phrase shāstra-yoga ("Yoga of the textbooks"). By contrast, the *Yoga-Shikhā-Upanishad (1.4) warns of the "snare of textbooks" (shāstra-jāla), i.e., mere book learning. See also grantha.

SHATA RATNA-SAMGRAHA ("Collection of One Hundred Jewels"), compiled by *Umāpati Shivācārya, an anthology of quotations from the *Āgamas expounding the philosophy of *Shaiva Siddhānta.

SHAT-CAKRA-BHEDA ("piercing the six centers"). The most common model of psychoenergetic centers (*cakra) distinguishes six such centers, with a seventh center serving as the terminal for the ascending "serpent power" (*kundalinī-shakti). On its upward path, the kundalinī is pictured as piercing (bheda) the six lower centers or "lotuses" (padma), as a string pierces the flowers of a garland.

SHAT-CAKRA-NIRŪPANA ("Investigation of the Six Centers"), the sixth chapter of Pūrnānanda Svāmin's Shrī-Tattva-Cintamani, a late voluminous treatise on *Tantrism consisting of twenty-five chapters. The Nirūpana, which comprises fifty-five (or fifty-six) stanzas, is the best-known work dealing with the process of *shat-cakra-bheda.

SHAT-KARMA ("six acts"), the first step of *ghatastha-yoga, according to the *Gheranda-Samhitā (1.12). It consists of the following practices: (1) *dhauti ("cleansing"), which has four constituent techniques; (2) *vasti ("bladder"), which is the yogic equivalent to an enema; (3) *neti (untranslatable), which is nasal cleansing; (4) *naulī, laulī, or laulikī ("to-and-fro movement"), consisting in rolling the abdominal muscles; (5) *trātaka (untranslatable), which is steady conscious gazing; and (6) *kapāla-bhāti ("skull luster"), which has three constituent techniques. The *Hatha-Yoga-Pradīpikā (2.21) recommends these six practices specifically for initiates who suffer from an excess of fat or phlegm (*kapha).

The term shat-karma can also refer to the following six *Tantric magical practices: (1) marana ("killing"); (2) uccātana ("repelling"); (3) vashī-karana ("bringing under one's control"); (4) stambhana ("arresting"), such as arresting a storm, for instance; (5) vidveshana ("creating enmity"); and (6) svastyayana ("causing welfare"). Most of these practices belong to black *magic. See also ashta-siddhi, siddhi.

SHAT-STHĀLA ("six stages"), a central doctrine of *Vīra Shaivism (or *Lingāyata). It refers to the six levels of spiritual maturation: (1) *bhakti ("devotion"), as expressed in ritual *worship at the temple or in the home; (2) mahesha (mahā-īsha or "great Lord"), the phase of disciplining one's *mind; (3) *prasāda ("grace"), the peaceful stage in which the *devotee recognizes the *Divine working in and through everything; (4) *prāna-linga ("phallus of the life force"), the stage at which the devotee begins to experience the Divine within the *body (as a consecrated temple); (5) sharana ("[taking] refuge"), the phase in which the devotee becomes a "fool of God," longing for *Shiva as a woman yearns for her lover; and (6) *aikya ("union"), the consummate stage at which ritual worship is at an end because the devotee has become the Lord (*īshvara).

In some contexts, shat-sthāla refers to the six psychoenergetic centers (*cakra) of the *body.

SHAUCA ("purity" or "cleansing"), one of the techniques of self-discipline (*niyama*), according to *Classical Yoga. It is also listed in some scriptures of *Postclassical Yoga as one of the ten practices of moral observance (*yama*). The *Yoga-Sūtra* (2.40) states that when *purity is perfectly cultivated, it leads to aversion (*jugupsā*) toward one's own *body and a desire to avoid contamination through contact with others. The *Yoga-Bhāshya* (2.32) notes that cleansing is twofold: external (*bāhya*) and internal (*abhyantara*). The former is effected by the use of *water, *earth, and other similar substances, as well as the consumption of pure *food. Inner cleansing is the washing away of the blemishes (*mala*) of the *mind. According to the *Bhagavad-Gītā* (13.7), *shauca* is a manifestation of knowledge (*jnāna*) and (17.14) forms part of bodily asceticism (*tapas*). See also *dhauti, shodhana, shuddhi*.

SHAUNAKA, mentioned in the *Mahābhārata* (3.2.14) as a sage learned in both *Sāmkhya and *Yoga. His other name is Gritsamada. He is traditionally identified as the famous author of the *Rig-Veda-Anukramanī* and *Rik-Prātishākhya* and eight other explanatory texts on the *Rig-Veda. His principal disciple was Āshvalāyana, who wrote three major works. Āshvalāyana's main disciple, in turn, was Kātyāyana, who is said to have been the *teacher of *Patanjali the grammarian.

SHAVA-ĀSANA (*shavasana*, "dead posture"), a synonym for *mrita-āsana*.

SHAYITA-TĀNA-ĀSANA ("reclined stretching posture"), cryptically described in the *Hatha-Ratna-Āvalī* (3.67) as stretching in the sleeping position.

SHEATH. See *kosha*.

SHEPHERD. See *gopa*.

SHEPHERDESS. See *gopī*.

SHESHA. See Ananta.

SHIKHĀ ("crest" or "tuft"), the lock or tuft of hair worn by some ascetics in imitation of *Shiva's hairstyle.

SHIKHIN ("tuft wearer"), an epithet of fire (*agni*). According to the *Tri-Shikhi-Brāhmana-Upanishad* (2.56), the *shikhin* situated in the center of the human *body is "lustrous like molten gold." The location of the *shikhin* is generally envisioned as being of triangular (*trikona*) shape. This scripture further mentions that it is quadrangular in the case of quadrupeds, hexagonal in the case of snakes, octagonal in the case of insects, and circular in the case of birds. These ideas belong to the realm of esoteric *anatomy.

SHĪLA ("disposition" or "behavior"). The *Yoga-Bhāshya* (1.2) speaks of three fundamental dispositions of consciousness (*citta*), resulting from the predominance of one or the other of the three primary constituents (*guna*) of *nature: luminosity (*prākhya*), activity (*pravritti*), and inertia (*sthiti*).

SHĪRSHA-ĀSANA (*shīrshāsana*, "head posture"), the headstand described in modern manuals of *hatha-yoga. In the earlier literature of this school of *Yoga, it goes by the name of *viparīta-kāranī. Cf. *sarvaanga-āsana*.

SHISHYA ("pupil" or "disciple"). *Yoga is an initiatory tradition that, as a rule, calls for a period of apprenticeship or *discipleship during which a spiritual aspirant submits himself or herself not only to rigorous self-discipline but also to a teacher (*guru*). After a potential disciple has pre-

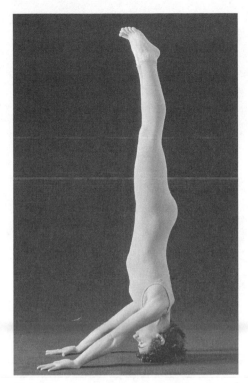

Shīrsha-āsana, the headstand, demonstrated by Donna Farhi. The position of the arms is a variation.

sented himself or herself to a master (*svāmin*), that *teacher applies certain personal and traditional criteria to the applicant to see whether he or she has the necessary qualifications or competence (*adhikāra*) for a life of spiritual *practice. A teacher might, of course, accept an unprepared student who displays promising potential.

The *Shiva-Samhitā* (5.10ff.) distinguishes four types of student, depending on the practitioner's commitment to spiritual life: (1) The weak (*mridu*) practitioner is unenthusiastic, foolish, fickle, timid, ill, dependent, rude, ill mannered, and unenergetic. He is fit only for *mantra-yoga. (2) The mediocre (*madhya*) practitioner is

endowed with even-mindedness, *patience, a desire for *virtue, kind *speech, and the tendency to practice moderation in all undertakings. He is fit for *laya-yoga. (3) The exceptional (*adhimātra*) practitioner demonstrates firm understanding, an aptitude for meditative absorption (*laya*), self-reliance, liberal-mindedness, bravery, vigor, faithfulness, the willingness to *worship the teacher's lotus *feet (both literally and figuratively), and delight in the practice of *Yoga. He is capable of practicing *hatha-yoga. (4) The extraordinary (*adhimātratama*) practitioner displays energy, enthusiasm, charm, heroism, scriptural knowledge, the inclination to practice, freedom from delusion, orderliness, youthfulness, moderate eating habits, control over the *senses, *fearlessness, *purity, skillfulness, generosity, the ability to be a refuge for all people, general capability, stability, thoughtfulness, the willingness to do whatever is desired by the teacher, *patience, good manners, observance of the moral and spiritual law (*dharma*), the ability to keep his struggle to himself, kind speech, *faith in the scriptures, the willingness to worship *God and the teacher (as the embodiment of the *Divine), knowledge of the vows (*vrāta*) pertaining to his level of practice, and, lastly, the practice of all types of Yoga.

Traditionally, the student has been expected to live with, and serve, the *teacher during the period of pupilage. Such a student is known as an *antevāsin* ("one who dwells near"). The reason for this is undoubtedly to give the teacher frequent opportunity to challenge the student's egocentric attitudes and behavior. Additionally, discipleship gives the student the opportunity not only to see the teacher's good example but also to benefit from the *adept's psychophysical "radiation," which is a primary form of spiritual *transmission. This is why the scriptures recommend the great principle of "contact with the Real" (*sat-sanga). The disciple assimilates the teacher's state of being, both by intention and by physical contagion, until—ideally—the disciple reaches *liberation, or at least the same level of spiritual accomplishment as the teacher, if the teacher happens to be not yet liberated. It is widely held that only a teacher who is fully *Self-realized, or *enlightened, can guide the student to Self-realization. See also *dīkshā, guru-yoga*.

SHISHYATĀ. See Discipleship.

SHĪTALĪ ("cooling"), one of the eight types of breath control (*prānāyāma) taught in *hatha-yoga. It is described in the *Gheranda-Samhitā* (5.73f.) thus: Draw in the *air by means of the (extended and curled) *tongue and gradually fill one's abdomen. Retaining it there for an instant, exhale again through both nostrils. This is said to cure indigestion and disorders arising from an imbalance of bile (*pitta) and phlegm (*kapha).

SHĪT-KRAMA ("process [causing the sound] *shīt*"), one of the three processes of *kapāla-bhāti, as described in the *Gheranda-Samhitā* (1.59f.). It gets its name from the sound produced when *water is sucked up through the mouth and expelled through the *nose. This practice is said to make one as beautiful as the god Kāma, the *Hindu equivalent of Cupid. According to the *Shāndilya-Upanishad* (1.7.13.3), which calls this practice *sīt-karī*, the practitioner should, after inhalation, retain the air for as long as possible. Here it is also stated that *shīt-krama* defeats *hunger and *thirst as well as *sleep and *languor.

SHIVA, the personification of the static, masculine form of the *Divine. The word

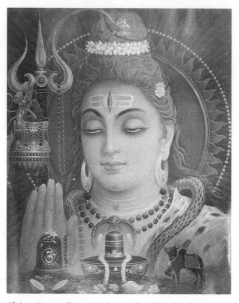

Shiva in meditation (popular Hindu representation)

means "benevolent"; paradoxically, Shiva is generally conceived as the destroyer of the universe. From a spiritual perspective, however, his destructive power is the essential process of breaking down (deconditioning) the ego personality so it becomes pervious to the divine *light. In countless myths, told in the *Mahābhārata and the *Purānas, Shiva emerges as the god of *yogins par excellence. He combines within himself the possibilities of both fierce asceticism (*tapas) and orgiastic excess. See also Aghora, *deva, shakti*.

SHIVĀGRAYOGIN, author of the *Shaiva-Paribhāshā* and other Sanskrit and Tamil works on *Shaiva Siddhānta; the main disciple of Shivakkolundu Shivācārya, whom he succeeded as head of the Suryanārkoil Ādhīnam in South India. His *Shaiva-Paribhāshā* is an excellent manual in which he expounds the epistemology, metaphysics, and ethics of Shaiva Siddhanta.

SHIVA-JNĀNA-BODHAM ("Illumination of the Wisdom of Shiva"), a Tamil work by *Meykandar that consists of only twelve verses, introducing the essentials of the philosophy of *Shaiva Siddhānta.

SHIVA-JNĀNA-SIDDHI ("Perfection of Shiva Wisdom"), a classic exposition of Southern *Shaivism (*Shaiva Siddhānta) by Arulnanda, the foremost of *Meykandar's forty-nine disciples. It has a brilliant commentary by *Jnānaprakāsha.

SHIVA-LINGA. See *linga.*

SHIVA-MANTRA, the most revered sacred *mantra of *Shaivism: om namah shivāya, or "*Om. Obeisance to *Shiva!" The *Shiva-Purāna (3.5.6.25f.) gives the text of the full *mantra: om namah shivāya shubham shubham kuru kuru shivāya namah om, or "Om. Obeisance to Shiva! Do [us] good! Do [us] good! To Shiva [be] obeisance! Om."

SHIVANANDA, SWAMI. See Sivananda, Swami.

SHIVA-PURĀNA, one of the major works of the *Purāna genre, comprising seven chapters with over 24,000 stanzas. As the title suggests, this scripture belongs to *Shaivism. *Yoga is defined as restraint in all one's activities and concentration on *Shiva. In section 17 of the first chapter, *mantra-yoga is introduced, involving the recitation (*japa) of the *shiva-mantra. Adherents of this type of Yoga are said to be of three kinds: the kriyā-yogin, who engages in sacred rites (*kriyā); the tapo-yogin, who pursues asceticism (*tapas); and the japa-yogin, who, in addition to observing the practices of the other two kinds of *yogin, also constantly recites the shiva-mantra. Yoga is again dealt with at length

in sections 37–39 of the seventh chapter. Five types of Yoga are differentiated: (1) mantra-yoga; (2) sparsha-yoga ("tangible Yoga"), a form of mantra-yoga coupled with breath control (*prānāyāma); (3) bhāva-yoga ("Yoga of being"), a higher form of mantra-yoga, where contact with the *mantra is lost and *consciousness enters a subtle dimension of existence; (4) abhāva-yoga ("Yoga of nonbeing"), the *contemplation of the *world in its entirety, associated with the transcendence of object-related awareness; and (5) mahā-yoga ("great Yoga"), the contemplation of *Shiva without any limiting conditions.

SHIVA-SAMHITĀ ("Compendium of [the Wisdom of] *Shiva"; prob. late 17th or early 18th cen. CE), one of the principal manuals of *hatha-yoga, consisting of 645 stanzas distributed over five chapters. It begins with a review of various schools of thought that are judged to be inferior to nondualist *Yoga. It is clear from this opening section that the author was thoroughly familiar with the metaphysics of *Advaita Vedānta. The second chapter deals with esoteric *anatomy, a subject taken up again in the concluding chapter in regard to actual yogic practice. The third chapter describes the five types of life force (*prāna) and the means of its regulation, including breath control (*prānāyāma) and several postures (*āsana). The fourth chapter treats the bodily "seals" (*mudrā). The fifth chapter appears to be a later appendage. It is presented as a discourse between *Ishvara (the Lord) and *Devī (the Goddess). Its content is mixed, ranging from definitions of different types of Yoga to descriptions of various esoteric practices. In several places this work emphasizes that even householders (*griha-stha) can obtain success in Yoga through diligent practice.

SHIVA-SŪTRA ("Aphorisms of *Shiva"), a source text of Kashmiri (or Northern) *Shaivism. It was composed ("discovered") by *Vasugupta in the early ninth century CE and has given rise to an extensive literature of commentary, the most important commentary being *Kshemarāja's *Vimarshinī*. Vasugupta's work consists of three sections with a total of seventy-seven *sūtras*. Similar to *Patanjali's *Yoga-Sūtra*, the *Shiva-Sūtra* can be regarded as an extremely terse exposition of *Yoga, with a fully developed technical vocabulary. See also Pratyabhijnā.

SHIVA-SVARODAYA ("Production of *Shiva's Sound"). The Sanskrit word *svarodaya* is composed of *svara* ("sound") and *udaya* ("rising," "production," or "success"). The "production of sound" refers specifically to the sound made by the *breath; *svara* is thus almost synonymous with *prāna. The *Shiva-Svarodaya*, a late work of 395 stanzas, deals with the flow of the life force (or breath) through the three principal pathways: the *idā-nādī on the left, the *pingalā-nādī on the right, and the *sushumnā-nādī in the middle. *Yogins have noted that the flux of the life force alternates between the left and the right channel (*nādī*) and that, when switching from the one to the other, it flows for a short period of time through the central pathway. This can be determined by checking which nostril is blocked. When both are open, the life force is thought to flow through the *sushumnā-nādī*. The cycle is said to last for approximately one hour per nostril. The flow can be changed in a few minutes by lying on the opposite side of the nostril that is blocked. Each flow is associated with certain auspicious and inauspicious moments. The *Shiva-Svarodaya* is largely concerned with divination on the basis of the breath.

SHIVA-YOGA, equated in the *Shiva-Purāna* (7.1.33.25) with *pāshupata-yoga*. According to this work (1.3.27), *shiva-yoga* is painful at first but subsequently auspicious. It consists of *shravana ("listening"), *kīrtana ("chanting"), and *manana ("pondering").

SHIVA-YOGA-RATNA ("Jewel of Shiva-Yoga"), an important treatise on the theory and practice of Southern *Shaivism consisting of 192 stanzas and a short prose appendix. It is one of the nine works ascribed to *Jnānaprakāsha. The *Yoga taught in this work closely resembles *asparsha-yoga*, but unlike *Gaudapāda, Jnānaprakāsha also outlines the practical techniques of *breath control and *meditation.

SHIVA-YOGA-SĀRA ("Essence of Shiva-Yoga"), one of the works of *Jnānaprakāsha. It is a digest of the yogic teachings of Southern *Shaivism.

SHODASHA-CAKRA ("sixteen[-petaled] center"), mentioned in the *Yoga-Kundalī-Upanishad* (1.69), is better known as the *indu-cakra.

SHODHAKA ("purifier"), in *Shaivism, the divine power (*shakti), which is ultimately responsible for the *purification of the spiritual *aspirant. That which is to be purified—the *ego personality—is known as *shodhya*.

SHODHANA ("cleansing" or "cleanliness"), the first member of the sevenfold discipline (*sapta-sādhana). According to the *Gheranda-Samhitā* (1.10), it is accomplished by means of the "six acts" (*shat-karma). See also Purity, *shuddhi*.

SHOKA ("grief"), one of the defects (*dosha). The teaching about the futility of grief figures prominently in the *Bhaga-vad-Gītā, where Prince *Arjuna is depicted as grieving at the thought of having to slay his kinsmen who had joined the enemy on the battlefield. *Krishna instructs him in the secret of the indestructibility of the *Self and encourages him to practice *karma-yoga.

SHONITA ("reddish"), a synonym for *rajas, the female sexual secretion.

SHOSHANA ("desiccation"), generally regarded as the essence of asceticism (*tapas). In *hatha-yoga it sometimes signifies the "drying up" of the life liquid (*rasa), as effected through the practice of the "great seal" (*mahā-mudrā). See also upavāsa.

SHOULDER STAND. See sarva-anga-āsana; cf. viparīta-kāranī-mudrā.

SHRADDHĀ ("faith"), which is sometimes deemed one of the practices of self-discipline (*niyama), is crucial to spiritual life. Already in the ancient *Rig-Veda (10.151) *faith is presented as an integral aspect of Vedic ritual and life. In this hymn, faith is even personified and called upon to establish itself in the pious worshiper who seeks to kindle the fire, offer oblations, and practice *generosity.

Faith is often explained as a "positive attitude" (āstikya-buddhi). The *Yoga-Bhāshya (1.20) defines the word as "mental repose" (cetasah samprasādah) and likens faith to a caring mother, since it protects the *yogin. As such, faith is the exact opposite of the mood of doubt (*samshaya), which saps a person's energies and disrupts the spiritual process. "Faith," states *Vācaspati Mishra in his *Tattva-Vaishāradī (1.20), "is the root of *Yoga." The *Yoga-Sūtra (1.20) treats faith

as a prerequisite for the induction of the supraconscious ecstasy (*asamprajnāta-samādhi). The *Bhagavad-Gītā (4.39) speaks of the "faithful" (*shraddhāvāms), who wins first wisdom (*jnāna) and then peace (*shānti). The same scripture (17.2f.) declares that faith can be of three kinds, depending on the prevalence of one or the other *guna.

The faith of embodied ones (*dehin) is threefold, springing from [their] very being (*sva-bhāva): *sattva-natured, *rajas-natured, or *tamas-natured. Hear [more about] them.

The faith of everyone is in accordance with his essence (*sattva), O Bhārata. This person (*purusha) is of the form of faith. Whatever his faith is, that verily is he.

Cf. Reason.

SHRAVANA ("listening"), an aspect of *bhakti-yoga. The term also stands for attentive listening to the sacred teachings, which is followed by pondering (*man-ana). In some contexts, shravana denotes auditory phenomena associated with *meditation practice, and as such is sometimes considered to be one of the obstacles (*upasarga or *vighna) on the spiritual *path. See also siddhānta-shravana.

SHRĪ ("blessed" or "holy"), a prefix to personal names; also a part of the titles of certain scriptures, such as *Shrī-Bhāshya. See also tiru.

SHRĪ is one of the names of the great *Goddess as the spouse of *Vishnu. The name emphasizes her auspicious and beautiful nature.

SHRĪ-BHĀSHYA ("Blessed Commentary"), the principal work of *Rāmānuja, in which he gives his original interpretation of the metaphysics and ethics implicit in the *Brahma-Sūtra.

SHRĪ-CAKRA ("blessed wheel"), another name for *shrī-yantra.

SHRĪLA PRABHUPĀDA (1896–1977), earlier known as A. (Abhay) C. (Caranaravinda) Bhaktivedanta Swami, the founder and spiritual head of the International Society for Krishna Consciousness (ISKCON), an offshoot of the ancient tradition of *Vaishnavism as taught in the first half of the sixteenth century by the ecstatic *Caitanya. Shrīla Prabhupāda was born Abhay Charan De and, deeply influenced by his father's devotional worship of *Krishna, showed an early interest in religion and spirituality. He first met his teacher, Bhaktisiddhanta Sarasvati Thakura, in 1922 and formally became his disciple ten years later, though he did not renounce the world until age fifty-six. Concurrent with his renunciation (*sam-nyāsa), he resolved to translate the entire *Bhāgavata-Purāna into English. After encountering numerous obstacles in India, in 1965 he arrived in the United States with twenty dollars in his pockets and nowhere to go. Entirely entrusting his life to divine guidance, he quickly found overwhelming support for his mission to revive "God consciousness" in the people of the *kali-yuga, especially Americans. In the following twelve years he wrote sixty books and opened 100 centers. Founded in 1966, ISKCON has particularly distinguished itself for publishing new translations of many ancient *Vaishnava scriptures, notably the *Bhagavad-Gītā and the *Bhāgavata-Purāna (in fifteen volumes). Also, its renouncers made the "*Hare Krishna" *mantra famous in the Western hemisphere. Teaching a form of *bhakti-yoga, Shrīla Prabhupāda's succeeded in a relatively short span of time to bring about a renaissance of the path of Krishna devotion.

SHRĪNIVASA BHATTA (7th cen. CE), the author of the *Hatha-Ratna-Āvalī, a work on *hatha-yoga. He appears to have also been an expert on the *Vedas, *Vedānta, *Tantra, and *Nyāya. He may have invented, or at least be a major advocate of, the *cakrī-karma technique.

SHRĪ-VIDYĀ ("blessed knowledge"), the most important esoteric tradition of *Goddess worship in South Indian *Shaktism (*Tantrism). The term also refers to this tradition's most sacred *mantra, which begins with a concatenation of seed syllables (*bīja-mantra): ham-sa-ksha-ma-la-va-ra-yūm ānanda-bhairavāya vashat tarpayāmi svāhā.

SHRĪ-VIDYĀ, the personification of the sacred knowledge, or gnosis, at the core of

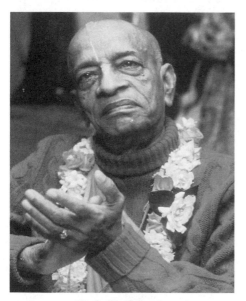

Shrīla Prabhupāda

South Indian *Shaktism. She is the divine *Reality manifesting in the *yogin as the awakened "serpent power" (*kundalinī-shakti). See also Devī.

SHRĪ-YANTRA ("blessed device"), also called shrī-cakra ("blessed wheel") or shrī-pura ("blessed city"), the best-known *yantra employed in Hindu *Shaktism and Tantric *Buddhism. It is composed of nine interlocking triangles, commonly depicted with five triangles pointing downward and four pointing upward. These represent the feminine principle (*shakti) and the male principle (*shiva) respectively. The arrangement of these interpenetrating triangles is such that they yield a total of forty-three small triangles, which house the deities (*devatā) associated with particular aspects of existence. This is sometimes indicated by inscribing in Sanskrit letters (see *alphabet) the names of the deities or their appropriate "seed sounds" (*bīja-mantra). This complex geometrical structure is usually enclosed by two circular lotus patterns of eight and sixteen petals respectively, as well as four concentric circles. The whole design is placed in a square

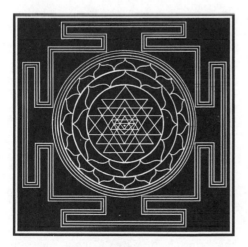

Shrī-yantra

surround of three parallel lines, forming what is known as the protective "world house" (bhū-griha). Cf. mandala.

SHRUTA ("what has been heard"), in *Classical Yoga, a synonym for "tradition" (*āgama).

SHRUTI ("revelation"; the fem. form of the past participle shruta), the sacred literature of *Hinduism, comprising the four ancient *Vedas and the *Upanishads. As opposed to the *smriti literature, the revealed scriptures are thought to be of non-human, or divine, origin. They have been "seen" or "envisioned" by the sages (*rishi, *muni) during extraordinary states of *consciousness. See also āgama.

SHUBHA-ICCHĀ (shubhecca, "desire for the splendid"), the first of seven levels of wisdom (*sapta-jnāna-bhūmi), on which the neophyte cultivates the will to attain *Self-realization. This corresponds to the Buddhist practice of cultivating the "enlightenment mind" (bodhi-citta). See also mumukshutva.

SHUBHA-NĀDĪ ("splendid channel"), extends from the "bulb" (*kanda) to the glans penis (medhra-anta); mentioned in the *Tri-Shikhi-Brāhmana-Upanishad (2.73).

SHUDDHA ("pure"). Cf. ashuddha.

SHUDDHI ("purity" or "purification"), a major concept of spiritual life. See also bhūta-shuddhi, Purity.

SHUKA, an *adept who is said in the *Mahābhārata (12.319.9) to have been able to fly through the air. According to the *Varāha-Upanishad (4.2.34), Shuka is a representative of instantaneous *liberation (*sadyo-mukti*) as opposed to gradual liberation (*krama-mukti*). See also Levitation, *mukti*.

SHUKLA ("white), a synonym for *shukra* ("semen"). See also *bindu, retas*; cf. *rajas*.

SHUKLA-DHYĀNA ("white meditation"), explained in *Upanishad Brahmayogin's commentary on the *Jābāla-Upanishad* as *meditation on the white brilliance of the *Absolute.

SHUKRA ("semen"), sometimes called *shukla*; a synonym for *bindu*. The *Shiva-Purāna* (5.22.49) notes that the strength of living beings depends on the semen.

SHŪNYA ("void"). The idea of the ultimate *Reality as the Void originated in Mahāyāna *Buddhism. It is also expressed in some *hatha-yoga scriptures, though is given a different meaning. In the *Hatha-Yoga-Pradīpikā* (4.56), the highest state of ecstasy (*samādhi*) is described as being void and full (*pūrna*) at the same time. The term is also occasionally employed to denote the suspension of the *breath after exhalation. The term *shūnyatā* ("voidness") is used in the sense of "absentmindedness" in the *Tejo-Bindu-Upanishad* (1.41) and is considered to be one of the obstacles (*vighna*). See also *sahasrāra-cakra*.

SHŪNYA-PANCAKA ("fivefold void"), mentioned in the *Vijnāna-Bhairava* (32), which refers to the sources of the five senses (*indriya*), i.e., the five *tanmātras*, upon which the *yogin must concentrate in order to realize the ultimate Void.

SHŪNYA-SHATKA ("sixfold void"). The *Svacchanda-Tantra* (4.288ff.) states that the divine power (*shakti*) manifests on six levels, which are associated respectively with the lower bodily center (*mūlādhāra-cakra*), the *heart, the region from the *throat to the "brahmic fissure" (*brahma-randhra*), the pervasive form of the divine power (called *vyāpinī*), and the *shakti*'s *samanā* and *unmanā* aspects. This must all be transcended in favor of the ultimate Void, which is the transcendental *Shiva.

SHŪRĀ-NĀDĪ ("valiant channel") extends, according to the *Yoga-Shikhā-Upanishad* (5.22), to the place at the middle between the brows (*bhrū-madhya*).

SHUSHKA-VASTI ("dry enema"), also called *sthala-vasti*; one of the two forms of *vasti. It is described in the *Gheranda-Samhitā* (1.48f.) thus: Assuming the *pashcima-uttāna-āsana*, gently push the intestines downward and then contract and dilate the sphincter muscle by means of the *ashvinī-mudrā*. This is said to cure constipation and flatulence and to stimulate the gastric fire (*jāthara-agni*). Cf. *jala-vasti*.

SHUSHRŪSHĀ ("obedience"). See *guru-shushrūshā*.

SHVĀSA ("inhalation"), a term used in *Classical Yoga both in the general sense of inhalation and the more specific sense of faulty breathing, being one of the obstacles (*antarāya*) on the yogic *path. The latter connotation is found already in the *Mahābhārata* (12.290.54), which lists *shvāsa* as one of the five defects (*dosha*) and states (55) that it can be conquered by a scant diet (*laghu-āhāra*). In another passage (12.266.6) *shvāsa* is said to be overcome by cultivating the "field knower" (*kshetra-jna*), i.e., by magnifying the principle of pure *Consciousness in one's life.

SHVETĀSHVATARA-UPANISHAD ("Whitest Horse *Upanishad*"; 3d or 4th cen. BCE or earlier), one of the more beautiful creations of the *Upanishadic genre. Consisting of six chapters with a total of 113 stanzas, this work is the earliest document of *Shaivism. Its curious title is left unexplained. According to *Shankara's learned commentary on this scripture, *shveta-ashva-tara* ("most white horse") is the title of a sage whose *senses (also esoterically referred to as "horses") are purified and under control.

In its theistic metaphysics, this work is rather similar to the *Bhagavad-Gītā*. It says nothing about *karma-yoga, however, and its yogic teachings center on meditation (*dhyāna). It introduces a sixfold *path (*shad-anga-yoga) that has the god *Rudra-*Shiva-Hara as the priceless goal of the spiritual aspirant. The following stanzas capture the orientation and tone of this early *Yoga scripture:

Following the Yoga of *meditation, they perceived the self-power (*ātma-shakti*) of the *god hidden by his own qualities (*guna). He is the one who presides over all the causes connected with time and self (*atman). (1.3)

The Lord (*īsha) supports this universe, composed of the perishable and the imperishable, the manifest and the unmanifest. The [individuated] self, [which is] not the Lord, is bound by [its notion of] being the enjoyer. But on knowing God, it is released from all fetters. (1.8)

The "foundation" (*pradhāna) [i.e., Nature] is perishable. Hara [= *Shiva] is immortal and imperishable. The one god rules over the perishable and the selves. By meditating on him, by uniting with and becoming the Real (*tattva), there is finally the cessation of all illusion (*māyā). (1.10)

By knowing God, the falling away of all fetters [is swiftly accomplished]. Upon the waning of the afflictions (*klesha) [i.e., spiritual *ignorance and its results], the falling away of *birth and *death [is accomplished]. By meditating on Him, there is a third [state], universal lordship, upon separating from the *body. [Thus the *yogin becomes] the solitary (*kevala) [Self], whose *desires are satisfied. (1.11)

The meditative process, which involves *recitation of the sacred syllable *om, is described as a kind of churning by which the inner *fire is kindled, which then leads to the revelation of the *Self's intrinsic splendor. Successful meditation (*dhyāna) inevitably gives rise to a variety of inner visions that, warns the text, must not be confused with *enlightenment. This is how the anonymous author of the *Shvetāshvatara-Upanishad* (3.8) describes the ultimate realization: "I know that great Self (*purusha) who is effulgent like the sun beyond darkness. Realizing him alone, one passes beyond *death. There is no other way for passing [beyond the cycle of repeated births and deaths]." This work has in rough outline all the basic elements of the yogic *path, and even includes the devotional (*bhakti) aspect.

SIDDHA ("accomplished" or "adept"; fem. *siddha-anganā*, "adept's companion"), a spiritual master who is generally held to be *enlightened, or to have reached perfection (*siddhi). According to the *Yoga-Shikhā-Upanishad* (1.159), an *adept can be recognized by his possession of paranormal powers (also called *siddhi). In the same work (1.50) it is also stated that the grace (*prasāda) of an adept is essential for a practitioner of *jnāna-yoga (or *jnānin) of inferior standing in order to become a full-fledged *yogin. See also *maha-siddha*, *shakti-pāta*.

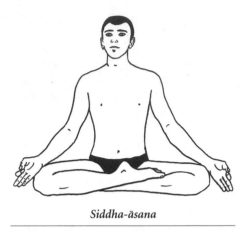

Siddha-āsana

SIDDHA-ĀSANA (*siddhāsana*, "accomplished posture"), a *meditation posture described in the *Gheranda-Samhitā* (2.7) as follows: Place the (left) heel at the anus and the other heel above the *genitals, while resting the chin on the chest and gazing at the spot between the eyebrows (*bhrū-madhya*). This posture (*āsana*) is said to lead to *liberation. The *Hatha-Yoga-Pradīpikā* (1.40) promises perfection in twelve years through the proper *practice of this technique. It also mentions (1.36) an alternative version in which the left ankle is placed above the genitals. This practice is also sometimes referred to as *vajra-āsana*, *mukta-āsana*, and *gupta-āsana*. In the *Yoga-Mārtanda* (5) it is also called *svastha-āsana*.

SIDDHA CULT (fl. 800–1200 CE), the recognition and *worship of a group of perfected beings known as the *siddhas*. The North Indian tradition recognizes eighty-four great adepts (*mahā-siddha*) who not only enjoy the superlative condition of liberation (*moksha*) but are also in possession of great paranormal powers (*siddhi*). They are venerated as deified humans. Best known among these extraordinary beings are *Matsyendra (known as Luipā in Tibet) and *Goraksha. As this roster of eighty-four spiritual notables makes clear, the Siddha cult straddled both *Hinduism and *Buddhism. The South Indian tradition knows of a pantheon of eighteen such adepts, notably *Agastya, *Tirumūlar, and *Civavākkiyar. This second list also includes several non-Indian individuals, of Chinese, Singhalese, and even Egyptian origin. Countless legends have been woven around the lives and miraculous deeds of these figures. Their teachings have been only imperfectly preserved, however. In addition to some writings—mostly of dubious authenticity—there are also numerous didactic songs (*doha*).

The *veneration of spiritual personages, as focal points of sacred presence or power, is of course a time-honored practice, dating back thousands of years, as is evident from the *Mahābhārata* and other early works. Teacher worship (*guru-pūjana*) is an aspect of this practice.

Integral to the Siddha cult or movement was a concern for bodily perfection, even physical *immortality. This orientation of "cultivating (the potential of) the body" (*kāya-sādhana*) led to the creation of *hatha-yoga. However, the historical connections between the Siddha cult and *hatha-yoga, *Nāthism, and *Kaulism are still rather obscure.

SIDDHA-DARSHANA ("vision of the adepts"). According to the *Yoga-Sūtra* (3.32), one can induce a visionary experience of the *adepts by practicing ecstatic "constraint" (*samyama*) on the "light in the head." The *Shiva-Samhitā* (5.87) states that this vision can be obtained through *contemplation of the heart center (*anahāta-cakra*).

SIDDHĀNTA ("doctrine," from *siddha*, "accomplished" or "established," and *anta*, "end" or "conclusion"). The teachings, or doctrines, are a "settled matter" because they are based on the experiences and realizations of *adepts. See also Shaiva Siddhānta.

SIDDHĀNTA-SHRAVANA ("listening to the doctrines"), one of the ten components of self-discipline (*niyama*), according to the *Darshana-Upanishad* (2.9). It is defined as the study of "the true, infinite knowledge (*jnāna*), the supreme bliss (*ānanda*), the supreme certainty, and the 'innermost' (*pratyanc*)." The *Yoga-Tattva-Upanishad* introduces it as one of the constituent practices of *hatha-yoga. Listening to the esoteric teachings creates right understanding and instills faith (*shraddhā*) and thus motivates the student to devote himself or herself to the ordeal of self-discipline and *self-transcendence. See also *shravana*.

SIDDHAPĀDA, mentioned in the *Hatha-Yoga-Pradīpikā* (1.6) as a master of *hatha-yoga.

SIDDHA-SIDDHĀNTA-PADDHATI (lit. "Tracks of the Doctrines of the Adepts"), an important work of early *hatha-yoga. Ascribed to *Goraksha, it consists of six chapters with a total of 353 stanzas. The text develops the philosophy of *Nāthism, especially the teachings about the body (*pinda*). In the first chapter six types or levels of *embodiment are distinguished, beginning with the transcendental (*para*) *body and ending with the "embryonic" (*garbha*) or physical body. Subsequent chapters deal extensively with esoteric *anatomy. In one verse (2.32) the genuine *yogin is defined as someone who knows firsthand the nine centers (*cakra*), the sixteen props (*ādhāra*), the three signs (*lakshya*), and the five ether spaces (*vyoman*). The nine psychoenergetic centers include the well-known series of seven, except that the *sahasrāra-cakra* is here called *nirvāna-cakra. The eighth center is the *tālu-cakra, which is situated at the *palate and is the location of the mysterious "bell" (*ghantikā*), or uvula, or "royal tooth" (*rāja-danta*), the point from which the divine nectar (*amrita*) drips. The ninth center is the *ākāsha-cakra, which is described as having sixteen spokes and is situated at the "brahmic fissure" (*brahma-randhra*) at the crown of the *head.

The fourth chapter introduces the "serpent power" (*kundalinī-shakti*), which is stated to exist in two forms, unmanifest (cosmic) and manifest (individuated). In the former state it is known as *akula, in the latter as *kula. This scripture further distinguishes between the lower, middle, and upper force (*shakti*), respectively located at the base of the spine, the *navel, and the crown of the *head. In the fifth chapter, the important point is made that success in *Yoga depends on the teacher's grace (*prasāda*). It empowers the practitioner to renounce all the paranormal powers (*siddhi*) that he or she has obtained and to proceed to the "nonemergent" (*nirutthāna*) state where the *body unites with the "supreme estate" (*parampāda*), or *Shiva.

Another work by this name consists of 100 stanzas and is attributed to a certain Parameshvara Yogin.

SIDDHA-SIDDHĀNTA-SAMGRAHA (lit. "Compendium of the Doctrines of the Adepts"), ascribed to Balabhadra, a work of 306 stanzas purporting to be a summary of the *Siddha-Siddhānta-Paddhati* of Nityanātha.

SIDDHI ("accomplishment"), a term used in the yogic scriptures in a number of ways. In the most general sense, it means "attainment" or "success." More specifically, the term is equivalent to *samsiddhi*, signifying "*perfection," i.e., *liberation. This is also occasionally referred to as the "great accomplishment" (*mahā-siddhi*). The *Shiva-Samhitā* (3.18) speaks of six specific preconditions for success in Yoga: (1) *vishvāsa*, confidence that the spiritual *path and one's efforts are fruitful; (2) *shraddhā*, faith; (3) *guru-pūjana*, *worship of the *teacher; (4) *samatā-bhāva*, the sense of *equanimity, the condition of psychic balance; (5) *indriya-nigraha*, control of the *senses; and (6) *pramita-āhāra*, moderate *diet.

A third, important connotation of the term *siddhi* is "paranormal attainment" or "magical ability." As we read in the *Yoga-Bīja* (54): "The *yogin is possessed of unthinkable powers. He who has conquered the *senses can, by his own will, assume various shapes and make them vanish again." Since ancient times *yogins* have been not only venerated as saintly folk but also feared as thaumaturgists, whose powers were many and whose curses are potent. The word *siddhi* stems from the same root as the word for "adept" (*siddha*). An *adept is someone who is master of his own *body and *mind as well as master of the forces of *nature.

The *yogin*'s powers are considered a by-product of the spiritual process, especially of ecstatic "constraint" (*samyama*). The *Yoga-Shikhā-Upanishad* (1.151ff.) speaks of two fundamental types of paranormal powers, those that are artificial (*kalpita*) and those that are nonartificial (*akalpita*). The former are produced by herbs (*aushadhi*), ritual (*kriyā*), magic (*jāla*), *mantra practice, and alchemical elixirs (*rasa*). In an aphorism that is possibly an interpolation, the *Yoga-Sūtra* (4.1) similarly explains that the powers can

spring from five possible causes: birth (*janman*), herbs (*aushadhi*), *mantra recitation, asceticism (*tapas*), and ecstasy (*samādhi*). They are deemed transient and have little efficacy. The second kind of *siddhis*, however, spring from self-reliance (*svatantrya*) and are permanent, greatly efficacious, and pleasing to the Lord (*īshvara*). They manifest naturally in those who are free from desire (*vāsanā*) and are the mark of a true adept (*siddha*). These powers are encountered in the course of one's spiritual *practice, just as a pilgrim on the way to the sacred city of Kāshī (modern Banaras) passes by a number of sacred spots (*tīrtha*). The *Yoga-Shikhā-Upanishad* (1.160) observes that the person lacking such powers is bound.

The literatures of *Hinduism, *Buddhism, and *Jainism are filled with references to, and examples of, paranormal abilities. Best known is the set of eight "great powers" (*mahā-siddhi*), which are thought to accompany *liberation. According to the *Yoga-Bhāshya* (3.45), these are *animan ("miniaturization"), *mahiman ("magnification"), *laghiman ("levitation"), *prāpti ("extension"), *prākāmya ("[irresistible] will"), *vāshitva ("mastery"), *īshitritva ("lordship [over the universe]"), and *kāma-avasāyitva ("fulfillment of [all] desires"). Some scriptures provide a slightly different list of *mahā-siddhis*. The *Purānas often group them according to the five material elements (*bhūta*) that serve as props for *concentration and ecstatic "constraint" (*samyama*). Thus the *Linga-Purāna* (1.9.30ff.) furnishes a detailed catalog of paranormal powers, including the ability to make oneself bulky or lean, to prophesize or see the future, to produce *fire from the body, to assume any form at will, and even to dissolve the entire *cosmos.

So long as one has a fickle *mind, advises the *Yoga-Shikhā-Upanishad (5.54), one should not dwell on the attainment of paranormal powers. The *Yoga-Tattva-Upanishad (75) regards them as one of the obstacles (*vighna) on the spiritual *path. The *Varāha-Upanishad (3.29) notes that they are not important to the aspirant who seeks to realize the *Self. The "seers of the Self" (ātma-darshin), announces the *Laghu-Yoga-Vāsishtha (6.14.4), do not long for them. The *Linga-Purāna (1.9.14) states that the initial hindrances (*antarāya) disappear through devoted spiritual practice, but then new obstacles (*upasarga) arise, i.e., the magical powers. According to the *Yoga-Sūtra (3.37), certain paranormal powers, called *pratibhā, are to be looked upon as obstacles in attaining ecstasy (*samādhi). *Patanjali, however, was obviously favorably inclined toward the use of the siddhis to gain a higher understanding of oneself and the cosmos, or else he would not have dedicated the entire third chapter of his work to what he calls *vibhūtis, or "manifestations (of power)." The *Tattva-Vaishāradī (3.55) declares that the siddhis are not necessary for attaining liberation (*kaivalya) but neither are they completely useless, because they can strengthen the practitioner's faith (*shraddhā).

Many texts, e.g., the *Yoga-Tattva-Upanishad (76f.), state that these powers should not be demonstrated but be kept secret. The reason for this is that any public display would interfere with the *yogin's life of quietude and, if he is not fully *enlightened, possibly ensnare him in *pride, causing all kinds of *karmic entanglements. Indian folklore and mythology knows of numerous stories in which ascetics or yogins have come to fall through their misuse of magical powers. Rarely do they end as happily as the story of Tibet's favorite adept, Milarepa, who in his youth used his magical abilities with devastating results, which is why his discipleship under Marpa was particularly difficult. *Secrecy is therefore enjoined more for the protection of the practitioner than for the innocent bystander. The widespread and consistent claims for the existence of paranormal powers in *Yoga deserve careful study through the empirical means available to *parapsychology. Given the extraordinary understanding and also control of the workings of the nervous system and the *mind demonstrated by *yogins, we should not be surprised if at least some of the paranormal phenomena claimed in the spiritual literature of Yoga and indeed of other traditions are based in reality. Still, how much of the traditional claims are pious fiction and how much solid fact remains to be discovered. See also cihna, pravritti.

SIDDHI, mentioned in the *Hatha-Yoga-Pradīpikā (1.6) as an *adept of *hatha-yoga.

SIGHT. See darshana, drishti.

SIGN. See arishta, cihna, lakshya, linga.

SIKHISM, a spiritual tradition that represents a synthesis between the devotional approach (*bhakti) of *Hinduism and the mysticism of Muslim Sufism. It was founded by *Nānak (1469–1539 CE), the first of ten *gurus recognized by the Sikhs. The teachings of the first five spiritual masters is found codified in the Granth Sahib ("Book of the Lord"). This scripture is also known as the *Ādi-Granth ("First Book") to distinguish it from the Dasam-Granth ("Tenth Book"), which was compiled by the tenth guru, Gobind Singh (1666–1708).

Apart from the gurus themselves, the

Ādi-Granth is the most sacred focal point of Sikh devotion, and it is recited daily by pious followers of this tradition. Central to Sikhism are **guru-yoga* and **mantra-yoga* in the form of recitation (**japa*) of the divine name (a practice that is called *nāma-mārga*, or "way of the name"). Ever since Nānak, the teachers of Sikhism have emphasized spontaneity or naturalness (**sahaja*) over **asceticism and forced **celibacy.

SILENCE. See *mauna*.

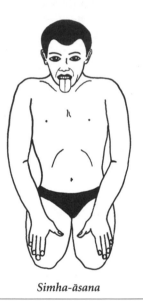

Simha-āsana

SIMHA-ĀSANA (*simhāsana*, "lion posture"), described in the **Gheranda-Samhitā* (2.14f.) as follows: Place the crossed and upturned heels under the scrotum, with one's knees on the ground and hands placed on the knees. Keeping the mouth open and applying the throat lock (**jālandhara-bandha*), gaze steadily at the tip of the nose (**nāsa-agra*).

SIN. See *pāpa, pātaka*; cf. *punya*.

SINGING. See *bhajana, kīrtana*.

SĪT-KARĪ ("making the [sound] *sīt*"), one of the basic forms of breath control (**prānāyāma*). It is taught in the **Hatha-Yoga-Pradīpikā* (2.54) as follows: Make a hissing sound (i.e., *sīt*) during inhalation through the mouth, whereas the exhalation should be done quietly through the **nose. See also *shīt-krama*.

SIVANANDA, SWAMI (Sanskrit: Svāmin Shivānanda; 1887–1963), one of the great modern masters of **Yoga. After a successful practice as a physician, he renounced the world in 1923, founded his own hermitage in 1932, and four years later established the Divine Life Society, which has since won an international reputation. He has over 300 publications attributed to him. Among his best-known disciples are Swami Cidananda,

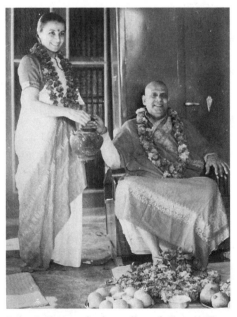

Swami **Sivananda** (seated) and Swami Sivananda Radha

who succeeded him as the head of the Divine Life Society, Swami Satyananda (whose *āshrama* is in Bihar), Swami Vishnudevananda (author of *The Complete Illustrated Book of Yoga*), Swami Satchidananda (founder of the Integral Yoga Institute in New York), Swami Venkatesananda (translator of the *Yoga-Vāsishtha* and other Sanskrit works), and Swami Sivananda Radha (1911–1995), a German-born woman who contributed significantly to translating traditional yogic wisdom into practical psychological terms for Western students.

SKULL. See *kapāla*.

SLEEP. See *nidrā, sushupti, svapna*.

SLOTH. See *ālasya*.

SMARANA ("recollection"), or remembrance of the *Divine, one of the aspects of *bhakti-yoga. It is the loving regard for one's chosen deity (*ishta-devatā*).

SMAYA ("pride") may, according to the *Yoga-Sūtra* (3.51), arise as a result of the flattering attention paid to the *adept by higher beings. It must be overcome to prevent renewed entanglement in worldly existence. See also Pride.

SMRITI (from *smri*, "to remember"). In the sense of "mindfulness," *smriti* is mentioned in the *Yoga-Sūtra* (1.20) as one of the factors that precede the supraconscious ecstasy (*asamprajnāta-samādhi*). In his commentary on this aphorism, *Vācaspati Mishra equates the word with *dhyāna* ("meditation"). A less specialized meaning of *smriti* in *Classical Yoga is that of "memory." As such it figures as one of the five types of mental fluctuation

(*vritti*). In some of *Patanjali's aphorisms the term is used in the sense of "depth memory," i.e., the deep structure of consciousness (*citta*), which is composed of the subliminal "activators" (*samskāra*) responsible for the *karmic continuity in one's *life and also between the present existence and future *embodiments.

A further connotation of *smriti* is "remembered (knowledge)," or authoritative traditional literature as opposed to revealed literature (*shruti*). See also *āgama*.

SNAKE CHARMING can be understood as a symbolic representation of *kundalinī arousal, whereby the snake is looked upon as a device (*yantra*) for focusing *attention.

SNĀNA ("bathing" or "ablution"), sometimes considered to be a component of self-discipline (*niyama), as in the *Hatha-Ratna-Āvalī* (3.3). The ritual of bathing is described in detail in the *Brihad-Yogi-Yājnavalkya* (7.1ff.). The *Garuda-Purāna* (50.8) distinguishes six types of ablutions: (1) *brāhma-* ("brahmic"), by means of sprinkling *water on oneself; (2) *āgneya-* ("fiery"), by means of smearing *ashes on the *body; (3) *vāyavya-* ("airy"), by means of the use of cow dung; (4) *divya-* ("divine, resplendent"), by means of bathing in sunshine; (5) *vāruna-* ("watery"), by means of bathing in water; and (6) *yaugika-snāna* ("yogic bathing"), by means of *meditation on the *Divine.

The *Shiva-Samhitā* (5.4) considers bathing one of the obstacles (*vighna*) but mentions (5.134) "mental bathing" (*mānasa-snāna*) at the sacred junction of the "inner rivers"—Ganges, Yamunā, and *Sarasvatī—which represent the three principal channels (*nādī*) through which the life force circulates and which come together at the *ājnā-cakra. This mental bathing is to be resorted to particularly at the time of *death.

SNEHA ("attachment"), a synonym for *rāga.

SOLAR POSTURE. See saura-āsana.

SOMA ("extract," from the root su, "to press out"), the draft of *immortality, used as a libation in the daily sacrificial *ritual of *Vedic times. Some scholars have identified it as an extract from the fly agaric mushroom, but this is doubtful, as the plant source of soma is often described as a creeper. During the era of *Tantrism, a new conception of the soma juice emerged according to which it is an inner secretion produced by the *body as a result of spiritual practice. It is also known as *amrita ("nectar of immortality") and sudhā ("well placed"). Some scriptures, however, make a clear-cut distinction between soma and sudhā, regarding the intoxication resulting from the latter as undesirable. The *Hatha-Yoga-Pradīpikā (3.44) claims that one who continually drinks the inner soma by means of the practice of *khecarī-mudrā conquers *death in fifteen days.

SORROW. See duhkha, shoka.

SORUBA-SAMĀDHI ("transformative ecstasy"), a Tamil term denoting the highest spiritual state of those *adepts who have succeeded in transubstantiating the *body. The Sanskrit equivalent of soruba is sarūpa (meaning "with form" but also "beautiful"), here standing for a condition that is deemed higher than the "formless" (*nirvikalpa) ecstasy. The luminous transubstantiated body of the great adepts is an expression of their mergence with the *Divine. They can assume any form at will

and do so in order to instruct others. See also Babaji, Ramalinga Swami.

SOUL. See jīva; cf. ātman, purusha, Self, Spirit.

SOUND. See dhvāni, nāda, shabda, svara, vāc.

SPACE. See ākāsha.

SPANDA ("quiver" or vibration"), a prominent technical concept in Kashmiri (or Northern) *Shaivism. It is the "throb" of utter *bliss of the ultimate *Reality. It is not movement as ordinarily understood but the transcendental cause of all motion. This philosophical notion is elaborated at length in *Vasugupta's ninth-century *Spanda-Kārikā, which is also often ascribed to his disciple Kallata.

SPANDA, one of the leading philosophical schools of *Shaivism, prominent in Kashmir.

SPANDA-KĀRIKĀ ("Composition on Vibration"), an independent commentary on the *Shiva-Sūtra, authored by either *Vasugupta or (less likely) his chief disciple Kallata. It explains the notion of divine vibration (*spanda), which is a central doctrine of Kashmiri *Shaivism. The Spanda-Kārikā has several significant commentaries, including a Vritti by Kallata.

SPARSHA ("touch"), one of the cognitive senses (*jnāna-indriya) related to the *water element. In the *Mahābhārata (12.232.21) the term denotes a superperception in the tactile field, which is a byproduct of *meditation.

SPARSHA-YOGA ("Yoga of contact"), a term in the *Shiva-Purāna (7.2.37.9) referring to *mantra-yoga coupled with *breath control. Cf. asparsha-yoga.

SPHOTA ("bursting forth"), an esoteric linguistic notion according to which the concept underlying a configuration of *sounds is eternal. This idea was taught by the grammarian *Patanjali and has traditionally been ascribed to the author of the *Yoga-Sūtra on the strength of aphorism 3.17, although a closer examination of this *sūtra does not lend support to such an interpretation. All discussion about the sphota is actually confined to *Vācaspati Mishra's commentary *Tattva-Vaishāradī (3.17). The word sphota is not even mentioned in the *Yoga-Bhāshya.

SPHURANA ("throbbing"), the pulsing of the life force (*prāna) as experienced by the *yogin. Sometimes this term is used synonymously with *spanda.

SPINE. See meru, vīnā-danda.

SPIRIT. See ātman, purusha, Self; cf. jīva, Soul.

SPONTANEITY. See sahaja.

SROTA ("stream" or "current"), a term traditionally used to classify the *Shaiva *Āgamas. Generally five streams are distinguished, related to the four directions and the center, though sometimes a sixth, "upper" stream is added, which is said to lead to instant realization through great force (*hatha). Cf. āmnāya, pītha.

STABILITY. See sthairya.

STAFF. See danda.

STAFF POSTURE. See danda-āsana.

STAMBHA ("stoppage"), in the *Yoga-Sūtra (3.21), the suspension of the *breath. This word also denotes the paranormal ability (*siddhi) to paralyze another being, as mentioned in the *Kaula-Jnāna-Nirnaya (4.14). See also kumbhaka.

STEADFASTNESS. See dhairya, dhriti.

STHAIRYA ("stability"), one of the practices of moral observance (*yama); the third member of the sevenfold discipline (*sapta-sādhana) of *hatha-yoga. According to the *Gheranda-Samhitā (1.10), it is also called sthiratā ("firmness"). The *Bhagavad-Gītā (13.7) treats it as a manifestation of wisdom (*jnāna), while the *Yoga-Sūtra (3.31) sees it as the fruit of ecstatic "constraint" (*samyama) upon the "tortoise channel" (*kūrma-nādī).

STHĀLA. See shat-sthāla.

STHALA-VASTI, a synonym for *shushka-vasti.

STHĀNA ("place" or "abode"), a synonym for *desha ("location"). Thus the *Gheranda-Samhitā (5.3–7) observes that one should not take up the practice of *Yoga in a far-off country, a forest, a metropolis, or in the midst of a crowd, since this would only frustrate one's endeavors. In a distant country, one loses faith (*shraddhā); in a forest, one has no protection; in the "wilderness" of the city, one is exposed to the public.

The term sthāna often refers to places in the *body that serve as props for *concentration and *meditation. Thus the *Goraksha-Paddhati (2.75f.) mentions nine such loci. Other scriptures mention five bodily regions governed by the five elements (*bhūta). According to the *Tri-Shikhi-Brāhmana-Upanishad (2.135f.), the area from the soles to the knees is the "earth place" (prithivī-sthāna); from the knees to the hips, the "water place" (ap-sthāna); from the hips to the center of the *body, the "fire place" (agni-sthāna); from the *navel to the *nose, the "air place" (vāyu-sthāna); and from the nose to the "brahmic cave" (*brahma-bila), i.e., the crown of the *head, the "ether place" (vyoma-sthāna).

The word sthāna also is a rare synonym for *āsana. See also marman.

STHITA-PRAJÑĀ ("he who is steadied in wisdom"), according to the *Bhagavad-Gītā (2.54), the sage who is content abiding in the *Self alone, who has repelled all desire (*kāma), and who is neither dismayed by sorrowful events nor elated by joyous experiences. Such an *adept is constantly immersed in the "vision of sameness" (*sama-darshana). He is also known as a sthita-dhī ("he who is steadied in visionary thought").

STHITI ("state" or "condition"), the mental disposition (*shīla) of inertia, as a manifestation of *tamas. The *Tattva-Vaishāradī (1.2) states that this term covers undesirable states such as heaviness, concealment, and dejection.

STHŪLA ("gross" or "coarse"), the outermost, or visible material aspect of a thing. Thus the "coarse body" (sthūla-sharīra) is the mortal physical frame, the "sheath composed of food" (*anna-maya-kosha). The opposite is *sūkshma. See also Cosmos.

STHŪLA-DHYĀNA ("coarse meditation"), *meditation on the "coarse" (*sthūla) aspect of a thing, such as the iconographic form of one's chosen deity (*ishta-devatā). Cf. jyotir-dhyāna, sūkshma-dhyāna.

STOTRA ("Hymn"), a literary category of poetic compositions in praise of the *Divine under its various *names.

STRĪ ("woman"), considered an embodiment or human representation of the feminine aspect of the Divine, or *Shakti. In the more ascetic schools of *Hinduism, however, women are often regarded as a threat to men. Sri *Ramakrishna, for instance, summarized the dangers of the *world in the phrase "woman and gold."

STUDY. See svādhyāya.

STYĀNA ("languor" or "sluggishness"), recognized in *Classical Yoga as one of the obstacles (*antarāya) on the spiritual *path. The *Yoga-Bhāshya (1.30) defines it as "inactivity of the mind" (akarmanyatā cittasya). It is a manifestation of *tamas. See also ālasya, tandrā.

SUBCONSCIOUS. Although the *Yoga tradition does not have a specific term for "subconscious," it clearly operates with this concept when explaining the automatic functions of the human *mind. Thus the entire teaching of the subconscious "activators" (*samskāra), which combine into concatenations called *vāsanā, presupposes an aspect of the mind that is less than fully conscious and yet has tremendous power over us. To achieve complete *freedom from suffering (*duhkha) and gain liberating *wisdom, the *yogin must disable these subconscious forces. Cf. Consciousness, Unconscious.

SUBJECT, TRANSCENDENTAL. See ātman; cf. Object.

SUBSTANCE. See dharma, dharmin, dravya.

SUBTLE. See sūkshma.

SUDHĀ ("well placed"), an intoxicating beverage, notably alcohol; in esoteric contexts is used as a synonym for the nectar of immortality (*amrita or *soma).

SUFFERING. See *duhkha*.

SUKHA ("joy," "pleasure," or "ease"). When used in association with the word *duhkha, the term sukha stands for "pleasure." Pleasure, as the *Yoga-Bhāshya (4.11) notes, gives rise to attachment (*rāga). The *Bhagavad-Gītā (18.36ff.) distinguishes three kinds of pleasure, depending on the prevalence of one or the other *guna: (1) Sāttvika-sukha is that which seems like *pain at first but then turns out to be nectar and generates serenity (*prasāda). (2) Rājasa-sukha is that which seems like nectar at first but then turns into poison; it springs from the contact of the senses (*indriya) with the sense objects (*vishaya). (3) Tāmasa-sukha is that which arises from *sleep, *sloth, and *inattention and simply leads one astray. According to the ascetic tradition of India, all forms of sukha—like all forms of duhkha, or suffering—must be overcome.

In *Tantrism pleasure need not be anxiously shunned, because it conceals or contains the ultimate bliss (*ānanda). Rather, the spiritual practitioner is advised to find the "great joy" (*mahā-sukha) in all ordinary moments of pleasure. See also *kāma, rati*.

SUKHA-ĀSANA (*sukhāsana*, "pleasant/easy posture"), identical with the *svāstika-āsana, according to the *Shiva-Samhitā (3.97). The *Tri-Shikhi-Brāhmana-Upanishad (2.52) describes it as that posture through which *steadiness can be gained. It is said to be suitable for those who cannot perform the other *āsanas. Generally, the sukha-āsana corresponds to the tailor's seat.

SŪKSHMA ("subtle"), the inner or psychic dimension of existence, which is not visible to the physical *eyes but can be experienced in *meditation. The subtle dimension extends all the way to the transcendental foundation (*pradhāna) of *nature. Cf. *sthūla*.

SŪKSHMA-DHYĀNA ("subtle meditation"), equated in the *Gheranda-Samhitā (6.9f.) with the *shāmbhavī-mudrā, the experience of the union of *Shiva and *Shakti. Cf. *jyotir-dhyāna, sthūla-dhyāna*.

SŪKSHMA-SHARĪRA ("subtle body"), the entire psychomental complex that, according to *Yoga metaphysics, can exist independent of the physical or coarse *body. This is the bodily "field" that remains after *death and that serves as the precondition for a future *embodiment. The existence of such a body is rejected by *Vācaspati Mishra in his *Tattva-Vaishāradī (4.10) on the grounds that there is no proper scriptural support for it and also because it is not necessary to postulate a subtle body in order to explain the process of rebirth (*punar janman). See also *ātivāhika-deha, deha, sharīra*.

SULABHĀ, a *yoginī mentioned in the *Mahābhārata (12.308.3ff.) who entered the *consciousness of King Videha in order to ascertain whether he was truly *enlightened.

SUN. See *ravi, sūrya*.

SUNDARADEVA, author of the *Hatha-Sanketa-Candrikā and *Hatha-Tattva-Kaumudī; he lived in Banaras (Varanasi), in Northern India. His teacher was Pūrnānanda.

SUNDARAR (Sanskrit: Sundara; early 8th cen. CE), one of the great Tamil saints of

*Shaivism, who came to be known as the "insolent devotee" because of his familiar (and to some offensive) behavior toward the *Divine. We know of his life and teachings primarily from his own passionate poetry. See also Crazy adept, Shaiva Siddhānta.

SUPERIMPOSITION. See *adhyāsa, upādhi*.

SUPPORT. See *ādhāra*.

SURĀ ("alcohol"). See *madya*.

SURĀNANDA, mentioned in the *Hatha-Yoga-Pradīpikā* (1.6) as a master of *hatha-yoga*.

SŪRYA ("sun"), an esoteric phenomenon or subtle anatomical structure that is thought to be situated in the region of the *navel. The scriptures of *hatha-yoga* describe it as devouring the "nectar of immortality" (*amrita*) that drips from the "moon" (*candra*) located in the *head. It turns the ambrosia that is naturally produced by the *body into poison, which then flows through the *pingalā-nādī*. Various techniques are proposed for stopping this solar generator and for enhancing and exploiting the lunar flow. See also Anatomy.

SŪRYA-BHEDA or SŪRYA-BHEDANA ("sun piercing"), one of the eight types of breath control (*prānāyāma*), described in the *Gheranda-Samhitā* (5.58f.) as follows: Energetically inhaling through the "solar channel" (i.e., the right nostril), carefully retain the *breath while performing the throat lock (*jālandhara-bandha*) until one perspires heavily. In another passage (5.66f.), the following technique is recommended: Raise from the navel (*nābhi*) the various forms of the life force (*prāna*) that are cut off from the solar channel, and then slowly exhale through the *idā-nādī (i.e., the left nostril). This should be done repeatedly for the awakening of the "serpent power" (*kundalinī-shakti*). See also *kumbhaka*.

SŪRYA-GRAHANA ("solar eclipse") occurs, according to the *Darshana-Upanishad (4.47), when the life force (*prāna*) reaches, via the right channel (or *pingalā-nādī*), the place of the "serpent power" (*kundalinī-shakti*), i.e., the *mūlādhāra-cakra*. Cf. *candra-grahana*.

SŪRYA-NAMASKARA ("obeisance to the sun"), a series of twelve dynamic postures (*āsana*) described in contemporary manuals of *hatha-yoga*. This series is so called because it should be practiced in the morning while facing the benign rays of the sun.

SUSHRUTA-SAMHITĀ ("Sushruta's Compendium"), one of two great texts on native Indian *medicine, the other being the *Caraka-Samhitā*. Since it draws on the philosophy elaborated in *Īshvara Krishna's *Sāmkhya-Kārikā*, this compilation belongs to the period after 350 CE. Its materials are in part considerably older, however, dating as far back as the time of the *Shata-Patha-Brāhmana. See also Āyur-Veda.

SUSHUMNĀ-NĀDĪ ("most gracious channel"), the central conduit through which the life force (*prāna*) flows from the psychoenergetic center (*cakra*) at the base of the spine to the crown of the *head. Already mentioned in the *Maitrāyanīya-Upanishad (6.21), this is the most important of all the *nādīs of the *body. The *Yoga-Vishaya (11) declares that it is of the form of delight (*sukha*). The reason for this is that the *sushumnā-nādī, in the words of the *Hatha-Yoga-Pradīpikā (4.17), "devours *time, which is created by the sun and the moon." That is to say, it is the secret pathway by means of which the *yogin transcends the polar dynamic between the left and the right psychoenergetic currents—the *idā-nādī and the *pingalā-nādī—and wins the immortal condition of *Self-realization. Hence it is called the "way to liberation" (*moksha-mārga) in the *Yoga-Yājnavalkya (4.30). The sushumnā-nādī, like all *nādīs, originates in the "bulb" (*kanda), but it alone proceeds to the "brahmic fissure" (*brahma-randhra) at the crown of the head. It runs along the spine, which is variously called *meru and vīnā-danda ("fiddlestick"). According to the *Shat-Cakra-Nirūpana (2), this axial channel is composed of several layers: the *vajrā-nādī, within which is the *citrinī-nādī, and within which is the *brahma-nādī.

The sushumnā must be purified of all defilements (*mala) so that the "serpent power" (*kundalinī-shakti) can ascend in it. This process is sometimes referred to as sushumnā-yoga or mahā-yoga ("great Yoga").

SUSHUPTI ("sleep"). See nidrā, svapna.

SŪTRA ("thread"), lit. the thread worn by male members of the upper three social estates of *Hinduism; also, a terse aphorism serving as a device for memorizing the sacred teachings. According to Kumārila Bhatta's Shloka-Vārttika (1.1.22f.), there are six kinds of such aphorisms, depending on their purpose: definition (samjnā), interpretation (paribhāshā), general rule (vidhi), restrictive rule (niyama), original statement (adhikāra), and analogy (atidesha). This style of writing is employed in the source books of the six systems (*darshana) of Hindu philosophy, such as the *Yoga-Sūtra of *Patanjali. In *Buddhism the term sūtra (Pali: sutta) refers to the memorable and memorized utterances of the *Buddha and other *adepts.

SŪTRA-ARTHA-BODHINĪ (Sūtrārthabodhinī, "Illumination of the Content of the [Yoga] Aphorisms") of *Nārāyana Tīrtha, an original commentary on the *Yoga-Sūtra consisting of about twenty-four folios. The same author also wrote the longer *Yoga-Siddhānta-Candrikā.

SVA-BHĀVA ("own being"), a person's inner nature, which he or she must honor in order to live life in a meaningful way. This important ethical concept is introduced in the *Bhagavad-Gītā together with the related concept of *sva-dharma. The sva-bhāva manifests in the "still small voice" of those who pause to turn their *attention within. See also sva-rūpa.

SVACCHANDA-TANTRA, an important and voluminous scripture (six volumes in the Sanskrit edition) that has a *kaula orientation. It expounds on *ritual and yogic practices, including *breath control and the recitation of the sacred syllable *om. It has a brilliant commentary by *Abhinava Gupta.

SVACCHANDA-YOGA ("Yoga of own will"), a phrase that occurs in *Kshemarāja's commentary on the *Shiva-Sūtra (1.11). It denotes the *yogin's perfect freedom after realizing the ultimate *Reality, which is also called svacchanda (from sva, "own," and chandas, "will"). This is another name for the state of absolute spontaneity (*sahaja).

SVA-DHARMA ("own norm"), the moral law or order (*dharma) as it applies to oneself. This concept plays an all-important role in the teachings of the *Bhagavad-Gītā (18.47), which has this memorable saying:

Better is [one's] own norm imperfectly [carried out] than another's norm well performed. By performing the action prescribed by [one's] own being (*svabhāva), one does not accumulate guilt (*kilbisha).

One should not relinquish "congenital" (*sahaja) action, defective though it be, O Kaunteya [= *Arjuna], because all undertakings are veiled by the faults (*dosha), as fire by smoke.

Here *Krishna instructs his disciple *Arjuna that a warrior (kshatriya) should defend the moral order by military force, if necessary. It would be inappropriate for a warrior to live the life of a merchant or a *brahmin, and vice versa. One must be true to one's innate (sahaja) obligations. According to the ethics of *Hinduism, these largely derive from one's place in society, which is determined by one's *karma. Sva-dharma has a double aspect. It is both the moral "categorical imperative" of one's essential being (*sva-bhāva) and the formalization of this inherent moral standard in terms of the caste laws. It is through the fulfillment of his or her sva-dharma that a person can actualize himself or herself. See also karma-yoga.

SVĀDHISHTHĀNA-CAKRA ("own-base center," from sva and adhishthāna) the second psychoenergetic center of the *body, in ascending order. It is depicted as a crimson six-petaled lotus situated at the *genitals. Its "seed syllable" (*bīja-mantra) is vam, pertaining to the water (*apas) element. The center's presiding deities are *Vishnu and the goddess Rākinī. The center is associated with the sense of taste (*rasa), the hands, and fertility, symbol-

ized by the image of an aquatic monster resembling a crocodile. This center contains an "inward-facing" phallus (*linga) shining like coral. Through *contemplation of this center, the *yogin becomes attractive to the *world, especially to the other sex, which can turn into a formidable test for him. See also linga-cakra.

SVĀDHYĀYA ("study"; lit. "one's own [sva] going into [adhyāya]"), mentioned in the *Yoga-Sūtra (2.1) as one of the constituent practices of *kriyā-yoga and (2.32) as one of the components of self-discipline (*niyama). The *Yoga-Bhāshya (2.1) explains it as the recitation (*japa) of the sacred syllable *om and other similar *mantras and as the *study of the sacred lore on *liberation (moksha-shāstra). This dual meaning has a historical explanation: in *Vedic times, study meant the memorization of the sacred tradition through repeated *recitation. Study was early on recognized as a viable means of self-understanding and *self-transcendence. This is borne out in the Shata-Patha-Brāhmana (11.5.7.1): "The study and the interpreta-

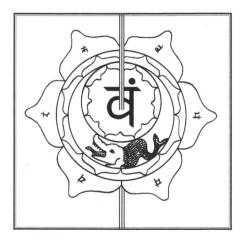

Svādhishthāna-cakra, the psychoenergetic center located at the genitals

298

tion [of the sacred lore] are [a source] of *joy. [The serious student] becomes mentally focused and independent of others, and day by day he gains [spiritual] power. He sleeps peacefully and is his own best physician. He controls the *senses and delights in the One. [His] insight (*prajñā) and [inner] glory (yashas) grow, [and he acquires the ability] to promote the world (loka-pakti) [lit. 'world cooking']."

Svādhyāya is more than mere intellectual learning. It approaches the quality of *meditation. It complements the practice of spiritual exercises, as the following passage from the *Vishnu-Purāna (6.6.2f.) makes clear: "From study one should proceed to *Yoga and from Yoga to study. Through perfection in study and Yoga, the supreme *Self becomes manifest. Study is one eye with which to behold that [Self], and Yoga is the other." See also grantha, shāstra.

SVĀMIN ("owner" or "lord"), a common title of respect for a spiritual personage; often written "Swami" in English. The svāmin is understood to be a master of himself (sva) rather than over other people, though he is popularly thought to possess all kinds of paranormal powers (*siddhi) as well. In *Classical Yoga the word also stands for the *Self, whereas sva signifies *nature.

SVAPNA ("dream") has been recognized since ancient times as a distinct state of *consciousness. Often the word means "sleep" in general and as such is a synonym for *nidrā or sushupti, but in numerous contexts it stands for "dream" in particular. The *Varāha-Upanishad (2.61) explains this condition as being the result of the mind's (*buddhi) traveling in the "subtle channels" (sūkshma-nādī). That is to say, the *dream state is based on the

focusing of *attention on the inner environment of the *body. The *Hamsa-Upanishad (8) states that dreams result when the psyche (*jīva) enters the pericardium of the *heart, while deep sleep (sushupti) comes about when it is focused on the "phallus" (*linga), *Shiva's sign, in the heart.

In the *Mahābhārata (12.232.4) svapna is regarded as one of the defects (*dosha). But according to the *Yoga-Sūtra (1.38), dream sleep can yield useful insights that may be suitable for *meditation. Also, the *yogin's dreams may contain important omens (*arishta).

SVARA ("sound"), sound in general; specifically, the sound made by the *breath. The *Amrita-Bindu-Upanishad (7) contrasts the svara with the asvara, the "soundless" *Absolute. This is a key concept of *mantra-yoga. See also shabda, Speech, vāc.

SVARA-CINTĀMANI ("Thought Gem on the Sound [of the Breath]"), a late work of twenty-four short chapters dealing with divination through the flow of the *breath. It is more detailed than the *Shiva Svarodaya.

SVARA-SAUSHTHAVA ("pleasantness of voice"), one of the signs (*cihna) of initial progress (*pravritti) in *Yoga, according to the *Shvetāshvatara-Upanishad (2.12); also referred to as "softness of the voice" (svara-somyatā). See also kind speech.

SVARGA ("heaven") or SVARGA-LOKA ("heavenly realm"), the domain of the *deities and, as the *Bhagavad-Gītā (9.20f.) reminds us, of virtuous folk who *worship the *Divine by means of sacrifices (*yajna) but who will nonetheless be reborn as soon as their merit (*punya*) is exhausted. *Heaven thus offers no permanent security from the pain of *change. It is not equivalent to *liberation.

SVARODAYA-VIJNĀNA ("knowledge of the rising of the sound [of the breath]," from *svara*, "sound," and *udaya*, "rising"), the art of diagnosing and predicting a person's *health and future well-being and *destiny by means of the *breath. This is thought to be possible simply because the breath is intimately connected with the *mind, and the mind is equally closely associated with the *body as a whole.

SVARODAYA-VIVARANA of Bhāva Shāstrin of Baroda (Gujarat), a late work of 125 verses on the subtle channels (*nādī*) of the life force (*prāna*).

SVA-RŪPA ("own form"), according to *Classical Yoga, the essential nature of a thing; solidity, e.g., is the characteristic property of the *earth element. The *Yoga-Bhāshya* (3.47) defines it as the conglomerate of the generic (*samānya*) and the particular (*vishesha*). An example of the generic would be audibility; of the particular, *sound. See also *sva-bhāva*.

SVASTIKA ("fortunate" or "auspicious," from *su*, "well," and *asti*, "it is"), an ancient symbol of the sun, which has entered the European consciousness as a symbol

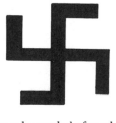

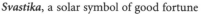
Svastika, a solar symbol of good fortune

of destruction. It came to be associated in *Yoga with the psychoenergetic center at the *navel, which is the place of the microcosmic "sun" (*sūrya*).

SVASTIKA-ĀSANA (*svastikāsana*, "fortunate posture"), mentioned already in the *Yoga-Bhāshya* (2.46) and described in the *Gheranda-Samhitā* (2.13) thus: Place one's *feet between knee and thigh (of either leg) while sitting straight (*riju-kāya*). The *Shiva-Samhitā* (3.96) notes that this posture wards off *disease and brings paranormal control over the wind (*vāyu*), presumably externally and internally (as the *breath). The *svastika-āsana* is specifically recommended in the *Shiva-Purāna* (7.2.16.55) for the *samaya* ritual, during which the teacher (*guru*) enters the *body of the *disciple. This posture is also called *sukha-āsana*.

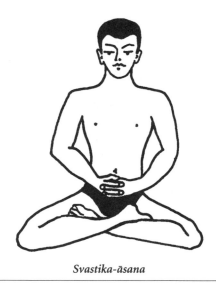

Svastika-āsana

SVĀTANTRYA ("self-reliance"), an important quality in a spiritual *practitioner. As the *Yoga-Shikhā-Upanishad* (1.154) asserts, self-reliance is essential in order to procure permanent perfection (*siddhi*).

At the same time, however, a student must not be so self-willed that he or she is incapable of *obedience to the teacher (*guru).

SVĀTMĀRĀMA YOGĪNDRA (prob. 14th cen. CE), the author of the *Hatha-Yoga-Pradīpikā. Although he venerates *Matsyendra and *Goraksha as his *gurus, he did not study with them personally.

SVAYAMBHŪ-LINGA ("self-existent phallus"), the phallic symbol associated with the *mūlādhāra-cakra. It faces downward and is encircled by the "serpent power" (*kundalinī-shakti). See also linga.

SVEDA or PRASVEDA ("sweat"), a phenomenon particularly associated with the initial stages of breath control (*prāṇā-yāma). The *Hatha-Yoga-Pradīpikā (2.13) recommends that one rub one's perspiration (jala) into the *body to give it "firmness" and "lightness." The *Tejo-Bindu-Upanishad (1.41) sees sweating as one of the nine obstacles (*vighna).

SWAMI. See svāmin. (Individual Swamis are listed under their personal names.)

SYMBOLISM Already in ancient *Vedic times, the sages of India availed themselves of symbol and metaphor to express the deeper truths of spiritual life. Thus many of the hymns of the *Vedas are composed in a symbol-laden *language that is only gradually being recovered by modern scholarship. For a long time, Western scholars thought that the Vedas were little more than primitive poetry containing no worthwhile knowledge. This assessment clashed with the veneration in which the Vedic scriptures have been held by the traditionalist Indians themselves. For them, the Vedas were revealed wisdom of the highest order. Today, Vedicists are beginning to be more appreciative of the level of literary sophistication found in the Vedic hymns, and some are even willing to entertain the view that these archaic compositions contain sophisticated thinking and deep wisdom.

Esoteric symbolism can also be found in the *Upanishads, which in many ways continue the *Vedic gnosis. The *Mahābhārata, too, is filled with pregnant symbols, as are the *Purānas. But spiritual symbolism reaches its peak in the *Tantras, which even employ a "twilight language" (*sandhyā-bhāshā) that is largely incomprehensible to the uninitiated. See also Mythology.

SYMPATHY. See dayā.

· T ·

TĀDĀGĪ-MUDRĀ ("tank seal"), described in the *Gheranda-Samhitā (3.61) thus: Assuming the back stretch (*pashcima-uttāna) position, make the belly like a water tank. In the opinion of the traditional commentators, this exercise is to be done while lying on one's back with the stomach made hollow. According to some contemporary authorities, however, this practice is to be performed by bending forward in the sitting position and inhaling so as to expand the stomach. This "seal" (*mudrā) is said to prevent aging and *death.

TAILOR'S SEAT. See *sukha-āsana*.

TAITTIRĪYA-UPANISHAD (*Taittirīyopanishad*), one of the earliest *Upanishads, belonging to the school of the ancient *Vedic teacher Tittiri, whose name means "partridge." This work contains many archaic notions, notably a primitive "ecological" interpretation of *life. According to this teaching, which is associated with the name of the sage *Bhrigu, everything is food (*anna*) for everything else: life feeding upon life in order to perpetuate itself. As one passage (2.21) has it: "From food, verily, creatures are produced—whatsoever [creatures] dwell on Earth. Moreover, by food, in truth, they live, and into it they finally pass." This potentially dreadful vision of life is balanced by another doctrine, according to which existence is inherently blissful (*ānanda*). The *Taittirīya-Upanishad* speaks of various levels of *bliss, from simple *pleasure to unexcelled bliss. Spiritual life consists in discovering the culmination of bliss, which is inherent in the Absolute (*brahman*). This scripture also contains the first reference to the doctrine of the five "sheaths" (*kosha*), of which the fifth and final sheath is composed of pure bliss. Here (2.4.1) we also find the first recorded mention of the word *yoga* in the technical sense, as the conscious control of the fickle senses (*indriya*).

TALKATIVENESS. See *prajalpa*.

TĀLU ("palate"), an important locus of the life force (*prāna*). Its yogic significance was recognized already in the *Taittirīya-Upanishad* (1.6.1), which mentions the "nipple"—i.e., the uvula—that hangs down from the palate and is "Indra's exit." Here the word *indra* stands for the individual psyche (*jīva*). Later works even

speak of a *tālu-cakra*, as the place of the "royal tooth" (*rāja-danta*) or the "bell" (*ghantikā*). Thus the *Saubhāga-Lakshmī-Upanishad* (3.6) states that from this psychoenergetic center (*cakra*) streams the "nectar of immortality" (*amrita*).

TĀLU-MŪLA ("root of the palate"), mentioned in the *Tri-Shikhi-Brāhmana-Upanishad* (2.132) as one of the eighteen sensitive zones (*marman*) of the *body. It also notes that this locus is associated with *consciousness in the state of deep sleep (*sushupti*).

TAMAS ("darkness"), the psychocosmic principle of inertia; in the *Yoga and *Sāmkhya traditions, one of the three primary constituents (*guna*) of nature (*prakriti*). As the *Bhagavad-Gītā* (14.8) declares, it springs from spiritual nescience (*ajnāna*) and deludes all beings, binding them by heedlessness (*pramāda*), sloth (*ālasya*), and sleep (*nidrā*). The *Tejo-Bindu-Upanishad* (1.41) counts it among the nine obstacles (*vighna*). The *Maitrāyanīya-Upanishad* (3.5) supplies a long list of characteristics of *tamas*, or *tamo-guna*. These include, among others, *fear, *confusion, *despondency, and *grief, as well as *hunger and *thirst. Cf. *rajas*, *sattva*.

TANDRĀ or TANDRA ("sloth"), listed in the *Yoga-Tattva-Upanishad* (12) as one of the defects (*dosha*). See also *ālasya*, *styāna*.

TANK SEAL. See *tādāgī-mudrā*.

TANMĀTRA ("that only," from the neuter pronoun *tad*, "that," and *mātra*, "only"), possibly a distortion of *tanu-mātra* ("fine matter"). According to the cosmology of the *Yoga and *Sāmkhya traditions, the term denotes the subtle (*sūkshma*) aspect of the material elements (*bhūta*): the potentials of sound (*shabda*), sight (*rūpa*, lit. "form"), touch (*sparsha*), taste (*rasa*), and smell (*gandha*). The *Sāmkhya-Kārikā* (38) describes them as being "nonspecific" (*avishesha*). In *Classical Yoga these five potentials pertain, together with *asmitā-mātra*, to the level of "unparticularized" (*avishesha*) existence. They arise from the *linga-mātra* and, in turn, give rise to the sixteen categories (*tattva*) of "particularized" (*vishesha*) existence: the mind (*manas*), the ten senses (*indriya*), and the five material elements (*bhūta*).

Tantra ("Loom," from the root *tan*, "to extend, expand"), most generally used as a synonym for *shāstra* ("textbook"). Specifically, however, the term refers to a work belonging to a genre of sacred writing in *Shaktism and *Shaivism but also in the tradition of *Buddhism. There are scores of *Hindu *Tantras*, which often take the form of a dialogue between *Shiva and his divine spouse, *Devī (or Pārvatī, etc.). The two best known *Hindu *Tantras* are the *Kula-Arnava-Tantra* and the *Mahā-nirvana Tantra*. Like the *Āgamas (of *Shaivism), the *Samhitās (of *Vaishnavism), and the *Purānas*, the *Tantras* cover a wide range of subjects. They contain accounts of psychocosmology and the history of the *world (divided into eons, or *yugas), descriptions of the *deities and their appropriate *rituals of worship, and of rites for the acquisition of a battery of *magical powers. There are also instructions about the esoteric process of activating the *kundalinī-shakti*, which is crucial to the spiritual *path of *Tantrism.

Tantra-Āloka (*Tantrāloka*, "Light on Tantra"), *Abhinava Gupta's *magnum opus*, which discusses in great depth the metaphysics and spiritual practice of *Tantrism from the viewpoint of Kashmiri *Shaivism. The Sanskrit edition with Jayaratha's *Viveka* commentary comprises twelve volumes.

Tantra-Sāra ("Essence of Tantra") by *Abhinava Gupta, a brilliant summary of the *Tantra-Āloka*.

tāntrika ("Tantric"), an adjective that is also used as a noun referring to the practitioner of *Tantrism.

Tantrism, the religious philosophy and culture expounded in the scriptures known as *Tantras*. The origins of Tantrism are still obscure. Some scholars trace the beginnings of Tantrism back to ancient

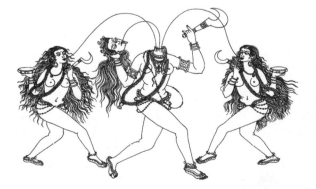

Tantrism makes use of sexual symbolism to express spiritual realities. The decapitated Goddess Chinnamastā, dancing ecstatically with her attendants, represents the spiritual law of self-sacrifice underlying all authentic spirituality.

cults current in the *Vedic period, while others detect Tantric elements in the allegedly pre-Vedic Harappan civilization (see Indus-Sarasvati civilization). Inasmuch as Tantrism avails itself of folk traditions, it is unquestionably extremely old. As a distinct cultural tradition, however, Tantrism emerged within *Hinduism, *Buddhism, and *Jainism in the early common era. The *Tantras* purport to expound a new teaching, or revelation (*shruti), that is particularly suited for the dark age (*kali-yuga).

Because of its long history and great diversity in the doctrinal and practical dimensions, it is very difficult to define or even generalize about Tantrism. What can usefully be said is that the pivot of most Tantric schools is the idea of *shakti, the feminine principle of cosmic existence, the *Goddess. The *tāntrika or *sādhaka seeks to enlist the help of this principle in the quest for *liberation. This is expressed in ceremonies of external worship (*pūjā) of the feminine *Divine but also in inner or symbolic rituals, notably the whole orientation of *kundalinī-yoga.

This rediscovery of the feminine cosmic principle was accompanied by a reappraisal of the human *body and bodily existence in general, which widely have a negative significance in the non-Tantric traditions. In contrast to the ascetic, world-denying schools of *Hinduism, the Tantric *adepts affirmed the body as the temple of the Divine and as an immensely valuable instrument for reaching *liberation. But this reevaluation of the body and *shakti-centered rituals also opened the gates to *occultism and *magic, which surprisingly parallels the contemporary renaissance of Goddess worship and the arcane arts.

Generally, three great approaches are distinguished within Tantrism: (1) the *dakshina-mārga, or right-hand *path; (2) the *vāma-mārga, or left-hand path; and (3) the *kula-mārga, or path of the prominent *Kaula sect. The first approach is the conservative mainline of Tantrism. The second approach, which has brought Tantrism into disrepute, involves the infamous *panca-tattva rite, which makes use of traditionally forbidden elements, especially sexual intercourse (*maithunā). The third approach can roughly be equated with *kundalinī-yoga, the exploitation of the *body's inherent psychospiritual potential. See also Aghorī sect, āmnāya, pītha, srota, vīra.

TAPAS ("heat" or "glow"), asceticism, which the *Yoga-Bhāshya (2.32) explains as the endurance of extremes (*dvandva). *Patanjali regards *tapas* as one of the three constituents of *kriyā-yoga, and he also counts it among the components of self-discipline (*niyama). He further states in his *Yoga-Sūtra (3.43) that *tapas* leads to perfection (*siddhi) of the *body and the *senses. This contradicts the characterization of *tapas* given in many scriptures, including the *Yoga-Yājnavalkya (2.3), which understand it as the "desiccation" (*shoshana), or emaciation, of the *body. Endorsing Patanjali's positive interpretation of asceticism, the *Tattva-Vaishāradī (2.1) notes that *tapas* should only be practiced so long as it does not imbalance the bodily humors (*dhātu).

Similarly, the *Bhagavad-Gītā (7.5f.) speaks against exaggerated asceticism, which springs from ostentation (*dambha) and selfishness (*ahamkāra) and which ignores the fact that the Lord (*īshvara) resides within the *body. According to this scripture (17.14ff.), *tapas* is threefold: (1) *shārīra-tapas*, or "bodily austerity," consisting of reverence (*pūjana) for the *deities, the "twice-born" (*dvija), the *teachers, and the sages, and comprising purity (*shauca), rectitude (*ārjava), chastity (*brahmacarya), and nonharming (*ahimsā); (2) van-maya-tapas, or "vocal austerity," consisting of speech that does not cause disquiet and that is truthful, kind, and pleasing, as well as study (*svā-dhyāya); and (3) mānasa-tapas, or "mental austerity," consisting of serenity (*pra-sāda), friendliness (saumyatva), silence (*mauna), self-restraint (atma-vinigraha), and purity of feeling (bhāva-samshuddhi). These three kinds of tapas are *sāttvika.

When asceticism becomes tinged with ostentation or the desire to win honor or fame, however, it is *rājasa. Finally, when tapas turns into self-torture or is performed to harm another being, it is *tā-masa. The *Uddhāva-Gītā (14.37), again, defines tapas as the abandoning of *desires (kāma-tyāga).

TAPASVIN, a practitioner of *tapas.

TAPO-YOGIN (masc.), or TAPO-YOGINĪ (fem.), a synonym for tapasvin.

TĀRAKA ("deliverer"), generally, the transcendental *Reality in its salvific aspect. In *Classical Yoga, however, the word designates not the *Absolute but the "wisdom born of discernment" (viveka-ja-jnāna), which appears at the culmination of the ecstatic (*samādhi) condition. The *Pāshu-pata-Brāhmana-Upanishad (1.32) uses the term to denote the sacred syllable *om. In *tāraka-yoga, again, it signifies the manifestation of the *Self in the form of *light.

TĀRAKA-YOGA ("Yoga of the delivering [sign]"), a *Vedānta-based Yoga taught in the *Advaya-Tāraka-Upanishad and the *Mandala-Brāhmana-Upanishad, which appears to have been widespread in medieval India. Central to this approach

are photistic phenomena that occur during *meditation and that are considered to be a manifestation of the *Absolute as "deliverer" (*tāraka). Three kinds of phenomena are distinguished: the *antar-laksh-ya ("inner sign"), the *bahir-lakshya ("external sign"), and the *madhya-laksh-ya ("intermediate sign"). The three "signs" (lakshya) are known as "corporeal deliverers" (mūrti-tāraka), whereas the higher realization of the *Self is styled "incorporeal" (amūrti) and "transmental" (*amanaska). The intermediate sign leads to the experience of the five types of luminous consciousness-space (*ākāsha).

TARKA ("reflection" or "pondering"), defined in the *Amrita-Nāda-Upanishad (16) as inference (ūhana) that is in keeping with tradition (*āgama). In the context of the sixfold *path (*shad-anga-yoga), however, this term may correspond to the experience of *savitarka-samādhi in *Classical Yoga.

TARPANA ("satisfaction"), one of the "limbs" (*anga) of *mantra-yoga. See also tushti.

TASTE. See āsvada, rasa.

TAT ("that"), a cryptic reference to the *Absolute, or *Self, in such doctrinal sayings (vākya) as "That art thou" (tat tvam asi).

TATTVA ("thatness"), *Reality; also, a category of cosmic existence. The relationship between these two connotations is well expressed in the *Shiva-Samhitā (2.54), which states that "when all the tattvas have disappeared, then the tattva itself becomes manifest." Classical *Sāmkhya distinguishes twenty-four such categories, which are the principal levels or principles of nature (*prakriti*): (1) *prakriti*, the transcendental ground of (insentient) existence; (2) *mahat* ("great one"), also known as *buddhi*; (3) *ahamkāra* ("I maker"), the principle of individuation; (4–14) the mind (*manas*) and the ten senses (*indriya*); (15–19) the five subtle elements (*tanmātra*); and (20–24) the five material elements (*bhūta*). Separate and above these categories is the principle of pure *Consciousness, the *purusha*.

In some schools of *Shaivism, thirty-six categories are recognized; the *Brahma-Vidyā-Upanishad* (62) hints at fifty-one, while the *Varāha-Upanishad* (I.7ff.) mentions as many as ninety-six. See also Cosmos, *shad-vimsha*.

TATTVA-VAISHĀRADĪ ("Autumnal Clarity on the Categories [of Existence]"), a major subcommentary on the *Yoga-Bhāshya*. Authored by *Vācaspati Mishra, this gloss is a work of considerable scholastic achievement that contains many illuminating philological observations. However, it does not match the appeal and authority of *Shankara's *Vivarana*.

TATTVA-VID ("knower of Reality"), an *enlightened being who, in the words of the *Bhagavad-Gītā* (5.8f.), knows that the *Self transcends all *action and yet engages in activities. Sometimes the appellation refers to someone who knows the categories of existence (*tattva*).

TEACHER. See *ācārya, guru, upādhyāya*.

TEJAS ("brilliance"), often cited as one of the effects of intense asceticism (*tapas*), expressed in the shining face of the saint. In the sense of overzealousness, *tejas* is listed in the *Tejo-Bindu-Upanishad* (1.41) as one of the nine obstacles (*vighna*) on the spiritual *path.

TEJO-BINDU-UPANISHAD (*Tejobindūpanishad*, "Radiance Point *Upanishad*"), one of the *Yoga-Upanishads*, comprising 465 stanzas distributed over six chapters. The clear break after the fourth chapter suggests that this is probably a composite work. The *tejo-bindu* or "radiance point" is said to be found in the *heart of the All-Self (*vishva-ātman*) during *meditation. This scripture, which is firmly grounded in the nondualist metaphysics of *Vedānta, puts forward a fifteenfold *path (*panca-dasha-anga-yoga*) and mentions nine obstacles (*vighna*) that foil spiritual *progress. The fourth chapter contains a description of the nature of living liberation (*jīvan-mukti*) and disembodied liberation (*videha-mukti*).

TEJO-DHYĀNA, a synonym for *jyotir-dhyāna*.

TEMPLE. See *deva-mandira*.

TERRIFYING POSTURE. See *ugra-āsana*.

THEISM. If theism is the doctrine affirming the existence of an ultimate *Reality, which can be called *God, then almost all spiritually based schools of thought in India may be described as theistic (*seshvara*, from *sa*, "with," and *īshvara*, "Lord"). Notable exceptions are certain schools of *Buddhism and the *Sāmkhya tradition within *Hinduism, but even here the attitude is more one of agnosticism than atheism. Only India's materialist philosophies—generically referred to as Cārvāka—espouse atheism in the strict sense of the word.

Within the category of theism, however, there is an enormous range of doctrinal variation both in *Hinduism and *Buddhism. At one end of the spectrum is the radical nondualism (*advaita*) of some schools, which regard all multiplicity as illusory, insisting that there is only the singular *Being. At the other end are schools such as *Classical Yoga that view *God (in the form of *īshvara) as one among many free transcendental *Selves, which logically must all coalesce in infinity. In the middle are the numerous schools subscribing to what can be styled "panentheism," which see the *cosmos with its countless *objects arising in the infinite body of the singular *Divine. See also Advaita Vedānta, Vishishta Advaita.

THOUGHT. See *cintā*, *dhī*; see also Mind.

THROAT. See *kantha*.

THROAT LOCK. See *jālandhara-bandha*, *kantha-samkoca*.

TILAKA (from *tila* or "sesame"), the small round dot of sandalwood paste painted on the forehead of *Hindu women and members of some ascetic sects as a sign of *devotion to the chosen deity (*ishta-devatā*).

TIME. See *kāla*.

TINTINI, mentioned in the *Hatha-Yoga-Pradīpikā* (1.8) as an *adept of *hatha-yoga.

TĪRTHA, a pilgrimage center. The *Darshana-Upanishad* (4.48ff.) distinguishes between external (*bahis-*) and internal (*antas-*) pilgrimage centers. The latter, which are deemed superior to the former, are also referred to as *bhāva-tīrthas*, the word *bhāva* meaning "mental condition." These inner *tīrthas* are various auspicious loci for focusing *attention, corresponding to the major psychoenergetic centers (*cakra*) of the *body.

TĪRTHA-ATANA (*tīrthātana*, "pilgrimage to a sacred site"), mentioned in the *Ud-*dhāva-Gītā* (14.34) as one of the twelve practices of self-restraint (*niyama*). This custom is also called *tīrtha-yātrā*.

TĪRTHANKĀRA ("ford maker"), the honorific title given to the twenty-four enlightened *adepts of *Jainism, notably the founder, Vardhamāna Mahāvīra, who revealed the spiritual *path.

TIRU ("sacred" or "holy"), a Tamil word found in many names of South Indian sages and literary works; corresponds to the Sanskrit term *shrī*.

TIRUMANKAI, an eighth-century chieftain who spent his wealth feeding 1,008 devotees of *Vishnu for an entire year as part of a pledge to a girl whom he wanted to marry. After depleting his own resources, he took to robbing the rich to feed the poor. Legend has it that one well-to-do brahmin couple who was waylaid by him turned out to be Vishnu and his divine spouse, Lakshmī, who revealed to him the sacred *mantra* "Obeisance to *Nārāyana" (*namo nārāyana*). As one of the *Ālvārs, Tirumankai traveled from temple to temple singing songs in praise of Vishnu. He composed more than 1,000 verses of the *Divya-Prabandham* and also authored the *Periya-Tirumoli*.

TIRU-MANTIRAM, the tenth book of the *Shaiva canon (see *Tiru-Murai*), composed in Tamil by *Tirumūlar. It consists of over 3,000 melodious verses on ethical, philosophical, and religious matters, including the yogic *path. Relying primarily on the *Āgamas and his own spiritual experience, Tirumūlar expounds the metaphysics of *Shaivism with great insight and lyrical beauty.

TIRUMŪLAR (1st cen. CE), one of the great *adepts of Southern *Shaivism, though not widely venerated today. He is the author of a remarkable Tamil work, the *Tiru-Mantiram*, which Kamil V. Zvelebil (1973) has praised as "the greatest treatment of *Yoga in Tamil literature." Tirumūlar was a proponent of the devotional (*bhakti*) approach. See also Nāyanmārs.

TIRU-MURAI, the sacred canon of Southern *Shaivism. It consists of twelve books featuring devotional poetry in praise of *Shiva, composed between the seventh and the twelfth centuries CE. See also Nāyanmārs, Shaiva Siddhānta.

TIRUPPAN, one of the *Ālvārs of South Indian *Vaishnavism. Born into a family of untouchable minstrels, he was denied entry into the local temple. Undeterred, Tiruppan stood at the banks of the Kaveri River all day singing songs in praise of *Vishnu in the form of Ranganātha. One morning, the temple priest came to the river to draw water for an offering to Vishnu. When Tiruppan, who was completely absorbed in ecstatic devotion to his beloved Lord, failed to step aside, the priest became so angry that he flung a rock at the untouchable, hitting him squarely in the forehead. Tiruppan humbly apologized and made room for the haughty brahmin. Witnessing the pain inflicted on his devotee, Vishnu resolved to teach the temple priest a lesson. When the priest entered the inner sanctum to make his offerings, he saw to his horror that the statue of Lord Ranganātha was bleeding profusely from the forehead. Not making the connection between this miraculous event and his own misdeed, the priest enlisted other brahmins and even the king to pray for this evil omen to disappear. Then Vishnu appeared to him in a dream, explaining how he had suffered intense pain because of the injury inflicted on his devo-

tee Tiruppan. He instructed the priest to go to Tiruppan and carry him on his shoulders into the inner sanctum of the temple, which he did. When Tiruppan at long last saw the image of his beloved Lord, he burst into a spontaneous song—the only one to have survived of all his numerous songs.

TIRU-VĀYMOLI of *Namm Ālvār, a long devotional poem in praise of *Vishnu that has been called the "Tamil *Veda." It consists of 1,102 verses, of which the closing words of one verse form the opening words of the following verse. It has several commentaries, the earliest being that of Tirukkurukai Pirān Pillān (early 12th cen. CE.

TITHI, a lunar day or station. See *amā-kalā*.

TITIKSHĀ ("forbearance"), defined in the *Uddhāva-Gītā* (14.36) as the "patient endurance of suffering" (*duhkha-sammarsha*). See also *kshamā*, *kshānti*.

TONGUE. The regular Sanskrit word for "tongue" is *jihvā*, but in the esoteric code of the scriptures of *hatha-yoga*, the tongue is also called *go* ("cow"), because it is "milked" to achieve elongation for the practice of *khecarī-mudrā*. The yogic act of inserting the elongated tongue into the nasal cavity is technically known as *go-mamsa-bhakshana* or "eating cow meat" (see, e.g., *Hatha-Ratna-Āvalī*, 2.145). See also *jihvā-bandha*, *jihvā-(mūla)-dhauti*.

TONGUE LOCK. See *jihvā-bandha*.

TORTOISE POSTURE. See *kūrma-āsana*.

TOUCH. See *sparsha*.

TRADITION. See *āgama, smriti*; cf. *shruti*.

TRANQUILLITY. See *prasāda, samatva, shānti*.

TRANSCENDENCE. See Self-transcendence.

TRANSFORMATION, COSMIC. See Change, Evolution, *parināma, vikāra*.

TRANSMINDEDNESS. See *amanaskata*.

TRANSMISSION, SPIRITUAL. See *shakti-pāta*.

TRANSUBSTANTIATION. Those traditions, such as *Tantrism and *hatha-yoga, that have a positive regard for the *embodiment regard *enlightenment or *liberation as an event that must include the *body in order to be complete. Instead of merely transcending physical existence, they aspire to transmute the *elements constituting the body to the point where a whole new body is created—a process otherwise known as "transubstantiation." This new body is known as "divine body" (*divya-deha*), which is endowed with all kinds of paranormal abilities (*siddhi*).

TRĀTAKA, also called *trotana* in the *Hatha-Ratna-Āvalī* (1.25), one of the "six acts" (*shat-karma*) described in the *Gheranda-Samhitā* (1.53f.) thus: Gaze steadily, without blinking, at a small object until tears begin to flow. This technique is said to cure all eye afflictions and to lead to clairvoyance (*divya-drishti*) and the *shāmbhavī-mudrā*. See also *drishti*.

TREE POSTURE. See *vriksha-āsana*.

TRIANGLE POSTURE. See *tri-kona-āsana*.

TRIDENT. See *tri-shūla*.

TRI-GRANTHI ("triple knot"). See *granthi*.

TRIKA ("Triad"), the principal spiritual tradition of Kashmir, which is a form of nondualist *Shaivism. Its name derives from the three philosophical categories of this system: *Shiva (standing for the ultimate *Reality), *Shakti (the Goddess or power aspect of Reality), and *nara* (the human being, representing the Spirit under the influence of ignorance, *karma, and *bondage). The Trika system was developed primarily by *Abhinava Gupta, who was initiated into this tradition by Shambhunātha from the city of Jālandhara in Northern India. The literature of Trika can be divided into three broad categories: (1) the *Āgamas (scriptures said to have been revealed directly by Shiva), notably the *Mālinī-Vijaya-Uttara-Tantra* (see Mālinī), *Svacchanda-Tantra, *Mrigendra-Tantra, Netra-Tantra, and the *Shiva-Sūtra; (2) the various texts on the doctrine of divine vibration (*spanda*), i.e., the *Spanda-Kārikā* and its several commentaries; and (3) the *Pratyabhijnā scriptures, such as Somānanda's *Shiva-Drishti and Utpala's *Pratyabhijnā-Sūtra*, together

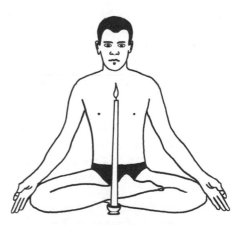

Trātaka, steady gazing as an aid to concentration

with their many commentaries. This final category also includes *Abhinava Gupta's *Tantra-Āloka* and *Tantra-Sāra*. See also Kaula school, Tantrism.

TRI-KONA-ĀSANA (*trikonāsana*, "triangle posture"), a posture described in contemporary manuals of *hatha-yoga* as follows: Standing upright with legs apart and arms outstretched, exhale and bend at the hip to one side. Repeat, bending to the other side.

TRI-KŪTA ("triple peak"), an esoteric designation for the spot between the eyebrows (*bhrū-madhya*), where the three principal channels (*nādī*) of the life force (*prāna*) meet, namely, the *sushumnā-*, the *idā-*, and the *pingalā-nādī*.

TRI-LAKSHYA ("triple sign"). See *lakshya*.

TRIPURĀ, one of the many names of the *Goddess in *Hinduism (more specifically *Shaktism). This name of the deity, who is the spouse of *Shiva, remembers her divine act of destroying the demon Tripura ("Triple City"), a well-known myth of Shaktism.

TRIPURĀ-RAHASYA ("Mystery of the Tripurā"), also known as the *Haritāyana-Samhitā*; a Vedānta text with strong leanings toward *Shaktism. It has a fascinating discussion of the various kinds of ecstasy (*samādhi*), favoring spontaneous ecstasy (*sahaja-samādhi*) over all other forms, including *nirvikalpa-samādhi*. This text was one of the favorite scriptures of the South Indian sage *Ramana Maharshi. The title celebrates the goddess *Tripurā.

TRI-SHIKHI-BRĀHMANA-UPANISHAD (*Trishikhibrāhmanopanishad*, "Triple Tuft Brāhmana-Upanishad"), one of the *Yoga-Upanishads. It gets its title from the recipi-

ent of the *Upanishadic wisdom, a *brāhmana wearing three tufts of hair. The text comprises 165 stanzas in two sections, which are an exposition of the nondualist metaphysics of *Advaita Vedānta. Its anonymous composer subscribes to an eightfold *path (*ashta-anga-yoga*), whose goal is union with the *Divine, identified with *Shiva and also with *Vishnu. The work begins with cosmological speculations, followed by an exposition of the four modes or states (*avasthā*) of *consciousness, which are related to the four "sheaths" (*kosha*). Two kinds of Yoga, *jnāna-yoga and *karma-yoga, are distinguished. The eightfold path described essentially corresponds to that of *Patanjali. This scripture also lists and describes seventeen postures (*āsana*) and provides details on esoteric *anatomy. Although the "serpent power" (*kundalinī-shakti*) is mentioned, it does not seem to play an important role in the prescribed approach. However, much attention is given to breath control (*prānāyāma*) and the purification of the channels (*nādī-shodhana*). Ecstasy (*samādhi*) is defined, in typical *Vedāntic fashion, as the merging of the psyche (*jīva*) with the *Absolute.

TRISHĀ or TRISHNĀ ("thirst"), often cited as one of the defects (*dosha*). Apart from its conventional meaning, the term is also employed metaphorically as the thirst for life. Already the *Mahābhārata (12.210.34) presents the thirst for conditional experience as the source of unenlightened or *karmic existence and all its attendant suffering (*duhkha*): "As a weaver inserts thread into a cloth by means of a needle, similarly the thread of conditioned existence (*samsāra-sūtra*) is secured to the needle of thirst [or desire]." As another stanza (12.173.25) of the great epic has it, this thirst cannot be quenched by a sip of water. It can only be eliminated through wisdom (*jnāna). See also abhinivesha; cf. kshudhā.

TRI-SHŪLA ("trident"), one of the emblems of *Shiva. To this day, it is carried by members of certain *Shaiva sects.

TRI-VENI ("triple braid"), a synonym for tri-kūta.

TRUTH. See rita, satya.

TURĪYA ("fourth"). See caturtha.

TURĪYA-ATĪTA (turīyātīta, "that which transcends the fourth"), according to the *Laghu-Yoga-Vāsishtha (3.9.124), the condition of living liberation (*jīvan-mukti), which is said to go beyond the seven levels of wisdom (*jnāna-bhūmi).

TURYA, a synonym for turīya.

TURYA-GA ("gone to the fourth"), one of the seven levels of wisdom (*jnāna-bhūmi).

TUSHTI ("contentment"), sometimes listed as one of the practices of self-restraint (*niyama). See also prīti, samtosha, tarpana.

TUTI, a spatial measure applied to the *breath. Thus the space between the inner and the outer *dvādasha-anta, the two end points of the movement of the *breath, is said to be sixteen tutis, which cover the sixteen vowel sounds from a to ah. The first fifteen vowels represent the *tithis or lunar days, whereas the sound value ah is changeless and represents the sixteenth digit (*kalā) of the moon (see amā-kalā). The *Yoga authorities constantly correlate the *microcosm with the *macrocosm.

TYĀGA ("abandonment"), the third "limb" (*anga) of the fifteenfold *Yoga (*pancadasha-anga-yoga) taught in the *Tejo-Bindu-Upanishad. In this work (1.19) tyāga is defined as the *abandonment of phenomenal forms (prapanca-rūpa), i.e., the *world, as a result of one's intuition (avalokana) of the *Self. A contrasting explanation is given in the *Bhagavad-Gītā (18.2), which understands tyāga as the relinquishment of the fruit (*phala) of one's *actions. This interpretation seeks to combat the popular understanding of tyāga as the total abstention from activities, which, according to the Gītā, is completely impossible. The *Laghu-Yoga-Vāsishtha (5.2.28f.) makes an important distinction between dhyeya-tyāga and jneya-tyāga. The former is characteristic of the liberated being (*jīvan-mukta), who continues to perform actions in the spirit of *play. The latter coincides with the dropping of the *body when all subliminal traits (*vāsanā) have been obliterated. See also samnyāsa.

TYĀGIN ("abandoner"), a practitioner of *tyāga.

311

· U ·

UDĀNA ("upbreath"), one of the cardinal currents of the life force (*prāna) in the *body. According to the *Tri-Shikhi-Brāh-mana-Upanishad (82), it circulates in all the limbs and joints and is responsible for digestion. But in the much older *Maitrāya-nīya-Upanishad (2.6) its functions are stated to be belching and swallowing. The udāna is also said to carry *consciousness up to the *head in the state of ecstasy (*sa-mādhi) and at *death. Several *hatha-yoga texts locate it in the *throat, while the *Siddha-Siddhānta-Paddhati (1.68) places it in the palate (*tālu). The *Yoga-Yājnavalk-ya (4.55) mentions that the upbreath is responsible for levitating the body. Mastery of the upbreath (udāna-jaya), states the *Yoga-Sūtra (3.39), leads to the paranormal power (*siddhi) of "nonadhesion" (asanga) and levitation (*utkrānti). According to the *Linga-Purāna (1.8.64) and other *Purānas, the udāna stimulates the sensitive zones (*marman).

UDDĀNA-KUMBHAKA ("upward pot"), breath retention (*kumbhaka) performed after exhalation in conjunction with *ud-dīyāna-bandha. It is prescribed in the *Gheranda-Samhitā (3.22) as a phase of the "great piercer" (*mahā-vedha).

UDDHĀVA-GĪTĀ ("Uddhava's Song"), an imitation of the *Bhagavad-Gītā that forms chapters 6–29 of the eleventh book of the *Bhāgavata-Purāna. It is a *Vedantic tract on Yoga and devotion (*bhakti), presented as a didactic dialogue between *Krishna and the sage Uddhāva.

UDDĪYĀNA-BANDHA ("upward lock"), also called uddāna; an important tech-nique of *hatha-yoga. This "lock" (*ban-dha) is described in the *Gheranda-Samhitā (3.10f.) as follows: Contract the abdomen above and below the *navel and toward the back. By this means the "great bird," the life force (*prāna), is constantly forced to "fly upward" (uddīna), i.e., ascend along the central channel (*su-shumnā-nādī). The Gheranda-Samhitā praises this practice above all the other "locks," calling it "a lion to the elephant of *death." According to the *Yoga-Shikhā-Upanishad (1.106ff.), one should perform the upward lock prior to exhalation, though most modern manuals insist that it should be practiced only after exhalation. The *Yoga-Kundalī-Upanishad (1.48f.) specifies that it should be done seated in the adamantine posture (*vajra-āsana) and while firmly pressing the "bulb" (*kanda) near the ankles. The *Varāha-Upanishad (5.8f.) warns that this

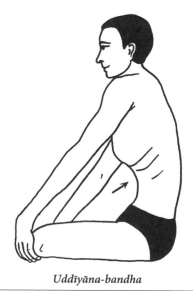

Uddīyāna-bandha

practice should not be attempted when one is hungry or is suffering from a weak bladder or bowels.

UDGĪTHA ("chant"), a synonym for *pranava.

UDYOGA ("effort" or "exertion"), in Kashmiri *Shaivism, the inherent transcendental activity of the ultimate *Reality in the form of *Shiva. This is a kind of creative tension, which is unleashed as soon as the divine power (*shakti) begins to stir, manifesting the various levels of existence. See also Effort, visarga.

UGRA-ĀSANA (ugrāsana, "terrifying posture"), described in the *Shiva-Samhitā (3.92ff.) thus: Stretching out both legs, firmly grasp one's *head with the hands and push it down onto the knees. This posture (*āsana), the text states, fans the bodily fire and is also called *pashcīma-uttāna.

UGRA BHAIRAVA, an *adept of the *Kāpālika tradition. According to a legend related in Mādhava's Shankara-Dig-Vijaya, Ugra Bhairava approached the great *Vedānta preceptor *Shankara, requesting that the sage sacrifice his life so that he, Ugra Bhairava, could achieve the ultimate goal of *liberation. He claimed that *Shiva had told him he could be liberated only if he could offer into the sacrificial fire either the head of an omniscient sage or the head of a king. His plea was so cleverly presented that Shankara was moved by compassion and agreed to sacrifice his own life, so that the ascetic could accomplish his desired objective. They met in secret, and Shankara prepared himself by entering into deep *meditation. As Ugra Bhairava was getting ready to sever the sage's head, Shankara's disciple Padmapāda, who had

certain paranormal abilities (*siddhi), suddenly realized what was about to happen. He too entered into meditation, became completely identified with *Vishnu in his form as Nara-Simha ("Man-Lion"), and, racing to the hiding place, attacked and tore Ugra Bhairava's chest open with his leonine claws.

UJJAYĪ ("victorious"), one of the eight types of breath control (*prānāyāma) taught in *hatha-yoga. It is described in the *Gheranda-Samhitā (5.69ff.) as follows: With one's mouth closed, inhale through both nostrils, while also drawing up the *breath from the *heart (i.e., the chest) and the *throat. Vigorously retain the breath in the mouth and simultaneously perform the throat lock (*jālandhara-bandha). Drawing the breath from the chest with a slight constriction of the throat causes a snoring sound, which is characteristic of this technique. According to the *Yoga-Shikhā-Upanishad (1.94), one should retain the breath in the abdomen and then expel through the left nostril. The texts mention a great number of curative benefits from this exercise, most of them relating to the respiratory system, but this exercise is also said to stimulate the digestive fire (*jāthara-agni).

UMĀPATI SHIVĀCĀRYA (14th cen. CE), an *adept counted among the fourteen principal teachers of *Shaiva Siddhānta. He was a disciple of *Meykandar and authored many Tamil works, including the Koyil-Purāna, Shiva-Prakāsham, and Paushkara-Āgama. He must be distinguished from the Bihari teacher Umāpati, who lived in the fifteenth century.

UNCONSCIOUS. *Classical Yoga and *Sāmkhya subscribe to the view that nature (*prakriti) is inherently unconscious (*acit) and that *consciousness or awareness (*cit) characterizes only the transcendental Self (*purusha). Thus the entire body-mind complex is thought to be insentient, and the phenomena of consciousness (*citta) are the product of material nature reflecting the "light" of the transcendental *Self. The *Vedantic schools of Yoga entertain a similar point of view, according to which all phenomena are (illusory) modifications of the same superconscious *Reality.

The modern psychoanalytical notion that the psyche includes areas that are not known, or known only indirectly, to the conscious mind is also not foreign to *Yoga. This idea is expressed in the teaching of the subliminal activators (*samskāra), subliminal traits (*vāsanā), and subliminal deposits (*āshaya), which are crucial to understanding the doctrine of *karma and reincarnation (*punarjanman). However, Yoga approaches these matters from an angle that is strikingly different from that of psychoanalysis. Psychoanalysis employs the concept of the unconscious in order to understand the irrational operations of the conscious mind and to integrate them in a rational manner and thus to lead from psychopathology to mental health. By contrast, Yoga has no particular interest in the unconscious aspects of our psyche, except insofar as these interfere with the spiritual process, i.e., prevent the stable acquisition of *meditation and *ecstasy and obstruct *liberation. Nor does Yoga seek to rationalize the irrational contents of the human mind but to transcend the entire mechanism by which unconscious *nature, in the form of the body-mind, obscures the fact of our intrinsic *freedom and *bliss. See also Subconscious.

UNENLIGHTENMENT, the condition of the ordinary individual, who has not realized his or her ultimate nature, the transcendental Self (*ātman, *purusha), and hence is enmeshed in the web of *karma. Cf. Enlightenment, Freedom, Liberation.

UNION. See aikya.

UNMANĪ ("exaltation"), or UNMANI-AVA-STHĀ (unmanyavasthā, "exalted state"), also often called manomanī (from mana and unmanī) or "mind exaltation." The *Gheranda-Samhitā (7.17) equates this condition with *sahaja(-samādhi), the state of perfect spontaneity. The *Hatha-Yoga-Pradīpikā (2.42), however, seems to equate this state with *nirvikalpa-samādhi, because for the duration of this condition the *body becomes rigid like a log of wood and the *yogin cannot hear even the sound of a large drum. It also defines the unmanī condition as the steadiness of the *mind, which is effected when the life force (*prāna) flows through the central channel (*sushumnā-nādī). In this context, it precedes the supreme ecstatic realization called *amanaskatā.

UNMANIFEST. See avyakta; cf. vyakta.

UNMESHA ("open [eyes]"), a technical term of Kashmiri *Shaivism denoting the externalization of the divine power (*shakti) through which the *creation of the *cosmos is set in motion. The term can also refer to the inner opening experienced by the *yogin who focuses on the transcendental *Consciousness. Cf. nimesha.

UNMĪLANA-SAMĀDHI ("ecstasy with open [eyes]"), in Kashmiri *Shaivism, the process of *evolution by which the *Divine creates out of itself the *cosmos in its many layers (see Vijñāna Bhairava 88). See also pratimīlana-samādhi; cf. nimesha, nimīlana-samādhi.

UNPARTICULARIZED. See *avishesha*; see *vishesha*.

UNSUPPORTED POSTURE. See *nirālambana-āsana*.

UPĀDHI ("superimposition"), a *Vedantic concept employed in some works on *hatha-yoga. It denotes a limiting attribution upon the singular *Reality, such as the life force (*prāna*), the mind (*manas*), the senses (*indriya*), the body (*deha*), or the sense objects (*artha*). Upon realization of *nirvikalpa-samādhi, all these distinctions vanish, and the *Self shines forth in its authentic singularity. The *Goraksha-Paddhati (2.81f.) notes that the *upādhis* cover up Reality and that they can be removed through constant spiritual practice (*sādhana*).

UPĀDHYĀYA ("instructor"), one who imparts exoteric and esoteric *knowledge but, as a rule, does not initiate the disciple (*shishya*) into the mysteries of practical spirituality. This is the function of the *guru. See also *ācārya*.

UPANISHAD BRAHMAYOGIN (18th cen. CE), also known as Rāmacandra Indrayogin, a pupil of Vasudeva Indrayogin famous for his commentaries on 108 *Upanishads*. His observations on the *Yoga-Upanishads contain many helpful explanations.

UPANISHADS, a genre of Hindu literature. The word *upanishad* is composed of the verbal root *sat* ("to sit") prefixed with *upa* and *ni*, and means "to sit down close to (one's teacher)." This is a reference to the mode in which esoteric *knowledge is transmitted by word of mouth from teacher (*guru*) to disciple (*shishya*). Traditionally, 108 *Upanishads* are spoken of, though well over 200 such works are extant. The earliest of them were composed prior to *Buddhism, dating as far back perhaps as the middle of the second millennium BCE. The youngest *Upanishads* were composed as recently as our century.

All *Upanishads* are looked upon as sacred revelation (*shruti*) and are regarded as belonging to the wisdom part (*jnāna-kānda*) as opposed to the ritual part (*karma-kānda*) of the *Vedic heritage. They represent a refinement of the spiritual teachings of the ancient *Vedas, characterized by the mystical internalization of the Vedic key notion of *sacrifice. The *Upanishads* wanted from the beginning to be understood as secret teachings (*rahasya*), and their metaphysical thinking revolves around four closely related themes: (1) the teaching that the transcendental core—the Self (*ātman*)—of one's being is declared identical with the transcendental core—the *brahman*—of the universe itself; (2) the doctrine of repeated embodiment (*punar-janman*) of human beings, or, as the earliest *Upanishads* put it, their repeated *death (*punar-mrityu*); (3) the doctrine of *karma and retribution, which seeks to explain the metaphysical effects of a person's *actions; and (4) the notion that the production of *karma* and future reincarnation can be prevented through spiritual practices, notably *renunciation and *meditation. In later periods the practical way to *liberation became identical with the approach of *Yoga, as is evidenced in the *Yoga-Upanishads. See also *Samnyāsa-Upanishads*; see also under individual *Upanishads*.

UPAPRĀNA ("secondary life force"). See *prāna*

UPA-PURĀNA ("Secondary *Purāna*"). See *Purāna*.

UPASARGA ("obstacle"). So long as one has not attained *enlightenment, or *liberation, one can always fall prey to a number of difficulties arising from the *ego. The yogic scriptures have detailed some of these obstacles on the spiritual *path. The *Maitrāyanīya-Upanishad (7.8) mentions constant joking, traveling, begging, earning a livelihood from skills, and wearing earrings or skulls out of spiritual hypocrisy as "obstacles to knowledge" (jñāna-upasarga). The *Mārkandeya-Purāna (40.1ff.) also furnishes a long list of obstacles, ranging from desire-bound *actions to magic (*māyā), knowledge, and paranormal abilities (*siddhi). To overcome these obstructions, this *Purāna (40.14) recommends that one focus one's *attention on the *Absolute, wearing a "white mental blanket." The *Shiva-Purāna (7.2.38.10) speaks of six obstacles: (1) *pratibhā (flash of illumination); (2) *shravana (auditory phenomenon); (3) *vārtā (superscent); (4) *darshana (visionary state); (5) *āsvāda (supertaste); and (6) *vedanā (supersensation). The *Yoga-Sūtra (3.37) applies the term upasarga specifically to flashes of illumination occurring in the five senses, which are obstacles to the ecstatic (*samādhi) state, which depends on sensory inhibition (*pratyāhāra). See also vighna.

UPASHAMA ("calmness"), sometimes regarded as one of the practices of moral observance (*yama).

UPASTHA ("that which stands up"), the male *genitals, which are traditionally considered a source of great power or vitality (*ojas). See also anga, linga.

UPASTHA-NIGRAHA ("genital control"), mastery of the sexual drive; occasionally listed among the components of self-discipline (*niyama). See also brahmacarya, ūrdhva-retas.

UPAVĀSA ("fasting"), sometimes counted as one of the practices of self-discipline (*niyama); also often considered to be a possible obstacle (*vighna) to spiritual *progress. The *Gheranda-Samhitā (5.31) specifically mentions that fasting should be avoided in conjunction with the practice of breath control (*prānāyāma). Already the *Mahābhārata (12.214.4) deems prolonged fasting as harmful and instead recommends abstention from eating between breakfast and the evening meal. The *Varāha-Upanishad (2.39) explains that true fasting consists in the proximity between the individual self (*jīva-ātman) and the transcendental Self (*paramaātman), and not the emaciation (*shoshana) of the *body.

UPĀYA ("means"), a technical term in Kashmiri *Shaivism. The *Shiva-Sūtra distinguishes between three means of approach to *Self-realization: (1) Shāmbhava-upāya ("means relating to *Shambhu") is alert passivity toward the *Divine; this is also known as "supportless Yoga" (nirālamba-yoga). (2) Shākta-upāya ("means pertaining to *Shakti") involves the agency of the mind (*citta), inquiring into its authentic nature (the true "I"). (3) Ānava-upāya ("individual means") is any of the many practices of *Yoga, such as *breath control and *meditation.

ŪRDHVA-RETAS, the psychophysiological process by which the semen (*retas) is made to flow upward (ūrdhva) rather than out through the urethra; also, the *yogin in whom this process is alive. First mentioned in the *Maitrāyanīya-Upanishad (2.3) as a practice of the vālakhilyas (a certain type of seer or *rishi), ūrdhva-retas has since ancient times been the esoteric reason for celibacy (*brahmacarya). It is the process underlying sublimation, by which the semen is transmuted into vital energy (*ojas*) that feeds the higher centers of the *body, notably the *brain.

USHTRA-ĀSANA *ushtrāsana*, "camel posture"), described in the *Gheranda-Samhitā* (2.41) as follows: Lying down, bend one's legs back and hold them with one's hands while energetically contracting the abdominal muscles and the mouth. A "camel seat" (*ushtra-nishadana*) is mentioned already in the *Yoga-Bhāshya* (2.46), though we do not know how it was practiced.

UTKATA-ĀSANA (*utkatāsana*, "raised posture"), described in the *Gheranda-Samhitā* (2.27) thus: Standing on one's toes with heels off the ground, place one's buttocks on the heels. This position is to be assumed particularly when doing the water enema (*jala-vasti*).

UTSĀHA ("zest"), one of the six factors that promote *Yoga, according to the *Hatha-Yoga-Pradīpikā* (1.16). A positive, energetic attitude toward spiritual practice is an essential prerequisite on the *path. Otherwise the *yogin cannot break his habit patterns and lay down new "tracks" that are conducive to wholeness and *liberation. See also *vīrya*.

UTTĀNA-KŪRMA(KA)-ĀSANA (*uttānakūrmakāsana*, "extended tortoise posture"), described in the *Gheranda-Samhitā* (2.33) as follows: Assume the "cock posture" (*kukkuta-āsana*) and then hold the neck with one's hands, assuming the pose of a tortoise with its limbs extended. It is generally thought that this complicated posture is done while lying on one's back. This appears to be similar to the "womb posture" (*garbha-āsana*) mentioned in modern works, where one balances on

one's buttocks. Some contemporary manuals of *hatha-yoga* contain a different description: Sitting on one's heels, arch backward until the *head touches the ground. One's hands are kept on the thighs. See also *kūrma-āsana*.

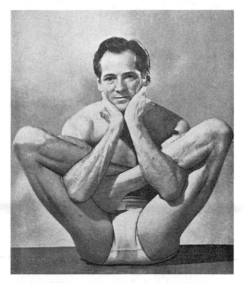

Uttāna-kūrmaka-āsana, demonstrated by Theos Bernard

UTTĀNA-MANDUKA-ĀSANA (*uttānamandukāsana*, "extended frog posture"), described in the *Gheranda-Samhitā* (2.24) thus: Seated in the frog posture (*manduka-āsana*), hold one's *head with the elbows and then stretch the *body like a frog. Some contemporary manuals of *hatha-yoga* describe this differently: Sitting on one's heels, arch backward until the head touches the ground. One's arms are folded around the head in such a way that the forearms serve as a cushion.

UTTANKA or **UTANKA**, a great *ascetic mentioned in the *Mahābhārata* and several *Purānas*. His teacher was Āpodadhaumya.

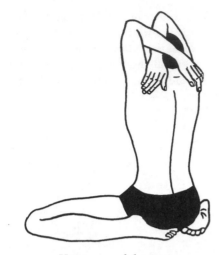

Uttāna-manduka-āsana

UTTHĀNA ("levitation"), a phenomenon experienced during the most advanced stage of breath control (*prāṇāyāma*). Some authorities understand this metaphorically rather than literally, whereby the practitioner's *consciousness is temporarily lifted out of the *body. See also *lāghava, siddhi*.

UTTHĀNA-ROMA ("erect hair"). The *Laghu-Yoga-Vāsishtha* (5.6.158) mentions the bristling hair of the sage Uddālaka as a phenomenon accompanying his ecstatic (*samādhi*) state.

· V ·

VĀC ("speech") sometimes stands for *sound in general. According to the *Yoga-Kundalī-Upanishad* (3.18ff.), there are four levels of sound—from the inaudible transcendental to the vocalized sound—which must be dissolved in reverse order until the supreme *Reality beyond all sound is realized. See also *shabda, vāk-siddhi*.

VĀC, the eternal Word, the *Goddess of divine speech mentioned in the *Rig-Veda* (10.71.3), where she is said to enter into the seers (*rishi*) for their inspiration.

VĀCASPATI MISHRA (mid-9th cen. CE), a *Shaiva *brahmin* of Mithila and a distinguished scholar who commented on all major philosophical systems of *Hinduism, with the exception of the *Vaisheshika school, which he treated in conjunction with the *Nyāya system. His expositions are marked by their great learning and exemplary lucidity. Among his many works is the *Tattva-Vaishāradī*, a subcommentary on the *Yoga-Sūtra*.

VĀHA ("flow"), the process of inhalation (*prāṇa*) and exhalation (*apāna*).

VAHNI ("fire"), a synonym for *agni*.

VAHNI-SĀRA-DHAUTI ("cleansing by way of fire"), also known as *agni-sāra-dhauti*; one of the techniques of inner cleansing (*antar-dhauti*) employed in *hatha-yoga. It is described in the *Gheranda-Samhitā* (1.20f.) thus: Push the *navel back against the spine a hundred times. This is said to cure all *diseases of the stomach, to fan the fire in the belly (*jāthara-agni*), and to yield a "divine body" (*divya-deha*). This text also enjoins great *secrecy about this practice.

VAHNI-YOGA ("fire Yoga"). See *agni-yoga*.

VAIKHĀNASA-SMĀRTA-SŪTRA ("Aphoristic Lawbook for Forest Dwellers"), as the title suggests, a work belonging to the *smriti* category that deals specifically with the duties of forest eremites, called *vaikhānasas*. It was composed some time in the fourth century CE and contains important references to *Yoga as practiced by certain ascetics (*tapasvin*). Thus chapter 8 speaks of hermits who live with or without wives and mendicants (*bhikshu*) who dedicate their lives to the quest for *liberation. Greatest among the last-mentioned ascetics are the "supreme swans" (*paramahamsa*). The same chapter also mentions three categories of yogic practitioners: (1) the *sāranga*- or "variegated" *yogins*, who comprise four kinds: those who do not practice *breath control but live with the conviction "I am *Vishnu"; those who practice *breath control and the other techniques of *Yoga; those who follow an eightfold Yoga (*ashta-anga-yoga*) beginning with *breath control (thus not *Patanjali's Yoga); and those who appear to practice an atheistic type of Yoga; (2) the *eka-rishya yogins*, who have a single *rishi ("seer"), the meaning of which is not clear in this context; five types are distinguished on the basis of their spiritual accomplishment; and (3) the *visarga-yogins*, who adopt various questionable means of self-mortification, sometimes even rejecting the practice of *meditation, and who can attain *liberation only in a future *life.

VAIRĀGYA ("dispassion"), also known as *virāga*, signifies the mood and practice of *renunciation, or the abandonment of passion (*rāga*); sometimes counted as one of the components of self-discipline (*niyama*). The *Yoga-Sūtra (1.15) defines it as the "awareness of mastery of him who is without thirst for seen (i.e., earthly) and revealed (i.e., heavenly) things." *Patanjali also speaks of a higher form of dispassion, consisting in one's nonthirsting for the primary constituents (*guna*) of *nature, resulting from the "vision of the Self" (*purusha-khyāti*).

Vairāgya is one of the two fundamental aspects of spiritual life, the other being practical application (*abhyāsa*) of the various techniques, especially *meditation. Unless practice is accompanied by an attitude of dispassion, one runs the risk of inflating rather than transcending the *ego. Dispassion without practice, on the other hand, is like a blunt knife: the psychosomatic energies released through dispassion are not channeled appropriately and thus may lead to confusion and possibly *delusion instead of *liberation. Hence the *Bhagavad-Gītā (6.35) enjoins their simultaneous cultivation. The *Uddhāva-Gītā (4.11) expresses the same conviction in the compound *vairāgya-abhyāsa-yoga*. See also Abandonment, Renunciation, *vītarāga*.

VAISHĀRADYA. See *nirvicāra-vaishāradya*.

VAISHESHIKA ("distinctionism"), one of the six philosophical systems (*darshana*) of *Hinduism. This school of thought, founded by Kanāda, is concerned with the differences (*vishesha*) between things. The Vaisheshika system offers an approach to *liberation through rational understanding of the categories of existence. Although primarily logical-cosmological in outlook, the *Vaisheshika-Sūtra* (5.2.16), which is ascribed to Kanāda but was probably composed between 200 BCE and 100 CE, mentions *Yoga, which it defines as "that which effects the cessation of suffering (*duhkha*)."

VAISHNAVA ("pertaining to *Vishnu"), an adjective also employed as a noun to denote a follower of *Vaishnavism.

VAISHNAVĪ-MUDRĀ ("seal pertaining to *Vishnu"), explained in the *Shāndilya-Upanishad* (1.7.14ff.) as one's external gaze (*bahir-drishti*) at an inner sign (*antar-lakshya*) while being unable to either shut or open the eyelids. The *Nāda-Bindu-Upanishad* (31) stipulates that this technique should be practiced for the manifestation of the inner sound (*nāda*). See also *shāmbhavī-mudrā*.

VAISHNAVISM, the religious culture centering on the *worship of *Vishnu; together with *Shaivism, one of the two great theistic traditions of *Hinduism. Originating in *Vedic times, the worship of Vishnu gained in popularity about the time of the *Buddha. The early phase of Vaishnavism is known as *Pāncarātra or the *Bhāgavata religion. The *Bhagavad-Gītā*, a part of the *Mahābhārata*, is the oldest available scripture of this tradition. The *Gītā*, which styles itself a "textbook of Yoga" (*yoga-shāstra*), gives us an excellent glimpse into the yogic orientation of early Vaishnavism. Fragments of the Pāncarātra teachings have also been preserved in other sections of the epic. The early common era saw the rise of a vast *Vaishnava literature known as the *Samhitās* ("Collections"), of which over 200 individual works are known to have existed. Only a few of these texts have been studied, one of them being the *Ahirbudhnya-Samhitā* (12.31ff.), which mentions a *Yoga-Samhitā* by *Hiranyagarbha. Concurrently with the creation of this literature, South India celebrated its own Vaishnava poet-saints, the *Ālvārs. Vaishnavism blossomed around the turn of the first millennium CE, receiving its greatest impetus through the teach-

ing and missionary activities of *Rāmānuja and his numerous disciples. This is also the period in which the highly influential *Bhāgavata-Purāna* was composed. The Yoga characteristic of Vaishnavism, which is strongly theistic, is *bhakti-yoga. This is tempered, however, by *karma-yoga. See also Krishna.

VAISHVĀNARA ("pertaining to all men"), the "fire" situated in the center of the human *body, which is responsible for digestion; also known as the *jāthara-agni.

VAITRISHNYA ("nonthirsting"), a synonym for *vitrishna*.

VAJRA ("thunderbolt," "diamond," or "adamantine"), a secret name for the *penis.

VAJRA-ĀSANA (*vajrāsana*, "adamantine posture"), described in the *Gheranda-Samhitā* (2.12) as follows: Tighten the thighs like a thunderbolt and place one's legs under the anus. This is said to yield paranormal powers (*siddhi*). This practice is also called "adept's posture" (*siddha-āsana*) in some works. The *Yoga-Sūtra* (3.46) speaks of adamantine robustness (*vajra-samhananatva*) as one of the aspects of bodily perfection (*kāya-sampad*).

VAJRA-DEHA ("adamantine body"), the transubstantiated *body of an *adept of *hatha-yoga, which is as indestructible as a diamond. The *Mahābhārata* (12.322.9) mentions a race of beings whose bones are like diamond (*vajra-asthi-kāya*), who were seen by the sage *Nārada when he ascended the sacred Mount *Meru. They are said to have a steady gaze, to live without eating, and to emit a beautiful scent. See also *divya-deha, dridha-deha*, Transubstantiation.

VAJRĀ-NĀDĪ ("adamantine channel"), a conduit inside the central channel (*sushumnā-nādī) of the *body. According to the *Shat-Cakra-Nirūpana (1), it extends from the *genitals to the *head. See also brahma-nādī.

VAJROLĪ-MUDRĀ ("vajrolī seal"), also spelled vajronī-mudrā; an important "seal" (*mudrā) of *hatha-yoga. The *Gheranda-Samhitā (3.45ff.) describes this technique as follows: Place one's palms on the ground and raise one's legs without letting the *head touch the ground. According to this manual, the vajrolī-mudrā is praised as the best of *Yoga practices, which awakens the "serpent power" (*kundalinī-shakti), causes longevity, and leads to all kinds of powers (*siddhi), notably control over the *semen (bindu-siddhi). The *Hatha-Yoga-Pradīpikā (3.85ff.), in contrast, understands this practice as the sexual technique of sucking up the female ejaculate (*rajas) with the *penis (mehana). In order to develop this ability, the *yogin is advised to blow into a tube that he has inserted into his penis. In his commentary on the *Yoga-Tattva-Upanishad (126), *Upanishad Brahmayogin describes the following technique: Dipping the penis into cow's milk poured into a bronze vessel, the *yogin sucks up the liquid with his penile shaft "resembling a thunderbolt" and then releases it again. When he has acquired sufficient control, he should ejaculate his semen (*retas) into the vagina and then draw it up again together with the woman's ejaculate (*shonita). Reflecting the antinomian spirit of left-hand *Tantrism, the *Hatha-Yoga-Pradīpikā (3.84) further observes that he who knows this technique may live as he pleases without detriment, and even disregard the practices of self-discipline (*niyama).

The practice of vajrolī-mudrā is also possible for women, according to the *Hatha-Ratna-Āvalī (2.101ff.). The woman is said to have her own *bindu (2.89). *Rajas is said (2.93) to resemble the essence of red lead (sindūra) and be permanently present in the female genitals (*yoni). Cf. amarolī-mudrā, sahajolī-mudrā.

VĀK-SIDDHI, or VĀKYA-SIDDHI ("power of speech"), often mentioned as one of the paranormal abilities (*siddhi) acquired by the *yogin. This is the ability of charging one's speech with numinous power so as to render it completely effective. See also vāc.

VĀMADEVA, a *Shaiva *yogin whose teachings are recorded in the *Shiva-Purāna (6.18.7ff.). An *adept by the same name appears in the *Varāha-Upanishad (4.2.35) as a representative of "gradual liberation" (*krama-mukti).

VĀMA-KRAMA ("left process"), one of the forms of *kapāla-bhāti. According to the *Gheranda-Samhitā (1.56f.), it is practiced by repeated and unstrained inhalation through the left nostril and exhalation through the right nostril. This is stated to cure disorders of phlegm (*kapha).

VĀMA-MĀRGA ("left path"), the left-hand approach in *Tantrism, which involves the literal enactment of the "five m's" (*panca-ma-kara). Mainstream practitioners of Tantrism regard this as a dangerous orientation, which leads those who are impure to ruin. Cf. dakshina-mārga, kaula-mārga.

VAMANA-DHAUTI ("cleansing by vomiting"), one of the forms of "heart cleansing" (*hrid-dhauti). The *Gheranda-Sam-

hitā (1.39) explains this technique thus: After meals, drink *water, filling up the stomach until it reaches the *throat. Then direct one's *gaze upward for a short while and finally vomit the water out again. If practiced daily, this is said to cure disorders of phlegm (*kapha) and bile (*pitta). See also *gaja-karanī*.

VANDANA ("prostration"), one of the aspects of the *Yoga of devotion (*bhakti-yoga*).

VARĀHA-UPANISHAD (*Varāhopanishad*), one of the *Yoga-Upanishads*, presented as a dialogue between *Vishnu and the sage *Ribhu. Comprising five chapters with a total of 273 stanzas, it begins with a description of the categories (*tattva) of existence and then proceeds to elaborate the metaphysical principles of *Vedānta. The text (2.55) takes a critical stance toward what appears to be *Classical Yoga, which, it argues, is based on a misconception about the Lord (*īshvara). This *Upanishad* (4.2.39) is also critical of *hatha-yoga, though it outlines that approach in the fifth chapter, which seems to be a later addition. Here *mantra-, *laya-, and *hatha-yoga are treated as stages of the eightfold path (*ashta-anga-yoga*). It favors *samputa-yoga* ("Yoga of the bowl"), which is essentially *kundalinī-yoga. The designation *samputa* is not directly explained but can be understood as the intersection of the three principal pathways of the life force (*prāna) in the *body—i.e., *sushumnā-, *idā-, and *pingalā-nādī*—and the *kuhū-nādī*.

VĀRI-SĀRA-DHAUTI ("cleansing by means of water"), one of the techniques of inner cleansing (*antar-dhauti) employed in *hatha-yoga. The *Gheranda-Samhitā* (1.17ff.) describes it as follows: Fill the mouth completely with *water and then swallow it slowly, move it into the stomach, and expel it through the rectum. This technique is said to be the foremost type of *dhauti, since it leads to a "divine body" (*divya-deha*).

VARNA ("coating" or "color"), the *Hindu system of four social estates: the priestly (*brāhmana), the warrior (*kshatriya*), the merchant (*vaishya*), and the servile estate (*shūdra*).

In the sense of "color," *varna* refers to the frequency of *light that characterizes the psyche (*jīva). Thus the *Mahābhārata* (12.271.33) mentions six colors: black, gray, blue, red, yellow, and white. These colors typify the *karma of a person, with black being the least favorable and white suggesting an advanced moral and spiritual level. "Clarity of color" (*varna-prasāda*) is mentioned in the *Shvetāshvatara-Upanishad* (2.12) as one of the signs of progress (*pravritti) in *Yoga. Color also plays a role in the visionary experiences associated with *tāraka-yoga.

Finally, the word *varna* is also employed to denote "sound" and "letter" in *mantra-yoga.

VARTAMĀNA-KARMA ("present *karma*"). See *karma.

VARUNA ("Coverer"), said to be related to the Greek Ouranos (Latin: Uranus), belongs to the oldest religious stratum of *Hinduism. In the *Rig-Veda* (6.48.14) he is described as the possessor of *māyā, or the mysterious power through which all forms (*rūpa) in the *cosmos are created. He also presides over the cosmic order (*rita) and metes out punishment to those who transgress it. In later Hinduism Varuna became the Lord of Death and the deity associated with *water, in particular the ocean.

VARUNĀ-NĀDĪ, or VARUNĪ-NĀDĪ ("Varu-na's channel"), one of the principal channels (*nādī) through which the *life force (*prāna) circulates in the *body. Most texts locate it between the *yashasvinī- and the *kuhū-nādī. According to the *Yoga-Shikhā-Upanishad (2.26), it is situated below the *navel and is responsible for the function of urination.

vāsanā ("dwelling"), desire; also, the subliminal trait left behind in the *mind by the exercise of *desire. As the Anna-pūrnā-Upanishad (4.78f.) declares: "So long as the *mind is not dissolved, so long the traits are not obliterated either. So long as the traits have not dwindled, so long the mind is not tranquil."

In *Classical Yoga, vāsanā is explained as a concatenation of subliminal activators (*samskāra). According to the *Yoga-Sūtra (4.24), the mind (*citta) is speckled with countless vāsanās. They depend on a person's stock of merit (*punya) and demerit (*apunya). The *Laghu-Yoga-Vāsishtha (1.1.10) distinguishes between pure (*shuddha) and tainted (mālina) vāsanās. The former are comparable to fried seed, which cannot sprout; the latter are the cause of reembodiment (*punar-janman). See also āshaya, karma.

VASISHTHA, or VASHISHTHA, the name of several illustrious sages. In the *Vedic era, Vashishtha was a seer (*rishi) who composed many of the hymns of the seventh book of the *Rig-Veda. In later times, a Vashishtha was a prominent sage in the *Rāmāyana and the *Mahābhārata, several *Purānas and *Upanishads, and not least in the *Yoga-Vāsishtha. According to legend, the rishi Vashishtha's personal quarrel with sagely King Vishvāmitra escalated into a feud between their respective clans. However, the story of their abiding enmity

is often taken to symbolize the clash of interest between the sacrificial ritualism of the priestly estate (*brāhmana) and the spiritual heritage of the warrior estate (kshatriya). See also saptarshi.

VĀSHITVA ("mastery"), one of the major paranormal powers (*siddhi) recognized in *Yoga. The *Mani-Prabhā (3.44) explains it as the "control over the elements" (bhūta niyantritva).

VĀSO-DHAUTI ("cleansing [by means of a] cloth"), one of the forms of "heart cleansing" (*hrid-dhauti). The *Gheranda-Sam-hitā (1.40f.) describes it thus: Slowly swallow a thick cloth four fingers wide and then draw it out again. This is said to cure abdominal *diseases, fever, enlarged spleen, leprosy and skin diseases, and disorders of phlegm (*kapha) and bile (*pitta). The *Hatha-Yoga-Pradīpikā (2.24) calls this technique simply *dhauti. According to this scripture, the cloth is four digits broad and fifteen spans long.

VASTI ("bladder"), one of the "six acts" (*shat-karma) of *hatha-yoga. According to the *Gheranda-Samhitā (1.45), it is of two types: *jala-vasti ("water enema") and *shushka-vasti ("dry enema"). The word is also sometimes rendered as "syringe," because the description given of this technique in the *Hatha-Yoga-Pradīpikā (2.26) involves the use of a tube inserted into the rectum by which *water is sucked up. The *Jyotsnā (2.26) mentions that the tube should be six fingers long and that two-thirds of it should be inserted.

VASUGUPTA (9th cen. CE), Kashmiri *adept and author of the *Shiva-Sūtra. According to one traditional account, the teachings encoded in this work were revealed to him by *Shiva in a dream. Ac-

323

cording to another account, he discovered them inscribed on the face of a rock on Mahādeva Mountain near Shrinagar, the modern capital of Kashmir. The rock, called shamkara-upala, is still a pilgrimage site.

VĀTA ("air" or "wind"), one of the five material elements (*bhūta) of the material *cosmos. Its symbol is the hexagon (shat-kona), it is associated with the color black and the "seed syllable" (*bīja-mantra) yam, and it is thought of as ruling the area from the navel (*nābhi) to the middle of the eyebrows (*bhrū-madhya). The word vāta is also employed as a synonym for *prāna ("breath"). It also signifies one of the bodily humors (*dhātu) and has the qualities of dryness, coldness, and mobility. See also tattva, vāyu.

VĀTA-SĀRA-DHAUTI ("cleansing by means of air"), one of the four techniques of inner cleansing (*antar-dhauti) employed in *hatha-yoga. The *Gheranda-Samhitā (1.15f.) describes it thus: Shape the mouth like the beak of a crow—in the manner of the *kākī-mudrā—and slowly suck in *air, filling the belly with it and moving it around, then slowly forcing it out through the rectum. This is stated to cure all *diseases and to increase the "abdominal fire" (*jāthara-agni).

VĀYAVĪ-DHĀRANĀ-MUDRĀ ("aerial concentration seal"), one of the five *concentration techniques described in the *Gheranda-Samhitā (3.77ff.). The practice consists in focusing one's *attention and *life force, through *breath control, on the *wind element for 159 minutes. This is held to stimulate the life energy and to enable one to move through space (khe-gamana). See also dhāranā, mudrā, panca-dhāranā.

VĀYU ("air" or "wind"), a synonym for *vāta and *prāna. Expressing a universal yogic sentiment, the *Shāndilya-Upanishad (1.7.6) declares that the breath (vāyu) should be tamed as one tames a lion, an elephant, or a tiger—step by step, lest it should kill one. Perfect mastery over the air element, known as vāyu-siddhi, culminates in the paranormal power of *levitation.

VĀYU-SĀDHANA ("discipline of the air"), a synonym for *prānāyāma used in the *Shiva-Samhitā (3.68).

VEDAS ("Knowledges"), the oldest portion of the sacred canon of *Hinduism, the four hymnodies: *Rig-Veda, *Atharva-Veda, *Yajur-Veda, and *Sāma-Veda. The hymns (sūkta, *mantra) of these collections are traditionally said to have been "seen" by seers (*rishi) and are regarded as revelation (*shruti). See also Upanishads.

VEDĀNTA ("Veda end"), a comprehensive term for the metaphysical ideas that originated with the *Vedas but found their classic expression in the *Upanishads, which are the esoteric continuation of *Vedic ritualism. Vedānta comprises a vast body of literature, both scholastic and popular. It is the dominant philosophy of *Hinduism, favoring a nondualist (*advaita) interpretation of existence: there is only the one *Reality, which appears manifold to the unenlightened *mind but which reveals itself as singular (*eka) and nondual (*advaya). As one of the six philosophical systems (*darshana) of Hinduism, Vedānta was systematized in the Brahma-Sūtra of Badārāyana (prob. 2d cen. CE). This concise treatment gave rise to a host of sometimes considerably divergent interpretations. The best-known and most influential school is the Kevala Advaita (absolute nondualism) of *Shankara (ca. 788–820 CE). Its great historical rival is the *Vishishta Advaita (qualified nondualism) of *Rāmānuja (1017–1137 CE). There is even a dualist school of Vedānta, the Dvaita school of Mādhva (1199–1270 CE). *Yoga played a varyingly prominent role in these schools and was interpreted differently by their protagonists, though no systematic study of the yogic materials present in the Vedānta tradition has as yet been undertaken. See also Advaita Vedānta, Ramakrishna, Vivekananda.

VEDĀNTA-SHRAVANA ("listening [to the teachings of] Vedānta"), one of the ten practices of self-discipline (*niyama), according to the *Tri-Shikhi-Brāhmana-Upanishad (1.34). See also shravana.

VEDANTIC, the anglicized adjective of *Vedānta.

VEDĀNTIN, a follower of the *Vedānta tradition.

VEDIC, the anglicized adjective of the Sanskrit word vaidika, meaning "pertaining to the *Vedas."

VEDIC YOGA, an analytical category referring to the protoyogic elements in the *Vedas, especially the *Rig-Veda and the *Atharva-Veda, some of whose numerous hymns may have been composed in the third millennium BCE or possibly earlier still.

VENERATION OF THE PRECEPTOR. See ācārya-upāsana; see also guru-bhakti.

VIBHŪTI ("manifestation"), in the *Bhagavad-Gītā (10.16), the "far-flung powers" by which *Krishna pervades the *world; in *Classical Yoga, a synonym for "paranor-

mal power" (*siddhi). The word also signifies the *ashes that *Shaiva ascetics smear on their bodies to indicate their status as world renouncers (*samnyāsin).

VICĀRA ("reflection"), one of the higher mental phenomena, or spontaneous thought processes, associated with a particular level of ecstasy (*samādhi), in which the object of *attention pertains to the "subtle" (*sūkshma) dimension of *nature. In *Vedānta and Vedānta-based schools of *Yoga, the word vicāra also can stand for existential pondering. Thus the *Laghu-Yoga-Vāsishtha (2.1.69) explains it as consisting of asking searching questions such as "Who am I?" and "Whence this universe?" This kind of inquiry is said to be a panacea for the "chronic disease of worldliness" (samsāra-roga). See also nirvicāra-samāpatti, savicāra-samāpatti; cf. vitarka.

VICĀRANĀ ("reflecting"), one of the seven levels of wisdom (*jnāna). See sapta-jnāna-bhūmi.

VICITRA-KARANI ("variegated procedure"), described in the *Hatha-Ratna-Avalī (3.68) as follows: In the position of *shayita-pashcimatāna, extend the hands while keeping the legs stretched out like sticks. This appears to be a variation of the *pashcimatāna-āsana, though the description is too cryptic for a precise identification.

VIDEHA-MUKTI ("disembodied liberation"), generally understood to be *liberation that coincides with the shedding of the *body at *death. Those who enjoy this condition are traditionally thought to roam the invisible or "subtle" (*sūkshma) dimensions of *nature. Vidyāranya offers a different interpretation in his *Jīvan-

Mukti-Viveka (2), however, arguing that the "disembodied" (*videha*) state refers to future embodiment only. Similarly, the **Tejo-Bindu-Upanishad* (4.33ff.) understands *videha-mukti* as the condition of perfect identity with the *Absolute to the point where all body consciousness has been lost. Cf. *jīvan-mukti*.

VIDHI ("rule"). The **Shiva-Samhitā* (5.4) lists the observance of rules and vows (**vrāta*) as a possible source of spiritual obstruction (**vighna*). This is meant to drive home the point that we benefit spiritually from what we do only if we are in right relationship to our *actions. So long as the *ego is involved, we are always in danger of mistaking the means (**upāya*) for the goal—e.g., keeping a *diet or practicing meditation (**dhyāna*) as if this was our ultimate concern.

VIDHŪNANA-ĀSANA ("shaking posture"), described in the **Hatha-Ratna-Āvalī* (3.70) thus: Alternately extend one leg and touch the big toe with the hand while holding the other leg by the ankle.

VIDYĀ ("knowledge" or "wisdom"), the antithesis of **avidyā*, or spiritual nescience. The ultimate condition of *Self-realization, or *enlightenment, is often characterized as one of gnosis, as opposed to the ignorance that marks the unillumined personality. As such, it is referred to as *bodha, *prajñā, and *jñāna. However, this *wisdom transcends the dichotomy between subject (consciousness) and *object (world) that is an integral part of conventional *knowledge. It is not a content of consciousness (**citta*), but the very nature of pure Consciousness (**cit*). In some contexts, the word *vidyā* stands for "technical knowledge," such as in the compound *khecarī-vidyā*, the technical

knowledge regarding the "ether-walking seal" (**khecarī-mudrā*). See also *brahma-vidyā, shrī-vidyā*.

VIDYĀRANYA TĪRTHA (prob. b. ca. 1314 CE), a learned *Vedānta scholar who composed such works as the *Panca-Dashī* (or at least the first ten chapters of it) and the **Jīvan-Mukti-Viveka*. He is often identified with Mādhava, the author of the *Sarva-Darshana-Samgraha* ("Compendium on All Systems"). He obviously had an intimate knowledge of *Yoga and appears to have followed the practical path of *ashta-anga-yoga*.

VIGHNA ("obstacle"). Spiritual life is uniformly characterized as being inherently difficult because it is based not only on critical self-understanding but also on the radical transcendence of the self, or *ego. This involves the constant willingness to drop habit patterns and adaptations that are not in keeping with one's growing understanding of the nature of one's authentic identity as the *Self rather than the personality complex, or limited body-mind. Some of these emotional and mental patterns can prove tenacious and become obstacles to change and maturation.

The *Yoga scriptures mention many different obstacles, or obstructions. The **Yoga-Tattva-Upanishad* (30f.), e.g., refers to the following obstacles that can occur at the outset of spiritual practice: (1) **ālasya* ("laziness"); (2) *katthāna* ("boastfulness"); (3) *dhūrta-goshthī* ("fellowship with rogues"); (4) *mantra-ādi-sādhana* ("cultivation of *mantras and so forth"), i.e., cultivation of such practices for the wrong reasons (e.g., to acquire magical *powers); and (5) *dhātu-strī-laulyaka* ("longing for a base woman"). These, the text states, should be avoided through the accumulation of merit (**punya*) and can be turned around through the practice of reciting the sacred *pranava (i.e., the syllable *om). Other works mention different remedies, but all imply that one should persist in one's spiritual efforts. In the *Yoga-Shāstra (101ff.) of *Dattātreya five obstacles are listed: *ālasya ("laziness"); prakatthāna ("gossiping"); mantra-sādhana ("cultivation of *mantras"); dhātu-vāda ("*alchemy"); and khādya-vādaka ("dicting"). The last three are included because they are often employed for the wrong reasons, such as the acquisition of magical powers (*siddhi).

The *Tejo-Bindu-Upanishad (1.40ff.) mentions the following nine obstacles: anu-samdhāna-rahitya ("lack of application"); *ālasya ("laziness"); bhoga-lālasa ("longing for enjoyment"); *laya ("inertia"); *tamas ("stupor"); *vikshepa ("distracted-ness"); *tejas ("overzealousness"); *sveda ("[excessive] sweating"); *shūnyatā ("voidness"), which probably stands for absent-mindedness. The *Yoga-Kundalī-Upanishad (1.56ff.) contains a similar catalog of obstacles on the spiritual *path, which include doubt (*samshaya) and sleep (*nidrā). A more extensive catalog is furnished in the *Shiva-Samhitā (3.32f.), which includes undesirable types of food, overeating (*atīva-bhojana), fasting (*upa-vāsa), misanthropy (jana-dvesha), cruelty toward animals (prāni-pīdana), female companionship (strī-sanga), and garrulousness (bahu-ālāpa). Elsewhere (5.3ff.) this scripture notes that obstacles can arise not only from pleasure (*bhoga) but also from one's practice of virtue (*dharma) and even from knowledge (*jnāna). Thus it refers to ablutions (*snāna) and rules (*vidhi) as instances of the second group, and knowledge about the subtle channels (*nādī) of the *life force and the ability to stop one's *breath as instances of the third group. This text (3.47) emphasizes that

even in the face of all these numerous difficulties, the *yogin should absolutely persist in his *efforts.

Morever, many scriptures state that the paranormal powers (*siddhi) are to be regarded as obstacles to the "great power" of *enlightenment. See also antarāya, dosha, upasarga.

VIJNĀNA ("knowledge"), secular *knowledge or intellectual understanding, as distinguished from wisdom (*jnāna). In some rare contexts, however, this word can also denote the ultimate liberating gnosis (*vidyā) and the transcendental *Reality itself.

VIJNĀNA-BHAIRAVA, also called Shiva-Vijnāna-Upanishad, by the great *adept and scholar *Abhinava Gupta; a central scripture of Kashmiri *Shaivism. The title refers to the supreme state of *Consciousness (vijnāna), which is none other than *Shiva (as *Bhairava). Its exact date is unknown, though it was well respected by the eighth century CE. The anonymous author claims this text to be the quintessence of the Rudra-Yāmala-Tantra, which is no longer extant. The Vijnāna-Bhairava describes 112 types of yogic techniques for achieving ecstasy (*samādhi). It is thus an important *yoga-shāstra.

VIJNĀNA BHIKSHU (1525–1580 CE), a *Vedānta monk and scholar who composed, in addition to several shorter works, authoritative commentaries on the Brahma-Sūtra, the *Sāmkhya-Sūtra, and the *Yoga-Sūtra (entitled *Yoga-Vārttika), and the digest *Yoga-Sāra-Samgraha. Vijnāna Bhikshu, an original thinker, promulgated a form of theistic Vedānta close to the Sāmkhya-Vedānta orientation of the *Purānas and the *Bhagavad-Gītā. In particular, he rejected *Shankara's more radical nondualist metaphysics for belief in the existence of a personal *God as the highest being, the multiplicity of Spirits (*purusha), and the reality of the *world. Though he was not a follower of the *yoga-darshana as such, Vijñāna Bhikshu was obviously well acquainted with *Yoga theory and technology. In his exegesis he tends to be more speculative than, for instance, *Vācaspati Mishra, another great Yoga savant, and often proposes interesting explanations where other commentators remain silent or merely reiterate previous opinions. His chief disciple was *Bhāva Ganesha.

VIJNĀNA-MAYA-KOSHA ("sheath composed of knowledge"), the bodily "envelope" (*kosha) formed of higher understanding, or what in some schools is called *buddhi.

VIKALPA ("conceptualization"), in *Classical Yoga, one of the five categories of mental "fluctuation" (*vritti), defined in the *Yoga-Sūtra (1.9) as *knowledge that is without perceivable *object and that follows verbal distinctions. This term is often also understood in the sense of "imagination" or "fantasy." All vikalpas are intrinsically impure and hence bind the individual to the finite *world. However, the tradition of *Shaivism recognizes the existence of a single pure (*shuddha) form of conceptualization: the thought "I am *Shiva" (shivo'ham).

VIKĀRA ("modification"), an important *Sāmkhya term, also often employed in the commentaries on the *Yoga-Sūtra. It signifies the transformations of the ground of nature (*prakriti) into distinct categories (*tattva) such as the ten senses (*indriya), the five sense objects (*vishaya), and the lower mind (*manas). See also parināma.

VIKĀSA ("expansion"). See adhyātma-vikāsa.

VIKSHEPA ("distraction"), in the *Yoga-Sūtra (1.30), a synonym for *antarāya ("obstacle"). It suggests that obstacles such as *sickness, *laziness, and *doubt distract one's consciousness (*citta) from the task of focusing on the spiritual process. These distractions are accompanied, according to *Patanjali, by pain (*duhkha), depression (*daurmanasya), tremor of the limbs (angam-ejatva), and faulty inhalation (*shvāsa) and exhalation (*prashvāsa).

VIMARSHA ("touching" or "examining"), the intrinsic self-apprehension of the transcendental *Being; in Kashmiri *Shaivism, one of the two essential aspects of the ultimate *Reality, the other being *prakāsha, or "luminosity."

VIPĀKA ("ripening" or "fruition"), the fructification of *karma, i.e, the visible results (in the form of advantageous or disadvantageous events) of former *actions, whether they were committed in this lifetime or previous embodiments. Cf. phala.

VIPARĪTA-KARANĪ-MUDRĀ ("inverse action seal"), described in the *Gheranda-Samhitā (3.33ff.) as follows: Place one's *head on the ground and, with one's hands spread out and legs raised, remain steady. This appears to be the original name for the headstand (*shīrsha-āsana). Some modern manuals interpret it as the shoulderstand, however, The idea behind this potent practice is to achieve a reversal of the the microcosmic "sun" (*sūrya) and "moon" (*candra). The "moon" oozes the precious ambrosia (*amrita), which trickles into the abdomen, where it is consumed by the "sun." Through this "seal" (*mudrā) the *yogin seeks to interrupt this process and save the nectar for higher purposes. Daily practice of this technique for up to three hours is said to greatly fan the "abdominal fire" (*jāthara-agni), which is why the practitioner should eat amply. This exercise is praised as a panacea for all ills and as a means of conquering *death itself. Cf. sarva-anga-āsana.

VIPARYAYA ("error"), one of the five categories of mental "fluctuation" (*vritti), defined in the *Yoga-Sūtra (1.8) as erroneous knowledge that is not based on the actual appearance of a thing. The *Yoga-Bhāshya (2.3) treats viparyaya as a synonym for the term *avidyā ("nescience"), which is "five-jointed." It is the arch error, as a result of which we misinterpret existence itself. Cf. pramāna.

VĪRA ("hero"), an important *Tantric category, referring to the spiritual practitioner who animates the "heroic" disposition (*bhāva), which is the only one suitable for the present age of darkness (*kāli-yuga). The *Kula-Arnava-Tantra (17.25) explains the term vīra as follows: "On account of being free from passion (*rāga), intoxication (mada), affliction (*klesha), anger (kopa), jealousy (*mātsarya), and delusion (*moha), and on account of being far removed from activity (*rajas) and inertia (*tamas), he is called a hero."

The above passage represents a fanciful etymological play on the words vīra ("hero"), vīta ("free"), and vidhūra ("far removed"), which contradicts other *Tantric scriptures that ascribe to the vīra a strong energetic (*rajas) quality. Often the vīra is understood to be the practitioner of the left-hand ritual involving the "five substances" (*panca-tattva), including sexual intercourse (*maithunā). The im-

plication is that the heroic practitioner risks everything in his or her struggle for *self-transcendence. See also vīrya.

VĪRA-ĀSANA (vīrāsana, "heroic posture"). Mentioned in the *Mahābhārata (12.292.8), this posture (*āsana) is described somewhat inadequately in the *Gheranda-Samhitā (2.17): Placing one leg on the (opposite) thigh, turn the foot backward. Modern manuals often describe this posture differently: Kneeling down, sit between the thighs.

VIRĀGA ("nonattachment"), a synonym for *vairāgya.

VIRAHA ("separation"), an important notion in the *bhakti tradition, where it stands for the temporary concealment of the *Divine, which serves to intensify the *devotee's love and longing for *union.

VĪRA SHAIVA SECT. See Lingāyata sect.

VIRTUE. See dharma, Morality, punya.

VIRŪPĀKSHA, mentioned in the *Hatha-Yoga-Pradīpikā (1.5) as a great *adept of *hatha-yoga. He may be the same as the author of the Virūpāksha-Pancashikhā, a work on *Yoga.

VĪRYA ("vitality" or "energy"), listed in the *Yoga-Sūtra (1.20) as one of the requisites of the yogic *path leading to superconscious ecstasy (*asamprajnāta-samādhi). Elsewhere in this work (2.38) vīrya is said to be acquired through the practice of chastity (*brahmacarya). In some contexts vīrya can mean "*semen." See also vīra.

VISARGA ("emission"), a cardinal concept in the philosophy of *Abhinava Gupta. It denotes the transcendental process of expansion (*vistara, vikāsa) and contraction (*samkoca), which is the movement of the vibration (*spanda) that forever characterizes the *Divine. Visarga is the union (*yāmala) of *Shiva and *Shakti; the Sanskrit letter also called visarga (a voiceless aspirant) is the symbolic expression of that metaphysical union. The centripetal force of the visarga draws the *adept into deeper and deeper meditative absorption, until he or she realizes the ultimate *Being.

VISHĀDA ("despair"). When Prince *Arjuna faced his family, friends, and teachers on the battlefield, he fell into a mood of confusion and despair. Although he knew that he was fighting for a just cause, he could not conceive of slaying them. Seeing Arjuna's despondency, *Krishna, who served as the prince's charioteer, instructed him in the secrets of *karma-yoga, the *path of self-transcending *action. The eternal order (*dharma), he taught in the *Bhagavad-Gītā, must be maintained. It was the duty of a warrior to fight for justice, and despair was an unmanly thing. This has often been interpreted as an allegory of the human situation in general.

Vishāda is occasionally counted as one of the defects (*dosha). The *Uddhava-Gītā (24.2) states that spiritual practitioners often tend to feel dejected, either from exhaustion or because of their failure to control the *mind properly, and recommends that they should then take refuge at the "lotus feet of the *Lord." The *Mārkandeya-Purāna (39.16) soundly suggests the practice of breath control (*prānāyāma) to overcome depression.

VISHAYA ("object"), the thing experienced through the senses (*indriya). The *Yoga-Bhāshya (4.17) compares *objects to a magnet because they bind conscious-ness (*citta) as if it had the properties of iron. Sensory awareness is the habitual condition of the *waking consciousness. In *Yoga, which typically endeavors to bring about the introversion of *attention, the sense objects are often regarded as the enemy. Thus in his *Tattva-Vaishāradī (2.55) the Yoga scholar *Vācaspati Mishra compares them to snake's venom (āshivisha), a sentiment echoed in numerous other works of different traditions. The *Bhagavad-Gītā (2.59) speaks of the "eating" (āhāra) of objects, and this notion is also present in the Sanskrit term *bhoga, meaning "experience" but being derived from the root bhuj ("to eat, consume, enjoy").

In some contexts vishaya stands for "worldliness," as in the *Yoga-Kundalī-Upanishad (1.60), where it is named as one of the ten obstacles (*vighna) and is contrasted with renunciation (virati). See also artha, lakshya, Subject.

VISHESHA ("special" or "particular"), in *Classical Yoga, the ontic level of the "particularized," which, according to the *Yoga-Bhāshya (2.19), is composed of the five elements (*bhūta), the ten senses (*indriya), and the lower mind (*manas). Cf. avishesha.

VISHISHTA ADVAITA, the *Vedānta school of "Qualified Nondualism," for which *Rāmānuja was the most distinguished spokesman. In contrast to the radical nondualism of *Shankara, this school of thought defends the view that the ultimate *Reality is not merely an unqualified (nirguna), impersonal *Absolute but the suprapersonal *Being in whom all qualities inhere. It appears that the early representatives of this school, such as *Nāthamuni and *Yamunācārya, practiced an eightfold *Yoga (*ashta-anga-yoga) with a strong devotional (*bhakti) orientation. Cf. Kevala Advaita.

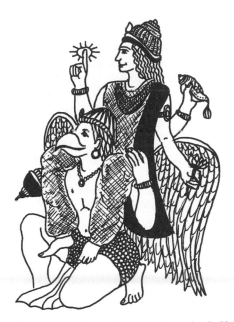

Vishnu mounted on his steed, Garuda, half man and half bird

VISHNU, originally a minor *deity of the *Vedic pantheon who, possibly because mythology endowed him with a carefully delineated personality and history, grew quickly into one of the principal deities of *Hinduism. His name means "pervader" and refers to his omnipresence. In the trinity (*tri-mūrti*) of medieval India, Vishnu stands for the principle of preservation, whereas *Brahma represents that of creation and *Shiva that of destruction.

Vishnu is the supreme Godhead worshiped in *Vaishnavism. His benign qualities invite a devotional (*bhakti) response, and *bhakti-yoga flourished in the religious culture of Vaishnavism. Vishnu's most significant aspect are his twenty-four "incarnations" (*avatāra) in different world ages (*yuga), among which

*Krishna is the most popular embodiment, *Rāma being a close second. The *Vaishnavas created many remarkable works extolling Vishnu and pointing out a *path to realizing unity or identity with that great god. Foremost among these scriptures are the *Bhagavad-Gītā* and the *Bhāgavata-Purāna*. See also *deva*.

VISHNU-GRANTHI ("Vishnu's knot"), the second of the "knots" (*granthi) or blockages in the *body, preventing the free flow of the life force (*prāna). It is located at the *throat, though some authorities place it in the *heart.

VISHNU-PURĀNA, one of the major works of the *Purāna genre. Its earliest portions predate the common era. It deals with *Yoga in the sixth canticle and understands it as the *path of meditation (*dhyāna).

VISHUDDHA-CAKRA ("pure wheel"), or VISHUDDHI-CAKRA ("wheel of purity"), the fifth psychoenergetic center (*cakra) in ascending order; also known as *jālan-*

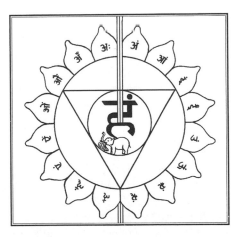

Vishuddha-cakra, the psychoenergetic center located at the throat

dhara-pītha and "great doorway to *liberation" (*mahā-moksha-dvāra*). It is located at the *throat or, as the *Yoga-Shikhā-Upanishad* (1.174) puts it, at the "throat well" (*kantha-kūpa*). It is generally depicted as a sixteen-petaled lotus of a smoky purple hue. According to the *Shat-Cakra-Nirūpana* (28), its pericarp is composed of the "circle of space" (*nabho-man-dala*), which resembles the full moon. This center is connected with the "seed syllable" (*bīja-mantra*) *ham*, the element ether (*ākāsha*), and the goddess Shākinī. The *Shiva-Samhitā* (5.92) states that by contemplating this *cakra*, one acquires an instant comprehension of the *Vedas* and all their mysteries.

VISHVA ("world"), the *cosmos in its entirety, which *Hindu cosmology pictures as a vast, multidimensional, dynamic being arising in the infinity of the *Divine and governed by the law of *karma*. The ordinary, unenlightened psyche (*jīva*) is entrapped in the processes of *nature and escapes this state of *bondage only through higher wisdom (*jnāna*, *vidyā*), i.e., realization of the transcendental *Reality. *Yoga is one of the spiritual avenues elaborated in *Hinduism by which the world-bound psyche can awaken to its true identity as the Self (*ātman*, *purusha*) and recover its essential *freedom. On the way to *enlightenment, or *liberation, the *yogin* may acquire all kinds of extraordinary insights and visions that reveal to him the immensity in space and time of the *cosmos. Such privileged knowledge, however, especially of the "subtle" (*sūkshma*) dimensions of the *world, must ultimately be renounced as well, so that the universe as a whole can be transcended.

For some but by no means all schools of Yoga, the world experienced by the unenlightened psyche is the great enemy of the spiritual process. They consequently regard transcendence of cosmic existence as the highest goal of human aspiration. This is the ideal of disembodied liberation (*videha-mukti*). A more integrated viewpoint looks upon the world as a potential aid to *enlightenment. According to this second view, after one has awakened from the dream of separate existence as a worldly *ego (a *subject confronting multiple *objects), one enjoys the world as a manifestation, or play (*līlā*) of the *Divine. This is the ideal of living liberation (*jīvan-mukti*).

VISHVĀSA ("confidence" or "trust"), mentioned in the *Shiva-Samhitā* (3.18) as a precondition for successful spiritual practice. See also *āstikya*, *shraddhā*.

VISHVA-UDARĀ-NĀDĪ (*vishvodarā-nādī*, "world belly channel"), also spelled *vishva-udarī-nādī* ("world-swelling channel"); one of the principal conduits (*nādī*) through which the life force (*prāna*) circulates in the *body. It is generally thought to be located between the *hasti-jihvā-nādī* and the *kuhū-nādī*. The *Yoga-Yājnavalkya* (4.44) places it in the middle of the belly (*tunda*), which would explain its curious name, since the *navel is the center of the *microcosm. This channel of the *life force is held to be responsible for the consumption of *food.

VISION. See *darshana*, *khyāti*.

VISMAYA ("wonder"), one of the ecstatic responses upon encountering the *Divine. See also *camatkāra*.

VISTARA or VIKĀSA ("expansion"), in Kashmiri *Shaivism, the outgoing phase of the divine heart (*hridaya*). See also *visarga*; cf. *samkoca*.

VITAL AREAS. See *marman*.

VITALITY. See *vīrya*.

VĪTA-RĀGA ("free from passion"), the condition of freedom from attachment (*rāga*); also, the person enjoying that state. The *Mundaka-Upanishad* (3.2.5) sees this as a precondition for *Self-realization, while the *Bhagavad-Gītā* (2.56) mentions it as a necessary qualification of the sage whose *wisdom is firmly settled (*sthita-prajnā*). The *Yoga-Sūtra* (1.37) speaks of such an individual as a fit object for one's *meditation. See also *vairāgya*.

VITARKA ("cogitation"), apart from its general application in the sense of "thought," has two basic meanings in *Classical Yoga. First, it stands for the spontaneous thought processes that occur in the state of conscious ecstasy (*samprajnāta-samādhi*) in relation to a "coarse" (*sthūla*) object of *contemplation. Second, *vitarka* denotes the kind of unwholesome deliberations that can arise in the course of the day, such as the idea to take revenge or to lie. For their extirpation, the *Yoga-Sūtra* (2.33) recommends that one dwell on the opposite idea, such as to bless and to speak the *truth regardless of one's emotional state. This practice is known as *pratipaksha-bhāvanā. See also *nirvitarka-samādhi*, *savitarka-samādhi*, *tarka*; cf. *vicāra*.

VITRISHNA or VAITRISHNYA ("nonthirsting"), a synonym for *vairāgya* ("dispassion").

VIVARANA, short for *Yoga-Bhāshya-Vivarana*; a remarkable subcommentary on the *Yoga-Bhāshya* of *Vyāsa. Its author is *Shankara Bhagavatpāda, whom Indian tradition identifies with the great preceptor (*ācārya*) of *Advaita Vedānta. In im-portance, this work ranks with *Vācaspati Mishra's *Tattva-Vaishāradī* and *Vijnāna Bhikshu's *Yoga-Vārttika* and is in fact more significant than either commentary. The *Vivarana* is noteworthy for its many original interpretations and metaphors, which show that the author must have been an intellectual giant.

VIVEKA ("discernment"), the recognition of the distinction between the real (*sat*) and unreal (*asat*), *truth and fiction, and particularly the transcendental *Self and the "nonself" (*anātman*); an important notion in *Classical Yoga, which insists on the eternal separation between the Spirit (*purusha*) and nature (*prakriti*). The *Yoga-Shikhā-Upanishad* (4.22), which is based on the nondualist metaphysics of *Vedānta, criticizes this view, stating that the *yogin's distinction between Self and "nonself" springs from *ignorance. See also *viveka-khyāti*, *vivekin*.

VIVEKA-KHYĀTI ("vision of discernment"), also called "wisdom born of discernment" (*viveka-ja-jnāna*) and "vision of otherness" (*anyatā-khyāti*); a key concept of *Classical Yoga. According to the *Yoga-Sūtra* (3.52), it is the direct means to *liberation and is said to be omniobjective (*sarva-vishaya*), omnitemporal (*sarvathā-vishaya*), and nonsequential (*akrama*). It is also referred to by *Patanjali as the deliverer (*tāraka*), which should make it clear that this is not mere intellectual understanding. Rather, *viveka-khyāti* occurs at the highest level of conscious ecstasy (*samprajnāta-samādhi*).

VIVEKA-MĀRTANDA ("Sun of Discernment"), a short tract on *Yoga, consisting of only eight couplets, apparently composed for a certain Sultan Ghiyās-ud-din. The text is attributed to Rāmeshvara Bhatta (14th cen. CE).

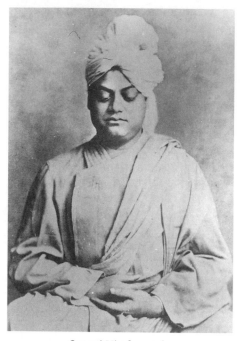

Swami **Vivekananda**

VIVEKANANDA, SWAMI. (1863–1902), the best known of the many disciples of *Ramakrishna. Born Narendranath ("Naren") Datta, he was educated at the Mission College in Calcutta, where he demonstrated a great talent for philosophy. He first met Ramakrishna at age eighteen and joined his *āshrama* two years later. He became the favorite pupil of the unsophisticated but wise Ramakrishna, who assured the young man that he had "seen" *God as clearly as they were seeing each other. Shortly after the death of his *guru* in 1886, Vivekananda renounced the world and, together with other close disciples, founded the Ramakrishna Order, which later developed into the Ramakrishna Mission, an organization that has done much to disseminate *Hindu teachings in the western hemisphere. Vivekananda gained world fame almost overnight by represent-ing *Hinduism at the 1893 World's Parliament of Religions in Chicago. He won the respect of such men as William James and Leo Tolstoy, and his teaching activity particularly attracted Aldous Huxley and Gerald Heard, who were instrumental in paving the way for *Vedānta in the West. Upon his return to India he was celebrated as a national hero. Vivekananda's numerous books, consisting primarily of his talks to small groups, include his widely read treatments of *rāja-yoga*, *karma-yoga*, *jnāna-yoga*, and *bhakti-yoga*. He interpreted *Yoga strictly from the viewpoint of the nondualist philosophy of *Vedānta.

VIVEKIN ("discerner"), according to the *Yoga-Sūtra* (2.15), a person who recognizes that sorrow (*duhkha*) lies hidden in everything, even in apparently pleasurable experiences. Such persons are said to be as sensitive as an eyeball, and yet, by virtue of their *concentration, they go beyond the pairs of opposites (*dvandva*). See also *viveka*.

Vow. See *vrāta*.

VRATA ("vow"), sometimes mentioned among the constituent practices of self-discipline (*niyama*). The *Yoga-Yājnavalkya* (2.11) explains it as one's holding fast to the spiritual means (*upāya*) in order to realize both virtue (*dharma*) and the *Self. The *Shāndilya-Upanishad* (1.2.11) defines it more conventionally as the steady performance of the regulations laid down in the *Vedas.

VRĀTYAS, sacred migrant brotherhoods of ancient India, held together by vows (*vrata*). They were connected with the earliest *history of *Yoga, and may have contributed significantly to the practice of breath control (*prānāyāma*) in connection with the presentation of the songs and melodies (*sāman*) composed by them. The literature of *Hinduism contains many references to these enigmatic groups, but the most reliable information about them is given in the *Vrātya-Khānda* (book 15) of the *Atharva-Veda*. The Vrātyas, it appears, were among those many communities that did not belong to the orthodox kernel of *Vedic society but had their own customs. In the eyes of the brahmic custodians of the Vedic sacrificial religion, they were despicable outcastes, and may even have been the occasional victims of human sacrifices. The Vrātyas worshiped *Rudra, the god of *wind (and *breath), who was later assimilated into *Shiva. The Vrātyas wandered primarily in the northeast of India, but in the course of time many converted to orthodox *Brāhmanism and became sedentary. Some of their members are said to have "quieted the penis" (*shamanica-medhra*), which suggests the pursuit of total celibacy (*brahmacarya*). Each group had a professional bard (known as *māgadha* or *sūta*) and a female called *pumshcalī* ("man mover"), who appears to have been a sacred prostitute. During the midsummer ceremony, bard and prostitute enacted the creative, erotic play between god and goddess, thus foreshadowing the *Tantric practice of ritual intercourse (*maithunā*).

VRIKSHA-ĀSANA (*vrikshāsana*, "tree posture"), a favorite posture (*āsana) among contemporary practitioners of *hatha-yoga; described in the *Gheranda-Samhitā* (2.25) thus: Standing straight like a tree on the ground, place the right foot on the left thigh. This is more than a balancing exercise, for it is thought also to stabilize the *mind.

VRISHA-ĀSANA (*vrishāsana*, "bull posture"), described in the *Gheranda-Sam-

hitā* (2.38) as follows: Placing one's buttocks on the right heel, place the left foot to the side of the right leg. See also *āsana*.

VRISHCIKA-ĀSANA (*vrishcikāsana*, "scorpion posture"), described in the *Hatha-Ratna-Āvalī* (3.74) thus: Place the two hands on the ground and then raise the ankles from the plow position. In contemporary *hatha-yoga manuals the scorpion posture is assumed from the handstand (steadying the *body either with the hands or the forearms). The legs are bent backward until the *feet touch the top of the *head.

VRITTI ("whirl"), a term that can signify a number of things, including "activity," "mode of life," "livelihood," and "rule." In yogic contexts, the term stands specifically for the "fluctuations" of consciousness (*citta). *Patanjali distinguishes five types of *vritti*: valid cognition (*pramāna), misconception (*viparyaya), conceptualization (*vikalpa), sleep (*nidrā), and memory (*smriti). These categories, though obviously not a comprehensive catalog of psychomental states, are all significant in the practice of *meditation and *ecstasy. As the *Yoga Sūtra (1.2) states, "Yoga is the restriction of the fluctuations of consciousness" (*yogash citta-vritti-nirodhah). According to aphorism 2.11, the fluctuations are to be restricted by means of meditation (*dhyāna). Their restriction (*nirodha) leads over into the state of conscious ecstasy (*samprajnāta-samādhi). The reason why the *yogin seeks to check these psychomental activities is that they obscure his true nature as the transcendental Self (*purusha) and thus embroil him in inauthentic existence and suffering (*duhkha), because they generate subliminal activators (*samskāra), which then give rise to renewed psychomental activity.

VYĀDHI ("disease"). The *Yoga-Sūtra (1.30) lists vyādhi among the obstacles (*antarāya) on the spiritual *path. The *Yoga-Bhāshya (1.30) explains the term as disorder of the bodily humors (*dhātu), secretions (*rasa), and organs (*kārana). Since *body and *mind form a unity, it is easy enough to appreciate that illness (*roga) may interfere with one's spiritual practice. It is difficult to concentrate and stay lucid when one has a fever or one's body is racked with *pain. It is therefore important that one should restore the body-mind to good *health, either through conventional means or, if possible, through yogic practices and the adoption of wholesome attitudes.

VYĀGHRAPĀDA ("Tiger-footed"), an *adept of the Nandinātha lineage who is said to have been a *disciple of both *Patanjali and *Tirumūlar.

VYAKTA ("manifest"), a frequently used concept of *Epic Yoga. The *Mahābhārata (3.211.12) has this instructive verse: "Whatsoever is created by the senses (*indriya) is called vyakta. That which is to be known as being beyond the senses and can be grasped [only] by symbols is the unmanifest (*avyakta)." In the *Yoga-Sūtra (4.13) the term refers to the properties (*dharma) of an *object existing in the present, in contrast to the properties pertaining to the past or future, which are technically known as "subtle" (*sūkshma). See also Cosmos, parvan.

VYAKTI ("manifestation"), the entire created *cosmos, which has evolved out of the transcendental ground (*pradhāna) of nature (*prakriti).

VYĀNA, one of the five principal forms of the life force (*prāna) circulating in the *body. As early as the *Maitrāyanīya-Upanishad (2.6), it is said to support the activities of inhalation (*prāna) and exhalation (*apāna). It is widely held to be diffused throughout the body, though some texts mention specific areas, such as the *eyes, *ears, *throat, and the joints, and is also often thought to make speech possible.

VYĀSA ("Arranger"), the name of several legendary sages. The *Vishnu-Purāna (3.3) mentions that there have been twenty-eight Vyāsas, since the *Vedas have been arranged as many times. Generally, however, *Hindu tradition treats Vyāsa as a single individual, who is also called Krishna Dvaipāyana, son of the seer Parāshara and the beautiful fisher girl Satyavatī, who, after miraculously regaining her virginity, married King Shāntanu.

Vyāsa is said to have compiled the four *Vedas, the *Mahābhārata, together with the *Bhagavad-Gītā, the vast *Purāna literature, and a host of other works. He is also credited with the authorship of the oldest extant commentary on *Patanjali's *Yoga-Sūtra, the *Yoga-Bhāshya. The *Mahābhārata (12.26.4) calls him the "foremost of *Yoga experts."

VYOMA-CAKRA ("ether wheel"), a psychoenergetic center (*cakra) located, according to the *Hatha-Yoga-Pradīpikā (4.45), at the "unsupported" (nirālambana) place between the *idā-nādī and the *pingalā-nādī. The *Yoga-Rāja-Upanishad (17) speaks of it as the ninth center, having sixteen spokes and being the abode of the supreme *shakti that bestows great *bliss. See also ākāsha-cakra.

VYOMAN ("ether" or "space"), a synonym for *ākāsha.

VYUTKRAMA ("inversion"), one of the three constituent practices of *kapāla-bhāti. According to the *Gheranda-Samhitā (1.58), it is practiced by slowly drawing *water up through the *nose and ex-pelling it again through the mouth. This is said to cure disorders of phlegm (*kapha).

VYUTTHĀNA ("emergence"). See Waking consciousness.

· W ·

WAKING CONSCIOUSNESS (Sanskrit: vyut-thāna), the predominant mode of *aware-ness, in which the ego identity (or psyche, *jīva) is either reinforced through habitual (karmic) responses to *life or gradually undermined through a spiritual reversal of one's values, attitudes, thoughts, and *ac-tions. For this reason it has special signifi-cance for the *yogin. The waking con-sciousness is by no means the only mode of awareness, however, and the yogin must learn to progressively discipline himself on all levels of possible experience. Thus he must conquer his dreams (*svapna) and even deep sleep (*nidrā, *sushupti). This means that he must cultivate Self-aware-ness (the consciousness of the *witness) in all states of *consciousness. Even the higher stages of awareness, as realized in ecstasy (*samādhi), are to be submitted to this discipline. See also jagrat, jāgarita-sthāna, sahaja-samādhi.

WALKING IN THE ETHER. See ākāsha-ga-mana.

WAR, or conflict, characterizes much of ordinary human *life. No comprehensive spiritual philosophy can afford to ignore this fact. Indeed, spirituality is often couched in terms of an endeavor to estab-lish psychic equilibrium (*samatva). Such a state of inner balance is typically sought to be cultivated through withdrawal from life. The *Hindu tradition of abandon-ment (*tyāga) or renunciation (*samnyā-sa) has generally taken this form. A dif-ferent orientation, however, has been es-poused in the *Bhagavad-Gītā, whose teachings are set against the backdrop of one of the greatest wars fought on Indian soil. It seeks to resolve the tension between doing one's duty (*dharma) by fighting for what is true and good, on the one hand, and striving for spiritual enlightenment (*bodha) or liberation (*moksha), on the other hand. In a crucial passage of the Gītā (2.18ff.) *Krishna offers his disciple Prince *Arjuna the following advice:

Finite, it is said, are these *bodies of the eternal, indestructible, incommensura-ble embodied being (*sharīrin) [i.e., the *Self]. Hence fight, O son of Bharata.

He who thinks of Him as slayer and he who thinks [that He can be] slain—they both do not know. He does not slay nor is He slain.

Never is He born or dies. He did not come into being, nor shall He ever come to be. This primeval [Self] is unborn, eternal, everlasting. It is not slain when the *body is slain.

*Krishna's ethics seems to fly in the face of the fundamental moral rule of nonhar-ming (*ahimsā). Hence his teachings about war have often been interpreted as being merely allegorical. Krishna, however, does not condone war in general. Rather, the war in which he and *Arjuna were involved was to reestablish the moral order (*dharma) that had been lost through the egotism of the Kurus, who had usurped Arjuna's kingdom. For only in a society where the moral order is intact are people free to devote themselves to the pursuit of the highest human aspiration, that of *self-transcendence or liberation (*moksha). Krishna's nonpacifist ethics cannot be properly appreciated apart from his spiritual philosophy.

WATER. See *ap, apas, jala.*

WAY. See *mārga,* Path.

WAY OF THE ANCESTORS. See *pitri-yāna.*

WAY OF THE DEITIES. See *deva-yāna.*

WHEEL. See *cakra.*

WHIRLS, MENTAL. See *vritti.*

WILL. See *icchā.*

WILL TO LIVE. See *abhinivesha.*

WIND. See *pavana, vāta, vāyu.*

WINE. See *madya.*

WISDOM, *knowledge that has sedimented in one's being to the degree that it transforms one's basic attitudes to *life and *death. It is a deep, lived understanding that individual human existence amounts to very little apart from the great *Being, or *Divine, in which it arises for a brief spell only to become dissolved again into that. Wisdom liberates one from the burden of the *ego consciousness and puts

one in touch with the essential identity that transcends the *body and the *mind. See also *jnāna, buddhi, prajnā, vidyā.*

WISH FULFILLMENT. See *prākāmya.*

WITHDRAWAL. See *pratyāhāra.*

WITNESS. Beyond the different states or levels of *consciousness lies the transcendental *Self, which is characterized as the witness (*sākshin*) of all psychomental phenomena. This witness, also called the "Fourth" (*caturtha*), is the single most far-reaching discovery of India's *seers and *sages, and undoubtedly their greatest contribution toward a universal *psychology.

WORK. See *karman.*

WORLD. See Cosmos, *bhuvana, loka, samsāra, vishva.*

WORLD AGES. *Hindu chronology operates with vast *time cycles. The manifest *world is thought to depend for its existence on the life of the creator god *Brahma, who is said to live for 100 brahmic years, corresponding to 311,040,000,000,000 human years. The universe is created concurrently with his birth, and upon his death it vanishes completely. After a period of latency, lasting 100 brahmic years, a new Brahma springs forth from the *Divine and with him a new universe. Thus the cycle of creation (*sarga*) and dissolution (*pralaya*) is repeated ad infinitum. There are also minor creations and dissolutions at the end of each brahmic day and night, corresponding to 8,640,000,000 human years. This period is known as a *kalpa, which is composed of 1,000 *mahā-yugas* ("great eons"). Each *mahā-yuga* is composed of 12,000 divine years, corresponding to 1,555,200,000 human years. The duration of each *mahā-yuga* is made up of four cyclic periods called *yuga*, which are marked by a progressive worsening of the moral order (*dharma*). These are the *krita-* or *satya-yuga* (lasting 4,000 divine years), the *tretā-yuga* (lasting 3,000 divine years), the *dvā-para-yuga* (lasting 2,000 divine years), and the *kāli-yuga* (lasting 1,000 divine years). Between each of these four *yugas* is a period of latency lasting 800, 600, 400, and 200 divine years respectively. Present humanity is thought to live at the beginning of a *kāli-yuga*, which is an age of darkness. With the collapse of the industrial myth of progress in the face of the far-flung ecological crisis precipitated by technology and consumerism, this traditional interpretation of contemporary history is believable enough.

WORLDLING (Sanskrit: *samsārin*), the individual trapped in conditional existence. Cf. *mukta, siddha.*

WORSHIP. See *arcanā, pūjā, pūjana.*

· Y ·

YAJNA ("sacrifice"). The notion of *sacrifice is one of the cornerstones of *Hinduism. Sacrificial *rituals played an all-important role already in the *Vedic age. Through sacrifice, the ancient Indians sought to win communion with and secure the blessings of the deities (*deva). As they saw it, the *world is built on the principle of sacrifice: the primordial *Being, or *purusha, sacrificed itself to bring forth the *cosmos. Similarly, *life perpetuates itself through the destruction of individual life forms.

Once this is understood, the only reasonable and mature response is to relate to existence as a continuous sacrifice. This idea was developed in the *Brāhmanas and the earliest *Upanishads. The *Chāndogya-Upanishad (3.16.1), e.g., declares: "Verily, man (*purusha) is a sacrifice." This recognition led to the notion of the inner or spiritual sacrifice, i.e., the dedication of one's life to a higher, cosmic purpose rather than the mere exoteric ritual offering of libations to the deities. Thus *karma-yoga* is essentially *action performed in the spirit of sacrifice, or self-surrender. In the *Bhagavad-Gītā (3.10) *Krishna draws a parallel with the unselfish *creation of the world by *Prajā-pati. In another passage of the same text (4.25ff.), various forms of sacrificial action are mentioned, from offerings to the deities to the surrender of the senses (*indriya) into the fire of self-restraint (*samyama), or the restriction of one's *diet, or controlled *breathing, etc. In one stanza (4.33) Krishna announces that the sacrifice of *wisdom (*jñāna-yajna*) is superior to material sacrifices (*dravya-yajna*), which captures the spirit of *Yoga in general. However, many yogic schools and *paths include material sacrifices in their daily practice (*sādhana). This is especially true of *bhakti-yoga.

YĀJNAVALKYA, the name of several teachers who lived in different periods. The best known Yājnavalkya is the revered *adept of the *Brihad-Āranyaka-Upanishad, who lived with his two wives in a forest hermitage (*āshrama). He taught the doctrines of

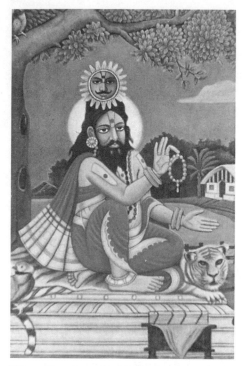

Yājnavalkya (popular Hindu representation)

YAJUR-VEDA ("Knowledge of Sacrifice"), the *Vedic collection (*samhitā*) that contains all the hymns relevant to the sacrificial rituals of the *brāhmanas. See also *Vedas*.

YAMA ("restraint"), the first "limb" (*anga*) of the eightfold yogic *path taught by *Patanjali. It stands for the moral observances, which form the very foundation of spiritual discipline. According to the *Yoga-Sūtra* (2.30), there are five *yamas*: nonharming (*ahimsā*), truthfulness (*satya*), nonstealing (*asteya*), chastity (*brahmacarya*), and greedlessness (*aparigraha*). These constitute the "great vow" (*mahā-vrata*) of the *yogin and are to be practiced on all levels irrespective of time, place, or circumstance.

The *Tejo-Bindu-Upanishad* (1.17), which has *yama* as the first "limb" of its fifteenfold *Yoga (*panca-dasha-anga-yoga*), defines it as the control of the *senses in the knowledge that "all is the Absolute (*brahman*)." The *Tri-Shikhi-Brāhmana-Upanishad* (2.28) explains it as dispassion (*vairāgya*) toward the *body and its *senses. The *Linga-Purāna* (1.8.10) interprets it as abstention (*uparāma*) in the form of asceticism (*tapas*). The *Kūrma-Purāna* (2.11.13) observes that the five disciplines of *yama* are conducive to the *purification of the mind (*citta-shuddhi*).

Many works of *Postclassical Yoga list ten practices under *yama*. Thus the *Tri-Shikhi-Brāhmana-Upanishad* (2.32) mentions the following: nonharming, truthfulness, nonstealing, chastity, sympathy (*dayā*), rectitude (*ārjava*), patience (*kshamā*), steadfastness (*dhriti*), moderate diet (*mita-āhāra*), and cleanliness (*shauca*). This series is repeated in several other *Yoga-Upanishads. The *Mandala-Brāhmana-Upanishad* (1.4), however, lists

rebirth (*punar-janman*) and *karma. Many centuries later, another Yājnavalkya authored the *Yājnavalkya-Smriti*, a work on law and ethics (*dharma*), written probably in the third century BCE. This text (1.8) notes that the highest teaching (*dharma*) is that which leads to the vision of the *Self (*ātma-darshana*) by means of *Yoga. This Yājnavalkya has also been credited with the authorship of the *Yoga-Yājnavalkya-Samhitā*.

Yājnavalkya is moreover the name of a Yoga *adept who is frequently mentioned or quoted in the later *Upanishads, and who may have been the author of the *Yoga-Yājnavalkya-Samhitā*, among other works. There is also a *Yājnavalkya-Upanishad*, which belongs to the genre of *Samnyāsa-Upanishads and may have been composed around 1400 CE.

the following nine practices: devotion to the teacher (*guru-bhakti*), adherence to the *path of truth (*satya-mārga-anurakti*), enjoyment of the Real (*vastu*) as it is glimpsed in pleasurable experiences, contentment (*tushti*), nonattachment (*nihsangatā*), living in solitude (*ekānta-vāsa*), cessation of mental activity (*mano-nivritti*), nonattachment (*anabhilāsha*) to the fruit (*phala*) of one's *actions, and dispassion (*vairāgya*).

The *Siddha-Siddhānta-Paddhati* (2.32) speaks of calmness (*upashama*), mastery of the senses (*indriya-jaya*), mastery of diet (*āhāra-jaya*), mastery of sleep (*nidrā-jaya*), and mastery of cold (*shīta-jaya*) as the constituent practices of *yama*, and makes the point that these have to be learned gradually. The *Yoga-Tattva-Upanishad* (28) treats scant diet (*laghu-āhāra*) as the single most important discipline.

YĀMA ("Restrainer"), the *Hindu deity of *death. In the *Katha-Upanishad* (1.1ff.) Yāma is introduced as the initiator of the young spiritual aspirant Naciketas. The story is a parable, which makes the point that we must first face our own mortality before we can hope to transcend the *fear of death and to win *immortality.

YĀMALA ("pair"), the union of *Shiva and *Shakti as *prakāsha and *vimarsha respectively. This term can also denote the physical union (*maithunā*, *samghatta*) between *yogin and *yoginī in certain schools of *Tantrism.

YĀMALA, a type of *Tantra*, such as the famous *Rudra-Yāmala-Tantra*, belonging to the *Tantric school of the same name. *Abhinava Gupta mentions eight such *Tantras*.

YAMIN ("restrainer"), a synonym for *yogin, the self-controlled spiritual practitioner.

YAMUNĀCĀRYA (918–1038 CE), one of the great *Vaishnava preceptors of the *Vishishta Advaita school of *Vedānta. The grandson of *Nāthamuni, he is said to have learned the eightfold *Yoga (*ashta-anga-yoga*) from the *adept Kurukanātha. He had numerous disciples, including *Rāmānuja. Yamunācārya wrote six works, the most important of which is his *Siddhi-Traya*.

YANTRA ("device"), a geometric representation of the levels and energies of the *cosmos and the human *body (as a microcosmic replica of the *macrocosm). *Yantras* are widely used in *Tantric worship, where they are treated as the "body" of one's chosen deity (*ishta-devatā*). They are drawn on paper, wood, and cloth, or inscribed on metal and other materials, or even constructed in three dimensions out of clay. They typically consist of a square surround, circles, lotus petals, triangles, and a central point known as the *bindu, representing the creative matrix of the universe and gateway to the transcendental *Reality.

In the higher stages of the *Tantric ritual, the *yantra* must be completely internalized, i.e., perfectly visualized. *Yantra-yoga* consists in the gradual dissolution (*laya*) of this inwardly constructed *yantra* together with the dissolution of the individuated *consciousness. If successful, this exercise will catapult the practitioner (*sādhaka*) into pure *Consciousness, beyond the subject-object distinction. *Tantrism employs a large number of *yantras*, and the *Mantra-Mahodadhi* (20) describes twenty-nine such geometric devices. The most famous *yantra* is the *shrī-yantra. See also *mandala*.

YASHASVINĪ-NĀDĪ ("splendid channel"), one of the principal channels (*nāḍī) through which the life force (*prāna) moves in the *body. Different scriptures mention different locations for this *nāḍī. Some place it between the *pingalā-nāḍī and the *pūshā-nāḍī, others between the *pūshā- and the *sarasvatī-nāḍī, and yet others between the *gāndhārā- and the *sarasvatī-nāḍī. It is widely thought to run from the "bulb" (*kanda) to the left *ear, though the *Shāndilya-Upanishad (1.4.11) specifies the big toes as its termination point.

YATI, any ascetic, including a practitioner of *Yoga.

YATNA ("effort"), exertion; according to the *Yoga-Sūtra (1.13), the very essence of spiritual practice (*abhyāsa): one cannot grow spiritually without applying oneself to the yogic disciplines. When spiritual striving becomes competitive, however, it is counterproductive. See also Effort, paurusha, prayatna; cf. Grace.

YĀTRĀ (from the root ya, "to walk"), pilgrimage. See also tīrtha-atana.

YAUGA ("yogic"), sometimes used as a synonym for *yogin, particularly in the *Nyāya and *Vaisheshika traditions.

YOGA (from the root yuj, "to yoke, harness"). The word yoga has a wide range of applications in the Sanskrit language, from "union" to "team," to "sum," to "equipment," to "conjunction," etc. Early on, it came to be applied also to "spiritual endeavor," specifically the control of the mind (*manas) and senses (*indriya). This usage is first found in the *Taittirīya-Upanishad (2.4.1), which dates back to the second millennium BCE.

By the time of the composition of the *Bhagavad-Gītā (3d or 4th cen. BCE), the word yoga was widely used to denote the *Hindu tradition of spiritual discipline, comprising different approaches to *Self-realization, or *enlightenment. In that formative period, Yoga was still closely allied with *Sāmkhya. This fact is reflected in the *Mahābhārata, which frequently employs the compound *sāmkhya-yoga. In subsequent times Yoga and Sāmkhya developed into separate philosophical schools, known as *Classical Yoga (*yoga-darshana) and Classical Sāmkhya respectively. The position of the former school was codified in the second century CE by *Patanjali in his *Yoga-Sūtra, while the latter's metaphysics was outlined one or two centuries later in the *Sāmkhya-Kārikā of *Īshvara Krishna.

If the schools of *Preclassical Yoga, as recorded in the *Bhagavad-Gītā, the *Moksha-Dharma, and other didactic portions of the *Mahābhārata, espoused a panentheistic philosophy, then *Patanjali introduced, as far as one can tell, a dualistic metaphysics. He appears to have rejected the idea that the *world is an aspect of the *Divine and made a radical distinction between nature (*prakriti) and the transcendental Self (*purusha). Hence *Bhoja, in his commentary *Rāja-Mārtanda (1.1), felt justified in characterizing yoga as vi-yoga ("separation").

Even though *Patanjali's system came to be regarded as one of the six classical schools of *Hinduism, however, its dualism prevented it from assuming greater cultural significance. The dominant philosophical orientation within the fold of Hinduism has always been nondualist (*advaita). Thus the schools of *Postclassical Yoga, as recorded in the *Yoga-Upanishads and the works of *Tantrism and *hatha-yoga, reaffirmed the panentheism of earlier times. This is also the essential position of the Integral Yoga (*pūrna-yoga) of Sri *Aurobindo. See also *abhāva-yoga, abhyāsa-yoga, adhyātma-yoga, agni-yoga, anna-yoga, ashta-anga-yoga, asparsha-yoga, bhakti-yoga, bhāva-yoga, dhyāna-yoga, hamsa-yoga, hatha-yoga, jnāna-yoga, karma-yoga, kriyā-yoga, kundalinī-yoga, lambikā-yoga, laya-yoga, mahā-yoga, mantra-yoga, nāda-yoga, pāshupata-yoga, rāja-yoga, sāmkhya-yoga, samnyāsa-yoga, sampūta-yoga, samrambha-yoga, sapta-anga-yoga, shad-anga-yoga, shiva-yoga, sparsha-yoga, svacchanda-yoga, tāraka-yoga, vahni-yoga*; Archaic Yoga, Epic Yoga.

YOGA, the name of a mythical sage mentioned in the *Mahābhārata* (13.150.45).

YOGA-AGNI (*yogāgni*, "fire of Yoga"), said in the *Yoga-Shikhā-Upanishad* (1.26) to "cook" the *body and bring it to sentience (*ajada*). This idea is fundamental to *hatha-yoga, which seeks to transmute the body into a "divine" vehicle with great paranormal capacities (*siddhi*).

YOGA-ANGA (*yogānga*, "limb of Yoga"). See *anga*.

YOGA-ANUSHĀSANA-SŪTRA-VRITTI (*Yogānushāsanasūtravritti*, "Commentary on the Aphorisms Expounding Yoga"), also called *Pradīpikā*; a subcommentary by *Bhāva Ganesha Dīkshita, a pupil of *Vijnāna Bhikshu. It seeks to elucidate his teacher's commentary on the *Yoga-Sūtra*.

YOGA-ARŪDHA (*yogārūdha*, "ascended in Yoga"). See *ārūdha*.

YOGA-ĀSANA (*yogāsana*, "Yoga posture"), described in the *Gheranda-Samhitā* (2.44f.) thus: Placing one's stretched (and crossed) *feet on the knees with upturned palms on the ground, inhale and fix one's gaze (*drishti*) at the tip of the nose (*nāsa-agra*).

YOGA-BALA ("power of Yoga"), a phrase often used in the literature of *Preclassical Yoga. Thus the *Bhagavad-Gītā* (8.10) observes that, at the time of *death, the *yogin should employ the power of *Yoga and devotion (*bhakti*) in order to steady the *mind, so that he may reach the *Divine. See also *bala*.

YOGA-BHĀSHYA ("Discussion on Yoga"), the oldest extant commentary on the *Yoga-Sūtra*, attributed to *Vyāsa. Probably composed in the fifth century CE, this work is the basis for all subsequent exegetical efforts in *Classical Yoga. While Vyāsa shows great familiarity with *Yoga, he does not appear to have belonged to the direct lineage of *Patanjali, the author of the *Yoga-Sūtra*. He seems, rather, to rely strongly on the ideas of the Sāmkhya teacher Vindhyavāsin (prob. 4th cen. CE). The argument of some *Hindu authorities, that the *Bhāshya* was composed by Patanjali himself, seems improbable, since the interpretations and terminology of the *Bhāshya* are occasionally at variance with the *Yoga-Sūtra*.

YOGA-BHĀSHYA-VIVARANA. See *Vivarana*.

YOGA-BHĀSKARA ("Illuminator of Yoga"), a no longer extant work on *Yoga by Kavīndrācārya Sarasvatī (1600–1675 CE), who also authored a number of works on *Vedānta.

YOGA-BĪJA ("Seed of Yoga"), a short modern treatise of around ten printed pages on the rules of yogic practice, especially *breath control. It is ascribed to *Shiva himself.

YOGĀCĀRA ("Conduct of Yoga," from *yoga* and *ācāra*), the idealist school of Mahāyāna *Buddhism founded by *Asanga in the fourth century CE. This school is criticized by *Vācaspati Mishra in his *Tattva-Vaishāradī* (2.15) for its concept of *liberation. It is sometimes thought that *Patanjali's *Yoga-Sūtra* (4.14–16) refers to Yogācāra as well, but the reference must be to an earlier Vijnānavāda tradition, such as the one represented by the *Lankāvatāra-Sūtra*.

YOGA-CINTĀMANI ("Thought Gem of Yoga"), a work by Shivānanda Sarasvatī comprising around 200 folios. It was probably authored in the late eighteenth or early nineteenth century CE.

YOGA-CŪDĀMANĪ-UPANISHAD (*Yogacūdamanyupanishad*, "Secret Teaching on the Crest Jewel of Yoga," from *cūdāmanī*, "crest jewel"), one of the *Yoga-Upanishads*, probably composed in the fourteenth or fifteenth century CE. Consisting of 121 stanzas, it expounds *hatha-yoga from a *Vedantic point of view. The anonymous author subscribes to the sixfold *path (*shad-anga-yoga*), paying particular attention to what he calls *prāna-samrodha* ("restraint of the breath"). The first 71 stanzas summarize the essentials of *hatha-yoga* theory and practice. This is followed by an excursus on ontogenesis, which is probably an interpolation. The text concludes with a description of sense withdrawal (*pratyāhāra*) and appears to be incomplete. Indeed, it is presumably a fragment of the *Goraksha-Paddhati*.

YOGA-DARSHANA ("Yoga view"), a phrase first found in the *Mahābhārata* (12.294.26), where it has a general meaning. Later it came to refer specifically to the philosophical system formulated by *Patanjali and elaborated by his commentators, also known as *Classical Yoga.

YOGA-GRIHA ("Yoga house"). See *matha*.

YOGA-KAKSHA ("yogic girdle"), a strap to secure the position of the knees while being seated in one of the postures (*āsana*); mentioned in the *Bhāgavata-Purāna* (4.6.39).

YOGA-KĀRIKĀ, an original Sanskrit commentary on the *Yoga-Sūtra* largely based on the explanations of *Vyāsa and *Vācaspati Mishra. This work, which comprises 346 verses, was composed together with an autocommentary entitled *Saralā-Tīkā* by *Hariharānanda Āranya.

YOGA-KĀRNIKĀ ("Ear Ornament of Yoga") of Aghorānanda, authored in the late eighteenth or early nineteenth century CE; a compilation of thirteen chapters comprising over 1,200 verses, whose value lies in the many quotations from other (including lost) works.

YOGA-KRITYA ("Yoga praxis"), a synonym for *sādhana that occurs in the *Mahābhārata* (e.g., 12.294.6).

YOGA-KUNDALĪ-UPANISHAD (*Yogakundalyupanishad*, from *kundalī*, a synonym for *kundalinī*), one of the *Yoga-Upanishads*, probably dating from the fourteenth or fifteenth century CE. It consists of three chapters with a total of 171 stanzas. As the title suggests, this work deals with *kundalinī-yoga*, which is expounded from the perspective of the nondualist metaphysics of *Advaita Vedānta. The first chapter outlines the spiritual *path; the second consists of a detailed exposition of the *khecarī-mudrā*; and the third describes the higher yogic processes and is interspersed with metaphysical speculations.

YOGA-MĀRGA ("Yoga path"). The metaphor of spiritual life as a *path or road (*mārga*) goes hand in hand with the image of the spiritual aspirant as an itinerant who progresses from one level of accomplishment to the next. The *Mahābhārata* (12.289.53) observes that it is a great *sin to abandon the yogic way simply out of comfort (*kshema*). More radical schools of nondualism reject the path metaphor since it merely reinforces the illusion that there is a separate entity, whereas, as they see it, only the one *Reality exists. Apart from such metaphysical objections, however, the path metaphor corresponds to psychological actualities and is useful to the degree that it does not serve goal-oriented striving.

YOGA-MĀRTANDA ("Sun of Yoga"), a work of 188 stanzas ascribed to *Goraksha; apparently a fragment of the *Goraksha-Paddhati*.

YOGA-MATA ("doctrine of Yoga"), *Yoga as a tradition or viewpoint; as such, a synonym for *yoga-mārga*.

YOGA-MUDRĀ ("seal of Yoga"), listed but not described in the *Hatha-Ratna-Āvalī*

(3.12) as one of the eighty-four postures (*āsana*). According to some contemporary works on *hatha-yoga, this posture is executed by bending forward while seated cross-legged, with the arms behind one's back and the hands folded. *Upanishad Brahmayogin, in his commentary on the *Tri-Shikhi-Brāhmana-Upanishad* (2.93), understands the *yoga-mudrā* as a hand gesture, equating it with the "seal of awareness" (*cin-mudrā*).

YOGANANDA, PARAMAHAMSA (1893–1952), one of the early *Yoga masters to come to the West. A pupil of Sri Yukteshwar (Sanskrit: Shrī Yukteshvara), he founded the Self-Realization Fellowship in 1920 and achieved world fame through his book *Autobiography of a Yogi* (first published in 1946). He taught Kriya-Yoga (Sanskrit: *kriyā-yoga*), a type of *kundalinī-yoga, and was eager to reconcile *Hinduism with Christianity. See also *parama-hamsa*. (See photo on p. 346.)

YOGA-NIDRĀ ("Yoga sleep"), an expression widely used in the literature of *Postclassical Yoga to denote the highest state of *consciousness. In Hindu *mythology *yoga-nidrā* is the state of *Vishnu at the end of a world age (*yuga*), when the universe is temporarily dissolved until the great god reawakens.

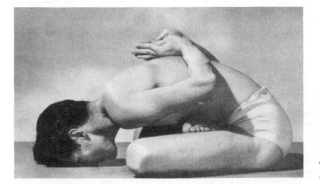

Yoga-mudrā, demonstrated by Theos Bernard

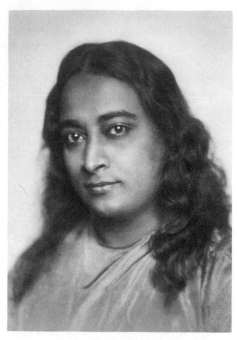

Paramahamsa **Yogananda**

Some contemporary *Yoga authorities employ the phrase *yoga-nidrā* to designate a state of deep *relaxation. The term is also applied to a yogic posture (*āsana) that is executed by interlacing the legs behind one's neck while resting on one's back with the hands clasped behind one's waist.

YOGA-PATTA, or **YOGA-PATTAKA**, a shawl; also, a contraption for resting the arms during *meditation. It is mentioned in the latter sense in the *Tattva-Vaish-āradī (2.46) and is also listed in the *Agni-Purāna (90.10) as one of the paraphernalia of the newly initiated *disciple and in another passage (204.11) as one of the utensils of a forest-dwelling ascetic (*vānapra-stha*). In some contexts *yoga-patta* denotes a kind of *ritual.

YOGA-PRADĪPIKĀ ("Light on Yoga") of Baladeva Mishra, a commentary on the

*Yoga-Sūtra composed in the twentieth century CE. It must be distinguished from the *Hatha-Yoga-Pradīpikā.

YOGA-RAHASYA ("Yoga Secret"), one of the lost Sanskrit works of the great South Indian adept *Nāthamuni.

YOGA-RĀJA-UPANISHAD (*Yogarājopani-shad*, one of the *Yoga-Upanishads. Consisting of only 21 stanzas, it speaks of *mantra-, *laya-, *rāja-, and *hatha-yoga, and deals particularly with the nine psychoenergetic centers (*cakra).

YOGA-SĀRA-SAMGRAHA ("Compendium on the Essence of Yoga"), also entitled *Jnāna-Pradīpā* ("Torch of Knowledge"); a concise summary of *Classical Yoga by the renowned scholar *Vijnāna Bhikshu.

YOGA-SHĀSTRA ("Yoga teaching" or "Yoga textbook"). See *shāstra*.

YOGA-SHĀSTRA ("Textbook of Yoga"), a medieval work of 334 stanzas attributed to *Dattātreya, expounding the principles of *hatha-yoga. This text has a *Tantric orientation, as is clear from its description of *vajrolī-mudrā, which involves sexual intercourse (*maithunā) in which both the male and female practitioner seek to absorb each other's "semen" (*bindu). Although the text knows of the tradition of 840,000 postures (*āsana), it describes only the lotus posture (*padma-āsana) and then proceeds to explain the more esoteric practices of the "seals" (*mudrā) and "locks" (*bandha).

YOGA-SHIKHĀ-UPANISHAD (*Yogashiko-panishad*, "Secret Doctrine of the Crest of Yoga"), one of the *Yoga-Upanishads, comprising six chapters with a total of 390 stanzas. The last chapter was probably appended later. This *Upanishad is presented in the form of a didactic dialogue between *Shankara (here *Shiva) and *Hiranyagarbha. On the basis of the nondualist metaphysics of *Vedānta, the anonymous author develops the outlines of a philosophy of the *body. The *yogin is asked to "energize" (ranjayet) his body (*deha) through the *fire of Yoga. The treatment that follows is a summary of *hatha-yoga lore, which ranges from brief instructions about rousing the *sarasvatī-nādī and the *kundalinī-shakti ("serpent power") to an original exposition of esoteric *anatomy. The fifth chapter repeats some of the information given in the first and also contains details about the psychoenergetic channels (*nādī). The concluding chapter deals specifically with the process of rousing the serpent power that lies dormant in the *body. Thus the approach favored in this work is that of *kundalinī-yoga.

YOGA-SIDDHI ("yogic perfection" or "yogic power"). See siddhi.

YOGA-SIDDHĀNTA-CANDRIKĀ ("Moonlight on the Yoga System"), also entitled Yoga-Sūtra-Gūdha-Artha-Dyotikā ("Illumination of the Secret Meaning of the Yoga Aphorisms"); a work by Nārāyana Tīrtha, who also authored the *Sūtra-Artha-Bodhinī.

YOGA-SUDHĀ-ĀKĀRA (Yogasudhākāra, "Mine of Nectar on Yoga"), a work by Sadāshivendra Sarasvatī (18th cen. CE).

YOGA-SŪTRA ("Aphorisms on Yoga"), the authoritative exposition of *Classical Yoga, ascribed to *Patanjali. This brief text was probably composed in the early common era, though some scholars place it into the second century BCE. Also known as Pātanjala-Sūtra, this work comprises four chapters (pāda) with a total of 195 aphorisms (some editions have one additional *sūtra). Attempts to dissect this composition into independent textual units have failed to convince, and *Patanjali's work appears to be relatively homogeneous. There is some evidence, however, that the author incorporated a series of existing definitions dealing with the eight "limbs" (*anga) of *Yoga (2.28–3.3 or 3.8). If this conclusion is correct, *Patanjali's Yoga should be more appropriately called *kriyā-yoga rather than *ashta-anga-yoga.

The first chapter, samādhi-pāda ("chapter on *ecstasy"), outlines the principal processes involved in the systematic transformation of *consciousness. The second chapter, sādhana-pāda ("chapter on the means"), introduces the basic concepts of kriyā-yoga practice. Then, at aphorism 2.28 the discussion switches over to the eightfold path. The third chapter bears the title vibhūti-pāda, as it deals with the paranormal manifestations of *Yoga (*vibhūtis or *siddhis). However, this section also contains important information about the higher stages of yogic practice. The final chapter, kaivalya-pāda ("chapter on aloneness"), introduces important philosophical notions and also treats of the terminal stages of Yoga, including *liberation itself, which is called *kaivalya.

Although *Patanjali understands his compilation merely as an "exposition" (anushāsana) of existing teachings, his work nevertheless does not lack originality. In his endeavor to formalize the yogic tradition, he has introduced new concepts and terms that clearly evince the autonomy of *Classical Yoga as one of the leading schools or philosophical systems (*darshana) of *Hinduism. In terminology the Yoga-Sūtra is close to Mahāyāna *Buddhism, and the connection between *Classical Yoga and Buddhism has often been noted by scholars, though no detailed study has hitherto been undertaken. Particularly the parallels between the *Yoga-Sūtra* and the *Abhisamayālankāra-Shāstra* (ascribed to *Maitreya) deserve closer scrutiny.

Given the importance of the *Yoga-Sūtra*, it is not surprising that it has given rise to a large number of exegetical works. The oldest available commentary is the *Yoga-Bhāshya*, which furnishes the key to our understanding of *Patanjali's work. Other important commentaries are *Shankara's *Vivarana*, *Vācaspati Mishra's *Tattva-Vaishāradī*, and *Vijnāna Bhikshu's monumental *Yoga-Vārttika*.

YOGA-SŪTRA-ARTHA-CANDRIKĀ (*Yoga-sūtrārthacandrikā*, "Moonlight on the Meaning of the Aphorisms of Yoga"), also entitled *Pāda-Candrikā* ("Moonlight on the Chapters [of *Patanjali's Work]"); a commentary on the *Yoga-Sūtra* by Ananta(-deva) (19th cen. CE).

YOGA-SŪTRA-BHĀSHYA-VIVARANA. See *Vivarana*.

YOGA-SŪTRA-GŪDHA-ARTHA-DYOTIKĀ. See *Yoga-Siddhānta-Candrikā*.

YOGA-SŪTRA-VRITTI ("Treatment on the Aphorisms of Yoga") a commentary on the *Yoga-Sūtra* by *Nārāyana Tīrtha.

YOGA-TARANGA ("Wave of Yoga"), a treatise similar to the *Yoga-Sāra-Samgraha* by Deva Tīrtha Svāmin, a disciple of *Vidyāranya Tīrtha.

YOGA-TĀRA-ĀVALĪ ("Sparkling Lines on Yoga"), a text attributed to *Shankara that, among other things, explains the practice of cultivating the inner sound (*nāda-anusandhāna*).

YOGA-TATTVA-UPANISHAD (*Yogatattvopanishad*, "Secret Teaching on the Principles of Yoga"), one of the *Yoga-Upanishads*. The anonymous author of this short tract of 142 stanzas seeks to integrate different forms of *Yoga on the philosophical foundations of *Advaita Vedānta. He emphasizes the interdependence of Yoga and gnosis (*jñāna*) and outlines the yogic *path, mentioning the four stages (*avasthā*), the five obstacles (*vighna*), the right environment (*desha*) for the practice of *breath control, rules about *diet, the paranormal powers (*siddhi*), the practice of concentration (*dhāranā*), techniques of *hatha-yoga, and the condition of living liberation (*jīvan-mukti*). This work decries intellectualism as well as ascetic torturing of the body (*kāya-klesha*).

YOGA-UPANISHADS (*Yogopanishads*), a group of twenty-one *Upanishads composed after the *Yoga-Sūtra and expounding *Vedānta-based yogic teachings, particularly *hatha-yoga and *kundalinī-yoga. Many of these texts belong to the fourteenth and fifteenth centuries CE. The following are generally listed among this group: *Advaya-Tāraka-, *Amrita-Nāda-, *Amrita(-Nāda)-Bindu-, *Brahma-Vidyā-, *Darshana-, *Dhyāna-Bindu-, *Hamsa-, *Kshurikā-, *Mahā-Vākya-, *Mandala-Brāhmana-, *Nāda-Bindu-, *Pāshu-Pata-Brāhmana-, *Shāndilya-, *Tejo-Bindu-, *Tri-Shikhi-Brāhmana-, *Varāha-, *Yoga-Cūdāmani-, *Yoga-Kundalī-, *Yoga-Rāja-, *Yoga-Shikhā-, and *Yoga-Tattva-Upanishad.

YOGA-VĀRTTIKA, also entitled *Pātanjala-Bhāshya-Vārttika*; an extensive commentary on the *Yoga-Sūtra* by *Vijnāna Bhikshu. It contains much original material and numerous quotations from *Hindu philosophical and religious literature. Next to the *Yoga-Bhāshya of *Vyāsa and the *Vivarana of *Shankara, this is the single most important commentary on *Patanjali's aphorisms.

YOGA-VĀSISHTHA-RĀMĀYANA, also designated *Yoga-Vāsishtha, Ārsha-Rāmāyana,* or *Jnāna-Vāsishtha;* a didactic poetic work of around 30,000 verses written in elegant Sanskrit and traditionally (though wrongly) attributed to Vālmīki, the composer of the *Rāmāyana. The Yoga-Vāsishtha is presented as a dialogue between Prince *Rāma and his teacher, *Vasishta. There has been much scholarly speculation about the date of this work, and estimates range from the ninth to the thirteenth century CE. It was probably composed after the *Laghu-Yoga-Vāsishta, which can be assigned to the early tenth century CE. There are a number of abridgments of this massive work, notably the *Yoga-Vāsishtha-Sāra-Samgraha.

The *Yoga-Vāsishtha* has inspired countless generations of spiritual aspirants. Its philosophical basis is *Advaita Vedānta: There is only the single *Consciousness (*eka-citta*), which is formless, omnipresent, and omniscient. The multifarious objects of the *world are present in it like innumerable images carved in stone or, as one passage (3.2.55) has it, like pictures in the artist's mind. The world, which is perceived as a result of our congenital nescience (*avidyā*), appears to the finite *mind as something external to itself. It is described as a dream or a bubble arising in the *Absolute. However, this metaphysical *truth is to be realized through unmediated experience rather than merely to be believed.

The spiritual *path outlined in the *Yoga-Vāsishtha* is that of *jnāna-yoga and has great similarity with the *buddhi-yoga of the *Bhagavad-Gītā, which is founded in a harmonious blending of wisdom (*jnāna*) and action (*karma*). Since, according to this work, the *mind creates its own *bondage and *liberation, there is no need to renounce the *world physically once the *truth of the single *Consciousness has been experienced. This is called the path of "mental liberation" (*cetya-muktatā*).

*Yoga is variously defined as "restraint of the fluctuations of *consciousness," "freedom from sensation," and "separation from the effects of the poison of passion." *Vāsishtha, who acts as a spokesman for this Yoga, teaches a discipline comprising seven stages (*bhūmi*), terminating in the *yogin's "abiding in the *Fourth" (*turya-ga*).

YOGA-VĀSISHTHA-SĀRA ("Essence of the *Yoga-Vāsishtha*"), an epitome of the *Yoga-Vāsishtha in forty-eight cantos, ascribed to *Gauda Abhinanda.

YOGA-VĀSISHTHA-SĀRA-SAMGRAHA (lit. "Compendium of the Essence of the *Yoga-Vāsishtha*"), a digest of the teachings of the *Yoga-Vāsishtha-Rāmāyana, compiled by *Vidyāranya.

YOGA-VID ("Yoga knower"), according to the *Yoga-Cudamani-Upanishad (64), one who knows about the harmonious identity (*samarasa-aikyatva*) of the two forms of human semen (*bindu*). This is a common esoteric explanation in the *hatha-yoga tradition. Elsewhere the term is often simply used as a synonym for *yogin.

YOGA-VISHAYA ("Object of Yoga"), a short work of thirty-three stanzas ascribed to *Matsyendra, though belonging to a later date. It covers such basic topics as the nine psychoenergetic centers (*cakra*), the three "knots" (*granthi*), and the nine "gates" (*dvāra*).

YOGA-YĀJNAVALKYA (full title: *Yoga-Yājnavalkya-Gītā,* or -Gītā-Upanishad), a work on *hatha-yoga consisting of 506 stanzas. It is written in the form of a dialogue between *Yājnavalkya and his wife, Gargi. P. C. Divanji (1954), the editor of this Sanskrit text, has placed it in the second century CE. This assignment is based on the identification of the author of the Yoga-Yājnavalkya with his namesake who composed the Yājnavalkya-Smriti and who in one stanza (3.110) recommends the study of "the Yoga teachings (*yoga-shāstra) promulgated by me." An analysis of the contents and terminology of the Yoga-Yājnavalkya suggests a much later date, however, perhaps the thirteenth or fourteenth century CE. There are many parallels between this work and the *Yoga-Upanishads, notably the *Shāndilya-Upanishad. Cf. Brihad-Yogi-Yājnavalkya.

YOGA-YUJ ("Yoga joined") the spiritual novice. In the *Vishnu-Purāna (6.7) the novice is enjoined to first contemplate the "coarse" (*sthūla) form of existence before proceeding to the more "subtle" (*sūkshma) aspects.

YOGA-YUKTA ("Yoga yoked"), a synonym for *yogin used particularly widely in the literature of *Preclassical Yoga. It denotes the practitioner who has brought his *senses and *mind under control by means of the techniques of *Yoga.

YOGI-DEHA ("yogin's body"), the transubstantiated *body of the *adept of *hatha-yoga. According to the *Yoga-Shikhā-Upanishad (1.41), this body is invisible even to the *deities. It is free from change and *bondage and is endowed with a variety of paranormal powers (*siddhi). It is described as resembling the ether (*ākāsha). See also divya-deha, Transubstantiation.

YOGIN, a male practitioner of *Yoga. The *Shiva-Samhitā (2.5) defines the yogin as someone who knows that the entire *cosmos is situated within his own *body. Similarly, the *Siddha-Siddhānta-Paddhati (2.31) states that he is called a yogin who fully knows the nine psychoenergetic centers (*cakra), the three signs (*lakshya), the fivefold ether (*ākāsha), and the "ambrosial shower" (dhārā) issuing from the *kāla in the *head.

There are different categories of yogins, depending on the type and rigor of their yogic disciplines, as well as their spiritual attainment. The *Yoga-Shikhā-Upanishad (1.75f.) distinguishes two kinds of yogins: those who pierce through the "sun" (*sūrya) by means of the various yogic techniques and those who break down the door of the central conduit (*sushumnā-nādī) and drink the *nectar from the cranial bowl. *Upanishad Brahmayogin explains the former type as samnyāsa-yogins (renouncers) and the latter as kevala-yogins (radical practitioners). The *Shiva-Purāna (7.2.38.25ff.) groups yogins according to their different paranormal abilities (*siddhi). The *Yoga-Bhāshya (3.51), again, offers the following fourfold classification: the *prathama-kalpika (neophyte); the *mādhu-bhūmika (who has reached the "honeyed level"); the *prajnā-jyotis (the advanced practitioner enjoying the *light of gnosis); and the *atikrānta-bhāvanīya (transcender). Cf. yoginī.

YOGINĪ, a female practitioner of *Yoga. According to the *Hatha-Yoga-Pradīpikā (3.99), a yoginī is more specifically a woman initiate who can preserve her own genital ejaculate (*rajas) and suck up the male semen (*bindu) by means of the practice of the *vajrolī-mudrā. In *Tantric contexts the term yoginī can also refer to the group of eight, sixteen, sixty-four or more female divinities, which are forms of the goddess *Durgā. The cultic worship of these *yoginīs* emerged in the ninth century CE and is related to the tradition of *Shaktism. Cf. *yogin*.

YOGI-PRATYAKSHA ("yogic perception"), another term for "direct apprehension" (*sākshāt-kārana*), which involves the *yogin*'s conscious identification with an *object. This is the basis of the practice of ecstatic "coincidence" (*samāpatti*) through which various paranormal powers (*siddhi*) can be acquired.

YOGI-RĀJ ("ruler of *yogins*"), also sometimes called *yoga-rāj* ("ruler of Yoga"); an honorific title granted to a spiritual master.

YOGYATĀ ("fitness"), a technical term of *Classical Yoga, introduced by *Vācaspati Mishra in his *Tattva-Vaishāradī* (1.4) to explain the special correlation (*samyoga*) between the transcendental *Self and the finite *consciousness or *mind, which is not spatiotemporal but a kind of "preestablished harmony." *Yogyatā* denotes a dual capacity (*shakti*), i.e., *nature's capacity to be experienced (*bhogya-shakti*) and the *Self's capacity for experience (*bhoktri-shakti*). See also *pratibimba, samnidhi*.

YONI (from the root *yu*, "to fasten, join"), lit. "holder." This word has a wide spectrum of applications, ranging from "source" to "home" to "vulva." In yogic contexts, it principally stands for the perineum or the vagina. Some texts describe it as being situated in the pericarp of the lotus at the base of the spine, known as the *mūlādhāra-cakra*. This area is also called *yoni-sthāna* ("perineal place") and *kāma-rūpa* ("desire-formed") and in the *Dhyāna-Bindu-Upanishad* (45) is said to be "adored by all *yogins*." It is thought to contain an inward-facing phallus (*linga*), which is a symbol of creativity.

YONI-BANDHA ("perineal lock"), a technique of *hatha-yoga, described in the *Yoga-Tattva-Upanishad* (120f.) as follows: Pressing the heels firmly against the perineum (*yoni*), force the *apāna* life energy upward.

YONI-MUDRĀ ("perineal seal"), occasionally used synonymously with *yoni-bandha*. Some authorities identify this practice with the *shāmbhavī-mudrā*, which they explain as the means for finding the source (*yoni*) within oneself. It is referred to but not described in the *Hatha-Yoga-Pradīpikā* (3.43). Brahmānanda in his *Jyotsnā* commentary, however, explains it as the "contraction of the penis" (*medhra-ākuncana*), equating this technique with the *vajrolī-mudrā*. The *Shiva-Samhitā* (4.1ff.) states that one should concentrate on the "prop" (*ādhāra*), i.e., the lowest psychoenergetic center (*cakra*) of the *body at the base of the spine, and contract the perineum while inhaling. The *Gheranda-Samhitā* (3.38) further specifies that inhalation should be done by means of the *kākī-mudrā*. The *yoni-*

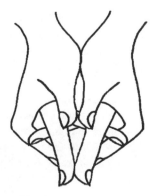

Yoni-mudrā, ritual hand gesture symbolizing the female generative organ

mudrā is widely praised in the scriptures of **hatha-yoga* and **Tantrism* for enabling the **yogin* to arrest ejaculation, even after the semen (**bindu*) has begun to flow.

Yoni-mudrā is also one of the symbolic hand gestures (**mudrā*) used in ritual contexts, especially in the worship of the Goddess (**Devī*). See also *mudrā, shakti-cālana-mudrā*; cf. *ashvinī-mudrā*.

YUGA ("eon"). See World ages.

YUKTA ("yoked"), often found in combination with other words, such as *yukta-āhāra* ("disciplined diet") or *yukta-svapna* ("controlled dreaming"). It is derived from the same root, *yuj*, as the word **yogin*. See also *yoga-yukta*.

YUKTA-ĀTMAN (*yuktātman*, "yoked self"), a common synonym in the scriptures of **Preclassical Yoga for the self-controlled **yogin* who, as the **Bhagavad-Gītā* (6.29) puts it, regards everything with the same calm indifference, or **sama-darshana*. The **Uddhāva-Gītā* (2.45) compares him to fire, for he has become bright through his **asceticism*.

YUKTI ("means"). The **Laghu-Yoga-Vāsishtha* (5.10.128f.) mentions the following four means of controlling the **mind: the acquisition of Self-knowledge (*adhyātma-vidyā-adhigama*), mixing with holy men (*sādhu-samgama*), abandonment of desire (*vāsanā-samparityāga*), and restraint of the motion of the breath (*prāna-spanda-nirodhana*). Elsewhere (6.1.58) it speaks of two principal means: Self-knowledge (**ātma-jnāna*) and **breath control (*prāna-samyama*).

· Z ·

ZEN. The Japanese word *zen* is derived from its Chinese equivalent, *ch'an*, meaning "meditation," which is a direct translation of the Sanskrit term **dhyāna* (in Pali, the language of the **Buddha: *jhāna*). Zen is Japan's form of **Yoga and is close in spirit to the spontaneous (**sahaja*) approach characteristic of certain schools of medieval **Tantrism. Through meditative sitting (Japanese: *za-zen*) and the use of attention-focusing devices known in Japanese as *koans*, the Zen practitioner endeavors to break through to the pure "Buddha mind" in sudden illumination (Japanese: *satori*). The state of *satori* must be distinguished from the typical yogic **samādhi*. Whereas the former occurs on the basis of the **waking consciousness, the latter is a mental transmutation that is preceded by sensory inhibition (**pratyāhāra*) in deep **meditation. Rather, the fleeting *satori* illumination is similar in nature to the permanent condition of **sahaja-samādhi*. Both reveal reality "as it is" (*yathā-bhūta*), free from all mental distortions.

ZEST. See *utsāha, vīrya*.

Bibliography

REFERENCES

Aurobindo, Sri. *Essays on the Gita*. Pondicherry, India: Sri Aurobindo Ashram, 1949.
———. *The Life Divine* (1955). 2 vols. Pondicherry, India: Sri Aurobindo Ashram, 1977.
———. *The Synthesis of Yoga* (1948). Pondicherry, India: Sri Aurobindo Ashram, 1976.

Bharati, Agehananda. *The Tantric Tradition*. London: Rider, 1965.

Divanji, P. C. "The Yogayājñavalkya." *Journal of the Bombay Branch of the Royal Asiatic Society*, new series, 28 (1953): 99–158, 215–68; 29 (1954): 96–128.

Eliade, Mircea. *Yoga: Immortality and Freedom*. Princeton, N.J.: Princeton University Press, 1969.

Hacker, Paul. "Śaṅkara der Yogin und Śaṅkara der Advaitin: Einige Beobachtungen." In *Beiträge zur Geistesgeschichte Indiens: Festschrift für E. Frauwallner*, special issue of *Wiener Zeitschrift für die Kunde Süd- und Ostasiens* (Vienna, 1968): 119–48.

Jung, Carl Gustav. *Psychology and the East*. Princeton, N.J.: Princeton University Press, 1978.

Krishna, Gopi. *Kundalini: The Evolutionary Energy in Man*. London: Robinson & Watkins, 1971.

Nowotny, Fausta. *Eine durch Miniaturen erläuterte Doctrina Mystica aus Srinagar*. The Hague, Netherlands: Mouton, 1958.

Radhakrishnan, Sarvepalli. *The Bhagavadgītā* (1948). London: Routledge & Kegan Paul, 1960.

Singh, Mohan. *Gorakhnath and Mediaeval Hindu Mysticism*. Lahore, India: Mohan Singh, 1937.

Van Buitenen, J. A. B. "Studies in Sāṃkhya." *Journal of the American Oriental Society* 76 (1957): 15–25, 88–107.

Wilber, Ken. "Are Chakras Real?" In *Kundalini, Evolution, and Enlightenment*, ed. John White, 120–31. Garden City, N.Y.: Anchor Books, 1979.

Woods, James Haughton. *The Yoga-System of Patañjali*. Delhi, India: Motilal Banarsidass, 1966.

Yogananda, Paramahamsa. *Autobiography of a Yogi* (1946). Los Angeles, Calif.: Self-Realization Fellowship, 1987.

Zvelebil, Kamil V. *The Poets of the Powers*. Lower Lake, Calif.: Integral, 1993.

RECOMMENDED READING

Aiyar, K. Narayanasvami. *Thirty Minor Upanishads* (1914). El Reno, Okla.: Santarasa, 1980. This volume contains renderings of a fair number of minor *Upanishads*, including some of the *Yoga-Upanishads*. The translations are not always accurate but are still useful.

Avalon, Arthur [Sir John Woodroffe]. *The Serpent Power* (1919). New York: Dover, 1958. A classic study of the esotericism and complex symbolism of *hatha-yoga*. It contains renderings of the *Shat-Cakra-Nirūpana* (Specification of the six centers) and the *Pāduka-Pancaka* (Five [verses] on the footstool).

Basham, A. L. *The Wonder That Was India: A Survey of the History and Culture of the Indian Sub-Continent before the Coming of the Muslims*. New York: Grove, 1954. The best general introduction to India's pluralistic culture.

Da Free John. *The Enlightenment of the Whole Body*. Middletown, Calif.: Dawn Horse Press, 1978. An excellent account of esoteric anatomy, founded in the author's personal experience and examined from the viewpoint of enlightenment.

Daniélou, Alain. *The Myths and Gods of India: Hindu Polytheism* (1964). Rochester, Vt.: Inner Traditions, 1985. A systematic, illustrated presentation of Hindu mythology, which is helpful to a proper understanding of Yoga.

Deussen, Paul. *Sixty Upaniṣads of the Veda* (1897). 2 vols. Translated from the German by V. M. Bedekar and G. B. Palsule. Delhi, India: Motilal Banarsidass, 1980. An English translation of Deussen's pathbreaking renderings of no fewer than sixty *Upanishads*, including many of the *Yoga-Upanishads*. Although the translations can now be improved upon, this compilation is still the most comprehensive attempt of its kind.

Eliade, Mircea. *Patanjali and Yoga*. New York: Schocken Books, 1975. A short illustrated account of Yoga theory and practice, culled from the author's classic study *Yoga: Freedom and Immortality* (see previous section).

Evola, Julius. *The Yoga of Power: Tantra, Shakti, and the Secret Way*. Translated by Guido Stucco. Rochester, Vt.: Inner Traditions, 1992. An informed introduction to Tantrism and Shaktism.

Feuerstein, Georg. *Holy Madness*. New York: Penguin/Arkana, 1993. An examination of antinomian behavior among spiritual adepts, particularly as manifested in the guru-disciple relationship.

————. *Introduction to the Bhagavad-Gītā: Its Philosophy and Cultural Setting*. Wheaton, Ill.: Quest Books, 1983. One of the few books to present the *Bhagavad-Gītā* in its historical and cultural context, without which the teachings in this important Yoga text are rather difficult to appreciate in depth.

————. *The Philosophy of Classical Yoga*. Rochester, Vt.: Inner Traditions, 1996. A scholarly monograph on the metaphysics and metapsychology of Patanjali's Yoga.

————. *Sacred Paths*. Burdett, N.Y.: Larson, 1991. Essays on various aspects of the yogic path.

————. *The Shambhala Guide to Yoga*. Boston: Shambhala Publications, 1996. A user-friendly introduction to Yoga.

————. *Wholeness or Transcendence? Ancient Lessons for the Emergent Global Civilization*. Burdett, N.Y.: Larson, 1992. A treatment of Yoga and Hinduism from the viewpoint of the evolution of human consciousness, using the model developed by the Swiss cultural philosopher Jean Gebser.

————. *The Yoga-Sūtra of Patañjali: A New Translation and Commentary*. Rochester, Vt.: Inner Traditions, 1989. A word-by-word translation of the *Yoga-Sūtra*, the textbook of Classical Yoga, together with a succinct commentary, based on the author's extensive philological and philosophical research on Classical Yoga.

Feuerstein, Georg, Subhash Kak, and David Frawley. *In Search of the Cradle of Civilization*. Wheaton, Ill.: Quest Books, 1995. A thorough review of the latest evidence and thinking about ancient India, notably the connection between the Indus-Sarasvati civilization and the Vedic Aryans.

Goswami, Syundar Shyam. *Layayoga: An Advanced Method of Concentration*. London: Routledge & Kegan Paul, 1980. A wide-ranging treatment of esoteric anatomy and *kundalinī-yoga*, based on the original Sanskrit scriptures of Yoga and Vedānta and featuring numerous quotations from the native Indian texts.

Iyengar, B. K. S. *Light on Pranayama*. New York: Crossroad, 1985. A masterful study of yogic breath control according to the traditional sources and from the author's personal experience.

———. *Light on Yoga: Yoga Dipika*. New York: Schocken Books, 1966. One of the most comprehensive and widely read presentations of *hatha-yoga* by a master of this branch of Yoga.

———. *The Tree of Yoga*. Boston: Shambhala Publications, 1989. An insider's introduction to Yoga, with many helpful and insightful comments about yogic practice.

Larson, Gerald James, and Ram Shankar Bhattacharya, eds. *Sāṃkhya: A Dualist Tradition in Indian Philosophy*. Princeton, N.J.: Princeton University Press, 1987. The single most comprehensive study of the Sāmkhya tradition, with numerous renderings from, or summaries of, the Sanskrit sources.

Leggett, Trevor. *The Complete Commentary by Śaṅkara on the Yoga Sūtras*. London and New York: Kegan Paul, 1990. The first English rendering of a little-known but important Sanskrit commentary on the *Yoga-Sūtra*.

Mishra, Kamalakar. *Kashmir Śaivism: The Central Philosophy of Tantrism*. Cambridge, Mass.: Rudra Press, 1993. A good introduction to one of the most remarkable philosophical schools of India, in which Yoga played a central role.

Olivelle, Patrick. *Saṁnyāsa Upaniṣads: Hindu Scriptures on Asceticism and Renunciation*. Oxford: Oxford University Press, 1992. An excellent rendering of the so-called *Samnyāsa-Upanishads*, together with a scholarly introduction about the tradition of renunciation in India.

Panikkar, Raimundo. *The Vedic Experience: Mantramañjari: An Anthology of the Vedas for Modern Man and Contemporary Celebration*. London: Darton, Longman & Todd, 1977. A penetrating, detailed study of the religiophilosophical ideas in the *Vedas*, the most ancient part of the canonical scriptures of Hinduism.

Radhakrishnan, Sarvepalli. *The Principal Upaniṣads*. London: Allen & Unwin, 1953. Basically sound renderings of eighteen major *Upanishads*.

Sannella, Lee. *The Kundalini Experience: Psychosis or Transcendence?* Lower Lake, Calif.: Integral, 1987. An introduction to the *kundalinī* phenomenon, based on clinical case studies of subjects who experienced spontaneous *kundalinī* awakenings. This book should be read in conjunction with the autobiographical account by Gopi Krishna (see under References).

Varenne, Jean. *Yoga and the Hindu Tradition*. Chicago: University of Chicago Press, 1976. An excellent introduction to the principal concepts of Yoga in the *Yoga-Upanishads*, including a rendering of the *Yoga-Darshana-Upanishad*.

Venkatesananda, Swami. *Vasiṣṭha's Yoga*. Albany: State University of New York Press, 1993. A free but very readable rendering of the author's abridgment of one of the finest Sanskrit scriptures on Vedantic Yoga.

Vivekananda, Swami. *Jnana-Yoga*. New York: Ramakrishna-Vivekananda Center, 1982.

———. *Karma-Yoga and Bhakti-Yoga*. New York: Ramakrishna-Vivekananda Center, 1982.

———. *Raja-Yoga*. New York: Ramakrishna-Vivekananda Center, 1982. All of Swami Vivekananda's works on Yoga are strictly from the point of view of Shankara's Advaita Vedānta. Their lasting value lies in the rich personal experience that the Swami brought to the subject matter.

Walker, Benjamin. *Tantrism: Its Secret Principles and Practices*. Wellingborough, England: Aquarian Press, 1982. A simple, short introduction to Tantrism.

For further references, the reader is referred to the extensive bibliography in Mircea Eliade's *Yoga: Freedom and Immortality* and the *International Yoga Bibliography,* compiled by Howard R. Jarrell (Metuchen, N.J.: Scarecrow Press, 1981). These works also contain references to editions of the Sanskrit texts cited or referred to in this encyclopedia.

Illustration Credits

The author gratefully acknowledges permission to reproduce the following illustrations: p. 25 (Āndāl), French Institute of Indology, Pondicherry; p. 34 (Yoga postures), Iyengar Yoga Institute of San Francisco; p. 43 (Sri Aurobindo), Sri Aurobindo Ashram, Pondicherry; pp. 47, 56, 85, 134, 161, 198, 215, 254, 262, 317, and 345 (Theos Bernard), G. Eleanore Murray; p. 48 (Nabani Das) and p. 94 (bhrū-madhya-dristhi), Richard Lannoy; p. 69 (cakra-āsana by Kay Bird), p. 115 (hala-āsana by Amy Cooper), and p. 277 (shīrsha-āsana by Donna Farhi), Bonnie Kamin, Fairfax, California; p. 84 (South Indian temple) and p. 256 (Hindu renouncer), Matthew Greenblatt; p. 106 (Swami Gitananda Giri), Meenakshi Devi Bhavanani and Yoga Jivana Satsangha, Pondicherry; p. 109 (grantha), p. 123 (Hindu religious ceremony), and p. 169 (shiva-linga), Himalayan Academy Publications, Kapaa, Hawaii; p. 122 (Hatha-Yoga-Pradīpika), Adyar Library and Research Center, Theosophical Society; p. 131 (priestly figure), S. P. Gupta; p. 145 (Kālī) and p. 270 (Shakti), Destiny Books, an imprint of Inner Traditions International, Rochester, Vermont, copyright 1986 Harish Johari; p. 158 (Gopi Krishna), Chuck Robison and Kundalini Research Foundation; p. 179 (Manikkavācakar), Munshiram Manoharlal Publishers, New Delhi; p. 240 (Ramakrishna) and p. 334 (Swami Vivekananda), Ramakrishna-Vivekananda Center, New York; p. 241 (Ramana Maharshi), Ramanashramam, Tiruvannamalai; p. 282 (Shrīla Prabhupāda), Clarion Call Publishing, Eugene, Oregon; p. 290 (Swami Sivananda and Swami Sivananda Radha), Yasodhara Ashram; p. 346 (Paramahamsa Yogananda), Self-Realization Fellowship, Los Angeles.

Every effort has been made to acknowledge copyright sources correctly. In the case of a few unidentified copyright sources—pp. 68 (Caitanya), 140 (Jnānadeva), 143 (Kabīr), 189 (Swami Muktananda), and 340 (Yājnavalkya)—the author and publisher would be glad to give full copyright acknowledgment in future editions of this work upon notification by the respective copyright holders.

The author holds copyright on the illustrations on pp. 2, 14, 22, 24, 49, 65, 85, 103, 104, 107 (both), 130, 173, 176, 179 (manipura-cakra), 180, 184, 190, 194, 197, 200, 206, 208, 216, 217, 249, 272, 273, 274, 278, 283, 286, 290 (simha-āsana), 298, 300 (both), 303, 309, 312, 318, 331 (both), and 351.